Applying the Roper–Logan–Tierney Model in Practice

For Churchill Livingstone:

Senior Commissioning Editor: Sarena Wolfaard
Project Development Manager: Mairi McCubbin
Project Manager: Ailsa Laing
Illustrations Manager: Bruce Hogarth
Designer: Judith Wright
Page Layout: Kate Walshaw (PTU Elsevier)

Applying the Roper–Logan–Tierney Model in Practice

Editor

Karen Holland BSc (Hons) MSc CertEd SRN
Senior Lecturer, School of Nursing, University of Salford, Salford, UK

Associate Editors

Jane Jenkins BA MSc SRN RNT
Senior Lecturer, School of Nursing, University of Salford, Salford, UK

Jackie Solomon MA PGDip SRN
Deputy Director of Nursing, Bolton Hospitals NHS Trust, Royal Bolton Hospital, Bolton, UK

Sue Whittam BA(Hons) RGN RCNT RNT
Assistant Director of Human Resources–Organisational Development and Learning, Education Centre, Bolton Hospitals NHS Trust, Royal Bolton Hospital, Bolton, UK

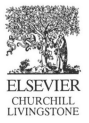

ELSEVIER
CHURCHILL
LIVINGSTONE

EDINBURGH LONDON NEW YORK OXFORD PHILADELPHIA ST LOUIS SYDNEY TORONTO 2003

CHURCHILL LIVINGSTONE
An imprint of Elsevier Limited

First published 2003
    Reprinted 2004 (twice), 2005

ISBN 0 443 07157 8

British Library Cataloguing in Publication Data
A catalogue record for this book is available from the British Library

Library of Congress Cataloguing in Publication Data
A catalogue record for this book is available from the Library of Congress

Notice
Medical knowledge is constantly changing. Standard safety precautions must be followed, but as new research and clinical experience broaden our knowledge, changes in treatment and drug therapy may become necessary or appropriate. Readers are advised to check the most current product information provided by the manufacturer of each drug to be administered to verify there commended dose, the method and duration of administration, and contraindications. It is the responsibility of the practitioner, relying on experience and knowledge of the patient, to determine dosages and the best treatment for each individual patient. Neither the Publisher nor the authors assumes any liability for any injury and/or damage to persons or property arising from this publication.

The Publisher

The publisher's policy is to use **paper manufactured from sustainable forests**

Printed in China

Contents

Reviewers

Graham Harris MA BEd(Hons) RGN RNT DipN(Lond)
Senior Lecturer, Division of Health Care in Middle
and Later Life, School of Health Care Practice,
Anglia Polytechnic University, Chelmsford, UK.

Nathalie Turville BSc(Hons) MSc DBN RGN RSCN
TeacherPractitioner, Senior Lecturer in Child Health,
Professional Development Team, Birmingham Children's
Hospital NHS Trust, Birmingham, UK.

Roper logan
ADL (Good)

Contributors

Karen Holland BSc (Hons) MSc CertEd SRN
Senior Lecturer, School of Nursing, University of Salford, Salford, UK

Helen M. Iggulden BA (Hons) MSc PGCE RGN
Lecturer, School of Nursing, University of Salford, Salford, UK.

Jane Jenkins BA MSc SRN RNT
Senior Lecturer (Adult), School of Nursing, University of Salford, Salford, UK

Debbie Roberts BSc(Hons) PGCert (Learning and Teaching) RGN
Lecturer in Nursing, School of Nursing, University of Salford, Salford, UK

Julia Ryan BA (Hons) MA RNT RN
Senior Lecturer, School of Nursing, University of Salford, Salford, UK

Jackie Solomon MA PGDip SRN
Deputy Director of Nursing, Bolton Hospitals NHS Trust, Royal Bolton Hospital, Bolton, UK

Susan Walker BSc(Hons) MA PGCE RGN
Lecturer in Nursing and Clinical Skills, School of Nursing, University of Salford, Salford, UK.

Sue Whittam BA(Hons) RGN RCNT RNT
Assistant Director of Human Resources – Organisational Development and Learning, Education Centre, Bolton Hospitals NHS Trust, Royal Bolton Hospital, Bolton, UK

Preface

The Roper–Logan–Tierney model for nursing has been widely used in practice areas in the UK, and as a consequence has been used within many UK schools of nursing to teach students how to link the theory and practice of nursing (Roper et al 2000).

This book has been written to enable students and their teachers (in higher education and clinical practice) to explore the different dimensions of the model through a variety of case studies and exercises. The case studies can be viewed as 'triggers' for student problem-solving skills in using the model, not just as a checklist for assessment, but as an approach to patient care. They will also enable students to identify and understand how the model can help them in caring for patients and clients in a variety of practice settings. The chapters focus mainly on caring for adults and older people, although the influence of childhood on adult health and illness is explored in the different chapters in keeping with the elements of the model itself.

We do not offer a critique of the model, an issue which Roper et al (2000, p.158) visit in their monograph. Rather we offer an exploration of how we believe the model can be used to guide practice in caring for patients, and to enhance student learning about varied patient-care situations. Like Roper et al (2000), we believe that its use in so many clinical practice contexts has established it as a valued framework for care delivery.

It is intended that the book will show, through each chapter and its associated case studies, exercises and information, how the Roper–Logan–Tierney model for nursing (Roper et al. 1996) can be used as a model for:

- understanding how we live in society
- nursing practice
- care planning
- teaching and learning.

This is not intended to be a 'recipe book' for caring for patients, but to offer students the opportunity to evaluate their own learning and understanding of different aspects of daily living, and to integrate the knowledge and skills into their practice as student nurses. Their mentors, as qualified practitioners, will also benefit through having a book that will enable them to 'unpack' the aspects making up the whole of their care practice, so that the students can clearly see the 'parts' that make up this whole.

In developing the case studies we have drawn both from our own experiences of clinical practice and from those of our students and colleagues. It is not an easy task to develop case studies that do not stereotype people and groups in society, but for the purpose of teaching and learning it is often unavoidable in order to illustrate different care contexts. We have made every attempt to avoid this, however, as well as trying not to sensationalise care situations. We welcome comments on these issues from readers.

This book offers pathways of decision-making supported by an evidence base. Each chapter will explore the model of nursing through focusing on each Activity of Living (AL) in turn, but demonstrating the interconnectedness of each one. We demonstrate that the model makes nurses aware of the importance of such integrated knowledge to a holistic approach to care.

The chapters themselves follow a similar pattern but allow for the individual nature of each activity. Each has a number of case studies through which that activity is explored, as well as a wide range of exercises, some of which encourage reflection on practice and others that will stimulate further learning and exploration by the reader. The book also encourages skills in literature searching and in using the internet as an information resource. Each chapter offers a list of useful websites related to the Activity of Living, as well as a list of further reading to enhance learning. Although the book is mainly focused on the health care system and nursing practice of England/UK, we have, whenever possible, integrated knowledge and exercises that enable readers in other countries to use it as a valued resource for learning.

Chapter structure

Each chapter is divided into two parts: the model of living and the model for nursing. Combined, they make up the Roper–Logan–Tierney model for nursing.

In Section 1 the authors illustrate how the model can be used to learn about the issues affecting lifespan and age, the factors affecting health and how the dependence–independence continuum can be affected by both health and illness. The use of the twelve ALs to illustrate the model's usefulness means that the book can be used as a single resource, through demonstrating the interconnectedness of such factors as physiological and psychological bases for care.

In Section 2 we use this knowledge, to strengthen this interlinking and to describe and explore the nursing care of individuals with health problems that mainly affect one particular Activity of Living. We also show how these impact on the other ALs. All chapters offer evidence to support rationale for practice and the underpinning knowledge base for care.

A brief summary of chapter contents

Chapter 1 An introduction to the Roper–Logan–Tierney model for nursing

This chapter is an introduction to the model for nursing and the basic principles underlying it. It also explores the use of the nursing process, which is then used in different ways in each chapter. The main focus is assessment of the patient using the model, which is used to plan, set goals (patient and nurse's) and implement and evaluate the care given.

Chapter 2 Nursing and the context of care

As nursing takes place in a social and political context, as well as a historical one, it is necessary to offer an introductory background into some of the issues affecting care delivery. This chapter focuses on issues such as the nature of nursing and health care, nursing practice, and international, professional and educational developments.

Chapter 3 Maintaining a safe environment

This chapter focuses on the AL 'maintaining a safe environment', and illustrates use of the model by focusing on such factors as the effects of stress and pollution on health and the importance of observations to maintain patient safety in the nursing care of patients undergoing surgical intervention.

Chapter 4 Communicating

This chapter highlights the importance of the AL 'communicating', not simply as an activity we all undertake in various ways, but also its relevance to how we undertake all the other ALs. There is a particular focus on neurological problems such as those caused by a cerebrovascular accident or stroke. The importance of understanding the communication needs of different cultural groups is also explored.

Chapter 5 Breathing

This chapter helps us to understand the impact on breathing of such factors as smoking and asthma. In particular, the interrelationship between breathing and the cardiovascular system. Both are illustrated through the use of a case study, which shows the impact of smoking and asthma on an individual's breathing and lifestyle.

Chapter 6 Eating and drinking

This chapter focuses on how what we eat and drink influences our lifestyles and health, and vice versa. Issues such as poor nutritional status of patients in acute care and the effect of illness on eating and drinking are explored in the case studies and exercises.

Chapter 7 Eliminating

Getting rid of waste products by our bodies is a necessary part of ensuring a balanced metabolism. Issues such as incontinence of urine are dealt with sensitively, as are the effects of various bowel problems. The main case study highlights the problems and care associated with recurrent urinary tract infections and enlarged prostate gland.

Chapter 8 Personal cleansing and dressing

The importance of how we dress and how we ensure personal cleanliness is linked to our society and culture, as well as our age and gender. It is influenced by many factors, explored in the chapter, as well as health problems, which can cause difficulties in maintaining our normal personal cleansing and dressing behaviours. The impact of such potentially debilitating skin problems as psoriasis, and the effects of lack of mobility on being able to care for oneself, are explored in the case studies.

Chapter 9 Controlling body temperature

Ensuring a normal core body temperature is imperative for survival and caring for people where this is compromised is an essential part of a nurse's work. This chapter illustrates potential imbalances through a case study, where a child's body temperature is raised, as well as the impact of such problems as heat stroke and hypothermia.

Chapter 10 Mobilising

This chapter focuses on the AL of mobilising and those factors that either help or hinder this. For some people being mobile means using a wheelchair and for others being able to walk using two legs. The main case study highlights the problems that arise when an 84-year-old lady living on her own has a fall, and the section on biological factors offers an understanding of the physiology of movement and joints to underpin the care offered to this lady.

Chapter 11 Working and playing

Being able to work and play is an essential part of maintaining the health and well-being of the individual. Being unable to do one or both of these can cause a variety of health and social problems. Examples in this chapter include a woman who becomes disabled due to a chronic back problem and a man who suffers from a myocardial infarction (heart attack) and is no longer able to be as physically active as he was. Again we see the importance of the model as a framework for assessing the potential factors influencing the care-planning cycle.

Chapter 12 Expressing sexuality

Expressing our sexuality occurs in different ways in different cultures and societies, and our sexual behaviour very often mirrors our social and cultural background. This chapter describes the physiological differences between men and women, and how their bodies function. The case studies focus on exploring how the model can help define sensitive nursing care for patients with health problems that have a direct impact both on the way in which they express their sexuality and on their sexual behaviour. Cultural issues related to expressing sexuality are also explored sensitively.

Chapter 13 Sleeping

Adequate sleep is essential for health and well-being. Being deprived of sleep can cause a variety of health problems and vice versa. This chapter explores a range of situations where sleep is compromised and the main case study focuses on the health problem of rheumatoid arthritis. Changes in sleep patterns and levels of consciousness are also explored, and how these are monitored, e.g. the Glasgow Coma Scale.

Chapter 14 Dying

The inclusion of dying as the final act of living (Roper et al 1996) illustrates the importance for nurses of understanding the way in which we manage this potentially distressing event in both our patients' and their families' and friends' lives. This chapter includes the sociocultural aspects of death and associated practices in relation to the dead and the dying, and the main case study focuses on the needs of a dying man, his partner and the nurses caring for him. It is an example of how the model can be used to highlight the different types of knowledge and care skills required to care for a dying person.

The appendices include a sample care plan document and a tool for using as a guide to assessing patients in each of the Activities of Living.

Writing this book has been a challenge, particularly in terms of the responsibility of demonstrating how a model for nursing, which has become part of nursing culture, can be applied in practice. Despite this, we have gained from the experience, learning more about the Roper–Logan–Tierney model for nursing and its potential for both practice and education, and learning about the evidence base for care and the different ways of helping student nurses and their teachers gain access to this evidence.

Karen Holland
Jane Jenkins
Jackie Solomon
Sue Whittam

2003

References

Roper N, Logan WW, Tierney AJ 1996 The Elements of Nursing: a model for nursing based on a model of living, 4th Edn. Churchill Livingstone, Edinburgh

Roper N, Logan WW, Tierney AJ 2000 The Roper–Logan–Tierney Model for Nursing: based on activities of living. Churchill Livingstone, Edinburgh

Acknowledgements

We could not have been able to complete the task of writing this book without some help.

We would particularly like to thank the contributors who have given us the benefit of their expertise and have delivered well-written and accessible information.

Graham Harris and Nathalie Turner deserve a special thank you. As our critical reviewers they have helped shape the book through their excellent feedback and questioning of rationale and chapter content. Their professional approach has been very welcome and has given us the confidence to know we were 'on the right track'.

We wish to thank all our colleagues in the School of Nursing at the University of Salford and Bolton Hospitals NHS Trust, who have lived this book with us. We especially wish to thank Jean Williams, the Head Librarian at the Post Graduate Medical Education Centre in the Bolton Trust, for her support with searching the evidence and Carolyn Wright, Chief Dietician, Bolton Hospitals NHS Trust, for her comments on Chapter 6.

All of us wish to thank our families for putting up with angst and elation, and also for ensuring that we were fed and suitably hydrated!

We especially wish to thank Mairi McCubbin, Project Development Manager at Elsevier, for her unstinting support throughout the project. She has been a supportive colleague and a critical friend. Thanks also to Sarena Wolfaard and Ailsa Laing from Elsevier, who have offered their expertise, reassurance and support during the publication period.

Finally we wish to thank Nancy Roper, Winifred Logan and Alison Tierney for the model for nursing on which this book is based. Their perseverance over time during its development and the promotion of its use in practice, and its standing value as a framework for care delivery, are commendable. It is, in our experience, an invaluable resource for nurses in practice and as a tool for helping student nurses link theory and practice. This book would not be possible without what has become known as the Roper–Logan–Tierney model for nursing.

A Model for Practice

CONTENTS

An introduction to the Roper–Logan–Tierney model for nursing, based on Activities of Living

Karen Holland

Introduction

The Roper–Logan–Tierney model for nursing was initially created as an education tool for 'beginning nursing students and their teachers' (Roper et al 2000, p. 1). Since then it has been used extensively within the United Kingdom and other countries throughout the world as a framework for nursing care and practice and teaching and learning.

To enable both students and qualified practitioners to apply the model in practice and for nurse educators to use the model as an educational tool, there is a need to revisit some of basic underlying principles of the model.

This chapter will therefore focus on the following:

- an overview of the Roper–Logan–Tierney model for nursing
- the model of living
- Activities of Living
- lifespan
- dependence/independence continuum
- factors influencing the Activities of Living
- the model for nursing
- individualising nursing care and the nursing process.

An overview of the Roper–Logan–Tierney model for nursing

The first model for nursing based on a model of living arose out of research undertaken by Nancy Roper in 1970. She sought to identify the core of nursing activities across any field of nursing practice, which could then be supported by knowledge, skills and attitudes required to work in the individual specialist fields, e.g. psychiatry, gynaecology, surgery, community or midwifery. As a result of this early work Roper, Logan and Tierney published 'The Elements of Nursing' in 1980, identifying the individual aspects of the model as a whole and how nursing could use it as a framework for the care of patients in a wide variety of situations.

The Model is divided into two parts: the model of living and the model for nursing.

THE MODEL OF LIVING

There are five components (concepts) in the model (see Fig. 1.1) namely:

- Activities of Living (ALs)
- lifespan
- dependence/independence
- factors influencing the ALs
- individuality in living.

Activities of Living (ALs)

Living is a complex process which we undertake using a number of activities that ensure our survival. Twelve such activities have been identified which are seen as the core of the model of living. These are:

- maintaining a safe environment
- communicating

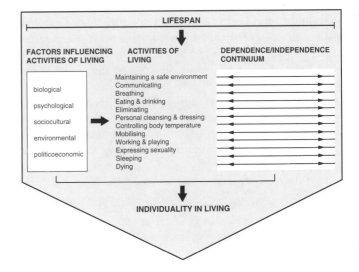

Figure 1.1 The model of living (from Roper et al 1996, with permission).

- breathing
- eating and drinking
- eliminating
- personal cleansing and dressing
- controlling body temperature
- mobilising
- working and playing
- expressing sexuality
- sleeping
- dying.

Although each of these activities will be examined separately throughout the text it is important to remember that we do not undertake one at the exclusion of others. For example, we cannot conceive of eating and drinking without elimination, or breathing. They are simply different dimensions of our lives and the impact of illness on one activity can have a major impact on another (see model for nursing and each Activities of Living chapter). In order to ensure that there is a common understanding of these Activities of Living when reading and using this book each one will now be described. More details in relation to these activities can be found at the beginning of every AL chapter.

Maintaining a safe environment

'In order to stay alive and carry out any of the other Activities of Living, it is imperative that actions are taken to maintain a safe environment' (Roper et al 1996, p. 21). These actions may include activities such as prevention of accidents in the home, driving carefully or washing hands after elimination.

Some of these activities, e.g. accident prevention, are not only the responsibility of the individual but of the society in which they live. They become shared responsibilities, which often need government legislation to ensure that they are carried out.

The environment in relation to the individual can also be thought of as having two elements, namely the external and the internal. For the purpose of this book the external is that which 'surrounds the body and provides the oxygen and nutrients required by all the cells of the body. Waste products of cellular activity are eventually excreted into the external environment' (Waugh & Grant 2001, p. 4).

Ensuring that this external environment does not cause a threat to life through pollution, or destruction of the rainforests are two examples of maintaining a safe external environment.

The internal safe environment is seen as:

the water-based medium in which the body cells exist. Cells are bathed in fluid called interstitial or tissue fluid. Oxygen and other substances they require must pass from the internal transport systems through the interstitial fluid to reach them. Similarly cell waste products must move through the interstitial fluid to the transport systems to be excreted. (Waugh & Grant 2001, p. 4)

This internal environment is maintained in a state of balance, i.e. homeostasis, which if threatened can pose a serious threat to the individual. A safe internal environment is therefore essential for survival (see Chapter 3).

Communicating

Roper et al (1996) see this activity in the following way.

Human beings are essentially social beings and a major part of living involves communicating with other people in one way or another. Communicating not only involves the use of verbal language as in talking and writing, but also the non-verbal transmission of information by facial expression and body gesture. (Roper et al 1996, p. 21)

The way in which we communicate will vary from culture to culture, especially in relation to nonverbal communication. Touching between men and women in public for example is not allowed in many cultures, e.g. Asian. To be able to communicate requires an individual to use their senses, such as sight, hearing and touch so that when they lose the ability to use these, e.g. become deaf or blind, they need to acquire other means of communicating (see Chapter 4).

Breathing

Breathing is an activity that is essential for life itself and all other activities are therefore dependent on us being able to breathe. Breathing ensures that oxygen is taken into the body and carbon dioxide (a waste product of cell metabolism) is removed. This process helps maintain the body's homeostasis. Breathing is an effortless activity and it is only when something happens to alter this, that we become aware of it. For example, the effect of running a race or climbing a mountain (see Chapter 5).

Eating and drinking

Eating and drinking, as with breathing, are essential to maintain the body's homeostasis, and we need to eat the right food and drink the right fluids that ensure the correct balance. Eating and drinking are dependent on being able to afford to buy food and drink, and it should be remembered that there are many people who cannot afford to do so. People are dying from starvation in many countries, and (even in hospitals) research has shown that patients are suffering from starvation as a result of inadequate observation of their in-patient diets. Eating and drinking are also very social activities, and what we eat and drink is very much influenced by the culture in which we live (see Chapter 6).

Eliminating

In this book elimination is both urinary and faecal, yet remembering that elimination also occurs through breathing (external respiration). The metabolic waste products of the body are removed via the process of elimination, that is urinary elimination gets rid of urine from the body (kidney function) and faecal gets rid of faeces (intestine function). Eliminating, like eating and drinking, is influenced by sociocultural factors. Many cultures have rituals and behaviours that govern these activities, and eliminating is a very private activity unlike eating and drinking which are very social ones (see Chapter 7).

Personal cleansing and dressing

Roper et al (1996) chose to call this activity personal cleansing rather than washing, and have included the activities of perineal hygiene, care of the hair, nails, teeth and mouth as well as hand-washing, body washing and bathing. As with many other Activities of Living it is influenced by socio-cultural factors. Dressing, i.e. clothing, is influenced by culture and also by circumstances such as climate or being in hospital. Age and gender will also influence how we dress or manage our personal cleansing activities (see Chapter 8).

Controlling body temperature

Human beings are able to maintain their internal body temperature at a constant level due to a heat regulation system, but extremes in external temperatures can cause this to endanger normal living. Severe cold and heat can cause hypothermia or heatstroke, which if untreated can cause trauma or death.

In normal circumstances we are able to control our environment, e.g. central heating in winter, or take steps to manage it when required, e.g. wearing thermal underwear if working or holidaying in freezing conditions (see Chapter 9).

Mobilising

Roper et al (1996) see the AL of mobilising as including:

> *The movement produced by groups of large muscles, enabling people to stand, sit, walk and run as well as groups of smaller muscles producing movements such as those involved in manual dexterity or in facial expressions, hand gesticulations and mannerisms: all of which are part of non-verbal communication.*
> (Roper et al 1996, p. 22)

Movement is essential for many other ALs, such as working and playing or eliminating and the effects of not being able to move, as can happen following trauma (e.g. spinal injury) or inflammatory disease (e.g. rheumatoid arthritis), can have a major impact on individual lifestyles and social activities (see Chapter 10).

Working and playing

Working for most people offers a way of obtaining income (money) to support how they live. Work can also be unpaid, as with housework or on a voluntary basis. For many women, housework and paid work are essential to maintain family life, but the social pressures on them undertaking both at the same time brings with it additional tensions. Unemployment can cause both health and social problems and both a lack of time and lack of money can prevent individuals from making time for 'play' activities. These can be varied, from visiting the theatre and cinema to exercising

in a health and fitness club. Physical and mental health is affected by work and play (see Chapter 11).

Expressing sexuality

Expressing sexuality encompasses more than sex and sexual activity. It relates also to how we see ourselves and our bodies in relation to each other and how we behave in society. Being a man or woman will influence how we express ourselves, which may not always be in keeping with what is considered 'normal' for the majority. For example being a gay man or lesbian woman in a society that does not allow such relationships to be publicly acknowledged can be very traumatic for individuals who love one another and who wish to express this to others (see Chapter 12).

Sleeping

Sleep enables the body to relax from the 'stresses of everyday living' and it is also during sleep that 'growth and repair of cells takes place' (Roper et al 1996, p. 22). It is therefore essential that individuals have enough sleep to ensure this takes place, although this does differ from person to person. Being deprived of sleep can have a marked effect on the individual and their health (see Chapter 13).

Dying

It is the process of dying that is included here not death 'which marks the end of life' and many people have to live with the fact that they face eventual death but not as an immediate event. This is not the same as the eventuality of death for all living things but having to live on a day-to-day basis knowing that there is no choice or prolonging of the event. For example, many individuals with cancer may have a short reprieve due to drug treatment, but will have to manage their daily lives with the knowledge that it is only temporary. Their family, friends and partners will also be affected by this knowledge. It is important to mention however that not everyone who has, or has had, cancer will necessarily die from its effects (see Chapter 14).

Exercise
1. Consider these Activities of Living and assess your own beliefs and/or practices in relation to each one.
2. How does this help you to understand the needs of others in relation to these activities? Discuss with a colleague.

Lifespan

The lifespan is a continuum (see Fig. 1.1) indicating movement of an individual from birth to death. Roper et al (1996, p. 23) state that:

> *As a person moves along the lifespan there is a continuous change and every aspect of living is influenced by the biological, psychological, socio-cultural, environmental and politico-economic circumstances encountered throughout life.*

The lifespan is therefore inextricably linked to age. Roper et al (1996) have identified five stages of life:

- infancy
- childhood
- adolescence
- adulthood
- old age.

Each of us will live through these stages in different ways and not always successfully. Infancy may be a period of great vulnerability for babies. Babies born prematurely for example are especially vulnerable to infectious diseases, and those born in countries where there are no facilities to manage their health status may well not survive. Lack of food will add to their vulnerability (World Health Organisation 2002a). Some babies are born with health problems that will require long-term care and support, necessitating numerous visits and stays in hospital, e.g. sickle cell anaemia. These problems can very often lead to other needs at other stages of the lifespan.

Childhood experiences will depend on the culture to which we belong as well as the environment in which we live. This is especially seen in how children are reared by their parents and others. Knowledge and understanding of child-rearing practice is essential to understanding adult behaviour, especially during illness. For example, Andrews (2000, p. 139) highlights the differences between cultures, such as Anglo-American, where 'children are socialised from a very early age to learn to control their feelings and emotions, especially in public places' and those where such expression is not repressed and is socially acceptable, e.g. Italian or Indian.

Adolescence is a Western society concept, dominated by the stages of puberty. In certain cultures the end of childhood and onset of puberty is marked by special rituals which ensure that there is a clear transition from childhood to adulthood. Once puberty is reached girls are very often married and become mothers themselves (La Fontaine 1985). Some adolescents experience psychological and emotional problems, some of which can require professional help and counselling. The outcome of these problems may well extend into adulthood.

Adulthood in Western society is identified by age rather than physiological body changes. Roper et al (1996, p. 39) state that 'early adulthood is considered to be a stage of relative stability, with both physical fitness and intellectual ability at their peak' but that 'with advancing age into the middle years of life, ill-health becomes more common'. They also state that 'there are two dominant areas of concern for all adults, namely work and family life'. The outcome of having neither can have a marked effect on an individual's life.

Old age is no longer seen as the end of one's active life, in either work or the home. A recent report on nursing older people (Department of Health 2001a: 9) states that:

> *People are living longer. The Office of Public Censuses and Surveys (1991) estimates that the average life span is increasing by 2 years per decade. Old age used to be defined as over 65, but now a large and growing proportion of the population is over 75, and the number of people over 85 has doubled since 1981. The population of older people is extremely heterogeneous and there is a great deal of debate in the academic literature about whether an increase in longevity means an extension of healthy active life or an extension of morbidity. The majority of those reaching old age are still in good health (Victor 1991) and it is clearly wrong to stereotype older people as infirm.*

Exercise

1. Consider this statement and what it could mean for future health care provision.
2. Consider the lifespan as it applies to your own family. How many life-groups are there?
3. Are you able to determine how your culture/society is influencing each age group?
4. Discuss your findings with a colleague from another culture/society and compare them in relation to each stage of the lifespan.
5. Consider how understanding the needs of different age groups will help you in your role as a nurse.

Many of these issues will be discussed at relevant points throughout the book.

One can see from the above that the lifespan is linked closely with dependence and independence, in both health and illness.

Dependence/independence continuum

Roper et al (1996) state that:

> *This component of the model is closely related to the lifespan and to the ALs. It is included to acknowledge that there are stages of the lifespan when a person cannot yet (or for various reasons can no longer) perform certain ALs independently. Each person could be said to have a dependence/independence continuum for each AL.*
> (Roper et al 1996, p. 23)

This relationship can be seen in Figure 1.1. Newborn and young babies can be seen to be very dependent on adults, as can those who may have sustained serious trauma resulting in being in a coma. Individuals may be dependent on equipment for their survival, for example artificial ventilation, or may be dependent on wheelchairs for their mobility. All of us are dependent on others in some way, for example transport or having somewhere to live and the effect of lack of transport or housing can be seen to have a detrimental effect on the health and wellbeing of individuals.

Without some kind of transport for example elderly people may become isolated in their communities. The devastating effects of lack of somewhere to live or shelter can be seen at the scenes of earthquakes or other natural or man-made disasters.

Dependence/independence status in each activity of living therefore is clearly linked to the factors which influence them.

Factors influencing the Activities of Living

Although Roper et al (1996) indicate that there are numerous factors that could influence our daily lives, they decided that five main groups were sufficient to avoid over-complicating the model. These groups are:

- biological
- psychological
- sociocultural
- environmental
- politicoeconomic.

Biological

> " *For the purpose of this model of living, the term biological relates to the human body's anatomical and physical performance. This is partly determined by the individual's genetic inheritance and although the influence of heredity is usually more obvious in facial appearance and physique, it also affects each person's physical performance. The individual's physical endowment is inextricably linked with other factors – psychological, socio-cultural, environmental and politico-economic.* "
> (Roper et al 1996, p. 25)

This link can be seen when considering the lifespan. For example, if there is a hereditary link to height, e.g. being short, then as the child grows and is measured against the normal percentile for his/her age this factor can be taken into account in the overall assessment of the child's development. However, should that child also be deprived of food or physical care then this could exacerbate the problems of a short height and normal development. The biological factors associated with an ageing body also cause problems and may restrict the person's independence. According to Rutishauser (1994, p. 617) 'however active a person has been and however regularly he or she takes exercise there is an inevitable decrease in physical performance with age' and suggests that 'this is due in part to decreased muscle mass, circulatory and respiratory efficiency'.

Psychological

Intellectual development begins in infancy as a result of stimuli via the sense organs. Later in childhood and adolescence this continues through 'formal education and the pursuit of personal interest and leisure'. In adulthood work and a career are important. Ageing however causes 'intellectual functioning to become gradually less efficient and may cause problems with Activities of Living, for example, there

may be difficulty with communication because the senses are less acute.' (Roper et al 1996, p. 26). 'Older people however are able to learn' as is evidenced by the number commencing Open University courses on retirement. They just have to adjust to different ways of learning (Wade & Waters 1996, p. 61). Emotional development is also closely linked to intellectual development and the lifespan – 'the need for love and belonging is crucial in young children; and from a stable and close relationship in infancy the child can grow with self-confidence and a feeling of worth' (Roper et al 1996, p. 26). One can see how an unhappy childhood and lack of emotional development could influence the way in which adults behave in relationships and when ill or needing care.

Sociocultural

The society and culture in which we live will also influence the intellectual and emotional development of an individual. What is considered the norm in one culture may be considered otherwise in another. Religion can have a major influence on lifestyle as can social class expectations and Roper et al (1996, p. 27) believe that 'where there is religious unity in a society, the culture and religion are almost inseparable.' It is however important not only to recognise the difference between culture and religion, but also how they are closely linked. Religion is a system of belief (a faith) whilst culture encompasses this and more. Leininger (1978, p. 491) for example defines it as:

> " *Culture is the learned and transmitted knowledge about a particular culture with its values, beliefs, rules of behaviour and lifestyle practices that guides a designated group in their thinking and actions in patterned ways.* "

Both culture and religion have an impact on individual lifestyle.

Exercise
1. Consider how your culture influences your dependence/independence on others.
2. How is social class or stratification illustrated in your culture?
3. Consider how religion influences your role and status in society?

Environmental

In Roper et al's model (1996), environment factors include atmospheric components, clothing, household environment, vegetation and buildings. They separate atmosphere into three components, namely:

- organic and inorganic particles
- light rays
- sound waves.

These are described in Box 1.1.

Box 1.1 Atmospheric components

Organic and inorganic particles

The atmosphere is in contact with exposed skin and outer garments on which it deposits inorganic matter such as particles, which are the products of combustion. Such particles can also be inhaled thereby relating it to the AL of breathing. In addition the atmosphere contains organic matter in the form of pollen, pathogenic microorganisms and vectors such as flies and lice. These can affect several ALs.

Light rays

Light rays are transmitted via the atmosphere; these can be from the sun providing daylight; from an electrically operated apparatus which provides light when natural lighting is inadequate or absent; from technological apparatus such as batteries and from burning candles. Light rays not only stimulate the sense of sight in normal eyes but also provide the ambience for such varied ALs as communicating, for example for hearing impaired people to maximise the visual input into a conversation.

Some of the sun's rays – ultraviolet – may burn the exposed skin or after long exposure, may even cause cancer and may require people to take preventative action by applying screening lotion or wearing clothes which cover the skin – a relationship to the AL of personal cleansing and dressing.

Sound waves

Sound waves are also transmitted by the atmosphere and in various ways can influence different ALs. For example those produced by speech are an essential part of communicating for most people. Those produced by professional vocalists could be said to relate to the AL of working while for the majority of people, singing would involve the AL of playing. Sound waves may of course contribute to an emergency warning such as a fire alarm, which would certainly influence the ALs of mobilising and maintaining a safe environment.

From Roper et al (1996), p. 28.

Politicoeconomic

Roper et al (2000, p. 71) state that:

> ❝ *For the purpose of this model of living the term politico-economic factors subsumes aspects of living which have a legal connection; frequently political and/or economic pressure and action is reflected in legislation.* ❞

They focus in particular on the state, the law and the economy. They conclude that 'in the modern world, every citizen is the subject of a state' and that 'the citizen is legally bound to obey orders of the state and to a large extent, the individual's ALs are influenced by its norms. These norms are the laws and the state has the power to enforce the law on all who live within its frontiers' (Roper et al 2000, p. 72). The state has a significant influence and its power is considerable. Although in some countries individuals and groups can register their outrage at certain issues without harm, in many others to do so could place the individual and in many cases their families, in danger of their lives. The effects of such power can be seen in the number of refugees across the world. It is therefore important that this aspect of world politics is understood, as many nurses will come into contact with displaced people requiring health care.

To be able to use the model for nursing in different countries requires its application to be context specific – a task which can only be touched upon in a book such as this.

Exercise

1. Identify how the State (Government) works in your individual society.
2. How is health and welfare managed?
3. Consider the effects of being a refugee and find out how many refugees, if any, the Government has accepted to stay in your country.

The world is becoming increasingly interdependent and this, according to Roper et al (2000, p. 74) 'appears to be leading the United Nations Organisation (UN) into a controversial sphere: the right to humanitarian intervention.' They believe that the 'UN lacks the money and trained personnel to enforce humanitarian operations everywhere they might be needed in the world, but the issue is creating international controversy and sometimes, acrimony'. The impact is also felt by health care services worldwide as the UN responds to major humanitarian disasters and ethnic conflict.

It can be seen from this overview of the five factors that they are inextricably linked and this needs to be considered when using the model as a framework for nursing care. This will be explored in each AL chapter.

Individuality in living

The fifth component is that of 'individuality in living' and stresses that each individual will experience and carry out the ALs differently. 'Each person's individuality in carrying out the ALs is, in part, determined by stage on the lifespan, and degree of dependence/independence, and is further fashioned by the influence of various biological, psychological, socio-cultural, environmental and politico-economic factors.' (Roper et al 2000, p. 75). They consider that a 'person's individuality can manifest itself in many different ways' (see Box 1.2).

Box 1.2 The Roper–Logan–Tierney model for nursing

- How a person carries out the AL.
- How often the person carries out the AL.
- Where the person carries out the AL.
- When the person carries out the AL.
- Why the person carries out the AL in a particular way.
- What the person knows about the AL.
- What the person believes about the AL.
- The attitude the person has to the AL.

From: Roper et al (2000), p. 75.

Summary points

1. The model of living has five components – Activities of Living, lifespan, dependence/independence continuum, factors influencing the ALs and individuality in living.
2. The five factors influencing the ALs are: biological, psychological, sociocultural, and environmental and politicoeconomic.
3. The lifespan is divided into five stages: infancy, childhood, adolescence, adulthood and old age.

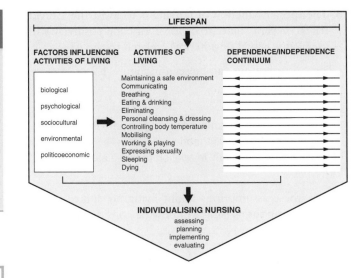

Figure 1.2 The model for nursing (from Roper et al 1996, with permission).

THE MODEL FOR NURSING

This section will focus on the model for nursing (see Fig. 1.2) which differs from the model of living in its fifth component – that of individualising nursing. Roper et al (2000, p. 77) state that:

> The objective in conceptualising living according to the first four concepts in the model of living is to identify each person's individuality in living, and this is the basis of our conceptualisation of nursing. The objective in conceptualising nursing according to the first four concepts in the model for nursing is to identify the individual's pattern of living (and actual or potential problems with any of the ALs) so that the nurse can individualise the nursing of that person taking account of that individual's lifestyle – and when appropriate taking account of family and/or significant others. Individualising nursing is accomplished by application to practice of the concept of the process of nursing comprising four phases. (Roper et al 2000, p. 78)

Assumptions on which the model is based

Nursing theorists who have developed model frameworks to explain and interpret the discipline of nursing make assumptions about how the world of nursing is viewed. They are indicative of the beliefs and values of the theorists. Roper et al (1996, p. 34) make the following assumptions in relation to their theory and model:

1. Living can be described as an amalgam of Activities of Living (ALs).
2. The way ALs are carried out by each person contributes to individuality in living.
3. The individual is valued at all stages of the lifespan.
4. Throughout the lifespan until adulthood, the individual tends to become increasingly independent in the ALs.
5. While independence in the ALs is valued, dependence should not diminish the dignity of the individual.
6. An individual's knowledge, attitudes and behaviour related to the ALs are influenced by a variety of factors which can be categorised broadly as biological, psychological, sociocultural, environmental and politico-economic factors.
7. The way in which an individual carries out the ALs can fluctuate within a range of normal for that person.
8. When the individual is 'ill' there may be problems (actual or potential) with the ALs.
9. During the lifespan, most individuals experience significant life events which can affect the way they carry out ALs, and may lead to problems, actual or potential.
10. The concept of potential problems incorporates the promotion and maintenance of health, and the prevention of disease; and identifies the role of the nurse as a health teacher, even in illness settings.
11. Within a health care context, nurses work in partnership with the client/patient who, except for special circumstances, is an autonomous, decision-making person.
12. Nurses are part of a multiprofessional health care team, who work in partnership for the benefit of the client/patient, and for the health of the community.

13. The specific function of nursing is to assist the individual to prevent, alleviate or solve, or cope positively with problems (actual or potential) related to the ALs.

These assumptions can be seen in Figure 1.2.

> **Exercise**
> 1. Consider these assumptions and compare them to other nursing models/theories.
> 2. How different are they in relation to these assumptions?

How these assumptions about living are linked to the assumptions about nursing will now be considered.

Activities of Living (ALs)

In Virginia Henderson's (1966) definition of nursing a link can be seen between the nurse and activities:

> *The unique function of the nurse is to assist the individual, sick or well, in the performance of those activities contributing to health or its recovery (or to peaceful death) that he would perform unaided if he had the necessary strength, will or knowledge. And to do this in such a way as to help him gain independence as rapidly as possible* (Henderson 1966, p. 15)

Henderson (1966) identified 14 activities where the nurse would help the patient by providing basic nursing care or provide conditions under which the patient could manage them unaided (see Box 1.3).

> **Box 1.3 Activities for helping patients through basic nursing care** (Henderson 1966, p. 16)
>
> 1. Breathe normally.
> 2. Eat and drink adequately.
> 3. Eliminate body wastes.
> 4. Move and maintain desirable postures.
> 5. Sleep and rest.
> 6. Select suitable clothes – dress and undress.
> 7. Maintain body temperature within normal range by adjusting clothing and modifying the environment.
> 8. Keep the body clean and well groomed and protect the integument.
> 9. Avoid dangers in the environment and avoid injuring others.
> 10. Communicate with others in expressing emotions, needs, fears or opinions.
> 11. Worship according to one's faith.
> 12. Work in such a way that there is a sense of accomplishment.
> 13. Play or participate in various forms of recreation.
> 14. Learn, discover or satisfy curiosity that leads to normal development and health and use of available health facilities.

Roper et al (1996) developed these activities further and arrived 'after lengthy debate' to their decision of 12 ALs as described in their Model (Roper et al 2000).

These ALs are:

- maintaining a safe environment
- communicating
- breathing
- eating and drinking
- eliminating
- personal cleansing and dressing
- controlling body temperature
- mobilising
- working and playing
- expressing sexuality
- sleeping
- dying.

It is important to note that these activities are interlinked in many different ways. For example, if an individual is having difficulties mobilising then this will also affect their need to eliminate, especially if the person is paralysed and unable to walk to the toilet or feel that they need to empty their bladder or bowel.

Each of these ALs will be examined in depth in each of the AL chapters, along with the other concepts of the model as they affect that individual activity. The ALs are the main focus of the model. Nursing in relation to the model is seen by Roper et al (1996, p. 35) as:

> *Nursing is viewed as helping people to prevent, alleviate or solve, or cope positively with problems (actual or potential) related to the ALs. Recognition of the fact that people's problems may be actual or potential means that nursing not only responds to existing problems but is also concerned with preventing problems, whenever possible.* (See Box 1.4.)

> **Box 1.4 Summary of the nursing function**
>
> | | | |
> |---|---|---|
> | **Prevent** | → | **Potential problems** |
> | | | From becoming actual problems |
> | | | This may involve the person carrying out the preventative activities |
> | **Alleviate or solve** | → | **Actual problems** |
> | | | Appropriate activities may be carried out by the nurse |
> | | | The person may be able to continue the activities with the objective of preventing a recurrence of the actual problem |
> | **Cope in a positive way** | → | Any problems that cannot be solved |
>
> From Roper et al (1996), p. 35.

The focus in the next section of this chapter will be on the concept of 'individualising nursing'. Before beginning to examine this in more detail it is important to acknowledge, within a nursing context, how the ALs are influenced by:

- stage of the lifespan
- level of dependence/independence and methods of coping with dependence
- factors which have influenced/are influencing individual lifestyle, i.e. biological, psychological, sociocultural, environmental and politicoeconomic.

Lifespan

> In a nursing context, the lifespan serves as a reminder that nursing is concerned with people of all ages; that an individual may require nursing at any stage of the lifespan, from birth to death

(Roper et al 1996, p. 37)

Young babies and children admitted to hospital will also require different nursing skills to that of adults and this is mirrored in the qualifications of nurses employed to nurse children. Involvement of the family is also encouraged, to avoid the adverse effects of separation. Infant and childhood death, whilst it does occur in countries with a developed health care system, is not as visible as it is in those where natural and man-made disasters occur on a regular basis, e.g. Southern African countries (World Health Organisation 2002b) and where health care often has to take place in hazardous environmental conditions. The nursing of adolescents requires an understanding of their physical and emotional development, in particular when they may be faced with serious illness, such as insulin-dependent diabetes (diabetes mellitus), which requires a significant alteration to their previous lifestyle. The nursing needs of adults and older people will depend on the reason they encounter health professionals. Three illnesses that have become more common in middle age are heart disease, cancer and stroke – all of which are responsible for an increase in the death rate in late adulthood (Roper et al 1996). Nurses will also come across older people in the course of their work either in hospital or in the community given that more people are living longer. The National Service Framework (NSF) for older people indicated that:

> The number of people (in Britain) aged over 65 has doubled in the last 70 years and the number of people over 90 will double in next 25 years

(DoH 2001b)

Knowing how to care for older people and what happens during the process of ageing is therefore an essential part of the nurse's role if they are to ensure that the care they plan and deliver is to meet individual needs.

Dependence/independence continuum

This continuum is an important component of the model for nurses. It reminds us that during our lifetime we can, depending on our health and life circumstances, move from the very dependent stage of infancy and childhood to the independent adult and older person stage. Ill health however could make us either partially and totally dependent in either one or more AL. The nurse will 'help people towards independence in the ALs and at other times help them to accept dependence' (Roper et al 1996, p. 42) This is indicated by arrows on the model framework (see Fig. 1.3), reminding us to assess the person's level of independence in each of the ALs and then 'judging in which direction, and by what amount they should be assisted to move along the dependence/independence continuum; what nursing assistance they need to achieve the goals set; and how progress in relation to these goals will be evaluated' (Roper et al 1996, p. 42).

Factors influencing the ALs

To be able to use the model effectively requires the nurse to have knowledge of the five factors and how they influence the ALs. In the model for nursing sections in each AL chapter you will see how this knowledge is applied to patient care and how the factors are interrelated when assessing a patient's needs. Knowledge of the structure and function of the heart (biological factors) for example, will help the nurse explain what happens during a heart attack (myocardial infarction) as will knowledge of the effects of smoking or obesity on the heart when promoting healthy living. Understanding the possible psychological effects of having a heart attack (psychological factors) will also make it easier to explain to patient relatives how their family member is likely to respond to their illness. Likewise understanding the patient's beliefs about health and illness and

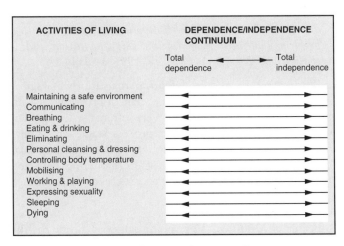

Figure 1.3 Dependence/independence continuum (from Roper et al 1996, with permission).

their cultural and religious beliefs (sociocultural factors) will enable the nurse to offer the appropriate pain relief or manage personal cleansing and dressing needs. Where and how the patient lives (environmental factors) will be essential knowledge when considering their discharge home from hospital as will knowledge of how the social services and the NHS work when discussing patient's rights with regards to treatment and care (politicoeconomic factors). As with the model of living the factors influencing the ALs interlink with the lifespan and the dependence/independence continuum to enable the nurse to adopt a holistic approach to nursing care.

Individualising nursing care and the nursing process

Each patient is unique, as is the nurse–patient relationship. The Roper et al (1996) model for nursing offers a framework for nurses to be able to ensure that this individuality is taken into account when undertaking nursing care. In order to ensure that all aspects of an individual's life are integrated into an effective plan of care, Roper et al (1996) use a problem-solving approach and the nursing process in conjunction with their model for nursing.

The nursing process

The nursing process is a systematic approach to planning and delivering nursing care. Yura and Walsh (1978) identified four main stages of this process, namely:

- assessment
- planning
- implementation
- evaluation.

Arets and Morle (1995) offer the following definition of the nursing process:

> 66 *The nursing process is an analytic problem-solving method whereby the attainment of pre-determined nursing goals by means of chosen nursing care strategies is attempted through a systematic application of assessment, problem identification, planning, implementation and evaluation.* 99 (Arets & Morle 1995, p. 311)

We can see from this definition that another stage is introduced into the approach, i.e. that of problem identification. In the USA, the term very often used instead is nursing diagnosis. The nursing process stages are similar to many other 'problem-solving' approaches, in particular the stages of research process, where gathering data and analysing them are fundamental to a successful outcome.

Assessment

Roper et al (2000, p. 124) point out that although 'the word assessment has generally been adopted for the first phase of the process of nursing', their view is that the word 'assessing' should be encouraged as it implies a more

cyclical activity rather a 'once only' one. They use the word to include:

- collecting information about or from a person
- reviewing the collected information
- identifying the person's problems with ALs
- identifying priorities among problems.

How is this information to be gained?

The main data (information) comes from the patient whenever possible (primary source) and any other data, for example from relatives, is a secondary source. It may not be possible however to obtain first-hand information from the patient, e.g. if they were unconscious, and 'second-hand' information thus becomes very important in helping the nurse and others to plan the care necessary.

Sources of data are:

- the patient
- family
- significant others
- health care professionals
- patient records/nursing notes.

Data can be collected in a number of ways, but whatever data are obtained it is essential that the nurse ensures that they are kept confidential in keeping with their professional code of conduct and that any recorded data are protected (Data Protection Act 1988).

As with the research process, observation and interview are two key methods of obtaining information. Observation of a patient however must be systematic in order to ensure that nothing is missed. It is here that a framework, such as the Roper–Logan–Tierney model for nursing is an essential tool. Other means of obtaining data are: physical examination of the patient, informal discussion with patient and significant others/family and medical records. Objective data are essentially those which can be observed and measured, while subjective data are how the patient defines or reports their own experience, symptoms and feelings.

Exercise

Imagine that you have tonsillitis.

1. What objective data (signs) would we be able to identify?
2. What subjective data (symptoms) may you describe?

You may habe considered these in relation to: 1. high temperature, red swollen tonsils, and for 2. having a sore throat, feeling very weak and 'dizzy'. We can clearly see the first but it is only the patient who is experiencing the second.

Roper et al (2000, p. 127) point out that biographical and health data are vital to ensuring effective assessment of nursing needs. This will include 'name, sex, age, usual place of residence and the person or people to contact when the client requires the assistance of a friend or family member, or when the client's health status is giving cause for concern'. Individual surnames and names are very important information and ensuring that individuals are recognised by the correct name is vital to avoid potential harm, for example when administering medication. Addressing the patient by their correct name is also important in different cultures, where naming systems often require the surname to be placed before the second name. It is important to note that titles such as Mr or Mrs may not always be appropriate. Similar or same surnames can also cause identification errors; hence it is essential that all names be recorded appropriately. How patients wish to be addressed needs to be determined. Nurses cannot assume that everyone wishes to be known by their first name nor that a request for formal address implies a lack of friendliness on the part of the patient (Holland & Hogg 2001).

The age of the patient is important as it indicates their position within the stages of the lifespan. Where someone lives can indicate the kind of community in which the patient lives, for example a small rural village or a flat in the middle of a large city. If they have no home, this can indicate that support services might be contacted in order to ensure care after discharge from hospital. Some health authorities in the UK employ community nurses to assess homeless patient's needs in the community and deliver care in a 'peripatetic' way, i.e. moving about from place to place to meet the patients. Of course it is not only those who are homeless that require the support of social services and other agencies.

The type of house/living accommodation the patient lives in will also be important if they are to be discharged home into the community from hospital, and may require a visit by the occupational therapist who will assess the suitability of the home for safety and accessibility for the patient. Some people may live in more temporary accommodation or travel about in caravans, e.g. nomadic people in some parts of the world, or gypsy travellers.

Making sure to record the name of a contact person and significant other is essential. Next of kin is required for legal purposes (Roper et al 2000) and for contact in case of emergency. It is also important to know of significant others, such as friends or neighbours, who are the patient's support network. Again such information will be useful for planning discharge home from hospital.

The occupation of a patient is useful, in that again it helps build up a picture of the person now requiring health care and will ensure a more holistic approach. If, for example, a young patient has had to have both legs amputated, it helps in the counselling process to know that he was previously a very active person, e.g. a sports teacher. This may affect his recovery, knowing that he is no longer able to do this work as he did previously.

Information about cultural and religious beliefs and practices is essential to providing holistic care. As part of daily living these will need to be accommodated into the plan of care, and will also have a significant effect on the assessment of their needs in all the ALs. For example, if a patient is a Jehovah's Witness, the nurse will need to be aware of the religious beliefs with regards to blood transfusion, and if a patient is a Muslim, that for many Muslims daily prayer is very important and helping the patient to undertake this in the hospital routine will be part of the care planned.

Any recent life events or crises that nurses need to be aware of can also help in the provision of holistic care, such as a recent bereavement that may have taken place in hospital. This could cause the patient to worry that they may not come out of hospital alive either. There is a need to be aware of the current health problems and how they have affected the patient's life, including how they have changed their daily Activities of Living. If they are being cared for in the home, how has their illness affected what activities they could previously manage safely, such as getting out of bed during the night to go to the bathroom which may be on a different floor. Planning for discharge home if they are in hospital should begin when they are admitted, taking account of this biographical and health data and the main assessment of needs in the Activities of Living.

Obtaining information from the patient and others however is not enough to ensure successful care planning and goal setting. The information needs to be relevant and interpreted accurately. Also all information does not need to be obtained immediately, as more often than not patients are in an anxious state on admission to hospital or making first contact with health professionals. It is also inappropriate in emergency situations. For example, a patient admitted with a heart attack (myocardial infarction) is not going to be able to answer questions as to their life style or social needs until they are in a stable condition. Recording the information obtained must also be accurate and clear – in order that patient care can be planned with confidence and based on substantiated data. Assessment is also a time for establishing a meaningful nurse–patient relationship, although as seen in Case Study 1.1 (Mr Davies) this may not be the most immediate action possible if the patient's health problem is critical. Roper et al (2000, p. 135) state that 'the objective therefore in collecting information about the ALs is to discover:

- previous routines
- what the person can do independently
- what the person cannot do independently
- previous coping behaviours
- what problems the person has, both actual and potential, with relevant ALs.'

Identifying the person's problems is in fact the final activity of the assessing phase of the nursing process. Roper et al (2000, p. 135) point out that:

    The nurse's role is to enable the patient/client to prevent, alleviate or solve, or cope positively with problems (actual or potential) related to the ALs. In many cases, the presence of actual problems (such as pain, bleeding, anorexia, pyrexia, acute depression, learning disability) may be obvious to the person and often is obvious to the nurse. But it has to be remembered that there may be a 'nurse-perceived' problem of which the patient is not aware (raised blood pressure being an obvious example) or a 'patient perceived' problem (such as a particular worry or obsessive behaviour or suicidal tendencies) of which the nurse is not immediately aware. Being alert to these possibilities will ensure that they are explored in the course of the assessment. 99

Identifying potential problems is very much dependent on the nurse's own knowledge of ill health, the possible complications and the underpinning cause including the altered physiology. In addition it is also dependent on the nurse's ability and skills to be able to use this knowledge to make, what are very often, critical decisions.

Assessment is the key stage of the nursing process and all other stages (including re-assessment) are dependent on how accurate this is in identifying patient needs and problems. Let us consider the kind of data that we need to obtain in relation to the 12 ALs (further information can be found in each AL chapter). It is acknowledged that using the model in practice will depend very much on the cultural and social context in which nursing exists. In some countries, the model framework will need to be adapted to allow for cultural differences as well as similarities and questions asked during the assessment will need to be adapted accordingly. It is also important to remember however that this takes into account both the nurse and patient's culture in this process. In New Zealand for example the concept of cultural safety has given rise to a complete change in how patient care is delivered and we can see how a definition of this recognises the importance of both the nurse and the patient culture in the case situation:

66 *The effective nursing of a person/family from another culture by a nurse who has undertaken a process of reflection on own cultural identity and recognises the impact of the own culture on own nursing practice. Unsafe cultural practice is any action which diminishes, demeans or disempowers the cultural identity and well-being of an individual.* 99
(Nursing Council of New Zealand 1996)

In 1996 the Nursing Council of New Zealand introduced guidelines for cultural safety (referring to safe and competent to practice) education for nursing and midwifery students. Through this education student nurses and midwives will:

- examine their realities and the attitudes they bring to each new person they encounter in their practice
- evaluate the impact that historical, political and social processes have on the health of people
- demonstrate flexibility in their relationships with people who are different from themselves' (Nursing Council of New Zealand 1996, p. 14).

Although the guidelines have been adopted to meet the specific cultural needs of people in New Zealand the principles of safe and competent practice in cultural care are of value to other similar multicultural communities worldwide.

Given this multicultural nature of many countries today, together with international travel, it must also be noted that an awareness of cultural differences when using language in communicating with patients is essential to an effective assessment of individual needs (see Chapter 4). In fact being able to communicate, either verbally, visually or through touch is an essential prerequisite for effective assessment of any patient or client. It is also important to consider the physical setting for the assessment, e.g. comfortable for the patient, and that the nurse has acquired the appropriate interviewing skills, e.g. listening and observing, to carry it out.

Assessment of patient's ability to maintain own safe environment Data here will be of two main kinds – namely physical observations and verbal information. It will be essential for care planning to identify if the patient/client has any difficulties (actual problems) with maintaining their own internal safe environment. For example, if they have been bleeding heavily (haemorrhage) they will probably be having difficulty in maintaining a balanced homeostasis and will require immediate fluid/blood replacement in order to survive. Assessment of blood pressure, pulse and respirations will be essential data for the nurse and the doctor to be able to plan care/treatment for the patient. The primary responsibility here is to maintain life and prevent deterioration by focusing on the physiological status of the patient.

It is also important to find out if the patient has any difficulties with their vision or hearing, which could compromise their physical safety. Questions such as 'Can the patient walk?' or 'How far can he/she walk?' may also be asked, and if the patient has a disability such as paraplegia (paralysed from waist down). Knowing this will also be important for ensuring that their skin integrity is maintained and that care can be instigated to ensure pressure sores do not develop. As well as its importance for patient care, the information is also very relevant for nursing practice. Knowing for example the patient is unable to move by himself also means that the nurse can plan for her own safe environment by ensuring that moving the patient is undertaken safely and with the right technique and equipment. The patient's relatives may also offer information here, if the patient is unable to do so. For example if a patient has had a stroke and their speech has been impaired, the information a relative can give may be crucial in determining the cause of their illness or their capability to manage their own safety (see Chapter 3).

Assessment of communication skills/needs Effective communication is an essential prerequisite for effective nurse–patient relationships (Robinson 2002). It is important for example to know whether a patient can hear what is being said, can understand the language in which a question is being asked and can actually answer by either speaking or sign language. We often assume also that people can actually read the written information given to them, and assessing this deficit is potentially a very sensitive issue. There are however ways of ensuring that direct questioning on this issue is avoided, through for example observing the patient reading diet sheets and asking if there is a need for explanation. These are cues to making an assessment (Arets & Morle 1995). Is the patient able to hear what you are saying? We cannot assume that because he or she is not wearing a hearing aid that they are not deaf. Does the patient normally wear a hearing aid and if so in which ear? Knowing this will help the nurse by ensuring that when speaking to the patient, they speak on the hearing side or speak more slowly and clearly.

Not speaking English for example can be a major communication barrier for patients and nurses working in a predominantly English-speaking society (and the same in other countries where another language is predominantly spoken) – but one that can easily be rectified through careful assessment of patient needs. Interpreters can contribute much to the assessment process, as can relatives. However in some cultures translating by men on behalf of women, or children on behalf of their parents, can cause untold embarrassment for all concerned and is to be avoided whenever possible. Very often accurate information will not be given, thus preventing a full assessment of patient needs (Holland & Hogg 2001). Other cues in assessing communication needs could relate to how the patient/client maintains contact with the nurse undertaking the assessment. For example, do they appèar reluctant to make eye contact? Do they seem withdrawn and not wanting to talk? These kinds of cues could indicate that the patient is worried about something or frightened to ask about their health problems. It could also be indicative of some kind of depression. All cues need to be assimilated and actual or potential problems then identified (see Chapter 4).

Assessing a patient's breathing needs

Observing a patient's breathing is the first stage in assessing needs, i.e. ensuring that the patient is able to breathe and that there is a clear airway. The way in which a person breathes may be indicative of a number of immediate and long-term health problems. For example if a patient has been admitted with an asthma attack, ensuring that they breathe effectively will be the nurse's first concern. Asking the patient to recall life history and other information will have to wait until their breathing has become more controlled and manageable for them. In some instances observing and then supporting an asthmatic's breathing could prevent them from requiring artificial mechanical support and ventilation.

As well as recording respirations per minute, the depth and regularity of their breathing is also important. They may be experiencing pain on breathing, resulting in their taking very shallow breaths. Long-term health problems affecting their breathing may have led the patient to adopt different positions in which their breathing becomes manageable – they may prefer to sit up using pillows or in a chair rather than a bed. Other questions such as 'Do they have a cough?' 'Is it productive or a very dry cough?' 'If they are producing sputum – what colour is it?' 'Do they smoke?' 'How many and how long have they smoked?' All these questions can lead to a picture of the patient's current and past health, and enable the nurse, doctor and other health professionals to plan care that will include realistic and manageable goals (see Chapter 5).

Assessing eating and drinking needs

Ensuring adequate hydration and nutrition is essential if health is to be maintained. Research has identified that patients suffer from malnutrition in hospital and that older people in particular are affected by lack of attention by nurses to their need for food and fluids (DoH 2001a). Assessment of individual eating and drinking needs will obviously depend very much on the patient's health problem or medical diagnosis. For example, a patient admitted to hospital for investigations of loss of weight and vomiting will need careful assessment of previous eating and drinking habits which will be important cues as to the reason for their current illness and symptoms. They may for example be alcohol dependent or may have a health problem such as anorexia nervosa. Past history of their patterns of eating and drinking are an essential part of the nursing assessment.

Have they likes or dislikes when it comes to food and drink? Are they eating a special diet? Do they have religious or cultural food and drink preferences? All these are questions that need to be determined during the assessment phase.

Other issues to take account of in order to ensure adequate hydration and nutrition are linked to physical activities. For example, can the patient cut up his or her own food? Have they got use of both hands? Are they able to swallow effectively?

All of these cues can then be examined as a group in order to be able to arrive at possible reasons for the patient's current problems, i.e. a diagnosis. The doctor will decide on a medical diagnosis which is inextricably linked to the nursing one – i.e. planning care requires an understanding of the underlying cause of the patient's illness in order to make sure that any care planned after the assessment will not further harm the patient (see Chapter 6).

Assessing a patient's elimination needs

Knowing about a patient's elimination habits is important, even if they are not experiencing problems directly linked to it. It is an aspect of living that some patients will find embarrassing to discuss and therefore requires sensitivity and sensitive questioning. For example, they may experience incontinence of urine when coughing or sneezing or they may have difficulty passing urine. This could be important information when patients have to go for surgery, especially postoperatively. It is important to know how often patients have their bowels opened in a day, if they take laxatives, especially if they are prone to constipation as this may require specific dietary measures, e.g. more fibre and fruit. If a patient has noticed any change from the normal bowel or urine output, it is necessary to determine what these are, for example colour, consistency, unusual smells. Some patients may have a colostomy or ileostomy from previous surgery and similar questions are just as relevant to them (see Chapter 7).

Assessing personal cleansing and dressing needs

Observation of the patient can provide a great deal of information about a patient's personal cleansing and dressing needs. For example if the community nurse has to undertake the assessment in the home, she can see what facilities are available for the patients to wash, bathe and dress themselves. In any situation the condition of clothing can be observed, is it clean or dirty? Has the patient been washing himself or herself or do they have a smell? This can also be linked to incontinence problems, especially in older people. Do they have skin problems such as psoriasis or eczema, which need additional care? Many patients will be embarrassed if they are no longer able to wash themselves and will need a great deal of reassurance that everything will be undertaken to ensure their privacy and dignity. In the community, day care services are available where people can be assisted with bathing on a daily or weekly basis.

If patients are not able to care for themselves they will be at a high risk of skin breakdown and pressure sores developing. Assessing their risk factor, by using a scoring system (Waterlow score for example) is an essential part of assessing personal cleansing and dressing needs (see Chapter 8).

Assessment of controlling body temperature needs

Assessing whether a patient has a normal or abnormal body temperature will entail both observation and measurement. Excessive perspiration or shivering for example could indicate a pyrexia (raised temperature), while the skin being very cold to the touch and white in appearance could indicate hypothermia (low temperature). Taking a patient's temperature using a thermometer of some kind, e.g. tympanic thermometer, will help to confirm this. Temperature is also affected by many factors that will indicate the treatment to be pursued (see Chapter 9). For example a raised temperature 7 days postoperatively could indicate a wound infection, which would require antibiotics.

Assessment of mobility needs

It will be immediately apparent if a patient admitted to hospital for example arrives in a wheelchair, that their mobility is either temporarily or permanently affected. Determining which will require very sensitive questioning of the patient or anyone accompanying them. Determining how dependent the patient is for help to move about will be essential if the care planned is to be effective and avoid the potential problems associated with immobility (see Chapter 10). Questions such as: 'Does the patient need mechanical aids to move about?' 'How restricted is their movement?' 'Is this restricted to one part of the body only?' 'Does this vary in different situations or times of the day?' Knowing that someone has rheumatoid arthritis or has suffered a stroke for example will immediately alert the assessor that the patient could be in need of both physical aids and human assistance. A less apparent problem may be that mobility is impaired due to fear of falling, rendering the patient dependent on the nurse for a whole range of daily activities such as going to the toilet. Again sensitive questioning and nursing management of the situation is essential.

Assessment of working and playing needs

Knowing about an individual's employment is essential when planning effective care, especially if their illness prevents them from returning to that work. It may be that the individual is unemployed, and that this may affect their feeling of self-worth. An awareness of their normal leisure activities or hobbies may also be valuable, for example in planning their discharge home from hospital. It may be necessary to communicate with other health and social care professions, such as the psychologist or social worker, to ensure that resources are available to enable them to manage not being at work due to their illness. Their work or leisure activity may have also contributed to their illness in some way. For example, they may have suffered a serious injury in the pursuit of rock climbing or been under stress due to working long hours (see Chapter 11).

Assessment of expressing sexuality needs

A discussion, rather than direct questioning, relating to expressing sexuality may be more appropriate and will need to be very sensitive and may not always be necessary for all patients. It is of obvious importance when patients are experiencing health problems related to sexual function, such as prostate or uterine cancer or termination of pregnancy. It is important to ensure however, even when such questions are necessary during the assessment that these are asked sensitively and appropriately. For some men and women their cultural or religious beliefs may prevent them from giving appropriate responses, especially if interpreters or members of their own families are asked to translate (Holland & Hogg 2001, Robinson 2002). There are many health problems that affect sexual feelings and function, and the nurse needs to be aware of these in relation to the patients they care for (see Chapter 12).

Assessment of sleep needs

Sleep is essential for healthy living and recovery from illness. How much sleep individuals need will vary, but adults, 'on average spend about one-quarter to one third of their lives sleeping' (Roper et al 2000, p. 47). It is important to assess therefore the usual sleep patterns of the patient and whether they take any medication or other activities, for example a hot drink, to promote sleep. Asking whether they wake often in the night, for example to go to the toilet is also important, especially if they are admitted to hospital where the environment is alien to them. Have they observed any change in their normal sleeping patterns? Do they need to sleep in the afternoon? These questions are very relevant when being admitted to a very busy surgical ward for example. Open visiting also means that the patient's day in hospital is now governed, not by patient needs necessarily but by convenience to their visitors. Restricted visiting times enabled patients who needed to rest and sleep the opportunity to do so without interruptions, and some ward areas still maintain this tradition. It is acknowledged however that open visiting is an opportunity to families to be involved in care. In Japan, for example, visiting a person who is sick in hospital is of cultural significance. It is a means of 'sustaining the identity of the patient as a social persona' and difficult to manage where there is restricted visiting to ensure adequate rest for the patient (Ohnuki-Tierney 1984) (see Chapter 13).

Assessment of needs in relation to death and dying

66 Dying is the final act of living. To die suddenly from natural causes in old age, and without loss of dignity, is what most people would regard as a "good death". However death is often preceded by a period of survival in a state of terminal illness, the duration of which may be prolonged, and perhaps accompanied by pain and distresses. 99 (Roper et al 2000, p. 51)

Assessing individual needs at such a time will require sensitivity and observation of both patients and their families, in particular will be any cultural or religious needs they may have. Assessing the needs of relatives or significant others may take priority in the case of a sudden death of a patient following admission to hospital for example, as will assessing the needs of the family to start the bereavement process (see Chapter 14).

It is essential when considering the assessment of patient's needs that there is no unnecessary duplication of information by different health and social care professions. Being asked the same or similar questions by a number of people could be both distressing and unnecessary. The introduction of the single assessment process as outlined in the National Service Framework for Older People (DoH 2001a) is an excellent example of how this can be avoided. This process:

66 recognises that many older people have health and social care needs, and that agencies need to work together so that assessment and subsequent care planning are person-centred, effective and co-ordinated. In particular, implementation will ensure that:

- *The scale and depth of assessment is kept in proportion to older people's needs*
- *Agencies do not duplicate each other's assessments and*
- *Professionals contribute to assessments in the most effective way 99* (DoH 2002).

Summary points

1. Each patient and their circumstances are individual and these need to be accommodated as much as possible into an individualised assessment.
2. There is no priority given in the assessment process to one specific activity of living, although the patient's illness will determine which activities are affected above others.
3. It is important to note that information about the patient is not only gained from the direct assessment itself. That is, information is also gained from other sources such as doctors' case notes and relatives.

Assessment framework in action Using a framework is essential to systematically gather information – in order to ensure accuracy and appropriateness of the data. It is also essential in order to be able to identify the actual or potential problems that the patient may experience. Consider the assessment stage in relation to the following patient (Case Study 1.1).

CASE STUDY 1.1

Assessment of patient's actual and potential problems

Mr Davies, a 50-year-old man, has been involved in a road traffic accident. He has been admitted to the ward with a head injury and is unconscious.

We can see immediately that obtaining information from Mr Davies himself is not going to be possible as he is unconscious, and the serious nature of his illness requires information which must be prioritised in order to ensure his safety and wellbeing. We can assume that, as we know his name secondary data from relatives and others will have been obtained or it may have been obtained from his wallet. Additional data such as information regarding his previous health, especially with regards to medication or illnesses that could contribute to his unconscious state, e.g. diabetes, will be essential. This first-stage assessment will have taken place in an accident and emergency unit or similar area. *(continued)*

CASE STUDY 1.1 (continued)

On arrival to the ward it will be essential to continue to assess Mr Davies and identify his needs and problems. For example, the first question the nurse may ask: can the patient maintain his own safe environment? Yes or No. If yes, he does not have an actual problem or a need to have it maintained for him. If no, then he does have a problem and therefore goals, nursing actions and evaluation of the care needs to take place.

Using the Roper et al (1996) model for nursing, what are Mr Davies's actual problems? (We can only assume some of those in a hypothetical situation such as that described but this exercise will give you some indication of problem-solving using both the nursing process and a nursing model framework.)

His main (actual) problem will be that: he is unable to maintain his own safe internal and external environment due to his unconscious state.

In order to meet this problem (problem is an unmet need) and to detect and prevent potential problems, some of the nursing actions (including continual gathering of certain types of data) and interventions will be as follows.

A safe internal environment (see Chapter 3) will be maintained by:

- Ensuring a clear airway is maintained to prevent the potential problem of asphyxia – by positioning of patient (allowing for the head injury).
- Observe pulse and blood pressure to detect the potential problem of raised intercranial pressure –indicated by a drop in pulse rate and a raised blood pressure.
- His temperature would be observed to detect the potential problem of damage to temperature control centre, indicated by high rise or severe drop in temperature.
- Observations need to be made of any head wound and any bleeding from the nose or ears which could indicate intercranial bleeding, and he is at risk of infection if he has an open head wound (potential problem).
- Neurological observations would be undertaken – using for example the Glasgow Coma Scale for observations – to detect potential problems of intercranial changes and consciousness levels (as indicated by possible restlessness and changes in levels of consciousness).
- A safe external environment will be ensured by careful positioning of Mr Davies in the bed, ensuring that equipment for emergency care is within reach and in

working order, for example oxygen, suction and emergency trolley with resuscitation equipment.

It is important when assessing a patient's needs/problems that priorities such as those above are determined. Other aspects of the model for nursing, such as lifespan, dependence/ independence and factors influencing his health will become more important as his health improves. One influencing factor however will be important at this time, that is the sociocultural. It is important, given the seriousness of Mr Davies condition, that his religious and spiritual needs are known. For example he may be a Jehovah's Witness and have strong beliefs about treatment requiring blood transfusion or he may be a Roman Catholic who attends mass regularly and would wish for a priest to visit him to offer prayers for his recovery.

Once we have ensured that his priority need is being met and his airway is clear and he is breathing normally, other actual problems can be assessed. For example:

- He will have an actual problem of immobility – due to his unconsciousness – and will therefore require his limbs to be moved and repositioned in order to ensure that the potential problem of breakdown in skin integrity (see Chapter 8) or deep vein thrombosis does not occur.
- He will have an actual problem of not being able to eliminate adequately or normally and he may be incontinent due to his unconsciousness or have urinary retention for the same reason (see Chapter 7).
- He will have an actual problem of not being able to eat or drink as he normally does. His nutrition and hydration needs will have to met by other means in order to ensure that the potential problem of dehydration and malnutrition does not occur (see Chapter 6).
- He will have an actual problem of not being able to meet his own personal cleansing and dressing needs (see Chapter 8).

Mr Davies will be constantly assessed and his care re-evaluated to an agreed care plan, and all members of the multidisciplinary team will make decisions about his care. His relatives/significant others will be included in his care whenever possible and he should be talked to at all times when care is carried out. Pemberton (2000) informs us that research has shown that there is a possibility that patients can still hear conversations and voices even though they are unconscious (Podurgiel 1990).

It can be seen from this small case study the way in which a problem-solving approach to Mr Davies care can be used, based on the data presented and also, most importantly, the knowledge of how to care for a patient with a head injury. In order to be able to ensure an accurate assessment of patient needs using the model for nursing, (see Appendix 3) it is essential that nurses have knowledge of the anatomy and physiology and potential problems associated with the presenting illness (each chapter will explore this in detail).

Once the patient's needs have been assessed, using the Roper et al framework, all information/data acquired must be documented in the nursing care plan (see Appendix 2). These will vary in their structure according to individual organisations' own policies and developments.

Exercise

1. Using a care plan of your choice undertake an assessment of a patient/client.
2. Note the kind of skills you used in the assessment process and how these influenced the responses you received from the patient and their families.
3. Identify actual and potential problems that the patient has.

Planning

Care is planned according to the nature of the actual and potential problems identified, and is dependent on the nurse's knowledge of appropriate care to be given for that health problem and taking account of the individuality of the patient.

According to Roper et al (2000, p. 137) the objective of the plan is:

- to prevent identified potential problems with any of the ALs from becoming actual ones
- to solve identified actual problems
- where possible to alleviate those that cannot be solved
- to help the person cope positively with those problems that cannot be alleviated or solved
- to prevent recurrence of a treated problem
- to help the person to be as comfortable and pain-free as possible when death is inevitable.

To achieve the plan requires the nurse and the individual to set goals, both short term and long term for the actual and potential problems identified. Some of these will be goals for the nurse to achieve in relation to the patient. For example if the patient has a raised blood pressure requiring medication, it is the nurse's task to ensure that the patient receives that at the appropriate times and in accordance with the doctor's prescription. On the other hand if the patient is very anxious about his blood pressure it could be their goal to try and reduce this anxiety by voicing their concerns and talking through any other activities they may have with the nurse. Roper et al (1996) point out these:

> ❝ *goals should be achievable within a person's individual circumstances, otherwise there is a danger of disheartenment. Whenever possible, goals should be stated in terms of outcomes which are able to be observed, measured or tested so that their subsequent evaluation can be accomplished. Whenever feasible, a time/date should be specified alongside a goal to indicate when evaluation should be undertaken.* ❞
>
> (Roper et al 1996, p. 57)

Kemp and Richardson (1994, p. 38) state that 'One of the advantages of goal setting is that it can act as a stimulus for the patient – something that gives him a sense of purpose, something to work for.' They cite the following example to illustrate this:

> ❝ *Mr John Brown, a patient with bone metastasis, was at home receiving terminal care. He was being cared for by his wife Anne and the district nurse. He had become withdrawn and was apparently not interested in anything and said as much. He just wanted "to get it over with". Anne and the nurse discussed how they could help him. Anne said that he had been a keen gardener until recently. It was suggested to John that he plan a flower garden with Anne and supervise her carry out the work. This they did together. He sat in a chair whilst she dug the garden and planted the seeds. There is no doubt that these activities, which were achieved through a series of goal steps, enabled the patient to reach the goal, 'Planned and supervised the planting of a flower garden by March 1988.'* ❞
>
> (Kemp & Richardson 1994, p. 38)

They concluded that 'by discussing a problem and identifying a person's strengths (in this case his love for his wife and his past interest) it was possible to motivate the patient and give him and his wife something to work for, which obviously helped them both.' (Kemp & Richardson 1994, p. 39). Goals can be either immediate, e.g. resuscitating a patient following a myocardial infarction; short term, e.g. for a diabetic patient to learn how to self-medicate and give their own insulin injection; or long term, e.g. in the case of alcohol dependence, not drinking any alcohol at the end of 3 years.

Kemp and Richardson (1994) offer the following advice on writing goal statements (based on Mager 1975):

> ❝ *A goal may contain the following:*
>
> - *Performance – the actual behaviour, communication or clinical features demonstrated by the patient, e.g. walks, recognises, and writes, reports, decreasing weight.*
> - *Condition – the environment or help required from a person and/or resources e.g. with the aid of the Zimmer frame; supported by daughter; in the hall*
> - *Criteria – the measurement of how well, how long, how far, how often, how much, e.g. walks with the Zimmer frame from the hall to the door twice a day; loss of weight – 1 kg in one week*
> - *Target – the predicted time by which the goal will be achieved and thus evaluated*
> - *Review – a checking time may be necessary for some long term goals, when an evaluation statement should be written.'* ❞
>
> (Kemp & Richardson 1994, p. 39)

Setting and achieving goals will be dependent on the patient, his health problem and 'the resources available, together with the nurse's skills and experience in dealing with the particular problem' (Kemp & Richardson 1994, p. 41).

In addition to planning care and setting goals through verbal/nonverbal interaction between patient and nurse, it is customary to record or document the care planned, indeed all the stages of the nursing process are documented. This is essential for continuity of care and also as a legal document, which records evidence of care and treatment given by health care professionals (Walsh 2002).

Exercise

1. Consider the issues raised in Box 1.5. What are your experiences of documenting care?
2. Discuss with colleagues how you would ensure confidentiality in multidisciplinary documentation and your views on patient-held records.

Nursing care plans can either be handwritten or as in some hospitals today, by inputting data into a computer (Walsh 2002). Some areas have standard nursing care plans, which although they appear to be contrary to the philosophy of nursing process and the Roper et al model for nursing, i.e. individualised care, can be used effectively. An example of their use would be in pre- and postoperative care where there are core nursing interventions to be undertaken in

---

Box 1.5 Documentation

All members of the healthcare team should share the patient's record. Increasingly care teams are developing multidisciplinary documentation that places all the different professions' records in a single document. This greatly improves communication between different members of the health care team. If a patient has a chronic condition that is managed largely in the community but still requires occasional admissions either for acute exacerbations or respite care, the patient care record can be held by the patient. Some health staff find this a rather radical suggestion but it is increasingly gaining acceptance. If involving patients as partners in care is to be meaningful why not let them look at their own notes? It means staff know exactly what community care has been given before admission and vice versa on discharge. It becomes a means of providing information about the patient's condition and the health professionals' nursing care plans, and contributes to continuity of care. Accurate and comprehensive written documentation facilitates collaboration and cooperation among members of the various healthcare professions to ensure optimal use of resources on the patient's behalf. The record is a confidential document; it is available only to those participating in the care by permission of the patient and employer.

From: Walsh (2002), p. 12.

---

order to ensure a safe environment for all patients undergoing surgery. Nursing care plans vary in their format in different countries and different hospitals and community settings. The model for nursing used, as a framework for the nursing process and nursing care plans will also vary. However most will reflect the stages of the nursing process, i.e. assessment, planning, implementation and evaluation.

Exercise

1. Find out what kind of care plan documentation is being used in the hospital or community where you work or are learning as a student nurse.
2. Identify what nursing model is being used as a framework for assessing, planning, implementing and evaluating care.
3. Discuss your findings with your colleagues and compare the use of these nursing care plans in practice.

Roper et al (2000) summarise the planning phase of the nursing process by stating that:

> ❝ *It involves producing a nursing plan that contains the following information:*
>
> - *Stated goals or desired outcomes for each problem*
> - *A date on which the goals are expected to be achieved*
> - *The nursing interventions (and patient participation) to achieve the goals*
>
> *The objective of the nursing plan is to provide the information on which systematic, individualised nursing can be based and implemented by any nurse.* ❞ (p. 140).

It is important to note here the need for any care planned to be based on best practice and best evidence in order to ensure quality care (Parsley & Corrigan 1999).

The development of integrated care pathways and resultant documentation may mean that the nursing care plan becomes an integral part of a multiprofessional document and care plan (Parsley & Corrigan 1999) According to Roper et al (2000, p. 143) documenting care can be seen to:

- be part of a monitoring programme related to the quality of nursing service
- provide factual information to managers when, because of staff shortages, items in the 'planned nursing' had to be omitted
- provide factual information to managers when a second best nursing intervention had to be planned because of lack of resources
- provide information that can be used in defence of patients'compliants in a legal context
- help nurses to describe nursing's contribution to the total health care programme, particularly important when submitting an application for adequate financial resources

- provide substantiation for adequate remuneration for nursing personnel
- contribute to a database for research in nursing.

Implementing

This is the third stage of the nursing process and is evidence of how the nurse intervenes to solve the actual or potential problems the patient/client may experience. The nurse plans and carries out the interventions by drawing upon a range of knowledge and skills and expertise in caring for patients in her own field of practice, as well as the expertise of nursing practice gained generally (see each AL chapter for examples of this 'expert practice' and intervention). An interesting example of how the Roper et al model for nursing was used to assess, plan and implement care in a very different environment to that of a Western hospital is seen in Heslop's (1991) care study of a sick Tibetan child (Tenzin) in a refugee settlement in Northern India. She used the model to work with the child's father (Sonam) to identify Tenzin's actual problems, discuss his management related to these problems and reassess them following implementation of the planned care. Despite the treatment and care however Tenzin eventually died from the diagnosed poliomyelitis but because of the collaborative approach between the nurse and the parent he was able to do so surrounded by his family at home.

> **Exercise**
> 1. Using the assessment of a patient already undertaken (see exercise on p. 19) identify the interventions you plan to undertake to ensure that actual and potential problems are solved.
> 2. Using appropriate documentation record these interventions and identify who will be responsible for their action.
> 3. Discuss with your mentor or preceptor how you will involve the patient and others in the care to be implemented.

Evaluating

Any care planned and implemented must have some outcome if it is to be worthwhile in terms of benefiting patients. Evaluating care also 'provides a basis for ongoing assessment and planning as the person's circumstances and problems change'. (Roper et al 2000, p. 141). It is an opportunity for nurses to evaluate whether the care they have either managed or delivered themselves has been effective in meeting the goals that were set by them or by the patient. If the goals have been met then interventions will have been successful. If they have not then the nurse might ask the following:

1. Is it partially achieved and is more information needed before reconsidering whether or not to continue or adapt the intervention?

2. Is the problem unchanged or static and should the goal and the planned intervention be changed or stopped?
3. Is there worsening of the problem and should the goal and the planned nursing intervention be reviewed?
4. Was the goal incorrectly stated or inappropriate?
5. Does the goal require intervention(s) from other members of the health care team? (Roper et al 2000, p. 141).

> **Exercise**
> 1. Using the nursing process and the Roper et al model for nursing as a framework undertake the total care of a patient. If you are a student ensure that this is supervised by a qualified nurse according to policy.
> 2. Analyse each stage of the nursing process undertaken and determine on what evidence was the care planned and delivered.
> 3. Summarise your learning needs following discussion with either your mentor or preceptor.

All four stages of the nursing process (including nursing diagnosis of actual or potential problems) are part of a cycle of care and should be responsive to change (see Fig. 1.4).

Summary points

> 1. The nursing process has four main stages, namely assessment (including nursing diagnosis of actual and potential problems) planning, implementing and evaluation.
> 2. Each stage is dependent on the effectiveness of the other in a cyclical process.
> 3. The Roper et al model for nursing is one framework that can be used to guide the nurse in the delivery of patient care and the design of the care plan documentation.

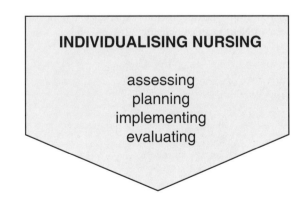

INDIVIDUALISING NURSING

assessing
planning
implementing
evaluating

Figure 1.4 Individualising nursing (from Roper et al 1996, with permission).

References

Andrews M 2000 Transcultural perspectives in the nursing care of children and adolescents. In: Andrews MM, Boyle JS (eds) Transcultural concepts in nursing care, 3rd edn. JB Lippincott Co., Philadelphia

Arets J, Morle K 1995 The nursing process: an introduction. In: Basford L, Slevin O (eds) Theory and practice of nursing, an integrated approach to patient care, pp. 304–396. Campion Press Ltd, Edinburgh

Department of Health 2000 Data protection Act 1998: Protection and use of patient information. (www.doh.gov.uk/dpa98/)

Department of Health 2001a Caring for older people: a nursing priority. DoH, London

Department of Health 2001b National service framework for older people. DoH, London

Department of Health 2002 The single assessment process – key implications for nurses. DoH, London (www.doh.gov.uk/scg/sap/nurses.html)

Henderson V 1966 The basic principles of nursing. International Council of Nurses, Geneva

Heslop P 1991 A preventable tragedy, Nursing Times 87(39): 36–39

Holland K, Hogg C 2001 Cultural awareness in nursing and health care. Arnold, London

Kemp N, Richardson E 1994 The nursing process and quality care. Arnold, London

La Fontaine JS 1985 Initiation – ritual drama and secret knowledge across the world. Penguin Books Ltd, Harmondsworth, Middlesex

Leininger M 1978 Transcultural concepts, theories and practices. John Wiley and Sons, New York

Mager RF 1975 Preparing instructional objectives, 2nd edn. Fearnon Pitman, Belmont, California

Nursing Council of New Zealand 1996 Guidelines for cultural safety in nursing and midwifery education. Nursing Council of New Zealand, New Zealand

Ohnuki-Tierney E 1984 Illness and culture in contemporary Japan. Cambridge University Press, Cambridge

Parsley K, Corrigan P 1999 Quality improvement in healthcare – putting evidence into practice, 2nd edn. Stanley Thornes, Cheltenham

Pemberton L 2000 The unconscious patient. In: Alexander MF, Fawcett JN, Runciman PJ (eds) Nursing practice, hospital and home (the adult), pp. 851–871. Churchill Livingstone, Edinburgh

Podrugiel M 1990 The unconscious experience: a pilot study. Journal of Neuroscience Nursing 22(1): 52–53

Robinson M 2002 Communication and health in a multi-ethnic society. The Policy Press, Bristol

Roper N, Logan W, Tierney A 1980, 1996 The elements of nursing, 1st edition, 4th edition. Churchill Livingstone, Edinburgh

Roper N, Logan W, Tierney A 2000 The Roper, Logan and Tierney model of nursing. Churchill Livingstone, Edinburgh

Rutishauser S 1994 Physiology and anatomy: a basis for nursing and health care. Churchill Livingstone, Edinburgh

Wade L, Waters K (eds) 1996 A textbook of gerontological nursing. Baillière Tindall, London

Walsh M (ed) 2002 Watson's clinical nursing and related sciences, 6th edn. Baillière Tindall, London

Waugh A, Grant A 2001 Ross and Wilson anatomy and physiology in health and illness, 9th edition. Churchill Livingstone, Edinburgh

World Health Organisation 2002a Child and adolescent health development. WHO, Geneva (www.who.int/child-adolescent-health)

World Health Organisation 2002b Health conditions aggravate South Africa famine. WHO Press release, WHO 63, 5th August. WHO, Geneva (www.who.int/mediacentre/releases/who6)

Yura D, Walsh MB 1978 The nursing process: assessing, planning, implementing and evaluating. Appleton, Century Crofts, New York

Further reading

Jamieson EM, McCall JM, Whyte LA 2002 Clinical nursing practices, 4th edn. Churchill Livingstone, Edinburgh

Robinson M 2002 Communication and health in a multi-ethnic society. The Policy Press, Bristol

Roper N, Logan W, Tierney A 1996 The Roper, Logan and Tierney model: A model in nursing practice. Chapter 12. In: Walker PH, Neuman B (eds) Blueprint for use of nursing models: Education, research, practice and administration. National League for Nursing, New York.

Roper N, Logan W, Tierney A 2000 The Roper, Logan and Tierney model of nursing. Churchill Livingstone, Edinburgh

Useful websites

www.culturediversity.org (Transcultural Nursing concepts)

www.doh.gov.uk (UK Department of Health)

www.icn.ch (International Council of Nurses)

Nursing and the context of care

Karen Holland

Introduction

Nursing takes place within a social and political context that is influenced by its history. Nurses need to be aware of the development of their profession in order to be able to understand the way in which factors outside their direct responsibility can have an influence on the care they give to patients and their families. This may be unique to each country in which that care is delivered. This care is also influenced by the way in which health care and nurse education is developed and managed.

Given the multicultural nature of societies throughout the world, and the way in which travel has made it easier for individuals from those countries to meet, it is important that some understanding of nursing practice in different countries is gained.

The essential requirement of nursing to be evidence based not only influences the way care is delivered but also the way in which students and qualified practitioners learn the skills of ensuring that the evidence is the best available.

To be able to use a model for nursing which has been developed over time to accommodate all manner of change, socially, politically and professionally, it is essential that the issues raised above be explored. The use of the model is dependent on understanding not only the factors influencing each Activity of Living, but more importantly the nature of nursing as practised by nurses and the context in which that care takes place. This chapter is only an introduction to nursing and the context of care and you will be directed to further reading to enhance your understanding of the issues raised. This chapter will therefore focus on the following:

1. The nature of nursing and health care
   - the role and function of the nurse
   - knowledge for nursing practice
   - skills for nursing practice
   - health care.

2. Health care and nursing practice
   - NHS in the UK
   - new roles for nurses in patient care
   - evidence-based practice in nursing
   - multiprofessional collaboration
   - delivery of care.

3. International perspectives in nursing and health care.
4. Professional issues influencing nursing practice.
5. Nurse education – its development and current context.

THE NATURE OF NURSING AND HEALTH CARE

Introduction

Nursing as an occupation takes place in a number of health care settings and is a universally recognised profession. According to Salvage (1993):

> ❝ *The mission of nursing in society is to help individuals, families and groups to determine and achieve their physical, mental and social potential, and to do so within the challenging context of the environment in which they live and work. This requires nurses to develop and perform functions that promote and maintain health as well as prevent ill-health. Nursing also includes the planning and giving of care during illness and rehabilitation, and encompasses the physical, mental and social aspects of life as they affect health, illness, disability and dying.* ❞ *(Salvage 1993, p. 15)*

The role and function of the nurse

The functions that a nurse has in society are seen to derive from this mission and should remain constant 'regardless of the place (home, workplace, school, university, prison, refugee camp, hospital, primary health care clinic or other site) or time in which nursing care is given, the health status of the individual or group to be served or the resources available' (Salvage 1993, p. 16). These functions can be seen in Box 2.1.

Box 2.1 Summary of the functions of the nurse

1. Providing and managing nursing care
   - Assessing the needs of the individual, family, group or community and identifying the resources required and available to meet them.
   - Identifying the needs that can be met most appropriately and effectively by nursing care and those that should be referred to other professionals.
   - Ranking the health needs that can best be met by nursing care in order of priority.
   - Planning and providing the nursing care required.
   - Involving the individual (and where appropriate, family and friends) in all aspects of care and encouraging community participation (if relevant and acceptable), self-care and self-determination in all matters related to health.
   - Documenting what is done at each stage of the nursing process and using the information to evaluate the outcome of the nursing care given, in terms of the individual, family, group or community, the nurse involved and the system within which the nursing care was given.
   - Applying accepted and appropriate cultural, ethical and professional standards.

2. Teaching patients or clients and health care personnel
   - Assessing the individual's knowledge and skills relating to the maintenance and restoration of health.
   - Preparing and providing the information needed at an appropriate level.
   - Organising or participating in health education campaigns.
   - Evaluating the outcome of such educational programmes.
   - Helping nurses and other staff to acquire new knowledge and skills.
   - Applying accepted and appropriate cultural, ethical and professional standards.

3. Acting as an effective member of a health care team
   - Collaborating with individuals, families and communities and other health workers to plan.
   - Acting as a leader of a nursing care team, which may include other nurses and auxiliary personnel as well as users of nursing services.
   - Delegating nursing activities and tasks to other nursing personnel and supporting them in their work.
   - Negotiating the user's participation in the implementation of his or her care plan.
   - Collaborating with other people in multidisciplinary and multisectoral teams in planning, providing, developing, coordinating and evaluating health services.
   - Collaborating with other health professionals in maintaining a safe and harmonious working environment that is conducive to team work.
   - Being actively involved in policy making and programme planning, in setting priorities and in the development and allocation of resources.
   - Participation in the preparation of reports to authorities and politicians at the local, regional or national level and when appropriate, to the mass media.

4. Developing nursing practice through critical thinking and research
   - Launching innovative ways of working to achieve better results.
   - Identifying areas for research to increase knowledge or develop skills in nursing practice or education and participating in such studies as required.
   - Applying accepted standards and appropriate cultural, ethical and professional standards to guide research in nursing.

From Salvage (1993).

Another more well-known definition of the role and function of the nurse is that of Virginia Henderson (1966):

> *The unique function of the nurse is to assist the individual, sick or well in the performance of those activities contributing to health or its recovery (or to peaceful death) that he would perform unaided if he had the necessary strength, will or knowledge. And to do this in such a way as to help him gain independence as rapidly as possible. This aspect of her work, this part of her function, she initiates and controls, of this she is master. In addition she helps the patient to carry out the total program whether it be for the improvement of health or the recovery from illness or support in death.*
> (Henderson 1966, p. 15)

Exercise

Consider these two descriptions of the functions and role of the nurse and discuss your responses with colleagues.

1. How does your own experience of nursing compare with Henderson's definition?
2. How many of Salvage's functions of a nurse have you undertaken in your role as either a student or qualified nurse?
3. What do you consider to be the most rewarding functions of your role as either a student or qualified nurse?
4. How does the society/culture in which you live influence how you carry out these functions?

In relation to Point 4 you may have considered the following issues:

- the status of nursing in different countries
- the health and illness beliefs of patients
- the health care system in which nursing exists.

For example, multiprofessional collaboration will be difficult to implement in a health care system which promotes a hierarchy of status, and where the medical team is considered to make all the decisions regarding patient care. Henderson's definition implies that nurses are only there to 'carry out the therapeutic plan as initiated by the physician', and this may still be the case in many countries. However certainly in the United Kingdom this is no longer the situation, with new roles enabling nurses to have much more of a lead in decision making regarding patients treatment and care (Humphris & Masterson 2000). These issues are explored later in the chapter.

Knowledge for nursing practice

As we can see from Salvage's description (Box 2.1) undertaking the role of a nurse will require an extensive knowledge and skills base with which to practice in an accountable way and this is drawn from a number of other disciplines as well as from the art and science of nursing itself. Those which have had a significant impact on nursing care include:

- sociology
- biological science
- psychology
- ethics
- anthropology
- health promotion
- politics and social policy
- research
- management
- economics.

We can see the influence of these disciplines in Roper et al's model itself, in particular the factors influencing the Activities of Living. For example, biological (biological sciences), psychological (psychology), sociocultural (sociology and anthropology), environmental (health promotion and social policy) and politicoeconomic (politics and economics). (Further details can be found in each AL chapter.) How has nursing used the source of knowledge from these disciplines? To be able to answer this question in its entirety is beyond the scope of this chapter. However a brief explanation of each discipline and a link to nursing will be offered.

Sociology

Jones (1994) defined sociology as follows:

> *Sociology is the systematic study of human society. It provides us with evidence and explanations of how society works, of the actions of individuals and groups, of patterns of similarity and difference between people*

(within a single society and between societies), of the distribution of social resources and economic and political power. Sociology is concerned both with studying individuals (social actors or agents) operating in the social world and with trying to understand how the social world "works" by investigating how social structures and relationships develop, persist and change.

(Jones 1994, p. 40)

Thinking of nursing, and the contexts in which it takes place, it can be seen that it offers a rich 'social world' for sociological investigation. Porter (1998) however notes that sociologists 'have not paid great attention to the actual work that nurses do'. In 1991 he chose to study effects of the nursing process on the working lives of nurses in an intensive care unit (Porter 1991) and one of his findings was that despite nurses having 'considerable informal input into decisions' that the most important ones 'about care were made by physicians, nursing care plans being constructed in response to those decisions' (Porter 1998, p. 79). It would be interesting to see if this still applied in 2002.

Biological science

Davey (1992, p. 42) stated that 'biology is the scientific study of the structure and function of living things and of the interactions of organisms with each other in the natural world and with their environment'. Roper et al (1996, p. 25) in the model for nursing, use the term as it relates to 'the human body's anatomical and physiological performance'. Knowledge of this is essential if nurses are to understand the nature of disease and patient symptoms as well as helping to promote healthy living. Examples of this interdependence are to be found in all AL chapters, e.g. in Chapter 5 it can be seen how a knowledge of gaseous exchange can help to understand the effects of smoking on breathing.

Psychology

Psychology considers the understanding of experience and behaviour of the individual, especially relevant to nursing considering that it involves caring for individuals. It includes understanding of emotional and intellectual development (Roper et al 1996). Knowledge of psychology would for example be important if you were to understand a child or adult's fear of hospitals, as would understanding how people behave when in stressful situations.

Ethics

Cooper (2001) states that 'ethics is the study of what is right or good'. She offers the following observations of its links to nursing:

> *Ethical nursing practice is based on general knowledge about ethical frameworks and principles, professional codes and guidelines, and particular knowledge of one's values and the values of the patient. Knowing about ethics however is not the same as developing*

ethical nursing practice. Moving from knowing about ethics to being an ethical nurse is similar to developing any other nursing skill. What is required is an intention to learn, self-reflection about values, as skilful teacher, dialogue with others and practice. "

(Cooper 2001, p. 46)

The Code of Professional Conduct (NMC 2002a, see p. 33) offers nurses an ethical framework in which to practice. Ethical principles guide nurses' actions and choices when faced with an ethical dilemma, for example not agreeing with the active resuscitation of a person who has told you they have no wish for this to happen. This may involve being an advocate for the patient. An advocate being 'one who supports or champions another, often because an individual, for whatever reason, is not in a position to speak adequately or effectively for him or herself' (Wallace 2002, p. 10).

Anthropology

Anthropology can be defined as the 'study of human nature, human society and human history' (Schultz & Lavenda 1990, p. 4) and a central concept is culture.

Madeline Leininger, an American nurse and an anthropologist has used this concept in the development of transcultural nursing which she states is a subfield of nursing, i.e. that it is:

" *the comparative study and analysis of different cultures and sub-cultures in the world with respect to their caring behaviour, nursing care, and health–illness values, beliefs and patterns of behaviours with the goal of generating scientific and humanistic knowledge in order to provide culture-specific and culture universal nursing care practices.* " *(Leininger 1978, p. 8)*

Other nurses such as Holden and Littlewood (1991) and Savage (1995) have used anthropology to view nursing very differently. Savage, in her ethnographic study of nurse–patient interaction, for example linked her finding of 'closeness' in nursing with kinship and family relationships. Littlewood (1991) discusses the way in which nursing is viewed as being 'polluting or dirty' work; a theme which is also developed in the work of Jocalyn Lawler (1991) on body care in nursing work.

Health promotion and education

Walsh (2002, p. 16) points out that 'given the difficulties surrounding the definition of health, there is little agreement about what constitutes health promotion and how it differs from health education'. He does offer however what he calls a very 'commonsense definition of health education' i.e. 'as teaching individuals about steps they can take to enhance their health (e.g. exercise) and avoid disease (e.g. use a condom during sex)'. If this is then linked to Tones (1993) definition, i.e. 'Health promotion = health education × healthy public policy' then he concludes that

'in this view health education is seen as empowerment which, when combined with a health-orientated public policy, leads to the promotion of health' (Walsh 2002). Nurses have a major role in promoting health and well-being, as well as preventing disease and Roper et al see this as being an essential factor in the model for nursing (Roper et al 2000, p. 102).

Politics and economics

Nursing exists in a political world, where the actions of Government affect the way in which it is delivered, e.g. setting down legislation as to what competencies nurses need, and also affect individuals who require nursing care, e.g. investing in new hospitals or making patients pay for their medication prescriptions. Roper et al (2000) explain the role of the state in a modern world and point out that:

" *the State is the apex of the modern social pyramid and has supremacy over other forms of social groupings, so, in general terms, the state regulates human activities of living. For example, in relation to the AL of mobilizing, traffic regulations are enforced by the state. However the state is dependent on the economic system that underlies legal order; only limited social progress is possible when a state has a precarious economic base.* "
(Roper et al 2000, p. 72)

Health economics is not a subject, in the past, that has been promoted in the nursing curriculum. However as Morris (1998, p. vii) points out this is now becoming increasingly important for nurses 'as efficient and cost-effective use of resources is seen as necessary for the provision of a high-quality nursing service'.

Research

The ability to understand research and critically appraise evidence is essential to taking forward the current NHS agenda in the UK (DoH 2000). Grant and Massey (1999, p. 117) state that 'the primary goal of nursing research is to develop a specialised, scientifically based body of knowledge unique to nursing' and in basic terms this research can either be quantitative (positivistic) or qualitative (interpretive), the former Grant and Massey (1999) define as 'research which examines specific phenomena' (e.g. testing hypotheses) and the latter 'research which explores human experiences as they are lived' (e.g. living with a chronic illness). Hamer and Collinson (1999) indicate that there are different forms of evidence arising from the above approaches and that it is essential that they are appraised, using set criteria, for their usefulness and quality (see p. 30).

Management

Watkins (1997, p. 15) stated that 'nurse managers require knowledge derived from the study of leadership, organisations and management if they are to provide managerial leadership in addition to the theory necessary for professional leadership'. Understanding how to manage change, how organisations function and how to ensure that the care being delivered is of a high quality are only three elements of the management role of a nurse. Others include managing conflict, decision making and effective communication. Management can occur at different levels of the organisation, from being responsible for managing individual patient care on a day-to-day basis to being responsible for directing a whole service such as a primary care trust. Changes taking place in health and social care in the UK, as in other countries, however now require that leadership and management are teased apart and leadership development has become a key component of the modernisation agenda with the launch of the NHS Modernisation Agency – National Nursing Leadership Project in April 2001 (Department of Health 2001 – www.nursingleadership.co.uk). The difference between managers and leaders can be seen in Box 2.2.

Exercise
1. Consider your normal 'working' day and map out the key areas of activity.
2. What knowledge did you use from any of the above disciplines to carry out nursing activities?
3. Discuss with colleagues or tutors how this knowledge was integrated into nursing practice and consider the value it had for patient care.

Skills for nursing practice

In order to carry out nursing care and related activities, nurses require a number of skills, ranging from practical and technical to problem solving and critical thinking. These could be seen as the key skills of nursing practice. The exact need for those skills have altered over time and nursing has had to respond accordingly. Let us examine what these skills are.

Exercise
Consider the extract from Lucy Seymer's book on the Nightingale Training School – 1860–1960 in Box 2.3.
1. What similarities can be seen between these expectations and those of your training and education?
2. What practical skills used by the probationers would still be appropriate in today's nursing practice?
3. Identify those duties that are no longer undertaken and consider what influenced their demise.

Box 2.3 Duties of a probationer under the 'Nightingale Fund'

You are required to be:

Sober, honest, truthful, trustworthy, punctual, quiet and orderly. Clean and neat.

You are required to become skilful:

1. in the dressing of blisters, burns, sores, wounds and in applying fomentations, poultices and minor dressings;
2. in the application of leeches, externally and internally;
3. in the administrations of enemas for men and women;
4. in the management of trusses, and appliances in uterine complaints;
5. in the best method of friction to the body and extremities;
6. in the management of helpless patients, i.e. moving, changing, personal cleanliness of feeding, keeping warm (or cool) preventing and dressing bed sores;
7. in bandaging, making bandages and rollers, lining splints;
8. in making the beds of patients, and removal of sheet whilst patient is in bed;
9. you are required to attend at operations;
10. to be competent to cook gruel, arrowroot, egg flip, puddings, drinks for the sick;
11. to understand ventilation, or keep the ward fresh by night as well as by day; you are to be careful that great cleanliness is observed in all utensils; those used for secretions as well as those required for cooking;
12. to make strict observations of the sick in the following particulars – the state of secretions, expectoration, pulse, skin, appetite; intelligence, as delirium or stupor; breathing, sleep, state of wounds, eruptions, formation of matter, effect of diet or of stimulants and of medicines;
13. and to learn the management of convalescents.

From Report of the Committee of the Council of the Nightingale Fund, for the year ending 24th June 1861. Seymer 1960, p. 151.

Box 2.2 Contrasting the roles of managers and leaders (adapted from Sofarelli & Brown 1998)

Role of the manager	Role of the leader
Create stability	Be proactive
Take control	Have integrity, an ethical approach and sound principles
Accomplish tasks	
Possess authority	
Hold power from their position	Thrive on change, challenge the status quo
Plan, organise and control human and material resources	Inspire followers
	Have vision
	Be willing to take risks
Enforce policy and procedures	Value people
	Develop relationships
Maintain hierarchical rule	Communicate effectively
Put the organisation before people	Not hold power through position or authority
	Empower others

Many of these prescribed duties have been replaced because of the influence of medical advances and technology, e.g. most nurses no longer have to make bandages or use poultices. Some duties however are unchanged, albeit carried out with more advanced resources. Skills such as observation, taking the pulse, wound care, preventing pressure sores remain an essential part of nursing work. (These skills and others undertaken by the nurse will be evident throughout each chapter.) Other skills such as application of leeches were abandoned but are now being reintroduced into main stream health care for a variety of conditions. One being in the treatment of osteoarthritis pain according to a small study being undertaken in Germany (Arthritis Research Campaign (ARC) 2001).

Health care

Proctor (2000, p. 58) notes that the term 'health care' is commonly used to describe the work of the health services, and the professions that carry out this care include medicine, nursing, physiotherapy, midwifery and occupational therapy (see Fig. 2.1 for other members of the team who assist the patient, their families and carers).

Wallace (2002, p. 69) points out that 'the health services require a range of healthcare professionals each with their own unique role, although partnership working is becoming more and more common as cross-boundary activity is increasing'. We can see the effect of this in the development of new roles in nursing in the UK (see p. 29). Integration between health and social care is also an influencing factor, in particular in the development of Primary Care Trusts

(PCTs) (DoH 1999b). The work of the health care professions has developed in response to the need of people and both have been influenced by the political and social context in which they exist. For example most of the health care needs of people in countries such as Ethiopia or India are very different from the health care needs of those in the USA or the UK. Africa for example 'has been hardest hit by the HIV/AIDS pandemic' whilst in the United Kingdom and the United States of America the effects of living style (e.g. high-cholesterol foods, smoking and alcohol) can be seen in the number of people with coronary heart disease (World Health Organisation 2001a). These needs are also affected by other conditions outside the control of people, with climate and weather being the most dramatic influence. Consider the devastating effects of the famine in Southern Africa where 'health conditions are putting 12–14 million people at particular risk during the ongoing shortage of food' (World Health Organisation 2002).

Advances in medicine and a significant improvement in the quality of life for people in many countries of the world have also brought with them one of the most significant influences on the future of health care generally. This relates specifically to the rise in the number of older people in the world. A World Health Organisation Press Release (1997) reported that:

> 66 *By 2020 the world will have more than 1 billion people age 60 and over, and 710 million of these will live in developing countries. Today there are an estimated 540 million people in the world aged 60 and over, 330 million of whom live in developing countries.* 99

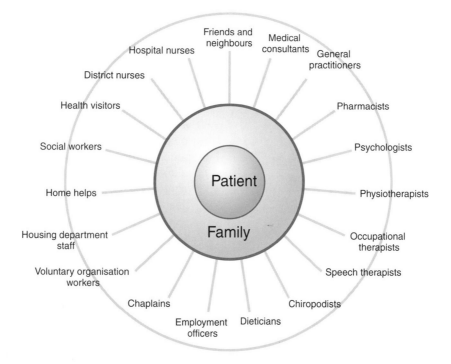

Fig. 2.1 Members of the team (from Roper et al 1996, with permission).

Ageing however does not mean ill-health. The WHO Global Movement for Active Ageing (WHO 2001c) suggest that 'if ageing is to be a positive experience, longer life must be accompanied by improvements of the quality of life of those who reach old age' and that it 'requires policies and strategies that value older people's contribution to their families, communities and economies and that enable them to maintain an optimal level of well being'. They suggest that 'Health is key to Active Ageing' and that 'maintaining good health throughout one's lifespan is essential to extend healthy life expectancy and maintain quality of life in old age' (WHO 2001c). Caring for the elderly person is a theme in many of the AL chapters, e.g. Chapter 10 (Mobilising) and Chapter 8 (Personal Cleansing and Dressing).

What significance therefore have all these issues for nursing practice? This will now be explored.

HEALTH CARE AND NURSING PRACTICE

Before the role of nursing in health care can be understood it is necessary to understand the health care system and its associated development in different countries. This section will initially focus on the health care system in the United Kingdom (UK).

The National Health Service in the UK

The National Health Service (NHS) was set up as a result of a series of post-World War II developments, the National Health Service Act 1946 and the birth of the Welfare State (Baly 1995). It came into operation on the 5th July 1948 and apart from some charges to prescriptions and appliances, the majority of treatments were free of charge. Its introduction necessitated a significant change to nursing and the resultant Nurses Act of 1949 saw a reconstituted General Nursing Council (GNC) and a new training scheme for nurses. The basic principles inherent in the setting up of the NHS remained until the new National Health Service and Community Care Act in 1990. This Act provided a framework for a closer working relationship between health and social care services, together with an increased consumer involvement in decision making about service provision. This would have a direct effect on how nurses for example, involved patients in their own care decisions – an important aspect when considering using a nursing model by which to assess, plan, implement and evaluate care. It also had an impact on where that care took place – in particular the shift to care in the community. There were however serious difficulties with the implementation of 'Government's new health market in the NHS' (Fatchett 1998, p. 29) but with the General Election of 1992 the election of the Conservative Government for another term of office ensured that the principles of the internal health market would be embedded in the UK

health care system. 1997 saw the Labour Government being elected into office and it was faced with a major challenge to reform the NHS. The White Paper – The New NHS Modern and Dependable (Department of Health 1997) set out this reform, which sought to keep what worked from the previous system, whilst ensuring that care delivery was improved for everyone who made use of the NHS. Improving health and reducing inequalities were cornerstones to its implementation, as was the need for 'quality' and its monitoring. The publication of A First Class Service – Quality in the New NHS (DoH 1998) provided the evidence of how this was to be undertaken, e.g. the setting up of the National Institute for Clinical Excellence (NICE), Clinical Governance and the Commission for Health Improvement. The impact of the NHS changes were to be significant to those who were employed to deliver the care as well as the organisations in which they worked. Some of the most significant for nurses in the UK and the way in which they delivered care to the patient have been:

- the introduction of new roles for nurses
- implementation of evidence-based nursing practice
- multiprofessional collaboration.

The introduction of new roles for nurses

Cameron (2000, p. 14) highlights two major initiatives that 'encouraged the development of new roles for nurses as well as for other health care professionals'. These were the waiting list initiatives and the reduction in junior doctors' hours.

For both the Conservative and Labour Governments the issue of long waiting lists has been problematic, and despite steps to reduce it, some patients were still having to wait 2 years or more for admission to hospital (Cameron 2000). However this trend has now changed, for a variety of reasons, with a reduction in waiting lists across the UK. In February 1999 for example, the Government announced a '£20 million boost to reduce waiting lists and waiting times' (DoH 1999a) by investing in new surgical equipment and facilities as part of modernising the NHS.

Long hours had been considered part of a junior doctor's working week but in 1991 the Government directed employers to begin to reduce them so that 'by the end of 1996 no junior doctor was supposed to be contracted to work more than 56 hours a week' (DoH 1991). To enable this to occur the Government allocated funding for the development of new clinical roles (Humphris & Masterson 2000). The reduction in junior doctors' hours meant that they would no longer be in a position to ensure continuity of care for patients, and there was a possibility of patients having to wait for assessment and treatments. Alongside this reduction in their hours was also a reduction in the number of doctors in employment. New roles for nurses were therefore encouraged and a plethora of specialist roles appeared. For example, night nurse practitioners, nurse-led services in preoperative assessment clinics and nurse endoscopists. The publication of the Scope of Professional Nursing Practice (UKCC 1992a) further enabled nurses, midwives and health visitors to expand their role beyond the boundaries of their professions, and Cameron (2000, p. 11) believes that:

> 66 *Without doubt such professional developments helped demolish unhelpful barriers between health-care professions with the result that nurses could develop their roles into areas that previously were firmly within the domain of medicine.* 99

It is important to reflect that in other countries nurses have been undertaking many roles and tasks that have been viewed as 'doctor's' in the UK. This is seen in the number of health initiatives reported by the WHO (2001b, p. 13), who also report that 'research conducted in North America and the United Kingdom on the nurse practitioner role supports positive results in patient outcomes, satisfaction and cost'.

Exercise
1. What new roles would help you as a qualified nurse to assess, plan, implement and evaluate the care given to patients?
2. Discuss with colleagues what impact new roles have had on how you deliver care to patients?

To facilitate your discussion you may wish to read Humphris and Masterson's book entitled: Developing new clinical roles – a guide for health professionals.

Implementation of evidence-based nursing practice

The need to provide evidence that the care you deliver is both effective and appropriate has arisen because of the changes within the health service, in particular successive Governments drive for quality and improvement in care delivery. Evidence can be from different sources and have different levels and forms (Hamer & Collinson 1999). Examples of evidence are audit findings and research. The University of York, NHS Centre for Reviews and Dissemination have set out a hierarchy of evidence, with well designed randomised controlled trials (RCTs) being number one. Hamer and Collinson (1999) state that:

> 66 *All research evidence is susceptible to variation and not all research is equal: the domination of the positivist, natural science paradigm as embodied in the medical sciences has placed it in a stronger position.* 99 *(p. 19)*

They identify the following research designs in their deliberations on the appropriateness of different forms of evidence: randomised controlled trials, case–controlled

studies, cohort studies, surveys, qualitative studies and professional consensus.

Exercise
1. Identify one area of nursing practice that you encounter in your workplace and determine what the underpinning evidence is?
2. How do you ensure that the care planned and implemented is underpinned by an evidence base?

In response to the latter you may have considered keeping yourself up to date professionally, undertaking a course of study to be able to review the evidence and its quality, or even setting up a journal club where you and colleagues can discuss evidence available and how you plan to implement this in your area of work.

It is now an important part of the nurse's role to ensure that the care she delivers is based on both evidence from nursing research and other sources (Hamer & Collinson 1999).

Multiprofessional collaboration

Fatchett (1998) states that 'the promotion of the concept of collaboration has been and remains an important theme underpinning current health policy activity' and offers the following reasons for 'the apparent surge' in its popularity:

- a growth in the complexity of health and welfare services
- expansion of knowledge and subsequent increase in specialisation
- a perceived need for the rationalisation of resources
- a need for lessening the duplication of care
- the provision of a more effective, integrated and supportive service for both users and professionals (Fatchett 1998, p. 135).

For nurses this means working in partnership not only with other health professionals but also with the users of health services. Despite the various debates about professional boundaries (Gabe et al 1994) there has been a major shift towards creating an integrated and collaborative approach to care development and delivery.

Examples of where this has been successful are in the development of pathways of care. Johnson (1997) explains these as:

> 66 *Pathways of care amalgamate all the anticipated elements of care and treatment of all members of the multi-disciplinary team, for a patient or client of a particular case-type or grouping within an agreed time frame, for the achievement of agreed outcomes. Any deviation from the plan is documented as a "variance"; the analysis of which provides information for the review of current practice.* 99 *(p. 11)*

Exercise

1. How could the Roper, Logan and Tierney model for nursing be used as a framework for documenting care as part of an integrated care pathway?

You may have considered that it would be invaluable as an assessment tool within an integrated care plan or you may decide to use it as a framework for ensuring that all aspects of an individual patient's life are considered. For example, if you were developing a pathway for caring for patients following a stroke the team would need to ensure that all the factors influencing the Activities of Living were included. To assess and plan the need for speech and language therapy would need a knowledge of the biological factors that have both led to the stroke and also why speech is impaired.

It is important to remember that multiprofessional collaboration is not about dissolving professional boundaries but about understanding and recognising the value each profession has to play in the care and wellbeing of the patient. This will then avoid the duplication of care practices and provide a more integrated and personalised service.

Delivery of care

Care is delivered in a number of different settings and in different ways. In many countries this setting can be divided into two main areas, namely hospital and community, with the latter encompassing a range of environments from care homes to health centres. In other countries care is delivered at the point of need and often in difficult and hazardous environments, e.g. refugee camps in war-torn countries.

In the UK there have been major changes to how care is delivered in the community, in particular through the developing integration of health and social care services. The setting up of the Primary Care Trusts is an example of how this collaboration and integration is being promoted (see Box 2.4).

INTERNATIONAL PERSPECTIVES IN NURSING AND HEALTH CARE

In 2001 the World Health Organisation (WHO 2001b) published their summary document – Strengthening nursing and midwifery: progress and future directions, which reported on the contribution that nursing and midwifery had made to health and development during the period 1996–2000 (WHO 2001b). The importance of these professions can be seen from their introduction:

> *Despite differences in local contexts, nursing and midwifery services are an essential foundation and support for every health system. These services are found*

Box 2.4 Devolution day for the NHS: Half a century of centralised healthcare is drawing to a close
(Milburn (2002) Press Release 1st April 2002, DoH Extracts)

Primary Care Trusts (PCTs) are free-standing, legally established, statutory NHS bodies that are accountable to their Health Authority. PCTs have the same overall functions as Primary Care Groups, thus allowing continuity with the strategic plans developed by them for their community. PCTs offer an unparalleled opportunity for local stakeholders – family doctors, nurses, midwives, health visitors, the professions allied to medicine, social services and the wider community they serve – to shape services to provide better health and better care.

PCTs will take responsibility for securing the provision of the fuller range of services for the local populations as Strategic Health Authorities step back from a hands-on commissioning role. They will take on responsibility for all family health services practitioners allowing a coherent view of the development of all the NHS services in the area. PCTs will have responsibility for the management, development and integration of all primary care services including medical, dental, pharmaceutical and optical. Primary Care Trusts bring a range of benefits to patients, the community and professionals:

- better support to practices
- better support to individual clinicians
- better integrated services
- better access
- better action to improve public health
- bringing decision-making closer to patients and local communities.

> *wherever health services are delivered, regardless of the service level, speciality area or service location.* (p. 1)

The report highlighted a number of challenges and strategic issues confronting nursing and midwifery services worldwide which need to be considered in the future as a result of their evidence. Some of these are:

- increasing case loads leading to stress and poor quality of services;
- increased mobility of health workers – likely to aggravate 'provider' shortages in some areas, exacerbated by increased consumer awareness of and demand for nursing and midwifery services (p. 5);
- knowledge explosion and access to technology solutions;
- epidemiological changes and service response – in particular the re-emergence of infectious diseases and increases in chronic health conditions. Women's health issues and an ageing population;
- poverty – nurses are not always recognised for what they can contribute to health care in different countries;

- human rights and gender – women are still systematically discriminated against in many countries – both as providers and users of health care services.

Nurses and midwives are very often the prime carers in health care, with no easy access to medical services. The WHO cite a number of initiatives where nurses have made a difference to health care.

1. In Senegal and South Africa nurses are involved in facilitating community participation as well as in supervising and implementing programmes to combat HIV/AIDS.
2. In Thailand, nurses and midwives provide a variety of mental health services including education, prevention and management of stress, conflict resolution, group and family therapy and community-based and mobile mental health clinics.
3. In Bahrain nurses run diabetic clinics and cardiac rehabilitation programmes (WHO 2001b, p. 12).

Exercise

1. Undertake a literature search to determine how nursing is developing in the various health care systems which exist in the world and determine if you can identify common themes emerging.

Some of the issues you may come across relate to the three universal themes that Salvage (1993) reports on, namely power, gender and medicalisation – which she states are all closely linked. **Power** is usually lacking even where there is a nursing voice at strategic level. **Gender** – women make up the majority of the nursing workforce and in many countries they 'suffer gender discrimination in both their personal and working lives'. **Medicalisation** – 'where medicine dominates every European health system to a greater or lesser extent' and nurses are seen as more or less assistants to the doctors. This can cause an undervaluing of nursing work and their caring role (Salvage 1993, p. 5).

Exercise

1. What would you have to consider if you wanted to implement the RLT Model in a country where nurses had no power to change practice, were discriminated against at work and in their personal life and were seen as 'assistants' to doctors?
2. Discuss the issues with colleagues or tutors and determine what would need to happen if nursing models were to be used as frameworks for care.

Some of the issues you may have discussed in relation to these questions may have included those surrounding the professionalisation of nursing, in particular the relationship between doctors and nurses. Understanding what it is to be a profession and a professional is essential if you are to be part of a team delivering care to those who are the vulnerable in society due to illness or other causes such as disability.

PROFESSIONAL ISSUES AND NURSING PRACTICE

So what is a profession? One sociologist who studied the sociology of professions was Talcott Parsons, and from his work arose the 'trait theory' of what a profession is. Jones (1994) noted that these were:

- theory of knowledge underlying and informing the practice of the profession
- code of ethics (accepted rules) regulating practice
- control of entry to the profession, through tests, training and so on, and through disciplinary powers
- professional authority over the layman, based on specialist knowledge
- confidential nature of the patient–client relationship
- existence of a professional culture: that is, an agreed way of behaving, which may be designed to exclude/impress.

Exercise

1. If these 'traits' are applied to nursing, can you decide if it is a profession? Discuss with colleagues and agree the basis for your decisions.

You may have considered that yes, nursing is a profession, based on the fact that there is a developing body of knowledge informing nursing practice, based on research and other forms of evidence. Yes there is a code of ethics or rather a code of professional conduct, entry to the profession is also controlled through registration with the NMC, nurses do have more detailed knowledge than the patient and there is confidentiality between the nurse and the patient (albeit within a sphere of accountability and 'doing the patient no harm'). The existence of a professional culture can be seen in the way nurses behave and practice but this may not be as easy to demonstrate in terms of evidence as the other 'traits'. Being a professional would encompass adhering to a code of professional conduct and ensuring that whoever called themselves a nurse had the right to do so (professional regulation). Let us consider some of these 'traits' and how they influence the care that you give to patients and work with colleagues.

Professional regulation

In the UK, up until 2002 the nursing profession was regulated by two professional bodies, namely the United Kingdom Central Council for Nursing, Midwifery and Health Visiting (UKCC) and the four National Boards in England, Scotland, Wales and Northern Ireland. The functions were different but they complemented one another. The UKCC set a code of professional conduct for registered nurses, midwives and health visitors to ensure that they maintained agreed standards of professional behaviour and practice (UKCC 1992b). This was revised in 2002 as part of the new Nursing and Midwifery Council (NMC) and came into effect in June 2002 (see Box 2.5).

For student nurses and midwives the NMC have guidance on clinical experience (NMC 2002b) which encompass some of the principles of the Code of Professional Conduct. For example in relation to accountability they state that:

> *as a pre-registration student you are never professionally accountable in the way that you will be after you come to register with the NMC. So far as the NMC is concerned, it is the registered practitioners with whom you are working who are professionally responsible for the consequences of your actions and omissions. This is why you must always work under the direct supervision of a registered nurse or midwife. This does not mean however that you can never be called to account by your*

university or by the law for the consequences of your actions or omissions as a pre-registration student.
(NMC 2002b, p. 4)

Full details of the Code of Professional Conduct as well as other professional body documents can be found at www.nmc-uk.org.

Codes of professional conduct are also found in other countries where there is a recognised training and education programme for nurses. In Australia for example they have both a code of professional conduct and a code of ethics. The Australian Code of Professional Conduct (ANC 1995) has eight standards – each of which is further divided into a series of explanatory statements (see www.anci.org.au/codeofconduct for full details). One can see the similarities with the NMC Code of Conduct.

Code of Professional Conduct (Australian Nursing Council 1995)

1. Provide safe and competent nursing care.
2. Uphold the agreed standards of the profession.
3. Practise in accordance with the laws relevant to the nurse's area of practice.
4. Respect the dignity, culture, values and beliefs of patients/clients and significant others in the provision of nursing care.
5. Promote and support the health and wellbeing and informed decision making of patients/clients in the provision of nursing care.
6. Promote and preserve the trust that is inherent in the privileged relationship between nurses and their patients/clients with respect to both their person and their property.
7. Treat as confidential personal information obtained in a professional capacity.
8. Refrain from engaging in exploitation, misinformation and misrepresentation in regards to health care products and nursing services.

The Australian Nursing Council (ANC 2002) have also developed a Code of Ethics for nurses, their rationale being that:

> *Nursing practice is undertaken in a variety of settings. Any particular setting will be affected to some degree by factors which are not within a nurse's control or influence. These include resource constraints, institutional policies, management decisions and the practice of other health care providers. Nurses also recognise the potential for conflict between one person's needs and those of another, or of a group or community. Such factors may affect the degree to which nurses are able to fulfil their moral obligations and/or the number and type of ethical dilemmas they may face.*
> (www.anci.org.au/codeofethics)

This Code consists of six broad value statements (with explanatory statements to support them). The purpose of the Code is to:

Box 2.5 Code of Professional Conduct (NMC 2002a)

As a registered nurse or midwife, you are personally accountable for your practice. In caring for patients and clients, you must:

- respect the patient or client as an individual
- obtain consent before you give any treatment or care
- protect confidential information
- cooperate with others in the team
- maintain your professional knowledge and competence
- be trustworthy
- act to identify and minimise risk to patients and clients.

These are the shared values of all the United Kingdom health care regulatory bodies.

1.1 The purpose of the Code of professional conduct is to:
  - inform the professions of the standard of professional conduct required of them in the exercise of their professional accountability and practice
  - inform the public, other professions and employers of the standard of professional conduct that they expect of a registered practitioner.

1.2 As a registered nurse or midwife you must:
  - protect and support the health of individual patients and clients
  - protect and support the health of the wider community
  - act in such a way that justifies the trust and confidence the public have in you
  - uphold and enhance the good reputation of the professions.

1.3 You are personally accountable for your practice. This means that you are answerable for your actions and omissions, regardless of advice and directions from another professional.

1.4 You have a duty of care to your patients and clients who are entitled to receive safe and competent care.

1.5 You must adhere to the laws of the country in which you are practising.

- identify the fundamental moral commitments of the profession
- provide nurses with a basis for professional and self reflection and a guide to ethical practice
- indicate to the community the values which nurses hold.

The six value statements are:

1. Nurses respect persons' individual needs, values and culture in the provision of nursing care.
2. Nurses respect the rights of persons to make informed choices in relation to their care.
3. Nurses promote and uphold the provision of quality nursing care for people.
4. Nurses hold in confidence any information obtained in a professional capacity and use professional judgement in sharing such information.
5. Nurses respect the accountability and responsibility inherent in their roles.
6. Nurses value the promotion of an ecological, social and economic environment which supports and sustains health and wellbeing.

Exercise

1. Consider both the NMC and ANC Codes of Professional Conduct and Ethics and identify the similarities between them.
2. How can the Roper et al model for nursing help you to ensure that the Codes are adhered to? For example, ensuring that cultural needs are taken account of in the assessment process or ensuring that informed consent is obtained prior to surgery as part of ensuring and maintaining a safe environment.
3. Access the ANC website and read the full code of professional conduct and code of ethics. Using the internet and other sources, search for other nursing codes of professional conduct in other countries and discuss them with colleagues.

This kind of regulation is termed 'self-regulation' but as Basford (1995, p. 137) outlines, this does not 'mean that a profession is totally autonomous and therefore totally self-regulating'. She states that all members of a profession are subject to 'the laws of the land' and that these include: criminal law, employment law, civil law and public law. An example of how a nurse came to break the law is seen in the case of Beverly Allit, convicted of murdering children in her care on a paediatric ward (Clothier et al 1994).

Patient care is therefore dependent on nursing practice that is based on a professional and ethical code. So how is it possible to ensure that those entering the profession are fit for taking on the title of nurse and will adhere to the code of professional conduct?

It is pertinent at this stage to look at the education and training of nurses, in particular the content of their 3-year programme which will ensure they are prepared for becoming a qualified nurse.

NURSING EDUCATION – ITS DEVELOPMENT AND CURRENT CONTEXT

In order to understand the present context, it is important to reflect on the past.

Nursing as a predominantly female occupation has been subjected to major changes since its origins in the late 1800s. The Nurses Registration Act 1919 ensured that the public were protected from untrained women who would no longer be able to call themselves 'nurse' without membership on the register. Since that time there have been numerous attempts to reform nursing and nurse education and training, with the result that in the UK in 1989, as a result of implementation of Project 2000 recommendations (UKCC 1987), all probationer nurses were recognised as students within the University (Higher Education) sector. In the USA however this had long been recognised as an essential prerequisite to ensuring professional status for nursing and the graduate nurse was well established within American health care.

Another major development taking place in the UK which is influencing the development of all the health and social care professions is interprofessional education (Barr 2002, Royle et al 1999, Miller et al 1999). To be able to deliver the current and future health and social care agenda requires a workforce that is interdependent as well as working interprofessionally (Audit Commission 2001).

Nurse education in the UK

The current provision of education for pre-registration student nurses in the UK is at two levels: graduate and diplomat, with the majority qualifying with a Diploma plus their registered nurse (RN) qualification. Prior to 2000 student nurse Diploma level education consisted of a 3-year programme, with an 18-month common foundation and an 18-month Branch in one of four areas of practice, namely; adult nursing, children's nursing, mental health nursing and learning disability nursing. At the end of that time students were expected to be able to meet the 13 competencies of Rule 18a (UKCC – 1989 – Amendment of Nurses Act 1979). These can be seen in Box 2.6.

As a result of a number of research studies into the effectiveness and appropriateness of the Project 2000 course (Jowett & Walton 1994, Macleod Clark et al 1996) and also a UKCC commission into preregistration education (UKCC 1999) Rule 18a was superseded by a new set of rules and competencies (Statutory Instrument 2000 No. 2554 – The Nurses, Midwives and Health Visitors (Training) Amendment Rules Approval Order 2000 – www.hmso.gov.uk) and a new course was proposed which had a 1 year foundation and 2 year Branch programme. The nursing competencies and guiding principles are more specific in what is expected of a student nurse after 1 year foundation and on qualifying. See Boxes 2.7 and 2.8.

Box 2.6 Statutory Instrument 1989 No.1456

Schedule 2 – The Nurses, Midwives and Health Visitors (Training) Amendment Rules 1989 – The Nurses, Midwives and Health Visitors Act 1979

Preparation for entry to Parts 12, 13, 14 and 15 of the register 18A

(1) The contents of the Common Foundation Programme and the Branch Programme shall be such as the council may from time to time require.

(2) The Common Foundation Programme and Branch Programmes shall be designed to prepare the nursing student to assume the responsibilities and accountability that registration confers, and to prepare the nursing student to apply knowledge and skills to meet the nursing needs of individuals and of groups in health and in sickness in the area of practice of the Branch Programme and shall include enabling the student to achieve the following outcomes:

(a) The identification of the social and health implications of pregnancy and childbearing, physical and mental handicap, disease, disability, or ageing for the individual, her or his friends, family and community.

(b) The recognition of common factors which contribute to and those which adversely affect physical, mental and social wellbeing of patients and clients and take appropriate action.

(c) The use of relevant literature and research to inform the practice of nursing.

(d) The appreciation of the influence of social, political and cultural factors in relation to health care.

(e) An understanding of the requirements of legislation relevant to the practice of nursing.

(f) The use of appropriate communication skills to enable the development of helpful caring relationships with patients and clients and their families and friends, and to initiate and conduct therapeutic relationships with patients and clients.

(g) The identification of health-related learning needs of patients and clients, families and friends and to participate in health promotion.

(h) An understanding of the ethics of health care and of the nursing profession and the responsibilities which these impose on the nurse's professional practice.

(i) The identification of the needs of patients and clients to enable them to progress from varying degrees of dependence to maximum independence or to a peaceful death.

(j) The identification of physical, psychological, social and spiritual needs of the patient or client; an awareness of values and concepts of individual care; the ability to devise a plan of care, contribute to its implementation and evaluation; and the demonstration of the application of the principles of a problem-solving approach to the practice of nursing.

(k) The ability to function effectively in a team and participate in a multiprofessional approach to the care of patients and clients.

(l) The use of the appropriate channel of referral for matters not within her sphere of competence.

(m) The assignment of appropriate duties to others and the supervision, teaching and monitoring of assigned duties.

From Her Majesty's Stationery Office (www.hmso.gov.uk).

Box 2.7 Nursing competencies – to be achieved for entry to Branch (after 1 year)

Domain – Professional and Ethical Practice

- Discuss in an informed manner the implications of professional regulation for nursing practice.
- Demonstrate an awareness of, and apply ethical principles to, nursing practice.
- Demonstrate an awareness of legislation relevant to nursing practice.
- Demonstrate the importance of promoting equity in patient and client care by contributing to nursing care in a fair and antidiscriminatory way.

Domain – Care Delivery

- Discuss methods of, barriers to and the boundaries of effective communication and interpersonal relationships.
- Demonstrate sensitivity when interacting with and providing information to patients and clients.

- Contribute to enhancing the health and social wellbeing of patients and clients by understanding how under the supervision of a registered practitioner:
  — contribute to the assessment of health needs
  — identify opportunities for health promotion
  — identify networks of health and social care services.
- Contribute to the development and documentation of nursing assessments by participating in comprehensive and systematic nursing assessment of the physical, psychological, social and spiritual needs of patients and clients.
- Contribute to the planning of nursing care, involving patients and clients and where possible their carers, demonstrating an understanding of helping patients and clients to make informed decisions.

(continued)

Box 2.7 *(continued)*

- Contribute to the implementation of a programme of nursing care, designed and supervised by registered practitioners.
- Demonstrate evidence of a developing knowledge base which underpins safe nursing practice.
- Demonstrate a range of essential nursing skills, under the supervision of a registered nurse, to meet individual needs which include: maintaining dignity, privacy and confidentiality, effective communication and observation skills, including listening and taking physiological measurements; safety and health, including moving and handling and infection control; essential first aid and emergency procedures, administration of medicines; emotional, physical and personal care, including meeting the need for comfort, nutrition and personal hygiene.
- Contribute to the evaluation of the appropriateness of nursing care delivered.
- Recognise situations in which agreed plans for nursing care no longer appear appropriate and refer these to an accountable practitioner.

Domain – Care Management

- Contribute to the identification of actual and potential risks to patients, clients and their carers, to oneself and to others and participate in measures to promote and ensure health and safety.
- Demonstrate an understanding of the role of others by participating in interprofessional working practice.
- Demonstrate literacy, numeracy, and computer skills needed to record, enter, store, retrieve and organise data essential for care delivery.

Domain – Personal and Professional Development

- Demonstrate responsibility for one's own learning through the development of a portfolio of practice and recognise when further learning is required.
- Acknowledge the importance of seeking supervision to develop safe nursing practice.

From: Requirements for preregistration nursing programmes (UKCC 2000).

Box 2.8 Nursing competencies – for entry to register

Domain – Professional and Ethical Practice

- Manage oneself, one's practice and that of others, in accordance with the UKCC's Code of Professional Conduct, recognising one's own abilities and limitations.
- Practice in accordance with an ethical and legal framework which ensures the primacy of patient and client interest and wellbeing and respects confidentiality.
- Practise in a fair and antidiscriminatory way, acknowledging the differences in beliefs and cultural practices of individuals and groups.

Domain – Care Delivery

- Engage in, develop and disengage from therapeutic relationships through the use of appropriate communication and interpersonal skills.
- Create and utilise opportunities to promote the health and wellbeing of patients, clients and groups.
- Undertake and document a comprehensive, systematic and accurate nursing assessment of the physical, psychological, social and spiritual needs of patients, clients and communities.
- Formulate and document a plan of nursing care, where possible in partnership with patients, clients, their carers and family and friends, within a framework of informed consent.
- Based on the best available evidence, apply knowledge and an appropriate repertoire of skills indicative of safe nursing practice.

- Provide a rationale for the nursing care delivered which takes account of social, spiritual, legal, political and economic influences.
- Evaluate and document the outcomes of nursing and other interventions.
- Demonstrate sound clinical judgement across a range of differing professional and care delivery contexts.

Domain – Care Management

- Contribute to public protection by creating and maintaining a safe environment of care through the use of quality assurance and risk management strategies.
- Demonstrate knowledge of effective interprofessional working practices which respect and utilise the contributions of members of the health and social care team.
- Delegate duties to others, as appropriate, ensuring that they are supervised and monitored.
- Demonstrate key skills.

Domain – Personal and Professional Development

- Demonstrate a commitment to the need for continuing professional development and personal supervision activities in order to enhance knowledge, skills, values and attitudes needed for safe and effective nursing practice.
- Enhance the professional development and safe practice of others through peer support, leadership, supervision and teaching.

From: Requirements for preregistration nursing programmes (UKCC 2000).

It can be seen throughout the competency statements that the Code of Professional Conduct and ethical practice are essential to being able to become a registered nurse with the NMC in the United Kingdom. Other countries have similar competencies to be achieved but there are no universally agreed competencies which would enable nurses to move freely across international boundaries. It is beyond the scope of this book to consider the reasons for this, however some of those could be attributed to the social, political, cultural and economic climate of each country and the lack of consensus internationally about the role and function of the nurse.

Nurse education worldwide

Nursing is a worldwide occupation and as such requires its education and training programmes to ensure that there are some commonalities between international boundaries. How nursing has developed in each country however will depend not only on its historical context, but most importantly on the social, political and economic needs prevalent at the time. Patient needs will also differ as a result of this. It can be seen how nursing has responded to change by the way in which its status as a profession has changed in different countries.

In Brazil for example, the introduction of undergraduate programmes for nurses 'elevated nursing to the status of a liberal profession, and the nursing faculty assumed major roles in nursing education' (Neves & Mauro 2000). However it took 14 years of lobbying the government for approval to be given for a new curriculum which was established in 1994 but 'was already outdated, and is failing to attend the societal demands of the nursing profession' (Neves & Mauro 2000, p. 4). The way in which nursing responds to changes in society is illustrated in Primomo's (2000) description of the way in which Japanese nurses are trying to manage the increasing ageing population and also the changing societal values in relation to family structure and women's roles. She states that:

> 66 *By increasing efforts to move nursing education into the university setting and by focusing curriculum on community-based care, nurses should be better prepared to meet the needs of its ageing society and function in autonomous roles. As the profession continues its efforts to become involved in health policy at the national and local level it is anticipated that nurses will have even greater opportunities to improve health and health care for the Japanese population.* 99
> (Primomo 2000, p. 15)

It can be seen from the examples cited that there is much in common between nursing in different countries and the importance of how society, politics and economics influence not only our understanding of patients needs but also to how nursing itself is developed, managed and delivered. The Roper et al model for nursing incorporates these dimensions in the model of living (see Chapter 1).

Summary Points

1. Nursing exists in a social, political and economic context.
2. To use the model for nursing requires an understanding of the role of the nurse as it exists across international boundaries.
3. The education of nurses is essential to the delivery of effective patient care that meets the needs of individuals and their families as appropriate to that society's needs.

References

Arthritis Research Campaign 2001 Leeches – a treatment for knee osteoarthritis? ARC (www.arc.uk/newsviews/press/aug20)

Audit Commission 2001 Hidden talents – education, training and developments for healthcare staff in the NHS. Audit Commission, London

Australian Nursing Council 1995 Code of professional conduct. (www.anci.org.au)

Australian Nursing Council 2002 Code of ethics. (www.anci.org.au)

Baly M 1995 Nursing & social change, 3rd edn. Routledge, London

Barr H 2002 Interprofessional education – today, yesterday and tomorrow. LTSN for Health Sciences and Practice, London

Basford L 1995 Professionalisation. In: Basford L, Slevin O (eds) Theory and practice of nursing, pp. 133–140. Campion Press Ltd, Edinburgh

Cameron A 2000 New role developments in context. In: Humphris D, Masterson A (eds) Developing new clinical roles, pp. 7–24. Churchill Livingstone, Edinburgh

Clothier C, MacDonald C, Shaw D 1994 Independent enquiry into deaths and injuries on the Children's Ward at Grantham and Kestoran General Hospital during the period February to April 1991 (Allitt Inquiry). HMSO, London.

Cooper C 2001 The art of nursing – a practical introduction. WB Saunders Co, Philadelphia

Davey B 1992 Biological perspectives. In: Robinson K, Vaughan B (eds) Knowledge for nursing practice, pp. 42–59. Butterworth Heinemann Ltd, Oxford

Department of Health 1991 Hours of work of doctors in training, the new deal. Executive letter 82. DoH, London

Department of Health 1997 The new NHS – modern, dependable. White paper, December 1997. DoH, London (www.doh.gov.uk/nhsind.html)

Department of Health 1998 A first class service – quality in the new NHS. DoH, London

Department of Health 1999a Waiting times – modernisation fund investment, £20 million boost to reduce waiting lists and waiting times. Department of Health Press Release, 22nd February 1999 (www.doh.gov/nhsexec/modfund.html)

Department of Health 1999b Primary Care Trusts – establishing better services. DoH, London (www.doh.gov.uk/pricare/pcts.html)

Department of Health 2000 Towards a strategy for nursing research and development, p. 10. DoH, London

Department of Health 2001 NHS national nursing leadership project. DoH, London (www.nursingleadership.co.uk)

Department of Health 2002 Devolution day for the NHS: half a century of centralised healthcare is drawing to a close. Milburn, Department of Health, Press Release 1st April 2002 (www.doh.gov.uk/pricare/pcts.html)

Fatchett A 1998 Nursing in the new NHS – modern, dependable? Baillière Tindall, London

Gabe J, Kelleher D, Williams G 1994 Challenging medicine. Routledge, London

Grant AB, Massey VH 1999 Nursing leadership, management & research. Springhouse Corporation, Springhouse, Pennsylvania

Hamer S, Collinson G (eds) 1999 Achieving evidence based practice. Baillière Tindall/Royal College of Nursing, Edinburgh

Henderson V 1966 The nature of nursing. Collier-Macmillan Ltd, New York

Her Majesty's Stationery Office 1989 Statutory Instrument 1989 no.1456, Schedule 2 – The Nurses, Midwives and Health Visitors (Training) Amendment Rules 1989 – The Nurses and Midwives and Health Visitors Act 1979. HMSO, London (www.hmso.gov.uk)

Holden P, Littlewood J 1991 Anthropology and nursing. Routledge, London

Humphris D, Masterson A 2000 Developing new clinical roles – a guide for health professionals. Churchill Livingstone, Edinburgh

Johnson S 1997 Pathways of care. Blackwell Science, Oxford

Jones LJ 1994 The social context of health and social work. Macmillan Press Ltd, Basingstoke

Jowett S, Walton I 1994 Challenges and change in nurse education – a study of the implementation of Project 2000. National Foundation for Educational Research in England and Wales, Slough

Lawler J 1991 Behind the screens – nursing, somology and the body. Churchill Livingstone, Edinburgh

Leininger M 1978 Transcultural concepts, theories and practices. John Wiley and Sons, New York

Littlewood J 1991 Care and ambiguity: towards a concept of nursing. In: Holden P, Littlewood J (eds) Anthropology and nursing, pp. 179–180. Routledge, London

Macleod Clark J, Maben J, Jones K 1996 Project 2000: Perceptions of the philosophy and practice of nursing. English National Board, London

Miller C, Ross N, Freeman M 1999 Shared learning and clinical teamwork: new directions in education for multiprofessional practice. English National Board, London

Morris S 1998 Health economics for nurses – an introductory guide. Prentice Hall, Hemel Hempstead

Neves EP, Mauro MYC 2000 Nursing in Brazil: trajectory, conquests and challenges. Online Journal of Issues in Nursing 5(2): 1–14 (http://www.nursingworld.org)

Nursing and Midwifery Council 2002a Code of professional conduct. NMC, London

Nursing and Midwifery Council 2002b An NMC guide for students of nursing and midwifery. NMC, London

Porter S 1991 A participant observation study of power relations between nurses and doctors in a general hospital. Journal of Advanced Nursing 16(6): 728–735

Porter S 1998 Social theory and nursing practice. Macmillan Press Ltd, Basingstoke

Primomo J 2000 Nursing around the world: Japan – preparing for the century of the elderly. Online Journal of Issues in Nursing 5(2): 1–20 (www.nursingworld.org)

Proctor S 2000 Caring for health. Macmillan Press Ltd, Basingstoke

Roper N, Logan W, Tierney A 1996 The elements of nursing. Churchill Livingstone, Edinburgh

Roper N, Logan W, Tierney A 2000 The Roper, Logan and Tierney model of nursing. Churchill Livingstone, Edinburgh

Royle J, Speller V, Moon A 1999 Exploring interprofessional education and training needs in public health. Wessex Institute for Health Research and Development, University of Southampton

Salvage J (ed) 1993 Strengthening nursing and midwifery to support health for all. WHO Regional Publications, European Series, No.48, World Health Organisation, Copenhagan

Salvage J 1995 Nursing intimacy. Scutari Press, London

Schultz EA, Lavenda RH 1990 Cultural anthropology, 2nd edn. West Publishing Co, St Paul

Seymer L 1960 Florence Nightingale's nurses – The Nightingale Training School 1860–1960. Pitman Medical Publishing Co. Ltd, London

Sofarelli D, Brown D 1998 The need for nursing leadership in uncertain times. Journal of Nursing Management 6: 201–207

Tones K 1993 Theory of health promotion; implications for nursing. In: Wilson-Barnett J, Clark J (eds) Research in health promotion and nursing. Macmillan, London

UKCC 1987 United Kingdom Central Council for Nursing, Midwifery and Health Visiting, Project 2000: the final proposals (Project Paper 9). UKCC, London

UKCC 1992a Scope of professional practice. United Kingdom Central Council for Nursing, Midwifery and Health Visiting, London

UKCC 1992b Code of professional conduct. UKCC, London

UKCC 1999 Fitness for practice. The UKCC Commission for Nursing and Midwifery Education, UKCC, London

UKCC 2000 Requirements for pre-registration programmes. United Kingdom Central Council for Nursing, Midwifery and Health Visiting, London

Wallace M 2002 A–Z guide to professional healthcare. Churchill Livingstone, Edinburgh

Walsh M (ed) 2002 Watson's clinical nursing and related sciences, 6th edition. Baillière Tindall, Edinburgh

Watkins M 1997 Nursing knowledge in nursing practice. In: Perry A (ed) Nursing – a knowledge base for practice, 2nd edn, pp. 1–32. Arnold, London

World Health Organisation 1997 Global movement for healthy ageing. Press release WHO/69 26th September 1997, WHO, Geneva (www.int/archives)

World Health Organisation 2001a Life course perspectives on coronary heart disease, stroke and diabetes – key issues and implications for policy and research. Summary report of a meeting of experts, 2–4 May 2001, WHO, Geneva

World Health Organisation 2001b Strengthening nursing and midwifery – Progress and future directions – 1996–2000. World Health Organisation, Geneva

World Health Organisation 2001c The global movement for active ageing. World Health Organisation, Geneva (www.int/hpr/globalmovement/index.html)

World Health Organisation 2002 WHO and the humanitarian crisis in South Africa. doc.4/8/2002 (www.who.int/disasters/emergency.cfm)

Further reading

Allen D 2001 The changing shape of nursing practice – the role of nurses in the hospital division of labour. Routledge, London

Baxter C (ed) 2001 Managing diversity and inequality. Baillière Tindall/Royal College of Nursing, Edinburgh

Bishop V, Scott I (eds) 2001 Challenges in clinical practice. Palgrave, Basingstoke

Chiarella M 2002 The legal and professional status of nursing. Churchill Livingstone, Edinburgh

Ewens A 2002 The nature and purpose of leadership. In: Howkins E, Thornton C (eds) Managing and leading innovation in health care, pp. 69–90. Baillière Tindall/Royal College of Nursing, London

Hyde J, Cooper F (eds) 2001 Managing the business of health care. Baillière Tindall/Royal College of Nursing, Edinburgh

Useful websites

www.nursingboard.ie (Irish Nursing Board, An Bord Altranais)
www.nursingcouncil.org.nz (Nursing Council of New Zealand)
www.nursingworld.org (Online Journal of Issues in Nursing – a free peer reviewed electronic journal – with links to other useful websites)
www.doh.gov.uk (United Kingdom Department of Health)

Nursing and the Activities of Living

SECTION

2

CONTENTS

Maintaining a safe environment

Susan Whittam

Introduction

Keeping ourselves safe is thought to be a basic survival skill, which all individuals possess, yet there are times when we are either unaware or unable to control the ability to do this. Throughout the world there are many differences in the types of hazards and risks that people are exposed to and just as many differences in the way that people manage their own safety. The inclusion of this AL in the Roper et al (1996, 2000) model is to draw your attention to the importance of being able to recognise the threats that exist to human survival and wellbeing and identify the impact that this may have upon any individual at any given time in their lives. The model helps us to develop our understanding by essentially focusing upon three key areas of concern as follows:

- the human body's ability to protect itself and the biological mechanisms that it employs to carry this out
- the ability that individuals have to make choices and take action to keep safe and free from danger
- the identification and understanding of the dangers and hazards that exist and how they pose a threat to individual safety and wellbeing.

These three areas of concern will be discussed throughout this chapter within the framework of the model and will help to develop an understanding of the AL and enable nursing interventions to be as individualised and effective as possible. Like most things in life it is not until something goes wrong do we seek to understand how our bodies or everyday life around us function. Often concern for our own health and safety only becomes heightened when we become ill, have an accident or hear about a tragedy or event that has had terrible human consequences.

By using the framework of the Roper et al (1996, 2000) model in the following way we can begin to examine and identify how complex and varied health and safety issues really are and also identify the interrelatedness that exists between the other ALs. This chapter will therefore focus on the following:

1. **The model of living**
   - maintaining a safe environment in health and illness across the lifespan
   - dependence and independence in the activity of maintaining a safe environment
   - factors influencing the activity of maintaining a safe environment.

2. **The model for nursing**
   - nursing care of individuals with health problems that are affecting their ability to undertake the activity of maintaining a safe environment.

THE MODEL OF LIVING

Maintaining a safe environment in health and illness across the lifespan

This component of the model describes the importance that safety plays at various stages of the lifespan. Safety is viewed as being a basic human survival skill and the model helps us to identify how this is achieved or compromised in normal everyday life. When applying the model in practice you will need to acknowledge that as people move across the lifespan they will encounter continuous changes in the way in which they ensure their survival and wellbeing, take risks and avoid hazards. This requires consideration of both the internal and the external environment. Essentially the internal environment considers the biological and psychological factors that may threaten safety and the external environment relates to the impact that sociocultural, economic and the surrounding environment may have upon health, for example:

- *Internal* Injuries and diseases causing physiological and psychological disturbances.
- *External* Accidents influenced by physical, psychological, sociocultural, environmental or politicoeconomic changes or limitations.

By understanding the basic needs and activities of individuals or groups there is the opportunity for the practice of nursing to become more supportive and effective. The life-span stages identified with the activity of maintaining a safe environment are as follows.

Childhood

Before birth, babies are totally dependent upon other human beings for their survival. In some cases there may be a known risk to the health and wellbeing of the unborn child, such as cystic fibrosis and Down syndrome (Wald & Hackshaw 2000). Through the provision of good antenatal care and increasing technological advances many physical and genetic disorders can be detected and in some circumstances babies can receive life-saving treatment prior to birth (Hubbard & Harty 2000).

Under normal circumstances the health of the unborn child is dependent upon the health and wellbeing of the mother in order to ensure the best chance of survival at birth and during the early weeks of life. To increase knowledge about common genetic disorders and the help and advice available to parents complete the following exercise.

Exercise

Down syndrome, heart defects, sickle cell anaemia and cleft palate are four examples of genetic/birth disorders.

1. What techniques are used for detection of these?
2. What advice and support can parents expect to receive?

It is important to know that support and availability of services will vary based upon demand, responsibility, personal finance, national wealth, geographical location, social class and the ability to seek out and understand information for oneself. In all cases advice and support need to be handled very sensitively and in accordance with individual need. You may also discover that there are huge variations across the world in the provision of screening programmes, treatment and care. This will be further discussed in the sections related to sociocultural, environmental and politicoeconomic influences upon the AL of MSE.

During birth the safety of the mother and the baby is critical as they are both at risk from a number of hazards and complications, many of which can be detected through a collaborative multiprofessional approach to good antenatal care (Sidebotham 1999). In the UK support for a healthy pregnancy and safe childbirth is provided by midwives whose practice is statutorily regulated to ensure optimum safety to both mother and child. Despite this the World Health Organisation's (WHO) Department of Reproductive Health and Research estimate that as many as 515 000 women die every year as a result of pregnancy and childbirth,

with women in the poorest countries being 300 times more at risk (WHO 2002b).

The responsibility for the safety of babies and toddlers within the home primarily rests with the family. The Royal Society for the Prevention of Accidents (RoSPA 2002) publish up-to-date information about a whole range of accidents and indicate that despite many years of safety campaigning the home continues to be one of the most hazardous places. The three most serious accidents being:

- impact accidents (bumps, falls and collisions)
- heat accidents (burns and scalds)
- ingestion and foreign body accidents (poisoning, choking and suffocation are most common in children under 4 years of age).

Exercise

1. To find out more about home safety browse through the RoSPA website (www.rospa.co.uk). You will find there are a series of projects that can help you to undertake home safety assessments.
2. Consider how you might use the information on the website to help patients and families improve safety within their own homes?

Despite medical advances in the treatment of common diseases, babies and toddlers continue to be at risk from childhood diseases, which even today can be life-threatening if not prevented or treated. Many countries are able to provide support for education and immunisation to reduce unnecessary health risks, but personal choices, beliefs, economic wealth, traditions and cultures all play a part in the extent to which the safety of young children can be assured.

When children start nursery and school they begin to experience an early and gradual independence. They become more adventurous and daring and increasingly exposed to outdoor school and play activities. Accident statistics show that from 0–14 years children require careful supervision in order to prevent many common accidents associated with road accidents, falls, fire, poisoning and drowning, as they are unable to adequately understand or deal with dangerous situations for themselves (Child Accident Prevention Trust 2000).

Exercise

In order to discover how children learn about safety:

1. Reflect on your own childhood. How did you learn about dangers within and outside the home?
2. Find out what personal safety topics are taught to primary school age children.

Schools play an important part in teaching young children about personal safety and even the safety of others. Teaching safety in the home is dependent upon the ability of family members to recognise and prevent accidents occurring and is rather more difficult to ensure.

Adolescence

Health and safety issues linked to adolescents are often associated with irresponsible behaviour. Increasing independence experienced at this stage of the lifespan can cause individuals to become more high-spirited and take more risks without realising the consequences. As a result, adolescents often compromise not only their own safety, but also risk the safety of others such as in road traffic accidents and accidents related to drug and alcohol misuse.

> **Exercise**
> 1. Identify the risks that you faced as an adolescent. Are they the same as those facing adolescents today?
> 2. List the dangers that currently face adolescents. What information or agencies are concerned with reducing risks to health?

Risk patterns change over time, resulting in new risks emerging continually. Often parents, as well as adolescents, are ill prepared for managing risks and this exercise should help to develop an understanding of why health and safety education is an important aspect of public health (see Chapter 12 for issues related to sexual risks and adolescents).

Adulthood

Independence and personal choice in adulthood expose individuals to a huge range of activities within the home, at work and in the pursuit of leisure, each activity carrying with it some degree of risk to safety. Young adults will perhaps be encountering many new activities for the first time and may be unaware of the threats to their own or other people's safety. At work there will be a number of specific risks associated with the type of work that is undertaken for which a joint responsibility for safety between the individual and the employer is expected. In this age group however it is the home that continues to pose the greatest threat to personal safety causing accidents associated with falls, fires, faulty appliances, poisoning, gardening and home improvement activities. In the UK home accident figures show that 3900 people are injured every week with one person per week being killed whilst carrying out home improvements, ladder accidents being the greatest cause of death. Despite having a greater awareness about personal safety, in each case it is known that carelessness, stress, absentmindedness, negligence, fatigue, illness and ageing contribute towards the cause (Department of Trade and Industry 2001)

> **Exercise**
> Explore how adults obtain information regarding safety.
> 1. Browse the Department for Trade and Industry website (www.dti.gov.uk) and determine the purpose of the Home Safety Network.
> 2. Determine how you could use the information contained within the website to:
>   * improve safety for yourself and your family
>   * support the specific needs of patients that you encounter.

The task of ensuring public safety is enormous, particularly when individuals and groups have different perceptions about what constitutes a safety precaution. It is important to appreciate this when helping patients to adopt different lifestyles. Because of different attitudes and perceptions some issues receive more public attention than others.

Old age

Today many people are living longer and as a result it is becoming more difficult to determine what constitutes a normal ageing process. Generally speaking ageing is observable by the onset of certain age-associated changes, however this can affect individual people in different ways, giving rise to the question of whether individual health changes as a result of old age or through the presence of disease (see Rutishauser 1994, Chapter 36). Nevertheless the physiological changes that are associated with ageing mean that elderly people become more prone to injury and ill health due to a deterioration in the functioning of body systems resulting in some common disorders, such as arthrosis, heart and lung failure and dementia (Health Education Authority 1999). Ultimately a deterioration in health leads to an increasing dependence upon others in order to maintain a personal level of safety.

> **Exercise**
> In order to increase your understanding of promoting safety in old age:
> 1. Find out what accidents elderly people are most likely to encounter.
> 2. Identify which of these occur (a) in the home, (b) outside the home.
> 3. List the most common disorders that affect older people.
> 4. Find out what agencies/services exist in your area to help elderly people avoid accidents.

In industrialised societies, through demographic and social changes, there is a greater need to provide public services to support the needs of elderly people. Often older people have to cope with living alone along with failing health and the increased risk of accidents, abuse and even attack. As a result in the UK there has been an increased demand for nursing and residential home accommodation and pressure to improve the systems for delivering health and social care. In recognition of the need to improve the care and support of older people in 2001 the government published a *National Service Framework for Older People* that includes specific targets concerning health and safety issues (Department of Health 2001a).

Dependency/independency

The degree of independence associated with the AL of maintaining a safe environment both internally and externally is essentially linked to age. Dependency is at its greatest in infancy, is affected by ill health, injury and disability and is expected to gradually increase in old age. The speed at which individuals achieve independence is essentially a gradual process, however dependency can occur gradually or suddenly. For example, an individual can be rendered unconscious instantaneously either by disease, injury or anaesthesia. However it is apparent that a person can never achieve complete independence within the AL, as there will always be a degree of dependency upon either other people or the surrounding environment in order to ensure safety. There are many examples of how events and the behaviour of others can compromise safety. For example individuals with mental health problems, learning disabilities, physical disabilities or those living where there is social unrest or risk of man-made or natural disasters. In relation to the body's internal environment independence is maintained through good health. There is however a risk to the body's normal ability to function at any stage of the lifespan, by the presence of disease, trauma or any other abnormal state.

Exercise

How does society value independence and what are its attitudes towards dependence? Ask three different people what their attitudes are in relation to the following:

1. A middle-aged adventurer who climbs Mount Everest or sails around the world single-handed.
2. A young person who backpacks around the world or takes a holiday in a resort notorious for excessive alcohol- and drug-taking.
3. A person with mental health problems living, with difficulty, in the community.
4. An elderly person with no family support remaining living in his/her own home.
5. Discuss your views with colleagues.

Attitudes to the above will vary, dependent upon personal experiences and beliefs. This will be further explored in the section of factors influencing the activity of MSE.

Factors influencing the AL of maintaining a safe environment

The AL of maintaining a safe environment is complex and multidimensional. This next section will help to develop an understanding of the complexity of the AL by discussing the importance that each of the factors plays in understanding the needs of patients. Each of the factors as described by the model will now be explored.

Biological factors

The function of keeping the body in a healthy state and correcting any disturbances relies upon several biological functions taking place, which are chiefly controlled by the nervous system. The systems work in conjunction with one another to carry out a series of very complex cellular processes that are triggered by changes either within the body (internal) or around it (external). In order to accurately assess and observe both the health and altered states of patients, it is vital that you understand what the systems are and how they work. For ease it is useful to identify the systems in relation to the functions they serve internally and externally as follows:

- the internal environment which is concerned with homeostatic balance, stability, protection and repair (autonomic nervous system, immunity and tissue repair)
- the external environment and the body's ability to avoid danger, and cope with changes (the sensory system or somatic nervous system).

Internal environment and related systems

Homeostasis To maintain the internal environment, the body relies upon an intricate and highly organised system of intercellular communication and control. The control process is known as homeostasis. In health the mechanisms are so efficient they are hardly noticeable, but in ill health states the mechanisms become disturbed and over time have difficulty in coping effectively. Dependent upon the underlying problem (pathophysiology) patients are often able (unless unconscious) to describe how unwell they feel. Together with patient accounts and a range of physiological observations it is possible to determine the root cause of the problem and the extent to which the homeostatic mechanisms are coping. When control breaks down, if not detected, the body will eventually reach a stage where homeostasis cannot be restored and normal cellular function will become seriously affected. This state is referred to as shock, and it is important to be aware that not only seriously ill or injured patients are at risk from it. Early detection of shock is vital, for if not supported by external means, death is likely to occur.

Homeostatic control The overall process of homeostasis is controlled by the nervous system, and it is responsible for constantly detecting and reversing the effects of even the slightest changes in cellular activity (see Fig. 3.1). The

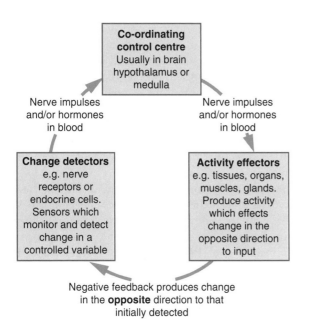

Fig. 3.1 Homeostatic feedback loop (from Hinchliff et al 2000, with permission).

role played by the nervous system is to initiate specific required responses in other parts of the body to achieve stability and balance. Communication with other parts of the body is achieved through the activation of nervous responses, chemical transmitter substances and hormones. Together the nervous (neural) and hormonal control systems complement each other to maintain homeostasis in many different ways. The responses occur at various speeds and are influenced by the nature in which the body needs to react and restabilise (see Rutishauser 1994, Chapters 3 and 10, Hinchliff et al 1996, Chapter 1.1).

Neural control Neural control of homeostasis is governed by the autonomic nervous system by transmitting fast electrical messages along nerve fibres to the internal organs. The system is divided into two distinct parts, the sympathetic and the parasympathetic, each having specific effects upon internal organs in order to control homeostasis (see Fig. 3.2).

Hormonal control Hormones are chemical substances secreted mainly by endocrine glands under the control of the hypothalamus. They each have a specific role to play in maintaining homeostasis and travel to their target via the

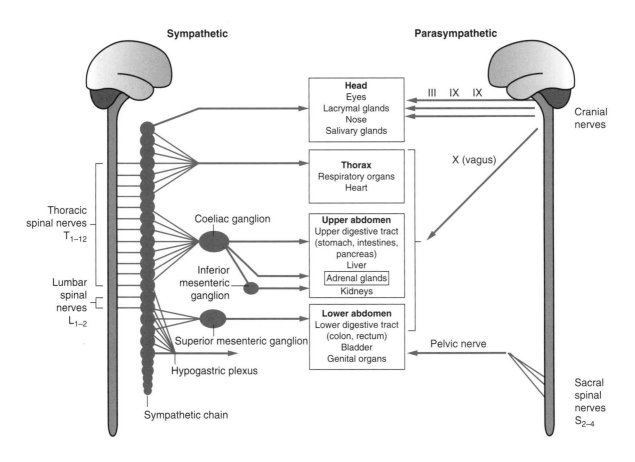

Fig. 3.2 Sympathetic and parasympathetic outflow (from Rutishauser 1994, with permission).

bloodstream. The response is much slower than that of the nervous system but more widespread (see Rutishauser 1994, Chapters 3 and 10). Figure 3.3 shows the position of the major endocrine sites.

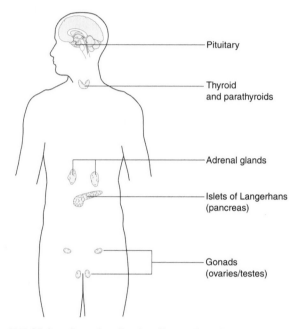

Fig. 3.3 Major sites of endocrine tissue (from Rutishauser 1994, with permission).

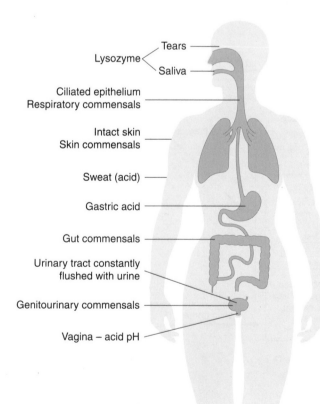

Fig. 3.4 Barriers to infection (from Alexander et al 2000, with permission).

Protective and defence mechanisms The human body provides a series of protective and defence mechanisms in many ways. The skeleton forms protective cavities for vital organs such as the brain, spinal cord and heart and lungs. The skin acts as a barrier to protect the body against potentially harmful microorganisms as well as being capable of interacting with the external environment through sensory nerve receptors. Other associated skin structures such as hair, nails, lymph, sweat and sebaceous glands all contribute towards protecting the body's inner and outer surfaces (see Fig. 3.4).

There are many potentially harmful agents that have the capacity to breech the body's defence mechanisms. When this happens the body relies upon the immune system to activate lymphocytes and destroy the invading organism (see Hinchliff et al 1996, Chapter 6.2, Rutishauser 1994, Chapter 15). The development of the immune system is based upon a process of exposure, recognition and response to particular harmful organisms throughout the entire lifespan, hence the immune system is as individual as the person (see Fig. 3.5).

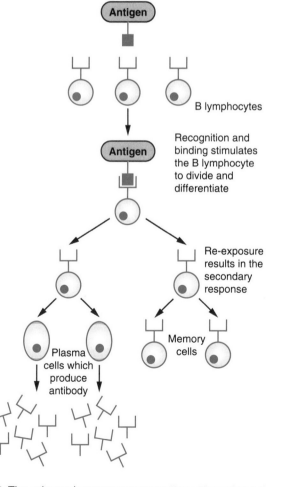

Fig. 3.5 The primary immune response (from Alexander et al 2000, with permission).

At birth the immune system is underdeveloped and new-born babies for the first few months of life have to rely upon the antibodies passed from the mother via the placenta. These are classed as natural ways to build up immunity, however the process can be artificially assisted through programmes of vaccination and immunisation (see Fig. 3.6). Disorders of the immune system are usually classed as being congenital or acquired and cause either a deficiency or over-activity resulting in a greater susceptibility to infections. Excessive hypersensitivity to foreign organisms causes an inappropriate reaction known as anaphylactic shock. This causes an acute inflammatory reaction that can develop within minutes and can be life-threatening as seen in asthma attacks and other allergic responses.

Inflammatory process and tissue repair The inflammatory process is a locally initiated defence mechanism that responds immediately following damage to tissue caused by injury or infection. The process involves the production and release of a variety of chemicals that serve to defend the affected area, remove dead cells and promote the process of healing. The inflammatory process is essentially the first stage of the tissue repair process and is characterised by a series of stages. If close to the surface of the skin the process can be directly observed as localised redness, swelling, reduced or loss of function, localised pain or irritation. Within a short space of time following the immediate inflammatory response the process of healing continues. The rate at which the process is completed depends upon the nature of the damage, which in some cases if chronic can take many years to be fully complete. The healing process is said to take place by primary and secondary intention (see Chapter 8).

Many factors play an important part in influencing the rate at which healing takes place, such as age, nutritional state, presence of infection and degree and location of the injury. For example, bones take considerably longer to heal and some tissue such as that found in the brain and spinal cord cannot repair itself leading to permanent disabilities.

Exercise

Consider the homeostatic processes involved in the following scenarios and determine what factors will influence recovery and return to normal function:

1. A child with a scald to his left arm.
2. An elderly lady with a fractured neck of the femur.
3. A middle-aged gentleman who has suffered a severe subarachnoid haemorrhage.
4. A middle-aged woman with an abdominal incision from a hysterectomy.
5. Make notes on each one and use diagrams to explain what is happening to normal physiological function.

In each case the human body would have instigated a common series of steps that would be observable either directly or indirectly towards reacting to the injury or intervention. The rate at which the individuals will recover is less predictable due to age, fitness, speed and accuracy of medical intervention to reduce complications and degree of vital organ involvement and damage.

External safe environment

The ability to interact with the external environment in order to avoid hazards and maintain safety is the concern of the somatic nervous system, which is made up of the following parts:

- central nervous system organisation and function
- skeletal muscle
- sensory organs.

Whilst each part has a distinctive role to play, together they provide a whole system that enables the body to be psychologically conscious of the surroundings and physiologically capable of responding to required changes. The system works by monitoring the external environment through sensory organs such as the eyes and ears, etc. By making sense of the information received the body is then able to protect itself by initiating the appropriate response (see Fig. 3.7).

The complexity of the system even today is not yet fully understood but Rutishauser (1994) gives a fascinating and detailed description of the system that also helps to understand how appropriate responses can also be suppressed either by disease, impairment or choice (see Rutishauser 1994, Chapters 20–29).

Understanding the systems in relation to the activity of maintaining a safe environment enables an appreciation of how important it is to preserve the ability to receive sensory information and how hazardous living can become when the ability to avoid danger is reduced either temporarily or permanently.

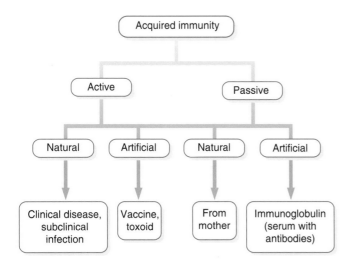

Fig. 3.6 Natural and artificial immunity (with kind permission from Kirkwood & Lewis 1989).

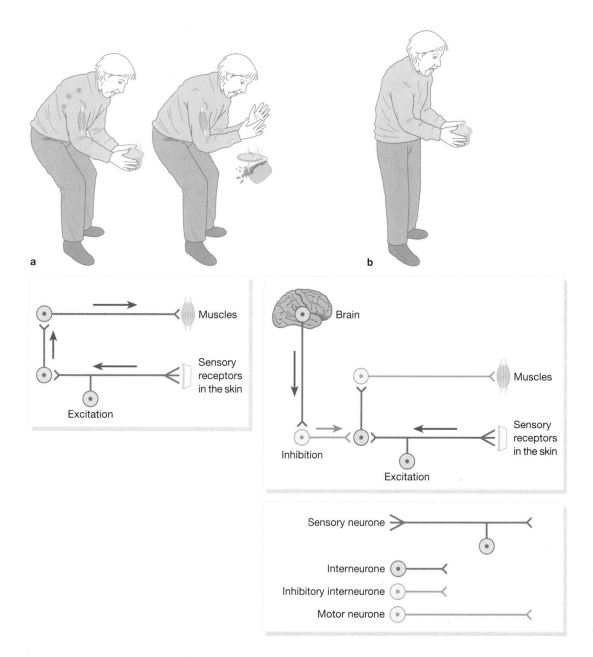

Fig. 3.7 An example of reflex response and how it can be inhibited (from Rutishauser 1994, with permission).

Exercise

Identify what hazards can be associated with a loss of sensation. What sort of hazards are the following people at risk from?

1. Through a works accident, Neil aged 38 years, has lost all sensation in his right foot.
2. Jenny is totally blind and needs to come into hospital for minor surgery.
3. Beverly has had meningitis and lost her sense of smell and taste.
4. John is profoundly deaf and is embarking on a sailing holiday.
5. Make notes about each one and consider other similar situations you may have come across in your nursing practice.

This exercise demonstrates the extent to which disorders of the body's control and defence can impact upon daily lives, wellbeing and safety, causing patients to alter their lifestyles either temporarily or permanently.

Psychological factors

It is well recognised that psychological health and wellbeing is just as important as our physical health. Here the model acts as a guide to help consider what issues may be affecting the patients' ability to support or improve their quality of life.

Psychological factors are associated with the extent to which individuals are able to control and influence their own safety and circumstances and central to the following:

- personality, mood and temperament
- knowledge, intelligence and competence
- attitude, motivation, confidence and personal experiences
- physical and mental impairment
- personal situations and stressors
- environment
- finances and resources.

This list demonstrates the complexity and the interrelatedness between the ALs and the factors affecting health (FAH), highlighting the importance of ensuring that all components of the model are carefully considered in relation to addressing the individual needs of patients. The extent to which risks can be avoided depends upon many factors, some of which could on reflection have been avoided and others that simply cannot be imagined or foreseen until after the event. When applying the model into practice it is useful to identify the extent to which individuals are able to control and influence their own safety by determining their level of understanding and/or experience. The ability to avoid or minimise risk is primarily based upon personal understanding, experience and motivation highlighting the importance that individual personality, intelligence, attitude and temperament play in the process. An analysis of common accident rates by McDonald & Davey (1996) showed that individuals with mental health problems are more likely to sustain accidents and that they are also likely to have a prolonged recovery period. The ability to avoid danger starts with being able to acknowledge that the potential for risk is present. Then the individual needs to be able to employ the appropriate actions and resources to avoid or minimise the risk. In doing so the individual will be influenced by a whole variety of other factors in order to ensure safety as shown in Figure 3.8.

The following exercise helps to develop a greater understanding of the complexity of health and interrelatedness of the components of the model.

> **Exercise**
>
> The following scenarios are examples of individuals whose psychological safety is compromised. Using the diagram in Figure 3.8 consider the extent to which the other factors affecting health would influence their ability to improve their safety.
>
> 1. A person with a physical disability accidentally sets the kitchen alight.
> 2. A woman who is suffering abuse.
> 3. An elderly person who is being intimidated by a group of children/youths.

In each case the degree of control is being influenced by a variety of factors such as physical ability, dependency and the environment. When caring for patients in clinical situations the nurse needs to consider the same factors.

Effects of stress

Stress is a term which everyone uses at some time in their lives, to describe a state of disruption, that is leaving them feeling threatened, uncomfortable or unwell, and this is known to contribute towards risks and accidents in all age groups. The subject of stress is hugely complex and has been studied from many perspectives (biological/physiological, psychological and sociological) in an attempt to understand the causes and various effects. As such there is a variety of models available which describe these phenomena (see Alexander et al 2000, Chapter 17). Fundamentally the concept of stress is related to an excessive pressure or demand upon any of the body's systems resulting in an effect upon emotional wellbeing, and thinking, reasoning

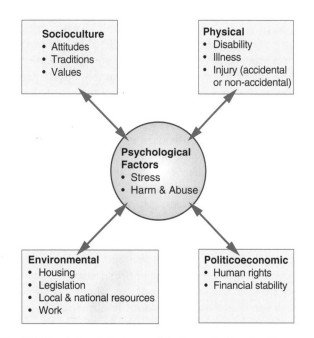

Fig. 3.8 The interrelatedness of factors affecting health.

and behaviour. A certain amount of stress is acknowledged as being a basic survival instinct that is followed by a process of recovery and adaptation. However when stress becomes too great or prolonged then the symptoms become observable.

Exercise

1. Think about how you react and feel if any of the following happened to you:
   - you lose your purse or wallet
   - you are alone in your car at night and break down on the motorway
   - you have very noisy neighbours.
2. What happens to you physically?
3. What happens to your behaviour and your thinking and reasoning processes?

Through this exercise some of the effects of stress can be readily recognised. Feeling nauseous, agitated, terrified or angry, resulting in you crying, shouting and not being able to 'think straight' are some examples. Try to remember those reactions and relate them to how patients may feel or behave in any given circumstance.

Irrespective of the cause, whether real or imagined, the body's defence mechanisms become affected, leading to a range of physical illnesses and diseases, poor coping mechanisms, behavioural changes and disturbances. Individuality means that some people are more able to manage their stress than others and this is closely linked to personality, experiences and support mechanisms. From a nursing perspective it is important for the concept to be fully understood if it is to be managed effectively, not only in relation to patient care but also for oneself.

Exercise

In order to determine the range of reactions that other people have towards stressful situations consider the following scenario.

A patient on the ward where you are working develops severe pain during visiting time. The patient's relative is shouting and demanding that the Consultant be called immediately. You are asked to stay with the patient, whilst your colleague who is in charge of the ward deals with the relative and tries to summon medical assistance.

1. Consider what physiological and psychological systems are reacting and describe how everyone might be feeling during this time:
   - the patient
   - the relative
   - your colleague
   - yourself
   - other patients.
2. Discuss your responses with colleagues.

Responses to this exercise will have illustrated that everyone would be acting differently to try and cope with the situation. Good communication skills are essential (see Chapter 4).

Nonaccidental injury (abuse and self-harm)

Nonaccidental injury (NAI) is a term that is used to describe deliberate injury and harm caused by the self or another person. It is known to exist in varying degrees in all ages, in all societies and from all walks of life. It has both physical and emotional consequences and is caused by many physical, psychological, sociocultural, environmental and politicoeconomic factors.

Abuse The problem of abuse is worldwide and over time, through a combination of media coverage and action from pressure groups, there has been increased public and professional awareness about the scale of the problem. In turn this has led to improvements in recognition and response mechanisms and support for victims through legal frameworks, statutory and voluntary services. The problem is known to exist across the lifespan and in a variety of environments such as the home, the workplace and unfortunately even professional care giving places such as residential homes and hospitals. Research into the problem has demonstrated that there is a direct link between abuse and dependency that has health and safety consequences for both victims and abusers (Wolf 1997). In an attempt to reduce the problem many national and international statutory and voluntary agencies exist to provide further research, awareness campaigns, literature, victim telephone helplines and support services.

Children and abuse The abuse of children is an international problem. It is found in all societies and results in general neglect, physical injury, emotional and sexual abuse and even death. There are many health and social factors that are known to contribute towards child abuse from victim and abuser perspectives. Despite this knowledge and understanding the problem remains of some magnitude particularly because it is almost always a closely guarded secret (WHO 1997). For an abused child there is a high risk that their emotional development will be disturbed and an even greater chance that they themselves become abusers in later life. In the UK many statutory and voluntary agencies such as Social Services departments and the National Society for the Prevention of Cruelty to Children (NSPCC) work together to provide services, information, child protection training and research in an effort to reduce the problem.

Women and abuse According to the WHO the abuse of women and girls is a major health and human rights concern, occurring throughout the entire lifespan and resulting in both physical and/or mental abuse. Abuse can take place either privately or publicly, within the home, at work or in the wider community and can consist of direct violence, coercion or deprivation of liberty (WHO 2000). The types of abuse women suffer encompass the following:

- battering
- sexual abuse
- dowry-related violence
- rape
- genital mutilation
- exploitation
- harassment and intimidation
- trafficking and prostitution
- punishments condoned by the state.

As a result women suffer a range of physical and mental health problems ranging from minor to severe injury, reproductive health problems, depression, anxiety and psychosomatic disorders. It is important to appreciate that abuse is not only associated with physical violence but also takes place in the form of preventing access to legal/human rights, education, personal incomes or even health care. Despite increased awareness of the problem some women will remain ignorant and powerless and unable to resolve or improve their situations. In many instances the women feel isolated and have a low self-esteem, living in fear of not only their own lives but also the safety of their children. As a result they are more likely to adopt unhealthy lifestyles or worst still become abusers themselves (Melies 2001).

Elderly and abuse Since the early 19th century, in the UK there has been a gradual increase in the number of older people and it is expected that this trend will continue to rise due to improved health and lifestyles. Unfortunately in some societies this has led to the development of a prevailing image that elderly people have low social autonomy and are a burden to society. This dangerous stereotyping has perpetuated social and political discrimination and highlighted that elderly people have been subjected to the following types of abuse (Webster 1999):

- financial exploitation (misappropriation of pensions and savings)
- physical abuse and neglect (withdrawal of food, fluids and overmedication)
- physical violence (by carers and intruders/thugs)
- psychological abuse (humiliation, ridicule and loss of dignity)
- sexual abuse.

It is important that the needs of a growing elderly population are recognised and that through good health and social policy professionals can appropriately support individual needs and maximise independent living (Dugmore 2002).

> **Exercise**
> Locate and browse the Age Concern website (www.ageconcern.org.uk) and consider how the information and links could help you support the needs of patients.

Disabled people and abuse Across the lifespan there are a range of disabilities that render people vulnerable to abuse, but individuals with learning difficulties, severe or chronic mental illness and physical disability are thought to be more at risk. The abuse arises from the dependency that is created by the disability and takes many forms ranging from withdrawing care, neglect or injury. For example Sullivan and Knutson (2000) identified that disabled school children were 3.4 times more likely to be abused than their non-disabled peers. The literature suggests that accident rates should be analysed more carefully in order to properly identify where nonaccidental rates might be obscured in general accident reporting.

Self-harm Self-harm is a term that is used to refer to injury that is inflicted either by the individual themselves or through their consent/agreement. For example a person who attempts to take their own life by cutting their wrists or taking an overdose of tablets would be considered to have harmed themselves, whereas tattooing and body piercing would be considered to be merely a fashion statement. In some cultures deliberate cutting or marking of the skin would signify a specific cultural/traditional rite. There is concern that the increasing incidence of self-harm is in relation to changing socioeconomic conditions (Gunnell et al 2000). Where the activity becomes extreme or inappropriate it is regarded as a sign of mental illness and the individual will require help and support to overcome the cause (Moffat 2000).

Sociocultural factors

Concern for safety differs throughout the world and the model urges us to acknowledge how social and cultural factors will influence the different behaviours that are found in societies. In the UK we take for granted the services that have been developed over many years to maximise personal and public safety. Indeed when those mechanisms fail to protect us we are at liberty to sue for compensation for any inconvenience or injuries sustained. The degree to which individual safety can be influenced is dependent upon two main factors:

1. The extent to which the individual can take responsibility for their own safety be that within the home, public places or the workplace.
2. The amount of financial, political and legal support that is available within society.

Not all countries are able to fully support the safety of individuals as in the UK and even in societies where concern for safety is fairly comprehensive, cultural differences can influence the types of hazards that exist and present inequalities in the way in which health is promoted and risks prevented. For example it is known that people of lower social economic groups and ethnic backgrounds are at greater risk of accidents (Eurens et al 2001).

At a basic level safety needs are met by the family, but in some instances cultural beliefs and values can be so strong that they actually compromise safety. In many countries throughout the world there may be little education or political support for safety and people are forced to accept the degree of danger that they face, such as people living in poor or war-torn countries. Within all societies the daily lives of people are at some point influenced by religious and spiritual beliefs. The extent to which this occurs depends upon the degree of openness and freedom of choice that exists. Some societies have to abide by strict codes and traditions that to the onlooker may appear inappropriate, especially in relation to safety. In some instances people become willing to risk the safety of themselves and others and even die for their beliefs, e.g. suicide bombers. When the outside world attempts to influence change or intervene in the interests of safety this can create turmoil, acts of terrorism and even wars. Acts of terrorism and war have, sadly, become a common feature of our lives.

The attack on America in September 2001 was one of the most extensive acts of terrorism the world has ever seen. It caused the loss of thousands of lives and was a startling reminder of how vulnerable even the most developed countries in the world are to the beliefs held by others. The scale of the attack and the devastation it caused heightened the safety awareness of people throughout the world.

Internationally a growing number of people are prepared to place themselves in great danger in order to escape persecution or seek out a better life in another country. The risks that asylum seekers take are a reminder of the lengths that people will go to in order to protect themselves from danger. In some cases this has resulted in people tolerating terrible conditions or facing death to escape from the dangers they faced in their country of origin. In relation to health it is important to recognise that many individuals will have been the victims of torture and organised violence and will have specific needs that will require expert attention (Burnett & Peel 2001, Dawood & James 2001).

Exercise

1. Examine your own views about health and safety and social differences.
2. Consider the risks associated with the practice of female circumcision.
3. Consider the risks in countries which do not have seat belt laws.
4. Compare your views with other colleagues.

Knowledge of the risks will influence actions, highlighting the importance that education plays in maintaining safety. However it is important to recognise how difficult it would be to change some of the practices that pose a risk to safety, because of tradition and strongly held beliefs.

As societies grow and develop it is inevitable that new hazards will emerge. Constant and rapid change, greater access to information and greater demand for services have seemingly speeded up the pace of life and work. As a result there appears to be a shortage of time and less tolerance, which is in turn creating new threats to our safety. In the UK alone recent railway tragedies, racial tensions, violent clashes and riots, and healthcare blunders are beginning to shake public confidence in the ability of the state to maintain safety. Rising crime rates involving theft, assault and murder have caused people to take greater action to protect themselves and their property. In the UK Victim Support is an independent national charity that offers free and confidential advice to over one million people per year who have been affected by crime. Even within schools and the workplace the antisocial behaviour of bullying is known to cause ill-health problems such as anxiety, depression and loss of self-esteem (Salmon et al 1998, Wolke et al 2001). As a result of an increased understanding of how people are affected by traumatic events it is now well recognised that victims, bystanders and rescuers can suffer from a range of physiological and psychological disturbances known as post-traumatic stress disorder (PTSD). In recognition of the problem, it has become necessary to provide a range of services to support the immediate and long-term effects that individuals may suffer such as mood swings, flashbacks, difficulty in sleeping or concentrating. As a result the issues of who should accept responsibility and blame for accidents and other traumatic events has become exceedingly complex and resulted in an increase in claims for compensation. Many legal firms now actively advertise their services widely to encourage individual claims.

Environmental factors

This aspect of the model is concerned with the surrounding (external) environment and the possible impact that certain conditions could have upon personal health and safety. The external environment can present many threats to public health at local, national and international levels and since the health of people is vital to the social economy, government initiatives are aimed at preventing and reducing risks wherever possible. In the UK, legislation exists to ensure that improvements are made to the environment in order to ensure public safety. Legislation outlines the responsibilities of governments, industries, groups and individuals in order to promote individual and public safety. Concern for environmental issues on a worldwide scale such as the depletion of the ozone layer, destruction of rain forests and reduction of food stocks such as fish, requires international agreement and commitment. The World Health Organisation (WHO) is instrumental in working with other intergovernmental agencies to encourage the development of strategies related to improving the health of people by improving the environment. In 2002 a joint United Nations and WHO report entitled *Children in the New Millennium: Environmental Impact on Health* published alarming facts that every day 5500 children the world over are dying from common preventable diseases such as diarrhoea (from polluted food and water) and acute respiratory infections (WHO 2002a). When issues are ignored pressure groups, such as Greenpeace, often form to draw attention to the problems.

The Roper, Logan and Tierney model recognises that nurses are well placed in their daily work with patients to reinforce and incorporate health and safety information into their care, in order to promote health and safety. To be effective however, nurses need to be able to present information in a creative and meaningful way and always ensure that the information is accurate, appropriate and up to date.

> **Exercise**
> Access the World Health Organisation website (www.who/int) and familiarise yourself with some of the current global environmental and health issues.

The subject of health and the environment is vast, but for the purposes of this chapter the following four areas will be used to explore the main health and safety issues:

- pollution
- accidents
- infection
- fire.

Pollution

Pollution is considered to be a by-product of modern living, which at some point through a lack of understanding and/or provision of resources becomes a hazard for health. For example, in some countries where effective sewage systems are not available there is a huge risk to public health whilst in industrialised countries there are risks from emissions which may find their way into the air or rivers. The growing number of pollutants worldwide is a cause for concern, some of which will now be briefly discussed.

Water pollution Water is vital to human survival and has a range of functions within the body with an essential role in maintaining health, therefore the provision of clean water is recognised all over the world as being a basic health requirement. On a global scale the contamination of drinking water poses the most significant risk to humans, and throughout history there have been countless disease outbreaks resulting from untreated, poorly treated or polluted water (Ritter et al 2002, Tibbets 2000). It is estimated that at least one-fifth of the Earth's population lacks access to safe drinking water and that the problem will worsen as the populations grow. Water becomes polluted by microorganisms and chemicals, which when swallowed may result in a whole range of ill-health problems, ranging from gastrointestinal diseases, infections, and tumours to genetic disorders (Barrell et al 2000, Cantor 1997). Today even wealthy nations struggle to ensure that water sources are pollutant-free, but for poorer countries that are unable to provide safe drinking water or access to health resources during disease outbreaks, the potential for death remains high.

Water contamination from industrial waste is a common factor of modern day living and can occur accidentally or

deliberately. When the risk of pollution is widespread it can affect the lives of not only humans but also marine life, wildlife and plant life. Ultimately there becomes a potential to disrupt the natural ecosystem, which in turn can interrupt the food chain. Humans who swim in polluted waters run the risk of contracting harmful infections and disorders such as viral hepatitis, skin reactions and oral thrush (Prieto et al 2001). As well as chemical substances finding their way into waters the tipping of glass, plastic and metal objects can cause injury and even death for both humans and animals. Together charitable, national and international agencies have raised awareness and introduced policies to reduce, prevent and reverse the damage caused by pollution.

> **Exercise**
> Using the World Health Organisation and Department of Health website as a source of reference (www.who.int/ith and www.doh.gov.uk/traveladvice) consider what advice you would give to someone who is travelling abroad in relation to:
>
> - drinking water
> - swimming.

Air pollution There are many pollutants that exist in the air and they have the potential to cause widespread damage. Many pollutants are invisible, which makes it difficult to deal with them, and often the first signs of air pollution will be changes in health patterns. The air naturally carries substances such as dust and pollen that are known to have an effect upon human health such as asthma. Chemicals emitted from cars, factories, agricultural pesticides, insecticides and household aerosols, which are responsible for damaging not only health, but also habitats, wildlife and even buildings, can also contaminate the air. When such substances travel in cloud form they can cause damage many miles away from the point of origin, by polluting in the form of acid rain. On a global scale there has been growing concern regarding the role that pollutants play in changing conditions within the Earth's atmosphere, potentially threatening the very life of the planet itself. This is often referred to as global warming, evidence for which is believed to be the form of floods, droughts, season changes and coastline alterations. It is believed that gases such as carbon dioxide, methane and chlorofluorocarbons (CFCs) are creating an imbalance in the Earth's natural ability to retain heat and protect itself via the ozone layer, from absorbing harmful rays from the sun. The dangers to human safety are thought to lie in relation to reductions in food production and emerging and changing disease patterns (McMichael et al 2000). For example, the thinning of the ozone layer enabling harmful ultraviolet rays to reach the Earth's surface has been linked to the increased incidence of skin cancer across the world. In the workplace a concentrated exposure to pollutants such as in the mining, nuclear and chemical industry is known to cause specific diseases and disorders raising the importance of acknowledging the public health issues associated with the work environment (the effects of the work environment upon health are discussed in Chapter 11).

At a personal level there has been a growing realisation about the number of hazards which people themselves can take action to avoid. Health promotion and prevention information have been influential in raising awareness, particularly in relation to the increased risk of carcinoma through exposure to sunlight and cigarette smoking (smoking is discussed in Chapter 5). Health professionals can play an important role in influencing public and individual safety by not only ensuring that patients have access to appropriate information and care, but also through influencing changes in health policy through research and practice developments.

Lead pollution Lead is a natural substance found in soil and water and was until recently used widely to make paint, plastics, petrol and water pipes. Today it is recognised as being a serious pollutant which can be ingested, inhaled or absorbed and capable of causing genetic disorders and further widespread damage to the immune, reproductive, renal, cardiovascular, musculoskeletal and haematopoietic systems (Johnson 1998). In many developed countries, recognition of the public health problem both occupationally and environmentally, has led to a decline in the use of lead-based products such as petrol, and lead water pipes have been replaced. Despite the known risks however only a few countries have introduced regulations governing the use of the metal (Tong et al 2000).

Noise pollution The subject of noise pollution is a difficult one to tackle because of individual acceptance and tolerance. Noise is a product of modern living brought about by the need for industrial, transport, communication, domestic and leisure requirements. Broadly, noise can have an effect on health in relation to the workplace where there has been growing recognition for the need to protect workers who are at risk from hearing loss or complete deafness. It has also been recognised that young people are at risk from damaging their hearing through prolonged periods of listening to loud music at dance clubs and through the use of stereo ear/headphones (WHO 2001). Damage to hearing however is not the only threat to health and safety. People who are subjected to noise that they have little control over can suffer from loss of sleep or concentration, which can lead to psychological disturbances and potentially increase the risks of injury from accidents.

Worldwide the increased use of mobile phones has created both concern and controversy. There are now international guidelines to ensure that the radio waves emitted from phones are kept low. In the UK, the Department of Health in recognition that health risks are still not fully understood have issued further information and advice to enable individuals, parents and employers to make informed choices about safety (Department of Health 2001c). More alarmingly there is sufficient evidence to show that use of mobile phones whilst driving is a contributing factor to some fatal road traffic accidents. In response to the growing problem RoSPA have issued a factsheet that outlines the dangers and guides best practice to individuals and employers which is available on the following website: www.doh.gov.uk/mobilephones.

Preventing accidents

The potential for accidents to occur exists in all aspects of daily life, in the home, at work, during travel and at play. Many accidents are actually preventable and in recent years increasing attention has been given to accident prevention because of the staggering costs associated with them. In the UK the Royal Society for the Prevention of Accidents (RoSPA) estimates that the current cost of accidents to the National Health Service is in the region of £450 million. This cost is increased by an additional £1750 million in loss of earnings, industrial output, pain, grief and suffering and does not include the cost of damage to property or the use of other emergency services such as the fire service (RoSPA 2002). The figures are kept up to date and are available on the RoSPA website (www.rospa.co.uk). Accidents are known to be responsible for 10 000 deaths per year across England alone. In response the government published a ten-year strategy to reduce death rates from accidents and save up to 12 000 lives (Department of Health 1999). The strategy outlines how health agencies and professionals can work together to reduce a range of accidents related to road, fire and home safety. To this extent it is vital that nurses keep themselves up to date in order to help achieve the targets, by providing patients with accurate information and helping them to make realistic and practical adjustments in their daily lives in order to prevent accidents.

Preventing accidents in the home It is known that people have more accidents in the home than any other environment; the kitchen, living/dining room, stairs, bedrooms and bathroom are extremely dangerous places. Accidents are related to everyday living activities such as playing, preparing food, carrying out household improvements or repairs or simply moving around the house. Different hazards can be linked to different family members, the most vulnerable groups being children, the elderly and those with learning disabilities and mental impairment.

Risks of accidents for children Accidents in childhood are known to pose the single greatest threat to life. Commonly children are known to suffer a range of accidents such as fractures, burns and scalds, drowning, choking and accidental poisonings, as a result of falls, road accidents, lack of appropriate supervision, secure storage and identification of risks, particularly when in unfamiliar environments. The prevention of many accidents in essence relies upon adult supervision and intervention to prevent them from occurring, particularly where very young children are concerned.

It is, however, difficult for those caring for children to be vigilant at all times and the natural curiosity of children to explore their environment means that not all potential situations can be predicted. The Child Accident Prevention Trust (CAPT) publish very detailed accounts of child accidents, capturing information from other accident-reporting bodies that would otherwise disguise child accident figures.

Research into accident patterns provides an aid into developing an understanding about accidents, which can help to maximise prevention. Surveys have also shown that the time of the day, days of the week and seasons also influence accident rates. Evenings, weekends and school holidays are known to record higher accident rates. Despite this knowledge accidents continue to happen, resulting in death, physical and psychological injury. To aid the prevention of accidents, health and social care professionals who work closely with families are able to assess dangers and offer guidance. In addition it is important to recognise that manufacturers of household items must play a part in maximising the safety of their products.

Risks of accidents in the elderly At the opposite end of the lifespan, elderly people over the age of 75 years are known to be more susceptible to accidents in the home, due to falls caused by poor mobility, failing sensory ability and general health. Falls in older people are known to be the major cause of death and disability as they have the potential to lead to other complications such as fractures, bronchopneumonia and pressure sores (Stuck & Beck 2001). Many elderly people live alone and are further at risk from not being able to summon for help, increasing the risk of complications such as dehydration and hypothermia in addition to their injury. Within the home, prevention can take the form of helping elderly people and their families assess the dangers that surround them and make the necessary changes to help them to live safely and independently. Simple measures such as removing obstacles, wearing sensible footwear, installation of alarm systems and ensuring regular communication with neighbours and family are vital in preventing and responding early to accidents in the home. Even within professional care environments such as care homes, day centres and hospitals, the prevention of falls should equally be given high priority (Gaze 2000). In the UK the National Service Framework (NSF) for older people published in 2001, specifically recognises the importance of reducing accidents as part of the overall strategy to improve the health of older people and urges professional and care agencies to work towards reducing accident rates (Department of Health 2001a).

Exercise

Identify how nongovernmental agencies contribute towards the health and safety of older people – browse the Age Concern website (www.ageconcern.org.uk) for information regarding the safety of older people and current campaigns.

Risks of accidents for people with disabilities In recent years more people with a range of disabilities have been encouraged to live independently within the community and gradual progress has been made to adapt living surroundings in order to maximise normality and safety. National statistics show, however, that accident rates are increasing, particularly for people with learning disabilities and mental health problems (Office for National Statistics 2000).

People with a range of disabilities require resources and support appropriate to their needs in order to help them live independently and remain safe. The Disability Links Alliance (DLA) provides information, advice, training and research and heads up campaigns to ensure that improvements in the standard of living for disabled people can be made. Many disabled people will require their homes to be redesigned to improve access and have living appliances, surfaces and accommodation height-adjusted to help reduce common household accidents that normal living accommodation would create. In the UK house-building firms are encouraged to build homes that make modification easier in order to encourage independent living at any time in life, but significant progress has been hampered by cost (Frain & Carr 1996). A range of resources is also available for the home to aid communication such as loop systems, personal emergency call systems and the use of flashing lights for telephones and door bells. Throughout the UK the Disabled Living Centre Council (DLCC) have a network of centres that provide free and impartial information and advice about products, solutions and equipment to enable easier living.

Exercise

Browse the Disability Alliance and Disabled Living Centre Council websites to increase your understanding of the resources that disabled people can access in order to promote safety (www.disabilityalliance.org and www.dlcc.org.uk).

Preventing accidents at work The importance of ensuring safety at work has two dimensions governed by the Health and Safety at Work Act 1974. One is the responsibility of the employer to protect employees and the other is the ability of the employee to act responsibly to ensure their own safety. In the UK the Health and Safety Executive (HSE) is a government agency that has statutory powers to record, monitor and investigate serious incidents. From this information the HSE are able to estimate the cost of accidents at work and publish reports and statistics on an annual basis (HSE 2001). Every job has some degree of risk ranging from injury to the development of diseases and disabilities.

Through programmes of training for employers and employees and the provision of safety equipment and workplace standards and policies, many associated problems can be prevented. The HSE is just one organisation that collects information related to a number of occupations across a variety of industries such as agriculture, construction, leisure services, health service, manufacturing and retail services. The information enables trends to be identified and strategies to be developed to reduce health problems in the workplace.

Exercise
Locate and familiarise yourself with the Health and Safety Executive website (www.hse.gov.uk). You will find useful information regarding the work of the HSE and specific information for health care-related topics.

In health care the risks associated with back injury, exposure to radiation and needlestick injuries are just a few examples of concern for accidents in the workplace, where both the employer and employee must take equal responsibility. In the UK there is a legal requirement for employers and self-employed people to report accidents and ill health at work under the Reporting of Injuries, Diseases and Dangerous Occurrences Regulations 1995 (RIDDOR 95). Not all countries have legislation to protect the safety of workers and worst still, may risk the health and safety of whole communities or even neighbouring countries. As a result pressure is brought to bear upon countries and companies worldwide by action groups and international agencies such as the International Labour Organisation (ILO) and the World Health Organisation (WHO) who work to establish international standards of safe practice in the workplace.

Preventing accidents in play, sport and leisure In the Western world, there has been a marked increase in the availability and pursuit of play, sport and leisure activities that, in turn, has brought about a variety of risks to health and safety. As a result it has become necessary to introduce new legislation in an attempt to prevent further injuries and deaths.

For children it is the responsibility of parents, schools and event organisers to assess the risks that may be present, whilst at the same time balancing the need for enjoyment and personal and social development. During normal play, injuries associated with climbing, tripping, colliding, fighting and falling result in minor injuries such as skin cuts and grazes, sprains and more serious injuries such as fractures and head injuries. However, for children road accidents remain the greatest cause of accidental death. In addition there has been growing concern for the safety of children at play, with an increasing number of reports related to street crime, drug taking, paedophile activity, abductions and even murders.

Prevention of accidents related to sport essentially rests with the individual, although companies and organisers would be expected to take responsibility for ensuring the safety of buildings and equipment. Nevertheless sporting injuries are known to account for a number of emergency hospital admissions, days off work and even deaths.

Exercise
1. How many everyday sports can you identify and what types of injuries are associated with them?
2. What would be the impact upon other daily living activities?

The most popular sports such as football or racquet sports result in many musculoskeletal injuries, such as bruises and sprains. Fractured limbs would result in altered dependency in other Activities of Living such as personal cleansing and dressing, eliminating and mobility. Some sports are even known to carry a high risk of injury or death and have been heavily criticised for the unnecessary cost of life and financial costs associated with ensuring safety or initiating rescue operations, for example outdoor pursuits such as mountain climbing, sailing, motor car and cycle racing and boxing. However it is not only sport participants who are at risk, so too are spectators, particularly when the sport attracts large crowds. Over the years the importance of crowd safety has been heightened following a series of serious incidents related to stadium safety and violent behaviour, resulting in many regulations being put in place by event organisers to both prevent and respond to incidents.

This section has shown that whilst the importance of play and leisure is important, it is not without risk, whether it is a family outing or a high-profile sporting activity. Whatever the activity, individuals and organisers must take equal responsibility to ensure that safety regulations around supervision, food hygiene, buildings and equipment have been adhered to.

Accidents related to travel The need to travel is an essential component of everyday living and changes in lifestyles over time have witnessed an expansion of travel methods and habits both for work and leisure purposes. As a result of a number of accidents and disasters related to air, coach, rail and sea travel, regulations have been enforced to establish standards of good practice in relation to safety checks and the provision of standard safety equipment. It is the responsibility of individual travellers, transport manufacturers and travel businesses to comply with safety standards. Failure to do so often leads to prosecution, which can result in the payment of fines or even a custodial sentence.

Although all types of travel carry an element of risk, road accidents in particular are commonplace in many countries. Over time a number of measures have been introduced in an attempt to reduce road accidents such as:

*   improved street lighting
*   traffic calming methods (e.g. speed bumps)
*   speed restrictions in accident black spots
*   breathalyser checks to reduce alcohol-related accidents
*   compulsory wearing of seat belts for front and rear seat passengers and correct fitting of baby seats
*   compulsory wearing of crash helmets for cyclists.

Despite these measures, with the number of vehicles on the roads ever increasing, the risk of road accidents and death remains high. In March 2000 the UK published an extensive Road Safety Strategy with the intention of dramatically reducing the number of deaths and serious injuries caused by all types of road accidents by the year 2010 (Department of Transport 2000). To this extent Roper et al (1996) point out the significance that changes in the law can have upon improving health and safety, highlighting the importance that pressure groups play in influencing government action. It becomes apparent that public safety is an extremely complex issue initially dependent upon the recognition and acceptance of personal responsibility. Nurses however have a variety of opportunities within their work at primary and acute care levels to support and influence individual behaviour in order to prevent accidents.

Preventing infection

Infection occurs when harmful pathogenic microorganisms invade the human body and cause disease and even death. Whilst not all microorganisms are harmful, under the right conditions infections can occur, highlighting the importance that preventing and controlling infection has in relation to the activity of maintaining a safe environment. To this extent advances in infection control need to be continuous in order to address infection control changes and challenges that are constantly occurring within the environment. Since the middle of the 20th century advances in infection control have led to the introduction of many national and international guidelines in order to safeguard public health, but individual responsibility and compliance is also essential.

In the UK every health care organisation has a responsibility to provide a range of services to ensure that national guidelines are implemented. In order to help maintain a safe environment against infection it is essential to have a basic understanding of how microorganisms behave, how infection is transmitted and how infection can be controlled. These can only be briefly described in this chapter and it is recommended that you use specialist texts (e.g. Ayliffe et al 2000), particularly when nursing patients with specific problems. It is essential that infection control care is always based upon an understanding of the patient's clinical care episode and informed infection control practice.

Microorganisms

Under normal circumstances the human body is host to many harmless microorganisms known as commensals, providing different parts of the body with protection against infection (see Table 3.1). Infection occurs when a disease-causing microorganism (pathogen) invades and damages body tissue. Microorganisms which cause infection do so by breaking through the body's defence mechanisms and affect specific body systems.

The chain of infection

The chain of infection illustrates the stages at which an infection develops and enters the body, outlining the sources of infection, sites of entry into

Table 3.1 Normal commensal microorganisms

Site	Organism
Skin	*Staphylococcus epidermidis* Diphtheroids *Corynebacterium* sp.
Mouth and throat	Staphylococci Streptococci Anaerobes *Neisseria* sp.
Nose	Staphylococci Diphtheroids
Gut	*Escherichia coli* *Klebsiella* sp. *Proteus* sp. *Streptococcus faecalis* *Clostridium perfringens* Yeasts *(Candida)*
Kidneys and bladder	Normally sterile
Vagina	Lactobacilli Streptococci Staphylococci Anaerobes

From: Alexander et al (2000).

and exit from the body, modes of transmission and host susceptibility (see Fig. 3.9). This simple cycle helps to identify the stages at which appropriate action and intervention contribute towards preventing and controlling infection.

Control of infection Effective infection control consists of a variety of activities related to the infection chain.

- *Destruction of microorganisms:* Preventing and destroying the cause of the infection is achieved with the use of antimicrobial agents which are used for sterilisation and disinfection processes. A range of techniques are utilised to minimise the spread of infection within the internal and external environment, through the use of chemicals such as liquids, gases and drugs and physical processes such as extreme heat and radiation. The use of antibiotics in modern medicine has revolutionised the control of infection, but misuse has encouraged the emergence of multiresistant strains of bacteria, which have brought about the need for careful monitoring and governance in the use of drugs and patterns of infections. To this extent it is now recognised that prevention of infection cannot rely on antibiotics alone and that prevention and control of infection techniques are of equal and vital importance.

- *Recognition of predisposing factors:* It is known that there are several factors which influence an individual's susceptibility and resistance to infection. Very young people and older people have diminished immune systems, which reduces the ability to combat infection. Likewise

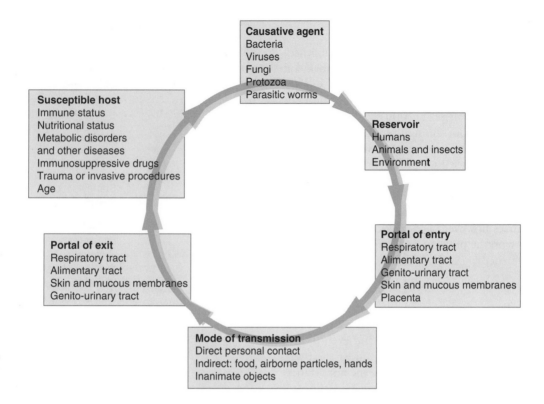

Fig. 3.9 The chain of infection (from Walsh 2002, with permission).

drugs and other diseases which alter the body's immune response mechanisms are known to increase the risk of infection. Prolonged exposure to cold and damp environments and lack of adequate diet and exercise reduce the ability of the body to maintain natural body defences against infection and there is also a known link between psychological stress and infections. Where tissue damage occurs through trauma, disease or surgical intervention infection becomes highly probable as skin defences are breached and tissue is exposed to microorganism invasion and multiplication.

- *Isolation:* Early isolation methods consisted purely of segregating and quarantining people in the belief that this would stop the spread of disease, as in the case of leprosy and bubonic plague sufferers. By the middle of the 20th century new understanding led to the development of more integrated approaches that concentrated upon prevention, treatment and cure and the provision of isolation hospitals were commonplace. As a result of new understanding and more integrated approaches many previously dangerous infective diseases such as smallpox have now been completely eradicated from the world and others have been dramatically reduced. Today it is well recognised that merely isolating the patient as a source of infection is insufficient, as it has implications for affecting individual mental wellbeing, confidentiality and human rights. The scope of informed control of infection is extensive. It begins with developing a greater understanding

about the behaviour of specific diseases and includes surveillance of contacts and sources and monitoring the spread and containment of the infection. As a result many countries, although not all, are able to protect public health by implementing best practice guidelines for the notification and isolation techniques of certain diseases.

Immunisation Immunity to disease can be achieved either naturally or artificially. Natural immunity is achieved through exposure to disease microorganisms (toxins) that enable the body to develop internal recognition and resistance mechanisms (antibodies). Artificial immunity is achieved by the deliberate introduction (vaccination) of a safe amount of modified disease toxin into the body enabling an immune response to be created without suffering from the effects of the disease (see Fig. 3.6).

Over time immunisation programmes have played a key role in reducing the incidence and risks of some of the worlds' most common and dangerous infectious diseases such as diphtheria, tetanus, poliomyelitis, whooping cough, measles, mumps, rubella and more recently meningitis. The aim of an immunisation programme is to target the most susceptible groups of people who are likely to contract the disease, such as children, women of child-bearing age, pregnant mothers, healthcare workers and travellers to foreign countries. In the UK a vaccination programme is recommended by the Department of Health and is available free of charge (see Chapter 9, p. 261).

Immunisation programmes vary throughout the world, but unfortunately not every country is able to afford the resources to prevent or treat some of the most common diseases, that for a relatively small cost would save millions of lives. By contrast in the UK, concern has shifted from the dangers of disease, to the risks associated with some vaccines, for example the Measles, Mumps and Rubella vaccine (MMR) (Moreton 2001). Without adequate protection, individuals increase the risk of contracting diseases, which may have serious consequences not only for themselves but also for whole communities. It is important to recognise however, that whilst immunisation provides added protection for maintaining a safer internal environment, this needs to be complemented with improved social and economic conditions to minimise the prevention and spread of infectious diseases.

Control of epidemics An epidemic occurs when there is a marked increase in the reported cases of a particular disease above the normal acceptable rate. Whilst each country must take responsibility for controlling its own epidemics, the WHO has a key role in monitoring infectious outbreaks, developing strategies to deal with them and encouraging international collaboration to prevent worldwide spread. If an epidemic does extend across the world then it becomes known as a pandemic. The risk of epidemics are far greater in modern times due to the relative ease that people and products can travel across land, sea and air, requiring the need for strict regulations to minimise the spread of infections.

The Foot and Mouth outbreak in the UK during 2001 highlighted how quickly the disease spread due to the fact that animals are transported long distances for sale and slaughter. The outbreak also highlighted how the world needs to be constantly alert to the development of epidemics and the risks they bring to public health. Worldwide there are always new concerns about emerging diseases and the threats they bring to public health linked to changing lifestyles such as hepatitis B and C and acquired immune deficiency syndrome (AIDS). More alarmingly, the use of disease microorganisms as a weapon of terror to threaten the safety of people en masse, as witnessed with the outbreaks of anthrax which followed the terrorist attacks in the USA in 2001.

Fire prevention

The devastating effects of fire are only too well known and increasingly, it has become essential to understand the importance of not only safety in the home but also in public places. The importance of information being available in many forms enables individuals to not only gain knowledge and understanding but also practical skills in relation to raising the alarm, the use of extinguishers and the planning of escape routes.

Fire in the home Despite major campaigns to increase public awareness house fires continue to cause many serious injuries and deaths. For children, house fires are known to be the biggest cause of accidental death within the home. (RoSPA 2002). The London Fire Brigade (2002) estimate that 81% of fires in the home are accidents caused by kitchen fires, smoking, candles and faulty electrical appliances. In the UK individual householders are expected to take responsibility for the safety of their own homes and insure their homes in order to replace items destroyed by fire as the costs can run into thousands of pounds. In the home the fitting of a smoke alarm is known to save many lives.

Fire in public places In public places such as the workplace, shops, hotels, restaurants and entertainment centres, there are obligations to reach legal safety standards. Despite this every year there are reports of terrible tragedies, resulting in severe injury and loss of life due to the fact that escape routes were blocked, locked or inadequate.

Fire control Having taken all necessary precautions to prevent a fire occurring, controlling a fire relies upon detection, raising the alarm, containing the fire and extinguishing it. Through community information programmes the Fire Brigade offer useful help and advice guiding people on how to prevent fires and ensure personal safety in the event of a fire both in the home and in public places.

Exercise
1. Find out how fire prevention is promoted within your community.
2. Locate the London Fire Brigade website and find out more about community fire safety programmes (www.london-fire.gov.uk).
3. Consider the devastating effects of fire on whole communities, e.g. forest fires in Australia.
4. Discuss with colleagues the impact on the health of communities which have experienced such devastation.

Individual effects of fire The effects of being injured in a fire can result in both physical and psychological trauma. Pain, stress, risk of infection and stigma from scarring are often long term. Loss of confidence may be encountered through a lack of desire to socialise or an inability to continue working during the healing process, which may cause additional anxiety for not only the individual but also for their family and social circle. Additional stress may be encountered where there has been a loss of property or an inability to make repairs either through physical disability or insufficient finances.

Politicoeconomic factors

Although the primary responsibility to maintain safety rests with the individual, this can be improved with the support of broader legislation and financial support.

Political responsibility

It is clear that action by governments to influence legislation and provide resources to promote the safety of the environment is crucial. In industrialised societies employers and service providers are expected to demonstrate regard for the safety of employees and customers. In developed countries public protection is supported through the provision of statutory and legal frameworks to such an extent that a public enquiry would seek to identify the cause and make recommendations to prevent further incidents. In some cases individuals are imprisoned under the charge of corporate manslaughter for failing to ensure that safety instructions were not followed. In the UK a series of railway disasters have resulted in a loss of public confidence regarding passenger safety, prompting major health and safety investigations and a review of the quality and safety management. Even in the NHS there have been a number of enquiries relating to public safety, quality of care and the accountability of practitioners such as the Bristol and Shipman tragedies (Mohammed et al 2001).

In a direct response to improve the quality, accountability and overall effectiveness of the NHS, the government have published plans for a ten-year programme of health and social care reform, not only to improve the delivery of services but also to ensure that standards and quality of clinical care can be effectively addressed and monitored through a process known as clinical governance (Department of Health 1998 & 2000). As a result all health care organisations are expected to have monitoring systems in place and all individual professionals and teams must be able to account for their actions (Crinson 1999).

Individual responsibility

At every stage of the lifespan there is a need for individuals to take some form of action to maintain safety. To a certain extent this is politically supported through legislation and the provision of public services. At some point the responsibility to ensure safety rests purely at an individual level, but this may have cost implications that become unaffordable and consequently safety can become compromised. For example, individuals and families on low incomes may be forced to go without safety equipment or obtain it second-hand and run the risk of additional hazards because the equipment is not entirely safe. Often within society action or pressure groups have been successful in drawing attention to issues that are in the interests of the safety of the public at large, forcing politicians to introduce legislation and appropriate services.

Conflict and war

Unfortunately the threat of conflict and war has become an ever-present factor in everyone's daily life at either a local or international level. Reports of new outbreaks and continuing conflict have become regular news items, to the point that we are in danger of becoming immune to the actual misery, death and destruction that has taken place. Since the USA terrorist attacks on September 11th 2001 there has been heightened awareness about the stability of world peace. The situation has created a longlasting concern for individual safety in the midst of not knowing what future threats may be or when they may occur. It is the responsibility of all governments and individuals throughout the world to remain vigilant but more importantly to seek ways in which to promote tolerance and understanding, enabling people to live without fear and in safety.

Conclusion

The framework of the model of living has been used to demonstrate how the Roper et al (1996, 2000) model can be used to guide your understanding of the individual differences that exist when carrying out the AL of maintaining a safe environment. When planning and delivering care to individual patients it is vital that individual differences are taken into consideration and in doing so there is an acknowledgement that no one activity takes place without being interrelated with any of the other 11 ALs. Throughout the chapter exercises have been designed to show how important it is to:

- keep up to date with information
- base the assessment of your patient upon their individual habits and needs
- be mindful of how your own experiences and values might influence nursing care.

The last exercises in this section will now provide two brief scenarios to help begin the application of the model into practice. These exercises will help you gain an appreciation of how the AL of maintaining a safe environment can be influenced and how this can impact upon the other ALs.

Factors affecting the activity of maintaining a safe environment

Exercise

Read through Case study 3.1 and consider how the activity of maintaining a safe environment is being influenced from a lifespan, dependency/independency and factors affecting health perspective.

Case study 3.1

Short case scenario to identify MSE issues relating to the factors affecting health

A 24-year-old mother of two primary school age children, has been discharged home from hospital following an assault by her husband where she sustained facial and back injuries.

You may have considered the following points:

Lifespan
- expectation that she should be in good health and be able to care for and protect herself and her children.

Change in dependency
- dependency may increase upon family and close friends to support immediate physical, psychological, social, environmental and economic needs.

Factors affecting health
Biological
- injuries will need to heal
- risk of infection, concussion and pain
- difficulty eating, drinking, mobilising
- vision may be affected.

Psychological
- anxiety, fear, anger and distress
- low self-esteem and risk of depression.

Sociocultural
- concern for safety of self and children
- concern regarding reactions of others (friends, neighbours, school, work colleagues).

Environmental
- concern regarding safety in the home
- concern regarding leaving the home.

Politicoeconomic
- May have immediate and long-term financial concerns.

Exercise

Read through Case study 3.2 and identify the impact that a change in health status would have upon the Activities of Living.

Case study 3.2

Short case scenario to identify MSE issues relating to the Activities of Living (ALs)

A 76-year-old lady who lives alone has been discharged home following hip replacement surgery.

Impact upon Activities of Living
MSE
- home safety issues to be considered to prevent further accidents.

Communicating
- concern for ability to summons help if required
- need to ensure has access to information and support to meet physical and psychological needs.

Eating and drinking
- may be unable to fully meet needs due to reduced mobility
- at risk from malnutrition and dehydration
- poor diet may affect healing process.

Eliminating
- may require assistance and aids to carry out activity safely.

Mobilising
- at risk from slips, trips and falls
- reduced mobility in short and long term may impact on independency/dependency and other ALs.

Maintaining body temperature
- reduced activity may lower body temperature.

Sleep and rest
- loss of sleep may increase risk of accidents.

Dying
- at risk from accident or injury leading to death.

Summary points

The two exercises have helped to demonstrate the following:

1. MSE can be affected by all the factors affecting health.
2. MSE can be affected by all other ALs.
3. The lack of ability to engage fully in this activity can have detrimental affects upon health and the quality of life.

THE MODEL FOR NURSING

Individualizing nursing for the activity of maintaining a safe environment

The application of the model for nursing is based upon integrating the components of the model of living (lifespan, dependence/independence and factors affecting health) with each of the four phases of the nursing process (assessing, planning, implementing and evaluating) as shown in Figure 3.10 (see also Chapter 1 for details of the model and the nursing process).

This part of the chapter will now concentrate on showing you how to link the framework of the model of living in relation to MSE, to nursing practice situations in order to determine individual patient needs. By using each of the components of the model of living as a main framework it becomes possible to appreciate how individuals normally carry out the activity of MSE. Whilst people are physiologically the same they may behave very differently depending

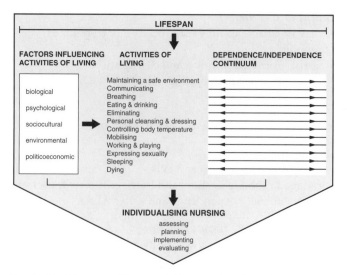

Fig. 3.10 Diagram of the model for nursing (from Roper et al 1998, with permission).

upon individual circumstances. The model of living in health is briefly summarised in Box 3.1. When applying the model for nursing it is necessary to transfer this knowledge

---

Box 3.1 Summary of the model of living in relation to MSE

Lifespan
Acknowledge what is considered to be normal development, physiology and lifestyle activities in accordance with age.

Dependence/independence
Recognition of temporary or permanent issues related to age and ill health states that create changes in independency.

Factors affecting MSE
Biological
- Internal – homeostatic systems are working correctly to ensure organ and system stability.
- External – there is ability to protect the body from external hazards.

Psychological
Emotional stability and intellectual capability affect the ability to cope with everyday life and identify dangers.

Sociocultural
Attitudes, beliefs and behaviour have a major influence upon maintaining safety.

Environmental
Dangers exist in the environment and measures can be taken to avoid them.

Politicoeconomic
Legislation, national and local resources and financial support is required to maximise safety.

---

and understanding to each individual patient in order to determine the extent to which the activity has altered as a result of injury or ill health. Only then can individualised care using the model be achieved.

This information will now form the basis upon which patients' needs can be assessed. By comprehensively and systematically integrating the MSE information within each stage of the nursing process, the individual needs of the patient can be identified in order to maximise the individuality of the care plan. Whilst using the book and when encountering individual patients in practice, you may find it useful to refer back to the information contained within the MSE model of living, recognising the importance of keeping up to date with related information in order to ensure that patients always receive a high standard of care. By using the model a broad range of nursing interventions will be identified that are appropriate to the AL such as:

- teaching patients about health and safety
- preventing accidents and ill health
- supporting patients to cope with altered health states
- providing care to support individual needs
- helping patients to adopt healthier lifestyles.

In order to help develop skills this section of the chapter will continue to provide a series of case scenarios and reflective exercises.

Assessment

Assessing the individual using the model for nursing

The aim of the assessment phase in relation to MSE is to utilise the components of the model of living to carry out the following:

- collect specific information related to the AL of MSE
- interpret information to determine the degree to which the AL is altered
- identify actual and potential problems related to the AL.

It is important to recognise that whilst the process of nursing begins with an initial assessment, it is a continuous activity, which supports the changing needs of patients through their entire period of care. This section of the chapter will now begin by describing how the model can be integrated to support the full range of patient assessment activities.

Collection of specific information related to the AL of MSE

Prior to the assessment
The assessment begins with using the components of the model of living to assess the patient's normal habits and routines in order to identify the extent to which ill health is influencing the ability to carry out the activity of MSE. When undertaking the assessment, it is important to

remember the interrelatedness of the AL of MSE in order to identify the following:

1. The actual or potential problems identified may be more readily aligned to another AL.
2. The extent to which other professional groups or agencies may be required to help solve or alleviate the problems.

What matters most is that through the assessment process, problems are firstly identified and that a realistic plan of nursing care is designed to meet the individual needs of the patient (see Chapter 1). It is important to remember that the accuracy of the assessment is based upon having a sound understanding of related normal health needs, particularly those related to vital body functions such as homeostasis and you are advised to make reference to other chapters and the recommended reading listed at the end of this chapter.

Identification of ill health problems associated with MSE

Before undertaking an actual patient assessment, it is important to have a good understanding of the range of ill health problems that are associated with MSE. The components of the model of living enable the identification of common illnesses that are associated with the activity of MSE and are shown in Box 3.2. When assessing patients this will enable a judgement to be made about the extent to which the activity of MSE can be altered in different ill health states and how this may manifest in individual patients.

Exercise
You may wish to check your knowledge and experience against the issues listed in Box 3.2 and consider them against your clinical experience to date. Consider what your learning needs might be, discuss these with your mentor and develop a learning plan.

The patient assessment

The ability to provide individualised nursing care is based upon the knowledge gained about a person's individuality in living. As demonstrated in the model of living, individuals carry out numerous activities to maintain a safe environment, some of which are similar and some of which are different. The purpose of undertaking an assessment of MSE is to determine what a particular patient's normal habits and routines are and identify where they may be vulnerable within the AL, given their current health state. Hence a thorough assessment is vital in order to ensure that the subsequent care plan is relevant to what the patient can realistically achieve and should reflect the following:

- how actual problems may be solved
- how to prevent potential problems becoming actual ones
- how to prevent solved problems from recurring
- how to alleviate problems which cannot be solved
- how to help the person cope with temporary or permanently altered states.

Box 3.2 To show identification of common ill health problems within the framework of the model

Lifespan
Consider ill health problems commonly associated with the stages of the lifespan, i.e. childhood illnesses and accidents, illness associated with lifestyle, disability and the ageing process.

Dependency/independency
Consider how dependency is altered in the presence of disease, trauma, medical intervention (i.e. anaesthesia or chemotherapy), trauma, disability and ageing.

Factors affecting health
Begin by identifying if the problem is being caused by an internal or external factor and consider the effect this may be having on other ALs. This demonstrates the interrelatedness and complexity of the AL.

Biological
- abnormality or damage to internal organs and systems that can lead to minor instability or life-threatening situations such as shock or haemorrhage
- problems associated with all known diseases affecting body organs and systems that are disrupted or failing
- infection

- trauma (haemorrhage, fractures)
- medical intervention (anaesthesia, surgery, reactions to investigations and treatments, i.e. pharmacological).

Psychological
- anxiety and stress
- disability
- abuse by self or others
- inability to recognise and avoid hazards.

Sociocultural
- trauma and injury associated with taking risks
- diseases associated with beliefs, behaviours or lack of understanding (infectious diseases).

Environmental
- trauma causing minor or major disabilities
- diseases associated with exposure to hazards, such as lung diseases, widespread tumours.

Politicoeconomic
- injuries and diseases associated with lack of ability to protect oneself in the home, in the workplace and in public places.

Data collection

In relation to MSE the assessment should be based on the following:

- What are the individual's attitudes to maintaining health and safety of self and others?
- What activities does the person engage in to maintain health and safety of self and others?
- What factors are influencing the individual's approach to maintaining a safe environment (ability, knowledge, experience, resources)?
- How the individual normally copes with the ability to maintain a safe environment?
- What identifiable problems or difficulties is the individual currently experiencing?

When undertaking an assessment ensure that the following skills are utilised:

- interviewing skills
- observation skills
- listening skills.

In addition there will also be a need to determine the extent to which the assessment is affected by physiological changes that are associated with MSE. For example, patients who are severely ill/injured, semiconscious or in a state of shock may be unable to provide information accurately, but this may also indicate that certain body systems are failing.

Exercise

Consider what assessment skills you have and the ones you need to develop when undertaking an assessment of MSE in the following areas:

Interviewing
- asking open and closed questions appropriate to the health status of the patient
- determine the priority of questions to be asked
- giving information and checking understanding
- involving relatives.

Observation
- verbal and nonverbal responses
- body language
- neurological and vital signs
- stress, pain and anxiety.

Listening
- act on verbal and nonverbal cues
- use of own body language to reassure and encourage the patient.

Using the components of the model of living in a systematic way will help structure the assessment. Regular use of the components will help to develop an effective assessment style and ensure that patients receive a thorough and professional assessment. The components of the model in relation to conducting an assessment of MSE will now be considered as shown in Box 3.3.

Box 3.3 MSE assessment guide

Lifespan
- At what stage of the lifespan is the patient?
- Does the patient have an understanding of risks/hazards associated with age and current situation?
- How vulnerable is the patient?
- By comparison with the expected normal lifespan how healthy/unhealthy is the patient?

Dependency/independency
- What constraints are influencing dependency (age, ill health)?
- Is the level of dependency high, average or low (upon other people or aids)?

Factors affecting health
Biological
- Is the patient in good physical health?
- Is there presence of a disability?
- Is there a risk of infection, shock, altered consciousness or haemorrhage?
- Are all senses responding appropriately?

Psychological
- Is the patient stressed or anxious?
- What is the patient's mood or temperament?

- Is the patient confident/motivated?
- Does the patient lack knowledge or understanding?
- What is the patient's experience or attitude to personal safety?

Socioeconomic
- What are the patient's personal beliefs/values regarding health and safety?
- Are there any social difficulties affecting health and safety?
- Is the patient at risk from exposure to any social hazards which may affect safety, health or recovery?

Environmental
- Is the patient able to recognise hazards within their environment (home, work and hospital)?
- Is the patient able to take appropriate action to maintain safety?

Politicoeconomic
- Are there any economic circumstances inhibiting the patient's health/lifestyle?
- Is a lack of resources/facilities compromising health, recovery and safety?
- Is the patient aware of support services that are available?

Patient assessment exercise

Using the assessment guide outlined in Box 3.3 consider the information that might gather from Case study 3.3. Record the information on the Patient Assessment Sheets provided in Appendix 2. This case scenario will be used as the main study for the chapter. Other short scenarios will be used to help transfer understanding of MSE to other individual patients.

Case study 3.3

Maintaining a safe environment

Frank is a 47-year-old man who has been admitted to the surgical ward following a diagnosis of a perforated gastric ulcer and is scheduled for emergency surgery. Frank has had a history of epigastric discomfort for some time and has been under the care of his GP, who has prescribed medication to relieve his symptoms. Frank has a hectic lifestyle and is under considerable stress at work. His eating habits are erratic, he smokes about 15 cigarettes a day and he admits to drinking heavily at times. Frank is married with two daughters who are both at university. On admission Frank is quite shocked, in pain and extremely agitated. His wife is upset as she has been trying to encourage Frank to slow down and change his lifestyle.

Using the knowledge and experience along with the assessment guide in Box 3.3 identify what Frank's individual MSE needs are as follows.

1. Identification of normal lifespan stage/lifestyle expectations, level of dependency and the factors which have led to the health breakdown.
2. Identify the actual and potential needs/problems associated with the AL of MSE.
3. Identify which other ALs are affected.

Assessment of lifespan, dependency and factors contributing to health breakdown

By using these three components of the model it is possible to determine the individual's normal habits and routines and identify where the patient is vulnerable within the AL. This aspect of the assessing MSE focuses upon the following:

- health expectation against stage on the lifespan
- usual routines and habits
- normal dependency capability
- previous coping mechanisms.

Box 3.4 outlines the kind of assessment information you might identify in relation to Case study 3.3.

From this exercise it is possible to determine that as an individual Frank has the following problems that have resulted in him becoming a surgical emergency:

Box 3.4 Assessment of lifespan, dependency and factors contributing to health breakdown

Lifespan
- common problem in adult life – exacerbated by adopted lifestyle
- under pressure at work and at home to provide for family needs
- need to identify why Frank has been unable to alter his lifestyle to prevent/reduce health breakdown.

Dependency
- currently in a high-dependency state – dependent upon surgical intervention to prevent life-threatening situation
- normally very independent with responsibilities for work and family.

Factors leading to health breakdown
Physical
- damage to digestive anatomy and function through poor eating habits, alcohol intake and smoking – has been taking antacid medication to relieve symptoms and visiting GP as required.

Psychological
- stress and anxiety affecting ability to adopt a healthier lifestyle
- has not been able to adjust lifestyle to cope with symptoms.

Sociocultural
- has strong values of being the family provider and need to achieve at work.

Environmental
- nature of work routine has not helped to improve eating and drinking habits – has support from wife to eat sensibly.

Politicoeconomic
- pressure to remain in employment and to fund mortgage and university fees.

- an acute shock and haemorrhage problem
- a longstanding peptic ulcer problem
- a health education need in relation to his diet, alcohol and smoking
- a health promotion need to adopt a healthier lifestyle.

Identification of actual and potential problems associated with MSE

Having identified the number of problems that are individual to Frank, the next stage is to determine which of the problems are actual and require solving and those which are potential and require prevention. By continuing to use the factors affecting health as a framework it becomes possible to apply knowledge of health to the patient's individual situation and determine the extent to which safety is threatened. Each of the factors will now be explored and Box 3.5 will illustrate how this can be applied to Case study 3.3.

Physical problems

As outlined in the model of living many activities associated with the AL of MSE are associated with mobility and sensory responses. When problems occur they can result in temporary or permanent changes. The degree to which the activity is altered ultimately has an effect upon complete independency and the ability to fully ensure safety. By considering the internal and external environments separately the nurse is able to plan in detail the care that is required to:

- detect and ensure early intervention for life- and safety-threatening situations
- prevent risks and accidents from occurring.

Prevention of life-threatening situations – shock Shock is one of the main causes of death in seriously ill patients and it is important that nurses have both the knowledge and the skills to ensure that appropriate and early interventions takes place. Caring for the patient with symptoms of shock requires an understanding of the pathophysiological processes that are taking place within the body and also the psychosocial effects that this may have upon the patient.

Shock occurs when the body's ability to distribute oxygen and nutrients to body tissues becomes diminished due to the following:

- a reduction of blood volume (hypovolaemic)
- damage to the heart (cardiogenic)
- altered vascular resistance (distributive) this includes septic shock, neurogenic shock, spinal shock, and anaphylactic shock.

Clinical signs and symptoms of shock The clinical signs of shock vary depending upon the underlying cause and are generally divided into four stages. Essentially the stages are indicators of the internal physiological mechanisms that are taking place in an attempt to restore homeostasis as described in the model of living (see p. 46). All types of shock are characterised by a fall in blood pressure, an initial increase in the pulse rate and a pale, cool and clammy skin. This is brought about by an early response by the sympathetic nervous system, triggered by a fall in blood pressure. Tissue hypoxia causes the heart rate to increase and a generalised vasoconstriction in an attempt to direct blood from less vital organs to the heart and the brain.

Stages of shock

1. *Initial stage* Initially there are no visible changes, but internally the cellular environment is changing producing a metabolic acidosis.
2. *Compensatory stage* At this stage the body is trying to correct the physiological disturbance.
3. *Progressive stage* The body enters this stage when the compensatory mechanisms begin to fail and start to produce adverse effects.
4. *Refractory stage* Damage to body tissues and organs cannot be stopped or reversed and death is imminent.

It is important to understand that the stages of shock are complex and it is not always possible to detect transition from one stage to another. It is recommended that you read further to increase your understanding around the distinguishing features of the different types of shock.

Haemorrhage A haemorrhage may be external and observable or internal and hidden. Where bleeding is external it may be arterial, venous or capillary. Arterial blood will be oxygenated and bright red, spurting rhythmically and blood loss can be considerable. Venous blood is bluish in colour and flows more evenly from the injured vessel, whilst capillary blood is reddish and tends to ooze from the area. When a vessel is injured the body initiates a response to reduce the bleeding (see Rutishauser 1994 Chapter 4). When bleeding is external, first aid treatment will be to apply pressure directly over the injured site. Where major vessels are involved surgical intervention will ultimately be required to repair the vessel. Where considerable blood loss takes place the patient will display signs of hypovolaemic shock.

Altered consciousness and mobility Through the onset of illness, injury or medical/surgical/pharmacological intervention consciousness and mobility can become altered. Even minor problems can create an increased level of individual dependency, which can result in an inability to maintain a safe environment either temporarily or permanently. These will be further discussed in Chapters 10 and 13, but because of the interrelatedness of the issues with MSE they are briefly outlined in this chapter. Unconsciousness presents a major threat to the patient's ability to maintain a safe environment. It is essential that the nurse is able to distinguish the difference between sleep and unconscious states which are indicative of altered physiology that can be potentially life-threatening.

Sensory impairment The model of living highlighted the importance that the five senses play in maintaining safety within the body's internal and external environment. Loss or impairment can be either temporary or permanent and will create a degree of dependency that requires adjustment. Loss of vision and hearing can be caused by ageing, disease or injury, which may not only affect the ability to communicate effectively but also increase the risk of accidents occurring. Loss of sensation means that individuals cannot feel pain, heat, cold or pressure. Paralysis is a term which describes a loss of sensation that is accompanied with a loss of movement and can cover large areas of the body as shown in Figure 3.11.

Different types of paralysis can make it difficult for patients to avoid hazards and ensure their own safety without the use of a range of living aids and resources to support

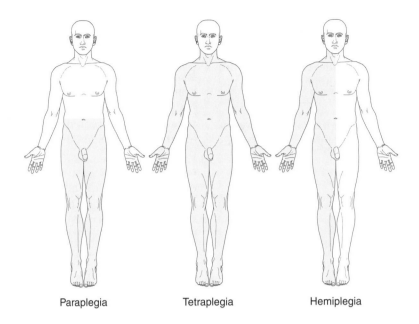

Paraplegia   Tetraplegia   Hemiplegia

Fig. 3.11 Motor and sensory loss in paralysis (from Roper et al 1998, with permission).

normal activity. Loss of smell and taste can be commonly experienced by individuals of all ages, caused by temporary minor ailments such as upper respiratory tract infections or through disease or ageing processes. Localised injury, medical treatment, medication and generalised disorders can also affect normal sensory function, putting patients at risk from a range of accidents such as burns and scalds, ingestion of poisons or an inability to smell fire or other noxious substances.

Risk of infection The risk of infection during illness is potentially greater due to a lowered resistance to infection and an increased exposure to a large number of micro-organisms. When patients are admitted to hospital the risk of exposure to an even greater number of microorganisms is further increased. It is vital that the spread of infection is rigorously controlled in order to prevent the patient from developing a nosocomial or hospital-acquired infection (HAI). A HAI is defined as an infection that was not present prior to admission to hospital and carries considerable costs for both patients and health care providers. For patients an infection becomes an added complication that can delay or even prevent recovery. Ultimately this leads to an increased hospital stay and costs for additional investigations, medications and provision of continuing care services. It is estimated that the cost of HAI to the health care sector is around one billion pounds per year (Public Health Laboratory Service 2000).

Psychological problems

When patients become unwell their mental health and intellect may become impaired due to infection, disease, injury or stress and anxiety. The effects of ill health may prevent the individual from being able to reason or make appropriate decisions regarding personal safety and it may be difficult to identify their normal individual state of dependency. It is important to recognise that patients who already have limitations, which are a part of their individuality, such as patients with learning difficulties or mental health illness, have these taken into consideration in order to ensure that their safety is maximised.

Sociocultural problems

Safety issues related to sociocultural needs are generally central to three areas of concern:

- the degree to which sociocultural issues may have contributed towards ill health
- the degree to which normal habits and routines may be disturbed by illness or injury
- the degree to which safety can be influenced due to individual beliefs and values.

Having established the issues that may have contributed to the health breakdown, it is also important to determine how the patient might be supported in the recovery phase. Assessment in this area may also give an indication of how the patient might manage their own personal safety during their stay in hospital and identify any specific individual needs that they may have in relation to personal beliefs and values. For example it may be important for the patient to carry out specific religious practices which if restricted may cause them anxiety.

Environmental problems

Unfamiliar environment When patients are admitted to hospital they are often anxious and frightened, indeed it may be the first time they have been an inpatient. They may not be familiar with the routine, equipment or the environment and this has the potential to lead to accidents. The age and dependency of the patient must be taken into consideration in order to provide the patient with the correct information, orientation, equipment, support or supervision.

Risk of accidents in hospital For the patient the care environment is unfamiliar and there are many potential hazards associated with the following:

- reduced mobility through age, illness, medication or medical intervention
- altered mental/conscious state
- impaired vision, hearing and speech
- lack of awareness or understanding of the need for safety precautions.

The hazards within the care environment can result in a number of accidents such as:

- slips, trips and falls
- drug administration errors
- medical negligence.

In the UK NHS organisations are required to have policies and procedures in place to assess, prevent and manage risks on behalf of both patients and employees. In 1995, the NHS introduced the Clinical Negligence Scheme for Trusts (CNST). The scheme is administered by the NHS Litigation Authority (NHSLA) and was created to protect Trusts against the effects of rising negligence claims, requiring trusts to have in place rigorous systems for preventing, monitoring and managing clinical risks (Sanderson et al 1998, Mission 2001).

Noisy environment Hospitals are known to be noisy environments which can create psychological disturbances for patients causing a lack of sleep, irritability, heightened arousal, impaired judgement, altered perception and thought processes and a reduced ability to hear. Noises originate from people within the environment such as staff, other patients and visitors talking, shouting out and moving around. Equipment such as telephones, trolleys, sinks, toilets, oxygen administration, ventilators, alarms and monitors create additional noises. Patients who have hearing loss or who are sedated seem least affected, but patients who are anxious, depressed or who have difficulty sleeping will be most affected.

Medication risks Under normal circumstances people take personal responsibility for correctly administering medications to themselves or to sick family members. Upon admission to hospital patients become dependent upon medical, nursing and pharmacy staff to prescribe and administer medication, except in places where self-medication schemes are in operation. Because of the potential dangers associated with medication, administration is strictly governed by legislation and nurses are required to adhere to various laws

(The Medicines Act 1968 and Misuse of Drugs Act 1971), local policy and professional standards (Guidelines for the Administration of Medicines NMC 2002b).

Risk of fire Hospitals are large buildings that have the potential for fire to break out. This is a serious matter since many patients may not be able to escape without help and some would also require continuing medical attention during the process. Some patients may express concern about their safety during their stay in hospital and will require reassurance in the form of being shown what to do in case of a fire. The Health and Safety at Work Act 1974 places the responsibility for organisations and their staff to take personal responsibility for observing and adhering to safety policy and keep continually up-to-date on how to raise the alarm and begin evacuation procedures.

Anaesthesia An anaesthetic is used to block any sensations of pain during surgery. It can be applied locally or regionally to a specific area of the body or generally. A general anaesthetic not only reduces pain but also induces unconsciousness as muscles become relaxed and reflexes are lost. During this time the patient will be unable to maintain an airway and dependent upon medical intervention to prevent risks occurring. Patient safety in the operating theatre is aimed at minimising the risks of infection, haemorrhage, allergic reactions, limb and posture damage, burns and retention of foreign bodies from the surgical procedure. It is vitally important to ensure that patients are correctly prepared for surgical procedures in order to minimise the risks from anaesthesia.

Politicoeconomic problems

Potential and actual problems related to MSE are often associated with the ability to afford the necessary resources to maintain health and prevent accidents, whether this is at a personal, community or national level. Without support, a lack of personal finances may reduce a person's ability to maintain health, or protect themselves from injury, for example the need to purchase medicines, special diets or home safety equipment. When advising patients about safety it is important to sensitively determine whether the advice is realistically affordable and where necessary support the patient's needs by making appropriate referrals to other agencies.

By using the factors affecting health as a framework, it has been possible to identify a range of actual and potential problems associated with MSE. Box 3.5 describes how the framework can help identify the problems related to Case study 3.3.

Identification of the impact on other ALs

In reality rarely would one AL be affected in isolation. Whilst this chapter concentrates upon MSE it is important to consider the impact that an altered dependency in MSE might have upon the other ALs, particularly in relation to the internal environment. Box 3.6 demonstrates how the problems identified from Case study 3.3 may impact upon the remaining ALs.

Box 3.5 Actual and potential problems identified for Case study 3.3

Maintaining a safe environment	Actual problems	Potential problems
Physical	The patient is shocked due to haemorrhage and peritoneal contamination from a perforation of the gastric wall caused by a peptic ulcer	The patient is at risk of loss of consciousness/cardiac arrest due to shock and haemorrhage The patient is at risk from injury due to bed rest, weakness and being in a strange environment
Psychological	The patient is agitated, anxious and in severe pain around the epigastric region	
Sociocultural		The patient may be concerned about his family and work
Environmental	The patient is at risk from accidents, being in an unfamiliar environment	The patient may be concerned about his ability to change his lifestyle
Politicoeconomic		The patient may have concerns about employment and financial commitments

Box 3.6 Impact of the MSE problem on other ALs

Activity of living	Actual problems	Potential problems
Communicating	• Has epigastric pain and is restless and anxious due to perforation • Has difficulty communicating due to oxygen therapy, nasogastric tube • Will be anxious about current health state and require information and reassurance	• May develop dry mouth and lips which may affect ability to communicate
Breathing	• Has difficulty breathing due to pain	• Respirations may deteriorate due to increased level of shock
Eating and drinking	Unable to eat or drink due to: • Nil-by-mouth requirement in preparation for surgery • Is nauseous and is vomiting • Has unpleasant taste in the mouth	• At risk of haemorrhage and haematemesis
Eliminating	• Unable to pass urine normally due to bed rest and urinary catheter	• At risk of diminished urinary output due to shock • May develop malaena due to gastrointestinal bleeding
Personal cleansing and dressing	• Has difficulty maintaining own hygiene needs due to current physical state	• At risk from developing pressure sores
Mobilising	• Unable to mobilise normally due to current physical state, pain, weakness and medical intervention	
Sleep and rest	• Experiencing difficulty due to pain and anxiety	
Work and play	• Unable to engage in normal activities due to current health state	
Expressing sexuality		• May be anxious about boo
Maintaining body temperature		• May develop an infection
Dying		• At risk of collapse due to sh

Exercise

Using the information presented so far in this chapter consider how different your assessment and identification of MSE might be in relation to the following scenarios.

1. A 72-year-old lady with diabetes and failing eyesight who lives alone has fallen at home and sustained a severe pretibial tear.

2. A 20-year-old man who has epilepsy has not been taking his medication regularly, he is admitted in a semiconscious state following a series of grand mal seizures over the last 3 hours.

3. A 36-year-old lady has developed MRSA following a routine surgical operation. Check your answers with the information in Boxes 3.7, 3.8 and 3.9.

Box 3.7 72-year-old lady with diabetes

Physical
- How long has she suffered from diabetes?
- How is the diabetes managed?
- When did the fall occur?
- How long has eyesight been poor?

Psychological
- What is the patient's mood?
- Does the patient seem alert?
- What are the patient's concerns regarding the injury?

Sociological
- What personal support is available?

Environmental
- Awareness of safety in the home?
- Availability of support/resources to promote safety?

Politicoeconomic
- Is there a lack of resources which have contributed to the problem?
- What might be preventing the patient from taking care of herself?

Box 3.8 20-year-old man with epilepsy

Additional information may need to be obtained from whoever is in attendance with the patient for example: family, friends, neighbour, work colleague or passerby.

Physical
- How long has he suffered from epilepsy?
- When did the seizures start?
- Has the patient experienced grand mal seizures before?
- Has the patient sustained any other injuries?
- What are the patient's neurological observations indicating?

Psychological
- How has the patient been behaving?
- What has the patient's mood been like?
- Has the patient been suffering from stress or anxiety?
- How compliant normally is the patient in taking his medication?

Sociological
- What support does the patient have at home?
- How does the patient normally cope with having epilepsy in everyday living (at home or at work)?
- Does having epilepsy restrict life and normal activities?

Environmental
- What are the risks for the patient at work?
- What are the risks of further injury by admission to hospital?

Politicoeconomic
- Does the patient require any resources to carry out normal living activities?
- Does the patient's health problem affect economic independency?

Box 3.9 36-year-old lady with MRSA

Physical
- What observable symptoms are to be recorded?
- What potential problems is the patient at risk from?

Psychological
- How is the problem affecting mood and personality?
- How is the patient coping with the situation?
- Is the patient irritable or anxious?

Sociological
- What restrictions/effects will isolation have upon lifestyle, individuality and independency?

Environmental
- Is the patient aware of the safety precautions required?
- Does the patient understand the reason for isolation?

[Politic]oeconomic
- [What ec]onomic difficulties might arise from prolonged [isol]ation?

Planning nursing activities

Planning nursing activities involves the following:

- identifying the priorities
- establishing short- and/or long-term goals
- determining the nursing actions/interventions required
- documenting the nursing care plan.

Planning nursing care accurately and effectively begins with exploring the actual and potential problems that have been identified and determining the nursing interventions that are required to achieve the following:

- to solve actual problems
- to prevent potential problems occurring
- to prevent solved problems from reoccurring
- to develop positive coping strategies for any problem which cannot be solved.

Throughout the planning phase it is important that the nurse remains focused upon the patient's problems and what is appropriate to the patient's recovery in the immediate, short and long term.

Factors influencing the planning stage

It is important to recognise that certain factors may exist to influence the planning stage. In relation to MSE these may be as shown in Box 3.10. Check the information contained within Box 3.10 to determine what your own personal development needs might be.

Identification of priorities

Having undertaken a comprehensive individualised assessment the next stage is to plan the nursing care. This begins by identifying the following:

- making a judgement about the priority order of the actual and potential problems.
- the impact that the health problem is having on all of the ALs.

By using the dependency/independency component of the model it is possible to develop criteria which describe the degree of altered dependency that the patient is experiencing particularly where this is causing a life-threatening situation. In clinical practice it is possible to use the criteria to score or measure individual patient or ward levels of dependency (see Box 3.11).

It is important to recognise that dependency/independency can change very rapidly and this requires continuous assessment. In relation to Case study 3.3 (p. 67) review the actual and potential problems identified and determine the priority against them (see Table 3.2).

The priorities identified amongst the other ALs are described as follows in Table 3.3.

From this exercise it can be identified that Frank's problems are not only serious, but are complex and initially much of the care he will require is central to the following:

- continuous observation of actual problems to detect for signs of his condition worsening prior to surgery
- supporting medical intervention to stabilise and improve his condition in preparation for surgery
- preventing potential problems from occurring.

This exercise demonstrates that by using the model it is possible to identify a number of problems and the effect these are having upon Frank as an individual. Planning care in this way also highlights that in some instances, preventing potential problems from occurring may take priority over actual problems, depending upon the threat that is posed to life. Tables 3.2 and 3.3 demonstrate how the main problem of shock is actually presenting, not only in relation to MSE but also by the impact this is having on all other ALs. The rationale for identifying problems using the model is to increase the understanding of the individuality in illness. By alleviating and supporting the main problem(s) it is also possible to observe the effect this has on other ALs. Coupled with a comprehensive assessment, focused upon the individual lifestyle, normal habits and routines of the patient, the setting of realistic short- and long-term goals becomes enhanced.

Box 3.10 Factors influencing planning nursing care for the AL of MSE

Nurses	Patients/clients
• Knowledge of normal physiology and specific pathophysiological processes	• Understanding of the need for safety
• Knowledge of normal living and dependency across the lifespan in various cultures	• Personal beliefs, values and experiences
• Knowledge and skill in required evidence base for nursing interventions	• Ability to communicate needs and describe symptoms and feelings
• Skill in observation and assessment	• Anxiety, pain and concern about coping mechanisms
• Skill in determining priorities	
• Staffing levels, skill mix, supervision and ongoing professional development	

Box 3.11 Dependency/independency priority criteria

Priority 1	Completely independent in the AL/independence maintained
Priority 2	Potential problem in the AL/remains mostly independent
Priority 3	Actual problems identified within more than one AL/some independency noted but remains mostly independent
Priority 4	Existence of actual and potential problems/a number of other ALs with associated increasing dependence
Priority 5	Life-threatening actual and potential problems/total dependence

Table 3.2 Prioritising MSE actual and potential problems related to Case study 3.3

Maintaining a safe environment	Actual problems	Priority	Potential problems	Priority
Physical	The patient is shocked due to haemorrhage and peritoneal contamination from a perforation of the gastric wall caused by a peptic ulcer	5	The patient is at risk of loss of consciousness/cardiac arrest due to shock and haemorrhage	5
			The patient is at risk from injury due to bed rest, weakness and being in a strange environment	4
Psychological	The patient is agitated, anxious and in severe pain around the epigastric region	4		
Sociocultural			The patient may be concerned about his family and work	3
Environmental			The patient may be concerned about his ability to change his lifestyle	2
Politicoeconomic			The patient may have concerns about employment and financial commitments	2

Table 3.3 To show identification of priorities in all other ALs

Activity of living	Actual problem	Priority	Potential problems	Priority
Communicating	Has epigastric pain and is restless and anxious due to perforation	4	May develop dry mouth and lips which may affect ability to communicate	3
	Has difficulty communicating due to oxygen therapy, nasogastric tube	4		
	Will be anxious about current health state and require information and reassurance	3		
Breathing	Has difficulty breathing due to pain	3	Respirations may deteriorate due to increased level of shock	3
Eating and drinking	Unable to eat or drink due to: • Nil-by-mouth requirement in preparation for surgery • Is nauseous and is vomiting Experiencing: • Has unpleasant taste in the mouth	4	At risk of haemorrhage and haematemesis	3
Eliminating	Unable to pass urine normally due to bed rest and urinary catheter	4	At risk of diminished urinary output due to shock	3
			May develop malaena due to gastrointestinal bleeding	3
Personal cleansing and dressing	Has difficulty maintaining own hygiene needs due to current physical state	3	At risk from developing pressure sores	2
Mobilising	Unable to mobilise normally due to current physical state, pain weakness and medical intervention	3	At risk from developing pressure sores, deep vein thrombosis	3
Sleep and rest	Experiencing difficulty due to pain and anxiety	3		
Work and play	Unable to engage in normal activities due to current health state	3		

Table 3.3 *(continued)*

Activity of living	Actual problem	Priority	Potential problems	Priority
Expressing sexuality			May be anxious about body image and self-esteem	3
Maintaining body temperature	Has difficulty in maintaining body temperature due to shock and haemorrhage	3	May develop an infection	3
Dying			At risk of collapse due to shock and haemorrhage	4

Table 3.4 **Short- and long-term MSE goals set for Frank**

Problem	Short-term	Long-term
The patient is shocked due to haemorrhage and peritoneal contamination from a perforated gastric ulcer	The patient's physical condition will be stabilised prior to surgery	The patient will recover from surgery without complications

Goal setting

Goal setting in relation to MSE can range from being immediate term (hourly), short term (less than 1 week) or long term (for a longer period). When setting goals, the seriousness of the problem and its identified priority must be taken into consideration. The goal statement is important, as it describes what the patient is expected to, or has agreed to, achieve (see Chapter 1). The more realistic, measurable and observable the goal the easier it becomes to monitor and evaluate the progress the patient is making. Table 3.4 gives an example of the short- and long-term goals that might be set for Frank. It is important to recognise that whenever possible, patients should be involved in the goal-setting process, as it provides an opportunity to promote independence, motivation and a greater understanding of personal health, safety and recovery (refer to Chapter 1 for further details on goal setting). Essentially the short- and long-term goals for Frank will be central to the following:

1. alleviate his immediate life-threatening problems
2. support his recovery from surgery
3. help him to adopt an altered lifestyle.

Table 3.4 shows the short- and long-term goals that could be set for Frank during his hospital stay in relation to MSE.

Once the short- and long-term goals have been set the appropriate nursing actions can be planned to enable the goals to be achieved.

Implementing care to meet maintaining a safe environment needs and problems

This section of the chapter will show how, by using the factors affecting health components of the model, nursing actions associated with MSE can be broadly outlined in order to guide professional nursing practice. It is essential that the nurse constantly updates knowledge and skills in the areas outlined in order to ensure that patients receive quality care.

Nursing interventions related to physical factors affecting ill health

The object of nursing actions related to physical factors affecting health are in relation to promoting and maintaining health and preventing disease irrespective of the health care setting. Nursing actions must be based upon full understanding of biological systems across the lifespan as described in the model of living, and linked closely to sound knowledge and understanding of anatomical and physiological systems.

Health education

Health education plays an important role in maintaining health and preventing disease. In order to ensure social and economic wellbeing, nurses should seize every opportunity to promote health where it is deemed appropriate to the individual needs of the patient. Health promotion should be aimed at:

- preventing diseases and reducing mortality rates
- reducing the risks associated with disease
- improving healthy lifestyles.

Observation of vital signs

As outlined in the model of living the human body is highly complex. For the purpose of understanding how the body functions, body systems are studied separately, and in the model the systems are aligned to specific ALs. In reality however body systems are very closely interrelated, hence the appreciation of why, during ill health, rarely is an AL altered on its own. The object of enabling the patient to maintain a safe internal environment depends upon being able to make accurate essential observations of the cardiovascular and neurological systems, as described within the model of living. In the model described by Roper et al (1996), vital signs are discussed under the AL of breathing (see Chapter 5) however it is important to acknowledge the importance of observation of vital signs as related to the AL of MSE. These include the measurement of vital signs that are related to the cardiovascular and central nervous systems as follows:

- blood pressure
- pulse rate
- circulation
- sensory and motor responses (neurological observations).

Vitals signs also include observation of respirations and body temperature and these will be discussed in Chapters 5 and 9. The process of diagnosing pathophysiological disorders will also involve many other specialised observations/investigations that will be specific to the preliminary diagnosis. For example blood tests, electro- and radiological investigations. When working in clinical practice it is important that nurses develop their understanding of specialised investigations and ensure patient's needs are fully supported and that practice is safe. When carrying out observations of vital signs, it is important that measurement is both consistent and accurate. Studies have shown that observation and recording techniques can vary considerably, leading to inaccurate recordings being made (Evans et al 2001). Since the patient's medical treatment and ultimate safety often relies upon vital sign information, the competency and accuracy of observation, recording and reporting cannot be stressed enough. In clinical practice it is important you are competent in the use of a variety of devices and ensure that observations are *always* accurately made and promptly recorded and reported.

Blood pressure Accurate recordings of the blood pressure and pulse provide information about changes in the patient's physiological state in relation to:

- diagnosis of the disease
- assessment of normal cardiovascular function
- assessment of cardiovascular recovery following disease, surgery or trauma.

The importance of making an accurate recording is essential in order to determine if homeostasis is being restored. Generally, alterations in systolic blood pressure indicate problems with cardiac output, whilst diastolic recordings enable venous return and cardiac inflow to be assessed. Individual patients can have very different blood pressure readings, therefore it is important to establish early each patient's normal reading. To ensure patient safety all staff should adhere to local policies and guidelines, which govern accurate recording (see Mallet & Dougherty 2000 for practice guidelines).

Pulse rate The purpose of assessing the pulse rate is to determine heart rate, rhythm and strength. The pulse rate is

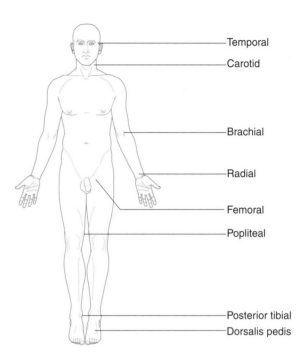

Fig. 3.12 Major pulse points (from Jamieson et al 2002, with permission).

most commonly assessed at the radial site but there are many other sites as shown in Figure 3.12.

The pulse can be measured either by palpation or by simultaneous sound and palpation, as used when measuring the apical-radial pulse. This requires two nurses to observe for deficits in the heart rate. It is important that the rate is measured for a full 60 seconds in order to ensure that an assessment of the following can be made:

- determine normal baseline range for lifespan
- estimate altered range caused by disease, medication, medical intervention
- correlate information with other observations, i.e. pulse and temperature.

Circulation Circulation can be visually observed or through palpation in several ways.

Capillary refill By applying pressure to the nail bed the skin becomes white (blanched). When the pressure is released quickly the skin should return to being pink within 3 seconds.

Temperature By touching the skin it is possible to detect areas of warmth and coolness.

Colour General observation of the patient's skin can indicate cyanosis, pigmentation, redness, pallor, jaundice or signs of bleeding such as bruising, petechiae or haematoma.

Moisture The skin can display signs of dryness and turgour caused by dehydration or sweating due to shock and anxiety.

Oedema Assessment of swollen areas around the feet, ankles, lower arms and sacrum can indicate circulatory dysfunction.

Neurological observations Assessment of the patient's conscious level is necessary in order to support the maintenance of a safe environment, particularly where there is increasing dependency caused by a variety of ill health states. Neurological observations are carried out in conjunction with blood pressure, pulse and respiratory rate measurement, enabling changes in the patient's condition to be detected and acted upon. In the UK the Glasgow Coma Scale observation chart (Jamieson et al 2002, Fig. 3.13) is used to record the full range of vital and neurological signs, incorporating three aspects of consciousness:

- visual responses
- verbal responses
- motor/sensory responses.

Preoperative nursing care
The aim of preoperative nursing care is to maximise the safety of the patient's internal and external environment in the days or hours prior to surgery. Surgical operations are classified as being either elective (planned) or an emergency. An emergency operation is carried out without delay in the interest of the patient's immediate survival. In either case, the aim is to ensure that the patient is as physically fit as possible, by conducting a thorough assessment of the patient through a range of medical and nursing observations and laboratory tests and investigations.

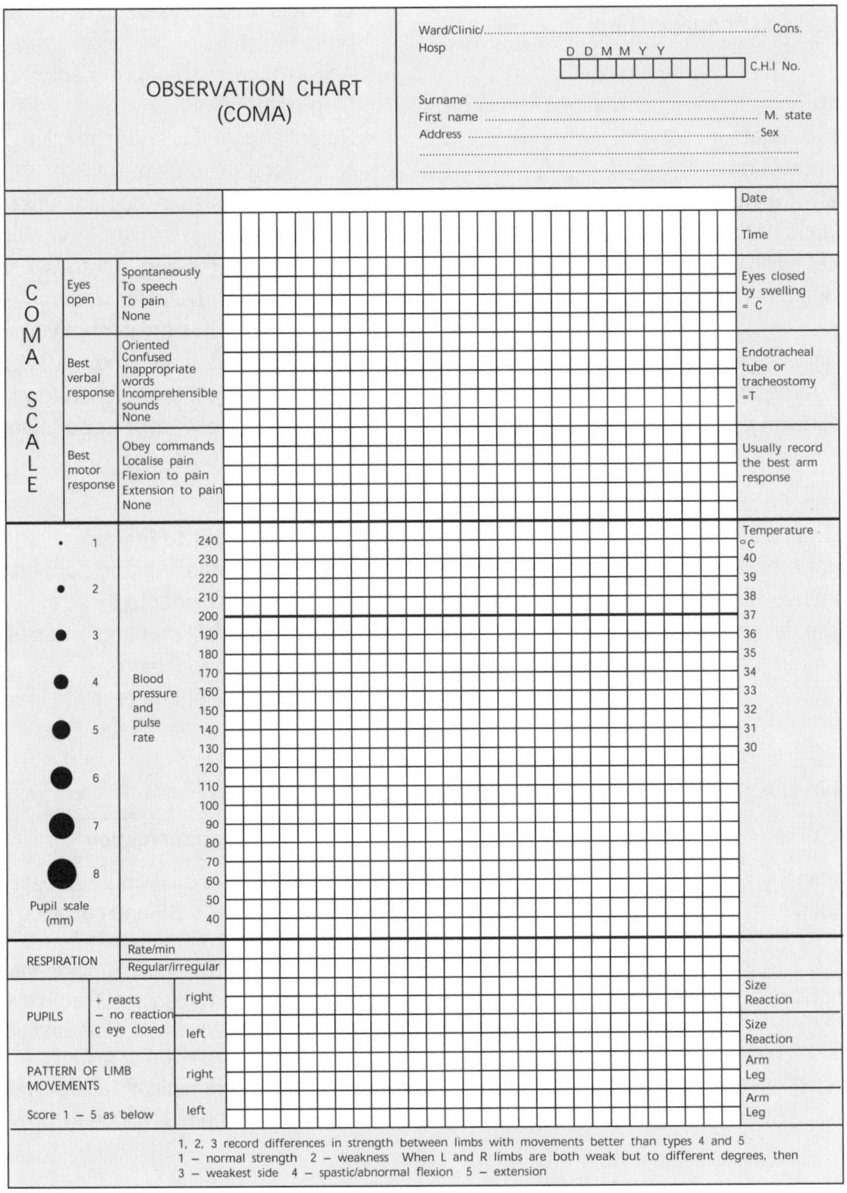

Fig. 3.13 Glasgow Coma Scale chart (from Jamieson et al 2002, with permission).

In preparing patients for surgery irrespective of the complexity of the surgery, a number of core procedures must be carried out in order to prevent potential risks/complications from occurring. The preoperative phase begins as soon as the decision for surgery has been identified and care is central to the patient being in the best possible health from a holistic perspective. The nurse must be constantly alert to any physiological changes that might occur in the preoperative phase for both emergency and elective patients, and report them promptly. Boxes 3.12 & 13 provide an overview of preoperative preparation, which whilst being essentially related to the AL of MSE, highlights once again, the interrelatedness to other ALs. Table 3.5 shows how this would relate to the care of Frank (Case study 3.3, p. 67).

Box 3.12 Overview of physical preoperative patient preparation

1. Patient history
- Information regarding lifestyle, normal health state and normal habits and routines specific to the individual that may be significant to surgery or recovery (i.e. history of previous illness and surgery)
- Drug history (prescribed and nonprescribed)
- Allergic reactions.

2. Physical assessment
- Cardiac, respiratory and renal functions
- Blood volume and composition
- Nutritional, fluid and electrolyte status
- Electrocardiogram, X-rays and laboratory tests
- Routine observations of temperature, blood pressure, pulse, respirations, conscious levels and circulation
- Urinalysis
- Other observations such as menstruation, diarrhoea, nausea, vomiting, dehydration, sore throat, bleeding gums or dental caries, discharges and wounds.

3. Health promotion
- Encourage patients who smoke to stop or reduce smoking to prevent complications
- Discuss pre- and postoperative safety requirements and rationale in relation to other ALs such as skin preparation, leg and chest, exercises, fasting, bowel and bladder preparation, premedication, bed rest, sleep, pain and identification checks.

Box 3.13 Example of preoperative checklist

- Pre- and postoperative procedures explained
- Check consent form has been signed
- Check preanaesthetic assessment has been undertaken
- Check operation site is correctly marked
- Record temperature, pulse, respirations and blood pressure (T, P, R & BP)
- Record urinalysis
- Administer bowel preparation
- Check if patient needs to micturate prior to premedication
- Administer preoperative medication
- Skin preparation
- Remove make-up and restrictive clothing
- Note dentures/crowns, etc.
- Note prosthesis, i.e. contact lenses, hearing aids, false limbs
- Ensure dentures and prosthesis are removed
- Tape/remove jewellery
- Ensure valuables are securely stored
- Check identification band
- Check when patient last had food or drink
- Ensure all investigation reports are present (i.e. blood and X-ray reports)
- Promote rest

Immediately prior to theatre
- Continue to reassure and support the patient
- Empty bladder prior to theatre
- Check identification band and case notes
- Escort patient to theatre
- Hand over patient correctly to theatre staff

Table 3.5 Preoperative nursing interventions for Frank (Case study 3.3)

Problem	Goal	Nursing intervention
Frank is to undergo abdominal surgery to repair a perforated gastric ulcer	Ensure Frank is physically fit for surgery to minimise the risk of complications	- Record baseline observation of vital signs (T, P, R & BP and conscious level) - Record urinalysis - Record results of blood tests, crossmatching - Record results of cardiovascular investigations - Record results of radiological investigations - Ensure Frank is fasted - Assess patient's allergic responses - Complete preoperative checklist
Frank is at risk from developing pre- and postoperative complications such as: - Shock - Haemorrhage - Chest infection - Thrombosis - Dehydration		

In order to ensure the safety of the patient immediately prior to going to theatre the checks listed in Box 3.13 would need to be undertaken.

Intraoperative care

Operating theatres are specifically constructed and operated to maximise patient safety at every stage of the patient's journey from reception through to the recovery room. Every aspect of care in the intraoperative phase is focused upon maintaining the safety of the patient from collapse, infection, complications and injury. Strict asepsis is maintained and precautions are taken to minimise the transmission of microorganisms from the air, equipment and personnel. Upon arrival at the operating theatre the following details are double-checked by the ward and theatre nurse in order to ensure safety:

- conscious level
- identification band, patient's notes and theatre list details
- operation consent from
- paired limb or organ site clearly marked and identified
- special problems highlighted, i.e. allergic reactions
- laboratory/investigation reports handed over
- preoperative medication amounts and effects
- vital sign status.

Throughout the time spent by the patient within the operating theatre from the induction of anaesthesia to recovery, the focus of nursing care is to maintain the patient's vital functions. The patient will only return to the ward when the vital functions are sufficiently recovered and the patient is no longer dependent upon life-supporting machinery.

Postoperative nursing care

All surgical interventions have a common series of problems that the patient may experience such as pain, tissue trauma, infection, shock and haemorrhage. As in the preoperative phase, MSE nursing actions focus upon supporting the vital body functions and minimising risks, to ensure that the patient makes a timely and uneventful recovery. Dependent upon the type and nature of the surgery there will be some general and specific physiological disturbances. Care of the patient must be central to the particular type of surgery and the ongoing individual needs of the patient. From the moment that the patient returns from the operating theatre nursing actions are central to constantly monitoring the patients recovery in terms of:

- monitoring vital physiological signs
- recording, interpreting and reporting any significant changes
- supporting patient comfort and pain
- providing information and encouragement to support recovery.

Table 3.6 illustrates the nursing interventions associated with the physical aspects of MSE care for Frank (Case study 3.3, p. 67).

All of the operative phases identified will have some kind of impact upon other ALs, depending upon the age, general fitness of the patient and type of surgery that is performed. This may lead to the identification of 'problems' that may be more suitably aligned to another AL. For example, pain may be described under the AL of communicating and wound care under the AL of personal cleansing and dressing. It is not the model's intention to be prescriptive, but to ensure that aspects of care are not overlooked. Through good clinical leadership, teams can agree how best key aspects of care should be aligned to the most appropriate AL.

Exercise

Impact of surgery on other ALs

In relation to Case study 3.3 (p. 67) consider what the postoperative care would be required in all other ALs.

Table 3.6 Postoperative nursing interventions associated with the physical aspects of MSE

Problem	Goal	Nursing intervention
Frank has undergone surgery for the repair of a perforated gastric ulcer and is at risk from: • Shock • Primary haemorrhage • Blood loss from the wound • Altered consciousness • Respiratory problems • Wound infection • Postoperative complications (chest infection, thrombosis, renal failure)	To return Frank to a normal conscious and physiological state and prevent the onset of postoperative complications	Monitor vital signs $1/2$ hourly until stable Monitor vital signs 2–4 hourly for 12–14 hours when stable Monitor conscious level Observe skin for signs of shock and circulatory problems Observe fluid intake and output for reduced output until normal intake resumes Provide oxygen as prescribed Position patient carefully to promote recovery to prevent injury and complications Record and report any significant changes Observe wound site for bleeding, drainage or swelling Maintain strict asepsis to prevent wound infection Encourage deep breathing and leg exercises to prevent postoperative complications

Day surgery

Day surgery involves admission, pre- and postoperative surgery and discharge all in 1 day and is gaining increasing popularity for both patients and health care providers. Success lies in transferring good practice from traditional pre- and postoperative care with a range of specific knowledge and skills in order to ensure the safety of the patient. Not all patients will be suitable for day surgery and some patients will require collaboration between multidisciplinary professionals in both the primary and acute care settings. Nurses working in day surgery units need to be flexible and have excellent assessment and communication skills to ensure effective patient care (Cahill 1997).

Administration of medicines

Administering medicines is an important role of the nurse and the practice is strictly governed by legislation, professional guidelines and local policy. In the UK, nursing practice is guided by the Nursing and Midwifery Council (NMC 2002a), whereupon individual nurses are personally accountable for their practice and responsible for keeping themselves up-to-date. Where mistakes are made there is a requirement for the employing organisation to investigate the incident and determine the cause of the error and if necessary refer the person to the NMC for professional disciplinary action. It is imperative that nursing care is focused upon the following:

- knowledge of the patient's condition and treatment regime
- knowledge of the patient's compliance and understanding
- knowledge of the medication action and potential side effects
- knowledge of legal, professional and local policy for checking and administration
- knowledge and skill in correct storage and preparation
- knowledge and skill in using the correct route of administration
- knowledge of correct procedure for recording administration
- knowledge of prescribing principles
- knowledge of the management and reporting of errors and incidents.

In the UK through the introduction of The Medicinal Products: Prescription by Nurses Act 1992 it is possible for some nurses to prescribe a limited number of drugs. The practice is strictly underpinned by an educational programme and employer approval (McCartney et al 1999, Humphries & Green 2000). Despite this occasionally mistakes are made which cause serious side effects and even death, therefore it is imperative that correct dosages are given, by the correct route and regular observations are made to detect side effects.

Nursing interventions related to psychological factors affecting ill health

The model of living highlighted the importance of nursing care being available to support the intellectual and emotional needs of the patients in relation to their individual needs. The range of support across the lifespan may require specific specialised nursing care for example Health Visitor expertise for children or mental health intervention for patients with specific disorders. As a basic survival instinct the human body is naturally equipped to cope with a certain degree of stress, but the extent to which individuals are able to cope varies immensely.

In relation to surgery, it is important to be able to determine the patient's level of understanding of pre- and postoperative procedures and identify any anxieties that are present. This helps the nurse to support the individual needs of the patient to provide information, relieve anxiety and ensure sufficient rest before surgery. Table 3.7 illustrates the nursing care that Frank would require to meet his psychological needs.

Nursing interventions related to sociocultural factors affecting ill health

Nursing actions in relation to sociocultural factors are central to integrating the patient's individual beliefs and values into the planned nursing care and providing support for any health inequalities that may have been identified. There is however a degree of complexity involved because of the vast differences that can exist between individuals. It is important that this is not overlooked at the expense of more medically orientated issues, as failure to do so can result in the following:

- unpleasant/uncomfortable care experience (leading to complaints)
- delayed recovery
- preventable risks/hazards not being identified.

Table 3.7 Illustration of psychological needs for Case study 3.3

Problem	Goal	Nursing intervention
Frank may be anxious about his ability to cope with: • Surgery and/or anaesthesia • Pain	Ensure Frank is psychologically fit for surgery	• Ensure Frank has sufficient information according to individual needs • Continuously assess the patient and family anxiety and provide information and support as required • Support patient rest and relaxation and report any difficulties/concerns • Administer sedatives as prescribed and monitor effectiveness

In a multicultural society it is increasingly important for nurses to consider how to preserve the individual patient's social, cultural, spiritual, religious and ethical needs in order to help the patient understand, agree and cooperate with any planned care. There are many traditions and beliefs associated with health and illness that can alter a person's behaviour when they become ill and the nurse must seek to understand how this may be observed in their patients. Every patient will have a different level of knowledge and understanding of their problems and different expectations regarding their treatment and involvement. For example, through the Internet a growing number of people have greater access to information regarding ill health and treatments and need to be informed and involved in their care. On the other hand other patients may have little understanding or no information. In relation to MSE it is important that the safety of the patient is ensured without infringing upon their personal beliefs, therefore nursing actions will be central to the following:

- determine the patient's level of understanding
- explain the rationale for procedures
- identify the difficulties this may pose for the patient/family
- report concern immediately
- negotiate and seek to provide an agreed safe level of care.

Informed consent

Prior to surgery or any other invasive diagnostic procedure, patients (or parents/guardians) are required to give their written consent. In the UK any person over the age of 16 years can legally give consent. In cases where the patient is unable to give their consent such as in an emergency, the doctor would obtain consent from the next of kin or guardian. Consent must only be given on the understanding that sufficient detail and information regarding the procedure has been received from the doctor. It is important that the details given enable the patient or guardian to understand the procedure and make an informed decision to proceed, having had the potential risks and complications pointed out. The purpose of gaining consent is to protect the patient from undergoing any unauthorised procedures and also to safeguard the medical practitioner and the health care organisation. The consent form is validated by the presence of signatures from the patient or guardian and the doctor.

There is a professional and legal requirement to ensure that consent is properly obtained in recognition of the individual needs of patients (Doyal 2001). The role of nursing actions is to support the patient and the doctor to ensure that the patient receives and understands the information being given and report any concerns that the patient may express at any time before the procedure.

Nursing interventions related to environmental factors affecting ill health

Safe practices in infection control

It is not always possible to immediately identify the presence of transmittable infections. Therefore as a precaution it is important to ensure that there are safe working practices in place to minimise crossinfection. All nurses have a professional responsibility to promote the control of infection at both a personal and patient level and take action to minimise the spread of infection through the use of safe up-to-date practice. It is also important to ensure that safe control of infection practice takes place in health as well as during times of illness. In the UK the prevention of healthcare-associated infections is such an important issue that safe practice is guided by national evidence-based principles (DoH 2001b), which govern the following:

- hospital environment hygiene
- hand hygiene
- the use of personal protective equipment
- the use and disposal of sharps.

Hospital-acquired infections (HAIs) commonly occur in surgical wounds, urinary and lower respiratory tracts caused by *Staphylococcus aureus* and Gram-negative bacilli, that are present in the nose and on the skin. The bacterium is spread by direct contact from people and equipment. To this extent it is imperative that the whole multidisciplinary team are aware of their individual responsibilities and are encouraged to cooperate in order to successfully control infection. It is important that within the care environment careful consideration is given to all aspects of cleanliness and control of infection such as:

- cleaning and disinfecting procedures for *all* patient, nursing and medical equipment (for example meal time utensils, toileting equipment, medicine pots, mattresses, bed linen and trolleys)
- correct disposal of clinical waste and spillages
- correct handling of specimens.

Failure to control infection effectively increases the opportunity for contamination either by direct contact or airborne routes, the most common being *Staphylococcus aureus*. There are a variety of *Staphylococcus aureus* strains, some of which are resistant to many antibiotics and referred to as methicillin-resistant *Staphylococcus aureus* (MRSA). MRSA are a problem in hospital because of the dangers they pose to vulnerable patients who already have a lowered resistance. MRSA is spread by unwashed hands, skin scales, dust and contaminated equipment or fabrics. Patients who are infected with MRSA are barrier nursed to prevent the spread to other patients and staff.

Isolation management This is a technique sometimes referred to as barrier nursing or source isolation, used to protect either a vulnerable patient from exposure to harmful microorganisms (reverse barrier nursing) or to prevent a known transmissible infection spreading to other patients or staff. Care of the patient is central to the following:

- determining the diagnosis
- determining the infective source
- determining the transmission modes
- determining the communicability of the infection.

In the UK as a minimum, universal blood and body fluid precautions must be followed and standard arrangements set in place as recommended by the Hospital Infection Control Practices Advisory Committee (HICPAC) (see Ayliffe et al 2000 for further information). In relation to individualising the care of the patient, isolation can be a very stressful experience requiring sensitive understanding. The nurse will need to address all the related factors affecting the care of the patient providing information to the patient and family and support to meet physical, psychological and sociocultural needs.

Hand hygiene Hands are known to be the main vehicle for the transmission of microorganisms between people and equipment and therefore good handwashing techniques are vital in controlling the spread of infection. Handwashing techniques have been the subject of many studies over time which have led to the development of guidelines for good practice (Ayliffe et al 2000, Pittet et al 2000, DoH 2001b). Handwashing guidelines are based upon the principle of seeking to reduce, remove or destroy potentially harmful microorganisms that may be present on the hands and are at risk of being transmitted to the patient. Every health care organisation will have specific guidelines governing handwashing technique and recommended cleansing agents. Box 3.14 provides an example of handwashing guidelines and Figure 3.14 shows the recommended standard technique that should be used (Horton & Parker 1997).

Use of gloves Gloves are used to protect both patients and staff in order to reduce the risk of crossinfection when carrying out a variety of procedures. They are made from a variety of different materials such as latex, vinyl and plastic, for specific purposes and can be coated inside with a powder to make application and removal easier (Russell-Fell 2000). The wearing of gloves is known to cause problems for some staff that may be allergic to either the material (such as latex), or the powder coating. Patients too are at risk from allergic reactions and there is some concern that the powder may increase the risk of wound infections (Dave et al 1999). In order to prevent risks occurring it is important that patients are accurately assessed and that gloves are appropriately selected for the task (Parker 1999). It is recommended that gloves are always used when handling blood and body fluids and that hands should still be washed after gloves have been removed.

Needle stick and risk from other injuries Essentially all patients are a source of infection and the nurse must

---

Box 3.14 Handwashing guidelines

Handwashing should be carried out
- on arrival and on completion of duty
- after using the toilet (self or assisting patients)
- before and after preparing, serving or eating food or medicines
- before and after attending each individual patient
- before and after aseptic procedures
- before and after removing protective clothing (masks, gloves or aprons)
- after handling contaminated laundry/equipment
- when hands are visibly soiled
- after contact with body secretions/excretions.

Procedure
- remove jewellery, wristwatches, bracelets and rings (except wedding rings)
- all surfaces of the hands must be washed
- pay particular attention to thumbs, fingertips and finger webs
- begin by wetting the hands with warm running water
- apply recommended soap/antiseptic cleansing agents
- use alcohol gel in situations where time or facilities inhibit hand washing
- use the technique outlined in Fig. 3.14 to rub agent into all areas
- rinse thoroughly under running water
- turn off taps with elbows or wrist or clean paper towel
- dry hands thoroughly using two clean paper towels.
- take care not to recontaminate hands when throwing paper towel away
- use hand creams provided to prevent skin irritation.

---

carefully balance the quality of individual care against the need to reduce the risks associated with the occupational transmission of infection. It is not always possible to know what the infection status of a patient is and all health care workers are advised to take universal precautions to minimise the risk of infection caused by either certain procedures or by patients themselves. These are categorised as being needle stick or sharp injuries or patient-related injuries, e.g. being bitten by a patient, which may result in contamination of the health care worker from bloodborne infections.

To protect staff all care organisations should have a policy and clear guidelines that must be followed governing the process for reporting and recording any incident irrespective of the patient's infection status. Policies will outline the action to be taken to ensure that appropriate attention is given to the injury site, blood investigations, prophylactic treatment, counselling and follow-up care. Through the occupational health department, staff should also have access to an immunisation programme in order to reduce infection amongst staff.

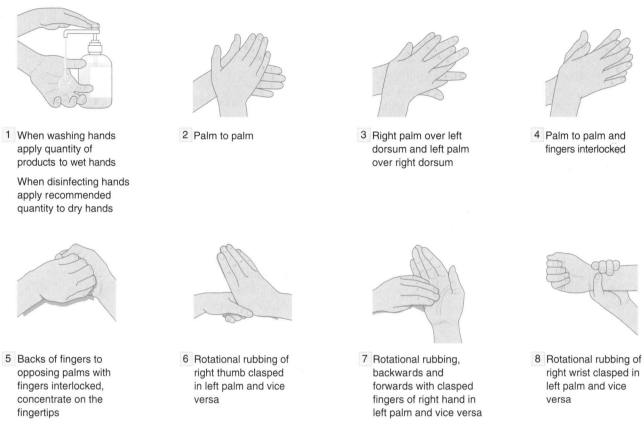

1 When washing hands apply quantity of products to wet hands

When disinfecting hands apply recommended quantity to dry hands

2 Palm to palm

3 Right palm over left dorsum and left palm over right dorsum

4 Palm to palm and fingers interlocked

5 Backs of fingers to opposing palms with fingers interlocked, concentrate on the fingertips

6 Rotational rubbing of right thumb clasped in left palm and vice versa

7 Rotational rubbing, backwards and forwards with clasped fingers of right hand in left palm and vice versa

8 Rotational rubbing of right wrist clasped in left palm and vice versa

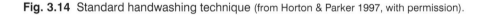

After washing, hands should be thoroughly rinsed

Fig. 3.14 Standard handwashing technique (from Horton & Parker 1997, with permission).

Control of infection environment Infection is known to spread more quickly in large open spaces and this understanding has influenced the way in which care facilities are being designed and provided. To reduce infection rates, consideration is now given to installing more single rooms with en-suite facilities, subdivided wards, more toilets and showers, hot hand dryers and dedicated rooms for wound dressing and invasive procedures and spaces for correct storage of equipment and substances.

Aseptic technique This is a technique which is used to reduce the risk of introducing pathogens into the body, based upon the principle that only uncontaminated objects or solutions make contact with the area and that the risk of airborne invasion is kept to a minimum. The technique should be carried out in a clean environment, using only sterile equipment and is used for dressing wounds, removing sutures, drains, etc., or carrying out other invasive procedures such as urinary catheterisation. It is important that hands are thoroughly washed, trolleys and surfaces correctly prepared and only sterile cleansing and dressing materials used (see Mallet & Doherty 2000 for practice guidelines).

Control of the external environment Nursing actions central to controlling the care environment in relation to MSE focus upon preventing accidents and ensuring that patients who are ill are able to receive sufficient rest and sleep. If it has been identified that a patient is at risk from falling or sustaining any other injuries because of their age or health state, then appropriate action should be taken. It is important to recognise that equipment used within the health care setting may have hidden dangers for patients such as trolleys and tubing. In addition unfamiliar environments and limited or shared facilities may cause the patient some anxiety and result in accidents. If the patient is receiving care as a result of a fall at home then the focus of care would be to discuss safety measures to be taken upon returning home, with a possible referral to another health or social care professional for further assessment. Controlling noise within the care environment can be difficult to achieve particularly when noises are coming from other patients. Increasing use of technology has resulted in a greater use of electronic equipment, which adds to the total volume of noise in any given environment. To this extent the nurse should consider regularly the effects this may have on individual patients and take appropriate individual or team action to minimise noises, particularly at night.

Nursing interventions related to politicoeconomic factors affecting ill health

It is important to recognise that for some patients an episode of illness or injury can create financial hardship. Not all patients enjoy the protection of employer sickness schemes. The nurse must be sensitive to the issue and consider that from the patient's perspective a financial anxiety may be greater than that of concern for physical wellbeing. To support patient care responsibly, it is important that nurses have a good understanding of how political and economic factors influence individual and community health. In doing so it is essential that nursing actions are central to the patient's individual circumstances and that the support of other health and social care professionals and agencies are sought in the most appropriate way.

Delivery of maintaining a safe environment nursing interventions

The delivery of quality care is dependent upon the quality of the information detailed within the care plan. In the care setting a variety of health professionals will need to refer to the care plan and it is essential that the plan is conducive to the delivery of consistency in care standards. Prior to the implementation of nursing activities the following must be in place:

1. A detailed written care plan and verbal handover to ensure that all staff are aware of patient progress, goals to be achieved and skills required to deliver the care.
2. Competent practitioners are identified to safely deliver the planned care.
3. Nursing actions and patient progress are recorded and goals are evaluated.

The nursing plan is a document that guides the required nursing activities to help the patient achieve the identified goals (see Chapter 1). The plan should be constantly reviewed and updated to record the following:

- when a goal/desired outcome has been achieved
- when nursing intervention has been changed to support goal achievement
- when the goal needs to be modified
- when the evaluation date needs to be changed
- when problems change or develop.

Factors influencing implementation of MSE nursing interventions

To ensure the effectiveness of implementing the MSE plan it is important to identify the factors, which can influence this.

Knowledge
- normal anatomy and physiology and pathophysiological states and processes
- related psychological effects associated with ill health
- social and cultural implications for poor health or recovery
- environmental influences and concerns
- political and economic influences and concerns.

Skill and competency
- philosophy of care and attitudes to patient care
- communication/interpersonal skills
- observation skills
- problem-solving skills
- technical/caring skills
- management/leadership skills (directing, coaching, delegating, supervising skills)
- teaching skills
- research skills.

Resources
- appropriate skill mix
- sufficient equipment
- sufficient support services.

MSE and medically derived care

In addition to the identified nursing care plan, it is also important to consider the impact that medical or other health care intervention can have and should where possible be integrated into the plan as shown in Table 3.8.

Evaluating care

The evaluation stage provides the basis by which to determine if the patient is making the desired progress and the mechanism to judge the effectiveness of the nursing actions. Evaluation of the patient's progress should be ongoing and undertaken on a continuous, hourly, per shift, daily or weekly basis, depending upon the patient's problem and timescale for achieving the goals. To evaluate effectively the following skills are required:

Table 3.8 Identification of medically derived care and its impact upon nursing care

Medically derived care	Nursing intervention/support
Specific medicotechnical intervention	Knowledge, skill and competency to manage equipment, observe results and report changes
Specific pharmacological intervention	Knowledge and skill regarding action and side effects
Specific nutritional intervention	Knowledge and skill to support patient information
Specific physiotherapy intervention	Knowledge and skill to provide 24 hour continuing care

- observing
- interviewing
- listening
- analysing
- measuring.

The steps in evaluating are detailed as follows. It is recommended that where possible the patient is involved in describing the progress/achievement made:

1. Check the identified goals against patient progress
   - Have the goals been partially or completely met?
   - Have the goals been unmet?
2. Is the timescale realistic?
3. Record the progress as follows:
   - goal completely met, state the evidence to support this and discontinue the problem
   - goal partially met then decide if there is a need to extend the timescale or modify the plan
   - goal not met at all then decide if there is a need to extend the timescale, change the plan or reassess the whole problem.

It is important to recognise that the evaluation stage can be influenced by a number of factors, which must be taken into consideration (see Box 3.15). Consider the skills that underpin these factors in relation to personal development needs.

Plan review

If the goals are achieved nursing actions effectively become redundant. Where goals are not achieved the following questions need to be asked:

1. Is more information required to determine goal achievement?
2. Should the nursing plan be adapted to enable the goal to be achieved?
3. Has the problem changed?
4. Can the nursing care planned be stopped?
5. Has the problem worsened?

Box 3.15 Factors influencing the evaluation of care

- Quality of the assessment and planning stages
- Accuracy of the goals set
- Standard and quality of the care delivered
- Timing of the evaluation(s)
- Knowledge and skills of the nurse
- Abilities of the patient

---

6. Should the goal and intervention be reviewed?
7. Was the goal inappropriate?
8. Does the plan require intervention from other health care professionals?

Upon discharge, there will usually be some continuing care needs that the patient requires. Often the patients themselves can meet the identified needs providing sufficient information is given. If the patient requires continuing health or social care support it is vital that information is transferred accurately to the appropriate professional such as general practitioner, community nurse, therapist or social worker. Table 3.9 illustrates the extent to which Frank in Case study 3.3 (p. 67) has achieved the goals set prior to discharge and indicates his continuing care needs.

Summary points

1. Maintaining a safe environment is essential for an individual's health and wellbeing.
2. Using a model framework together with the nursing process, the nurse can identify the way in which the AL is interdependent with all the other ALs.
3. Assessment of patient needs associated with the AL of maintaining a safe environment involves taking account of both internal (within the body) and external (outside the body) environments.

Table 3.9 Evaluation and plan review

Goal	Evaluation	Plan review
Frank's physical condition will be stabilised prior to surgery	Frank's physical condition was satisfactorily stabilised prior to surgery	No further preoperative intervention required
Frank will recover from surgery without complications	Frank made a successful recovery with no immediate complications noted	Continue to observe vital signs twice daily until discharge from hospital
Ensure Frank is psychologically fit for surgery	Frank is fully aware of the need for surgery and received information and support to reduce anxiety	Frank has some concerns regarding his recovery
Frank will need to adapt lifestyle to promote full recovery and prevent further problems following discharge	Frank will need further advice and support prior to discharge to help adjust lifestyle	Refer to appropriate health professionals • Dietitian • Counselling services • Medical team and GP

References

Alexander MF, Fawcett JN, Runciman PJ 2000 Nursing practice – hospital and home, 2nd edn. Churchill Livingstone, Edinburgh

Ayliffe GAJ, Fraise AP, Geddes AM, Mitchell K 2000 Control of hospital infection – A practical handbook, 4th edn. Arnold, London

Barrell RA, Hunter PR, Nichols G 2000 Microbiological standards for water and their relationship to health risk. Communicable Disease and Public Health 3(1): 8–13

Burnett A, Peel M 2001 Asylum seekers and refugees in Britain. The health of survivors of torture and organised violence. British Medical Journal 10(322)/(97286): 606–609

Cahill H 1997 Day surgery: principles and nursing practice. Baillière Tindall, London

Cantor KP 1997 Drinking water and cancer. Cancer Causes and Control 8(3): 292–308

Child Accident Prevention Trust 2000 Injury facts and figures 1999: some background. CAPT, London

Crinson I 1999 Clinical Governance: the new NHS, new responsibilities? British Journal of Nursing 8(7): 449–453

Dave J, Wilcox MH, Kellett M 1999 Glove powder: implications for infection control. Journal of Hospital Infection 42(4): 283–285

Dawood M, James J 2001 What are you afraid of? Nursing Times 97(40): 24–25

Department of Health 1998 A first class service: quality in the new NHS. HMSO, London

Department of Health 1999 Saving lives: our healthier nation. HMSO, London

Department of Health 2000 The NHS plan: a plan for investment – a plan for reform. HMSO, London

Department of Health 2001a National service framework for older people. HMSO, London

Department of Health 2001b The *epic* project: developing national evidence-based guidelines for preventing healthcare associated infections. Journal of Hospital Infection 47 (Jan 2001)

Department of Health 2001c Mobile phones and health. HMSO, London (www.doh.gov/mobilephones/ mobilephones.htm; last accessed June 2002)

Department of Trade and Industry 2001 Home accident surveillance system 23rd annual report: accident data and safety research, home, garden and leisure. DTI, London

Department of Transport, Local Government 2000 Tomorrow's roads: safer for everyone. The Government's road safety strategy and casualty reduction targets for 2010. HMSO, London

Doyal L 2001 Informed consent: moral necessity or illusion? Quality in Health Care 10:(i): 29–33

Dugmore I 2002 Developing a strategy to tackle elder abuse. Nursing Times 98(1): 42–43

Evans D, Hodgkinson B, Berry J 2001 Vital signs in hospital patients: a systematic review. International Journal of Nursing Studies 38(6): 643–650

Eurens B, Primatesta PP, Prior G, Bajekal M, Boreham R, Brookes M, Falaschetti E, Hirani V 2001 Health survey for England: the health of minority ethnic groups '99: a survey carried out on behalf of the Department of Health: Vol 1: Findings. Office for National Statistics, HMSO, London

Frain JP, Carr PH 1996 Is the typical modern house designed for future adaptation for disabled older people? Age and Ageing 25(5): 398–401

Gaze H 2000 Avoiding slips, trips and broken hips. Nursing Times 96(25): 12–13

Gunnell D, Sheperd M, Evans M 2000 Are recent increases in self harm associated with changes in socio-economic conditions? An ecological analysis of patterns of deliberate self-harm in Bristol 1972–3 and 1995–6. Psychological Medicine 30(5): 1197–1203

Health and Safety at Work Act 1974 (www.hmso.gov.uk/acts)

Health and Safety Executive 2001 Health and safety statistics 2001. Stationery Office, London

Health Education Authority 1999 Older people and accidents, Fact Sheet 2. HEA, London

Hinchliff SM, Montague SE, Watson R 1996 Physiology for Nurses, 2nd edn. Baillière Tindall, Edinburgh

Horton R, Parker L 1997 Informed infection control practice. Churchill Livingstone, London

Hubbard AM, Harty MP 2000 MRI assessment of the malformed fetus. Baillière's Best Practice and Research in Clinical Obstetrics and Gynaecology 14(4): 629–650

Humphries JL, Green E 2000 Nurse prescribers: infrastructures required to support their role. Nursing Standard 14(48): 35–39

Jamieson EM, McCall JM, Whyte LA 2002 Clinical nursing practices, 4th edn. Churchill Livingstone, Edinburgh

Johnson FM 1998 The genetic effects of environmental lead. Mutation Research 410(2): 123–140

Kirkwood E, Lewis C 1989 Understanding medical immunology, 2nd edn. John Wiley & Sons Ltd, Chichester

London Fire Brigade 2002 Fire safety in your home fact sheets. (http://www.london-fire.gov.uk/fire_safety/in_your_home; last accessed June 2002)

Mallet J, Dougherty L 2000 The Royal Marsden manual of clinical nursing procedures, 5th edn. Baillière Tindall, London

McCartney W, Tyrer S, Brazier M, Prayle D 1999 Nurse prescribing: radicalism or tokenism? Journal of Advanced Nursing 29(2): 348–354

McDonald AS, Davey GCL 1996 Psychiatric disorders and accidental injury. Clinical Psychology Review 16(2): 105–127

McMichael AJ, Haines R, Slooff R, Kovats RS 2000 Climate change and human health: impact and adaptation. Geneva, WHO (www.who.int/environmental_information/ climate/climchange.pdf; last accessed September 2002)

Medicinal Products Prescription by Nurses Act 1992 (www.hmso.gov.uk/acts/acts 1992)

Medicines Act 1968 (www.hmso.gov.uk/acts)

Melies A 2001 Small steps and giant hopes: violence on women is more than wife battering. Health Care Women International 22(4): 313–315

Mission JC 2001 A review of clinical risk management. Journal of Quality in Clinical Practice 21(4): 131–134

Misuse of Drugs Acts 1971 (www.hmso.gov.uk/acts)

Moffat C 2000 Self-inflicting wounding, part 2: identification, assessment and management. British Journal of Community Nursing 5(1): 34–40

Mohammed MA, Cheng KK, Rouse A, Marshall T 2001 Bristol, Shipman and clinical governance: Shewhart's forgotten lessons. Lancet 357(9254): 467

Moreton J 2001 MMR vaccination: the case for evidence-based practice. British Journal of Community Nursing 6(4): 4, 199–200

Nursing and Midwifery Council 2002a Code of conduct. NMC, London

Nursing and Midwifery Council (2002b) Guidelines for the administration of medicines. NMC, London

Office For National Statistics 2000 National health activity for sick and disabled people: accident and emergency, and acute outpatient and day cases 1981–98: social trends 30. The Stationery Office, London

Parker LJ 1999 Infection control. 1: A practical guide to glove usage. British Journal of Nursing 8(7): 420–424

Pittet D, Hugonnet S, Harbarth S, Mourouga P, Sauvan V, Touveneau S, Perneger TV 2000 Effectiveness of a hospital-wide programme to improve compliance with hand hygiene. Infection Control Programme 356(9236): 1307–1312

Prieto MD, Lopez B, Juanes JA, Revilla JA, Llorca J, Delgado-Rodriguez M 2001 Recreation in coastal waters: health risks associated with bathing in sea water. Journal of Epidemiology and Community Health 55(6): 442–447

Public Health Laboratory Service 2000 Press Release 000121 Hospital acquired infections cost to the health sector (www.phls.org.uk/news/pressrelease/00p/00012pr.htm; last accessed June 2002)

RIDDOR 1995 Reporting accidents at work, Reporting of accidents – the reporting of injuries, diseases and dangerous occurrences, regulations 1995 (www.waverley.gov.uk/environment/has_accidents.asp; last accessed June 2002)

Ritter L, Solomon K, Sibley P, Hall K, Keen P, Mattu Linton B 2002 Sources, pathways, and relative risks of contaminants in surface water and ground water: a perspective for the Walkerton inquiry. Journal of Toxicology and Environmental Health 65(1): 1–142

Roper N, Logan W, Tierney AJ 1996 The elements of nursing: a model for nursing based on a model of living, 4th edn. Churchill Livingstone, Edinburgh

Roper N, Logan W, Tierney A 2000 The Roper, Logan and Tierney model of nursing. Churchill Livingstone, Edinburgh

Royal Society for the Prevention of Accidents 2002 Home safety fact sheet: the RoSPA guide to home safety projects. RoSPA, Birmingham

Rutishauser S 1994 Physiology and anatomy: a basis for nursing and health care. Churchill Livingstone, Edinburgh

Russell-Fell RW 2000 Avoiding problems: evidence-based selection of medical gloves. British Journal of Nursing 9(3): 139–146

Salmon G, James A, Smith D 1998 Bullying in school: self reported anxiety, depression and self esteem in secondary school children. British Medical Journal 317(7163): 924–925

Sanderson IM, Annandale R, Over C, Ward S 1998 Clinical focus: the CNST 1: a review of its present function. Clinical Risk 4(2): 35–50

Sidebotham M 1999 Under the microscope. CESDI: the sixth annual report. British Journal of Midwifery 7(8): 477–479

Stuck A, Beck JC 2001 Preventing disability and death in old age. International Journal of Epidemiology 30(4): 900–901

Sullivan PM, Knutson JF 2000 Maltreatment and disabilities: a population-based epidemiological study. Child Abuse and Neglect 24(10): 1257–1273

Tibbets J 2000 Water world 2000. Environmental Health Perspectives 108(2): A69–73

Tong S, von-Schirnding YE, Prapamontol T 2000 Environmental lead exposure: a public health problem of global dimensions. Bulletin of the World Health Organization 78(9): 1068–1077 (www.who.int/bulletin; last accessed September 2002)

Wald NJ, Hackshaw AK 2000 Advances in antenatal screening for Down syndrome. Baillière's Best Practice and Research in Clinical Obstetrics and Gynaecology 14(4): 563–580

Webster S 1999 Recognising and tackling elder abuse. The Practitioner 143(1596): 164–173

Wolf RS 1997 Elder abuse and neglect: Causes and consequences. Journal of Geriatric Psychiatry 30(1): 153–174

Wolke D, Woods S, Bloomfield 2001 Bullying involvement in primary school and common health problems. Archives of Disease in Childhood 85(3): 197–201

World Health Organisation 1997 Child abuse and neglect. Fact sheet N150. WHO, Geneva

World Health Organisation 2000 Violence against women. Fact sheet 239. WHO, Geneva

World Health Organisation 2001 Occupational and community noise. Fact sheet 258. WHO, Geneva

World Health Organisation 2002a Pollution-related diseases kill millions of children a year. Press release WHO/36. WHO, Geneva

World Health Organisation 2002b Pregnancy exposes women in poor countries to a 200-fold risk of dying vs rich countries. Press release WHO/39. WHO, Geneva

Further Reading

Alexander MF, Fawcett JN, Runciman PJ 2000 Nursing practice – hospital and home, 2nd edn. Churchill Livingstone, Edinburgh

Ewles L, Simmnett I 1999 Promoting health: a practical guide, 4th edn. Baillière Tindall, London

Hinchliff SM, Montague SE, Watson R 2000 Physiology for nurses, 2nd edn. Baillière Tindall, Edinburgh

Rutishauser S 1994 Physiology and anatomy. A basis for nursing and health care. Churchill Livingstone, Edinburgh

Useful Websites

Age Concern (www.ageconcern.org.uk)
Child Accident Prevention Trust (www.capt.org.uk)
Department of Health (www.doh.gov.uk)
Disabled Living Centre Council (www.dlcc.org.uk)
Disability Alliance (www.disabilityalliance.org)
Department for Trade and Industry (www.dti.gov.uk)
The Health and Safety Executive (www.hse.gov.uk)
International Labour Organisation (www.ilo.org/)
National Society for the Prevention of Cruelty to Children (www.nspcc.org.uk)
Royal Society for the Prevention of Accidents (www.rospa.co.uk)
The World Health Organisation (www.who.int/peh/)

Communicating

Helen Iggulden

Introduction

Human communication has evolved over thousands of years, and has been influenced and motivated by survival and safety needs, bonding needs, social and cultural factors and technological changes. People communicate their thoughts and feelings by the actions of their nerves and muscles in speaking, writing, hearing, seeing, touching and gesturing in a range of different personal, social and formal situations.

The first part of this chapter (the model of living) will explore:

- the process of communication
- communication across the lifespan
- biological features of communication rooted in the nervous system
- the role of emotion and other psychological factors involved in the act of communicating
- the influence of social, cultural and educational factors in communicating in different situations
- how the environment influences our communication abilities and patterns
- how legislation and economic factors have influenced the development of human communication.

Each of these sections has exercises, activities and reflective triggers to help you to relate these general aspects to clinical situations.

The second part of this chapter (the model for nursing) then focuses on some case studies, highlighting how communication is affected when people become ill. The discussion uses the nursing process and the application of biological, psychological, social, cultural, environmental and economic aspects.

THE MODEL OF LIVING

To enable you to appreciate the different kinds of communication please undertake the following exercise.

Exercise
1. Think of a range of different words that you associate with communication.
2. Group or classify the words under different headings.

Your words may have included any of the ones mentioned below or any one of a hundred others not mentioned here: speak, talk, shout, whisper, hail, touch, frown, glare, grin, chuckle, write, type, listen, hear, sign, point, listen, read, touch, feel, describe, explain, media, information, telephone, email, praise, scold, internet, report or publish. The simplest way of grouping these words is under the headings of verbal and nonverbal. However, a different classification is suggested below because it demonstrates how complex and subtle communication can be when it involves many parts of the nervous system and when influenced by social and cultural factors, emotions, learned behaviour and skills and technology:

- vocal: shout, whisper, chuckle, talk, telephone
- facial: frown, glare, grin
- bodily gestures: point, shrug, touch
- written: write, type, publish, email
- electronic: internet, media, email
- communication: describe, explain, praise, scold
- perceiving/receiving: look, listen, read, touch, feel, taste.

This classification shows that words take on meaning when combined with nonverbal features, and the mode and purpose of communication. Receiving and perceiving account for a significant element of all communication acts. The Greeks were well aware of this and have a proverb to warn of it: 'Nature has given us two ears, two eyes and but one tongue. To the end we should hear and see more than we speak'.

Models of the process of communication

Models are flow diagrams of how communication takes place, which aim to draw attention to the features that are common to all situations. Communication models however, need to be treated as one useful tool rather than as a complete toolkit. Simply shouting, 'Help' requires a far less sophisticated model than one that seeks to represent the highly complex patterns that develop in families, communities and organisations. Consider the following examples.

Example 1

Laura is a Staff Nurse with an 8-month-old baby and she is keen to spend Christmas at home with her. Gina, the ward manager is finding it very difficult to cover the ward over Christmas.

Face-to-face communication

Laura: Hi Gina (smiles) Could we meet up sometime today to sort out the Christmas off-duty (pulls a face and laughs).

Gina: (Lips tighten, eyebrows lower, no eye contact with Laura, stares at the desk) Yes of course although I do not know what everyone wants (with sarcastic emphasis) yet.

In this situation Laura is getting nonverbal responses from Gina as she speaks and she will probably (assuming she has commonsense and empathy) modify her response when she realises how Gina is feeling about the issue of the Christmas off duty.

Email from Laura to Gina

Hi Gina, I would be grateful for an early Christmas Eve, day off Christmas and any shift you like on Boxing Day. Please could you let me know ASAP so I can make my arrangements? See you, Laura

In this situation the message is delivered instantaneously, and the receiver cannot give the sender simultaneous responses.

Thus, while a simple communication model will serve for the email communication, a transactional model is more suitable for face-to-face contact and more situations where the subtleties of communication become apparent.

A transactional model of communication shows how we make ongoing adjustments to the content style and manner of our communication. Laura's face-to-face communication with Gina enables her to receive, decode and respond to Gina's verbal and nonverbal behaviour, while at the same time Gina is responding to the fact that Laura has registered that she (Gina) is feeling bad tempered about the off duty. Laura is modifying her tone and facial expression as a result (see Fig. 4.1).

Written communication

Written communications can compensate for the absence of nonverbal indicators by using levels of formality, layout, vocabulary, certain conventions of greeting and leave-taking and punctuation. Both formal and informal writing also make use of features such as emboldening, underlining, and italicising to add emphasis. Consider how the meaning is made clear by the use of these conventions in the second of these sentences.

1. pleasedonothaveanythingtoeatordrinkaftermidnighthe
   nightbeforetheinvestigationbringaurinesamplewith
   youandbeawarethatyoumayfeeldrowsyafterthe
   investigationandmaynotbeabletodriveacarimmediately
   afterwards.
2. Please do **not** have anything to eat or drink after **midnight** the night before the investigation.
   Please bring with you a sample of urine.
   BE AWARE that you may feel drowsy after the investigation and may not be able to drive a car immediately afterwards.

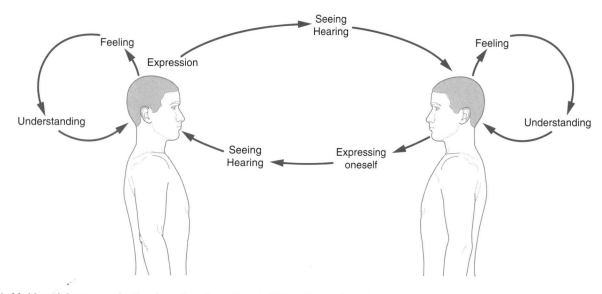

Fig. 4.1 Multimodal communication in action (from Moonie 2000, with permission).

Exercise

1. What do you think of the overall tone of these instructions?
2. Are they clear and unambiguous?
3. What questions might still be in the patient's mind?

Electronic communication

The more modern forms of written communication such as emailing and text messaging are already influencing and changing the formality and conventions of paper-written communication. However, the rules governing this form of communication are still in the making, although email packages will often give an e-etiquette guide in the Help menu.

Oral communication

The invention of the telephone created a new medium of communication that has developed a technique and style of its own to compensate for the lack of visual nonverbal information. On the telephone, we pay extra attention to the manner of speaking, the tone of voice, the pitch, and the breathing patterns to gain information about the person we are talking to. Telephone contact with patients and their relatives is a daily part of most nurses' lives, and experienced nurses will often perceive and respond to these nonverbal indicators. Blind people also become highly skilled in interpreting the more subtle qualities of voice, whilst someone who is deaf develops a keen eye for facial expression, gesture and lip movements.

Face-to-face communication

Face-to-face communication offers the richest scope for multimodal communication. However, the formal conventions governing board meetings or meetings between heads of state differs very much from those operating in the relationship that develops between nurses and patients. At its best this relationship balances human closeness and professional integrity and is the subject of many nursing theorists such as Hildegard Peplau, Patricia Benner and Pam Smith. Government legislation and regulation by the Nursing and Midwifery Council (2002a) ensure a level of formality and code of professional conduct that clearly indicate the professional role responsibilities (see Chapter 2). Thus, a professional relationship with a patient may be a close one, but clearly differs from the informal relationships with friends and family.

Universal and culture-specific communication

Verbal and nonverbal communication, oral and written communication involve several different parts of our nervous system that help us assimilate overall meaning. There are primitive, instinctive nonverbal behaviours such as crying, frowning, laughing or smiling in all human societies. In fact, some of these may also be seen in creatures fairly close to us in the evolutionary chain such as apes and chimpanzees. Nonverbal communication can also develop as an integral part of a specific culture within a social group. Some societies (e.g. Italians) use many gestures and facial expressions, while others (e.g. Japanese) use very few. Also and unfortunately, a nonverbal gesture may mean one thing in one society and something very different in another. For example, in France using a finger to pull down the eyelid means that the speaker is aware of something going on, whilst in Italy the same sign means that the listener must become aware. Cultural variations in facial expression, eye contact, gesture and body posture are among the first things a 'foreigner' notices, and it can be very difficult working out what they mean and even more difficult deciding whether one is permitted to use them.

Exercise

Consider the ways in which people communicate when they are angry, sad, confused or excited.

1. What kind of facial and body movements do they make in each situation?
2. Draw figures of facial expressions and body movements to represent these. Compare yours with fellow students/colleagues.

Exercise

Now consider the crying of babies.

1. Are there different kinds of crying?
2. How do mothers and others learn to interpret a baby's cry?
3. What aspects of communication do you think are innate and what is learned? Discuss your findings with colleagues and/or other students.

Transition from verbal to nonverbal communication

Although primitive man made simple sounds to convey simple messages, as human life became more complex, it outstripped the capabilities of this simple system and a pictorial writing developed. Later alphabetic systems developed which made economic use of symbols. Today there are over 100 major languages (each spoken by at least one million people), and thousands of other languages and dialects. Yet for political and economic reasons English has become the major world language. This is because of its dominance in its former empire outside England, in India, Africa and particularly because of the economic dominance of the English-speaking United States of America.

The activity of communicating across the lifespan

Childhood

Theoretical explanations of how babies learn to speak and communicate are mainly the province of psychology and linguistics, but the biological substrate is crucial. Before birth virtually all the neurones and some synapses are formed and in the first weeks of life babies use them to announce hunger or discomfort and to explore their own bodies. A little later babies explore two-way linguistic communication. This two-way language is acquired in stages.

The babbling stage occurs spontaneously and babies try out a variety of sounds, some of which are the sounds of human language. In the second stage single words appear, followed by a two-word communication, which can usually be understood by an adult. Longer 'telegraphic' sentences then emerge, which are refined in childhood, and depend on innate language ability and the richness of the child's communicative environment. Deaf children exposed to sign language show the same stages of language acquisition as do hearing children exposed to spoken language (Fromkin & Rodman 1983). Imitation theory argues that children learn their language by imitating an adult. Speech and reinforcement theory suggests that children are conditioned by positive, negative or corrective reactions to their attempts at speech. Neither on its own can fully explain this complex process.

Exercise

In the 13th century the German Emperor Frederick II, curious to know what language children would speak if they were raised without hearing any words at all, decided to conduct some empirical research. Seizing a number of newborn children from their parents, he handed them to nurses with strict instruction to feed them, but not to talk to them or to hold them. The babies never learnt a language. They all died before they could talk. Frederick's experiment whilst failing to find the answer to his desired question had nevertheless made an important discovery.

1. What do you think that important discovery was? Discuss with colleagues.

Adolescence

One of the marked features of many adolescents is a great need to communicate with their peers, and an increasing withdrawal from communicating with adults. During this phase of development, adults may see adolescents as increasingly 'uncommunicative', or sullen. Adolescents often need more privacy, yet need more social contact with their peers. They develop peer-bonding behaviour such as using their own 'crowd's' jargon, dress code and values. The use of slang, taboo words, and cursing reaches a peak in this period of development. Adolescents may take up extreme positions on certain issues and defend those positions with strong emotions, a combination with which it is difficult to reason. Adolescents also begin to learn decision-making through experience rather than someone telling them which way to do things to achieve the best outcome, their attention span grows and their intellectual curiosity strengthens.

Exercise

Greg is 17 and very bright in English, History and German, and he is expected to do well in his A levels. However, at the dermatology clinic, which he attends for treatment of his severe acne, he uses vague words, 'I've done what you said and stuff' and instead of answering the nurse's questions directly, he says 'Well you know what I mean like'.

1. What skills and techniques might elicit a more specific response? Discuss with colleagues.

Adulthood

In early adulthood people are more likely to interact with people of all different ages through their work, leisure and family activities. Communication skills develop from this as well as from formal training and from experience in applying for jobs and attending interviews. In addition, young adults meet for the first time the intricacies of completing commercial, social, governmental and legal documentation in relation to making claims, purchasing goods, taking out a mortgage and deciding on a pension scheme. It is estimated that 7 million adults who are native speakers have literacy problems, whilst another half a million adults need help with speaking and writing English as a second language (DfES 2001).

In early adulthood, the loss of the tremendous physical growth spurt is counterbalanced by the increased strength of maturity and experience and in many cases a liberating financial independence. Early adulthood is often a time when people will travel widely which may bring them into contact with a range of different cultures and values. In addition being able to use computers has become a basic requirement for employment in many jobs, and middle adulthood may be a time of mastering new skills. It is also in this period that pressures of caring for elderly relatives, supporting adolescents or child-minding grandchildren can reduce the time and opportunity to go to an evening class to learn a language or pursue hobbies that bring in social contact and interpersonal communication. Nevertheless, the communicative range of people in middle adulthood is probably at its peak, blending all the advantages of experience, education and work.

Later life

Growth and decline are such individual variables that it is unwise to make generalised or sweeping statements of the effects of ageing on communication ability. As a group however, elderly people are more vulnerable to stereotyping by others than any other age group. Carers may assume that older people have a far greater degree of hearing and comprehension impairment than they actually have. This can lead to inappropriate and mismanaged communication, with a corresponding decline in their psychological and physical wellbeing.

Social contacts often diminish as people get older, as relatives and friends become ill or die, or as other problems such as mobility limit an active social life. Even in residential care it can be difficult to form new relationships, although the social climate and the regular company of nurses and carers can considerably benefit an elderly person's quality of life.

Exercise

Margaret is 88 years old, lives alone and manages to get from the kitchen to the living room using two sticks. She has had a leg ulcer, which has now healed, and you are about to discharge her from community nurse visits. You feel that she might deteriorate emotionally and psychologically once the visits stop.

1. What kind of questions could you ask to help make a nursing assessment of her communication needs and abilities?
2. Consider how you would ensure that her communication needs are met following discharge from community nursing care services.

Factors influencing the AL of communicating

Biological factors

Despite differentiating cultural, psychological, social and political features, the basic biological equipment is similar in all humans. The nervous system provides the human organism with the ability to:

- survive
- express emotions
- exchange information
- develop and maintain interpersonal and social relationships
- enjoy and share creative and recreational activities.

Neurones

Along with all but the most primitive organisms, the basic communicative unit of the human nervous system is a nerve cell or neurone (see Fig. 4.2).

Some neurones are sensory (afferent) which transmit sensations such as heat, pain, pleasure, danger or discomfort. Other neurones are motor (efferent), which enable us to act, either consciously or unconsciously, in response to different sensations (see Fig. 4.3).

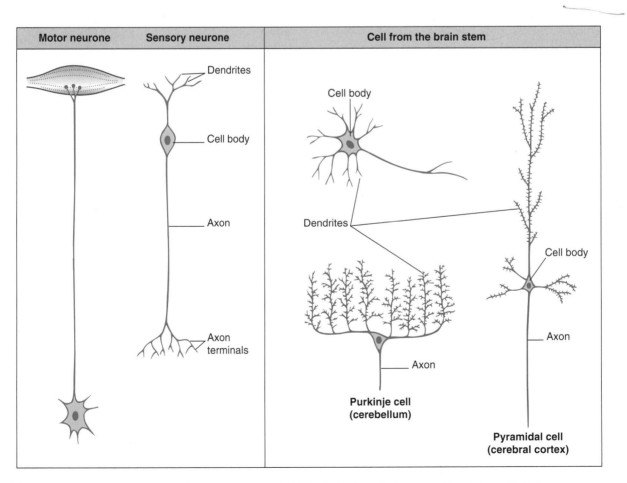

Fig. 4.2 Sensory and motor neurones – the basic unit of communication (from Rutishauser 1994, with permission).

The millions of neurones in the nervous system are organised into 'neuronal pools' and pathways and are connected by association or interneurones that help process information. These pools and pathways process and integrate incoming information from other pools or from simple sensory receptors in the skin, the eyes, the ears or the mouth (see Fig. 4.4).

Central nervous system

The central nervous system develops from the neural tube. It grows to form the spinal cord, lower brain, mid brain and higher brain. The most primitive reflexes emerge from the spinal cord and lower brain. The midbrain acts as a kind of relay station between the lower brain and the higher brain, and gives rise to emotions. The higher brain analyses symbolic information and gives rise to cognitive and intellectual abilities (see Figs 4.5, 4.6 and 4.7).

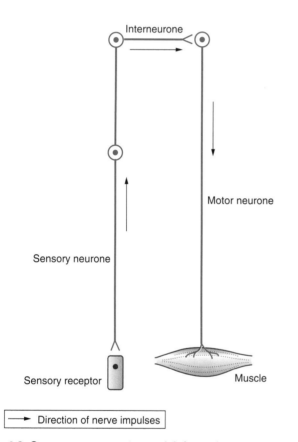

Fig. 4.3 Sensory neurones transmit information to motor neurones, which can then activate muscles (from Rutishauser 1994, with permission).

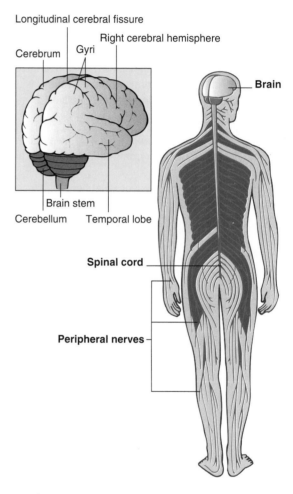

Fig. 4.5 Component parts of the nervous system (from Rutishauser 1994, with permission).

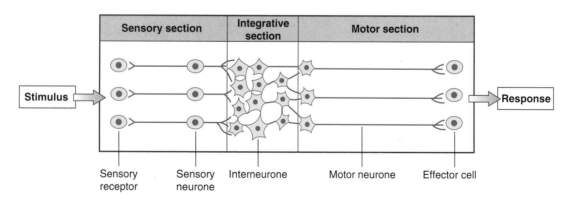

Fig. 4.4 Integrating information (from Rutishauser 1994, with permission).

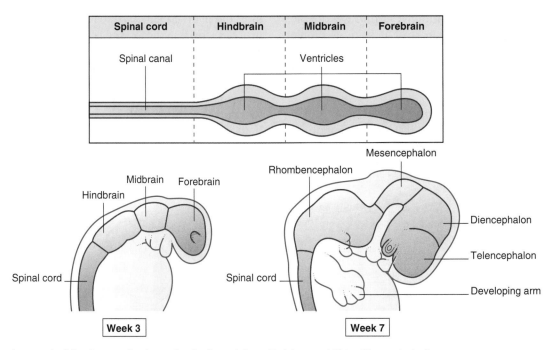

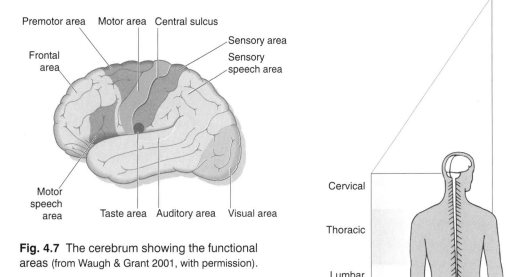

Fig. 4.6 Development of the human brain and spinal cord (from Rutishauser 1994, with permission).

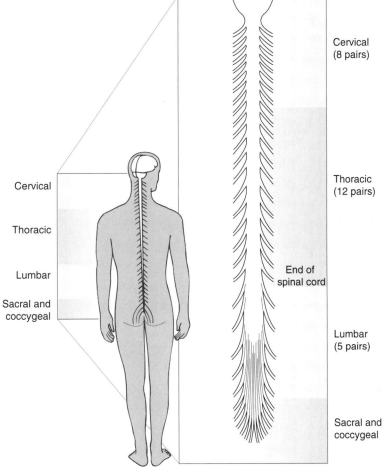

Premotor area   Motor area   Central sulcus

Frontal area

Sensory area

Sensory speech area

Motor speech area

Taste area   Auditory area   Visual area

Fig. 4.7 The cerebrum showing the functional areas (from Waugh & Grant 2001, with permission).

The peripheral nervous system

Communication between the brain, spinal cord, trunk and limbs of the body is achieved through the peripheral nervous system. It is made up of 12 pairs of cranial nerves and 32 pairs of spinal nerves (see Fig. 4.8). These nerves are sensory and motor and connect the limbs, trunk, head and neck with the central nervous system. They may operate as a reflex, such as the knee jerk elicited by a tendon hammer, or voluntarily for example when kicking a ball.

Cervical

Thoracic

Lumbar

Sacral and coccygeal

Cervical (8 pairs)

Thoracic (12 pairs)

End of spinal cord

Lumbar (5 pairs)

Sacral and coccygeal

Fig. 4.8 The spinal nerves (from Rutishauser 1994, with permission).

Thus the links may be very primitive at the level of reflex action (see Fig. 4.9) or may be part of a chain of complex responses that involve a whole range of neuronal pools and pathways as part of the 'decision tree'. This is best illustrated in Fig. 4.10.

The autonomic nervous system

The autonomic nervous system is part of the central nervous system and the peripheral nervous system, although it is often described separately. It regulates unconscious processes such as heart rate, smooth muscle contraction, blood pressure, respiration rate and glandular secretion, keeping these processes balanced. They do this by either increasing activity through stimulation of the structures by the sympathetic branch or by decreasing activity in the structures through inhibition by the parasympathetic branch. The main exception is that the parasympathetic branch actually stimulates digestive processes (see Fig. 4.11).

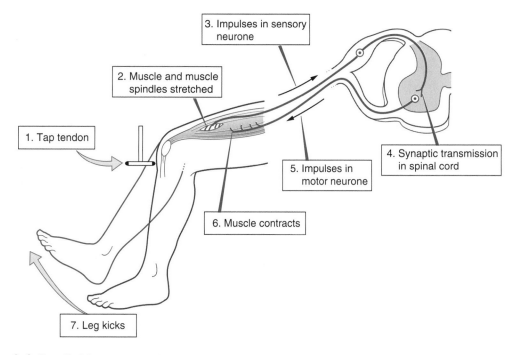

Fig. 4.9 The knee jerk (from Rutishauser 1994, with permission).

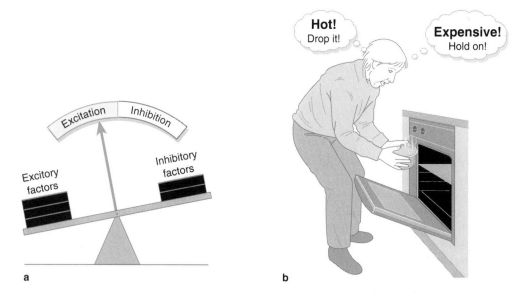

Fig. 4.10 How we respond to a stimulus depends on the balance between excitatory and inhibitory factors (from Rutishauser 1994, with permission).

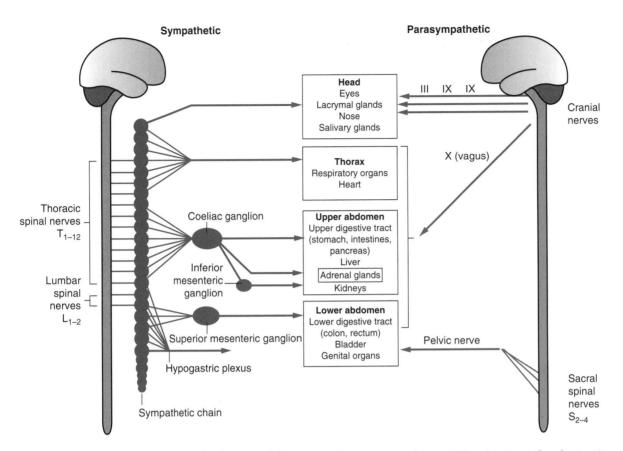

Fig. 4.11 The sympathetic and parasympathetic parts of the autonomic nervous system and the structures they innervate (from Rutishauser 1994, with permission).

Blushing is a good example of the autonomic system in action. When people are embarrassed they may find verbal ways of trying to alleviate the uncomfortable situation, but nothing can stop the sympathetic system from dilating the blood vessels in the face and neck, giving the tell-tale red hue.

Vision and the eye

The eyes allow us to learn more about the surrounding world than any of the other four senses and much of the brain is designed to interpret visual information. We see by processing the light that colours, shapes and objects give off, even in dim light (see Figs 4.12 and 4.13).

Exercise

Pain is the result of damage to or pressure on a part of the body and can be managed very effectively if the care team have a good understanding and a range of potential interventions to choose from.

1. On a scale of 1–10, with 10 being excellent, how good is your current understanding of pain theory, assessment, and management?
2. If you do not score yourself well, refer to the Further Reading list at the end of this chapter and compile an action plan to read and apply the principles and practices of pain management.
3. Undertake a literature search and review of the literature on pain assessment and management.

Exercise

Bill works for a local plastics firm and has done so for the last 4 years. He is checking some equipment when a pipe carrying corrosive material splits and the material sprays into his face and eyes.

1. Look up the structure and function of the eye and then explain briefly what a 'detached retina' is and how it might affect someone in the Activities of Living.
2. Write down ways in which nurses can help in communicating with him in view of his sudden loss of vision.

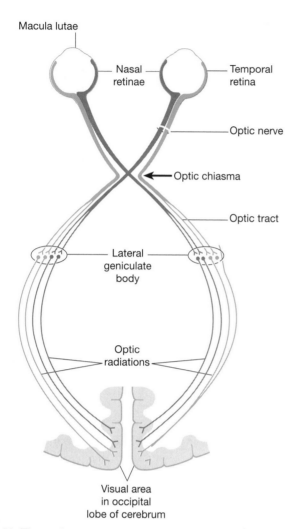

Macula lutae

Nasal retinae

Temporal retina

Optic nerve

Optic chiasma

Optic tract

Lateral geniculate body

Optic radiations

Visual area in occipital lobe of cerebrum

Fig. 4.12 The optic nerves and their pathways (from Waugh & Grant 2001, with permission).

An accident such as Bill's is particularly terrifying, although any loss of sight is very frightening. When nurses attend to people with an eye injury or problem they may need to overcome the fear many people have of having their eyes touched. Sudden loss of vision can make people lose confidence and feel vulnerable. They will also have lost visual aspects of nonverbal communication and need thoughtful and considerate help to compensate for this sensory loss. This can be done in simple ways:

- tell the person when you have entered the room or are about to leave
- say who you are
- don't raise your voice, but speak clearly
- approach and leave the patient from the side where vision is best
- put things at the side where the vision is best and in the same place each time
- at mealtimes use a clock face metaphor to describe where food is on the plate
- ask whether they would prefer to eat alone or with assistance.

Hearing and the ear

Although a huge part of the human brain is given over to analysing visual information, auditory information contributes to that analysis. Hearing is the sense used in decoding emotional messages conveyed through voice tone, modulation, pitch, and rhythm, which the brain then matches against visual information. Sound enters the system through the external ear (see Fig. 4.14) through to the brain where the sound is perceived, and either understood or not as the case may be. This whole process takes less than half a second. Consider the following case study.

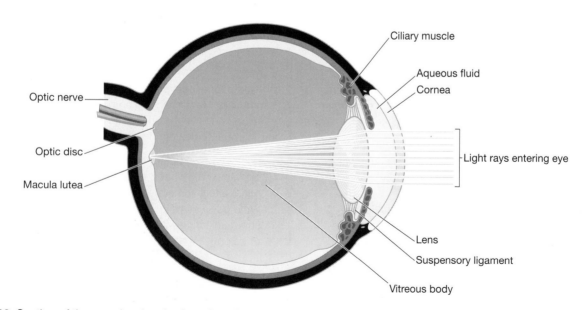

Ciliary muscle

Aqueous fluid

Cornea

Optic nerve

Optic disc

Macula lutea

Light rays entering eye

Lens

Suspensory ligament

Vitreous body

Fig. 4.13 Section of the eye showing the focusing of light rays on the retina (from Waugh & Grant 2001, with permission).

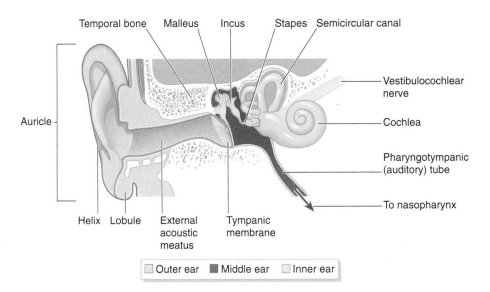

Fig. 4.14 Structures through which sound passes before entering the brain (from Waugh & Grant 2001, with permission).

Case study 4.1

Communicating with someone who uses British Sign Language

Hannah Jones is 16 years old and is considering embarking on her first sexual relationship with her boyfriend, Phillip. They have known each other for 2 years, are happy together, and are aiming to attend the same college after the summer break. Hannah, who is prelingually profoundly deaf, uses British Sign Language as her first and preferred language.

Hannah has been a patient at the same GP Practice since she was a child. Hannah has rarely needed to visit her GP, and her mother was always on hand to interpret for the GP and Hannah. Hannah now wants to discuss contraception with the Practice Nurse. Hannah has asked her mother not to be informed of the appointment and therefore mum is not available to assist in interpreting at the appointment. The Practice Nurse recognises there is a lot of information to convey to Hannah, and it is imperative that Hannah understands this information.

1. What rights does Hannah have in the situation that could assist her?
2. What ethical issues might arise when a mother interprets for her daughter in a situation like this?
3. What should the Practice Nurse do first?
4. Consider the barriers to effective communication in this case study. Discuss with colleagues and identify your learning needs in communicating with people who have hearing difficulties.

In this scenario the nurse has a responsibility to ensure that the communication environment takes into account Hannah's needs. Her first task would be to find a British Sign Language interpreter for the appointment. The interpreter's role is to enable the nurse and Hannah to converse. The interpreter has a responsibility to ensure that the communication meets the needs of everyone present. They also facilitate understanding across English-speaking and -signing cultures.

Using an interpreter is a process that some nurses find initially difficult because of the third party involvement. However, some fundamental guidelines can quickly assist the situation.

1. Make sure you can see everyone involved in the discussion.
2. Speak directly to the deaf person not to the interpreter.
3. Speak at your normal speed and in full sentences, do not raise your voice.
4. The interpreter will be signing what you are saying, just after you have said it, so there will be a time delay in the responses from the deaf person.
5. It is good practice to prepare the interpreter in advance of the session, inform them of what they will be interpreting, where it will be, and start and finish times.
6. Be gender aware, in health situations it is good practice to ensure gender-appropriate interpreters are used though the deaf person may have their own preference.

Using a family member for interpreting is not good practice; it places too much responsibility on the relative and may affect the quality of care given to the patient. In addition, the family member filtering the information or not having the requisite signing skills to provide sufficient information to the nurse, doctor or patient could seriously undermine the deaf person's access to their health information. Refer to the Further Reading for more sources on understanding the rights of deaf people, British Sign Language, the role of interpreters and the British deaf community (Sharples 2002).

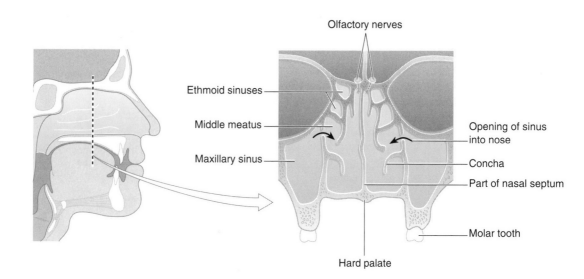

Fig. 4.15 Structures involved with sense of smell (olfactory receptors) (from Rutishauser 1994, with permission).

Smelling and the nose

Whilst seeing and hearing are highly prized sensory experiences, olfaction (smelling) also exerts a very powerful influence on communication activities at a very fundamental and primitive level (see Fig. 4.15). The sense of smell adds a richness to life that we aren't always conscious of, and as well as giving great pleasure, it can warn of danger, such as burning or leaking gas, or even in checking out food stuffs. Smells are processed very close to the 'emotional brain' (the limbic system) and can have strong emotional associations.

> **Exercise**
> 1. Think back over your life and jot down any smells that you can remember from your past.
> 2. With what do you associate these smells?
> 3. Are the smells pleasant or unpleasant?
> 4. Do you have a favourite perfume/aftershave?
> 5. Why is it a favourite and how does it make you feel?

The sense of touch

When changes occur in the external and internal environments sensory receptors are stimulated. These enable the experience of touch, temperature, pain and pressure from receptors in the skin (see Fig. 4.16).

All these sensations are processed by the brain through the limbic structures, which label them as pleasant, unpleasant, soothing or arousing. The sensation experienced then activates the sympathetic system if the experience is arousing or the parasympathetic system if the experience is calming. General senses are distributed throughout the body and include tactile ones of touch, pressure, vibration, tickle, itch, and thermal ones of hot and cold, and acute and chronic

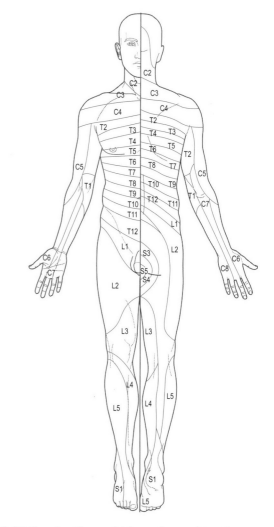

Fig. 4.16 Sensing the world through our skin – the dermatome area (from Rutishauser 1994, with permission).

pain receptors. Deeper sensory receptors enable the monitoring of the position of muscles, bones and joints (the sense of proprioception) (see Fig. 4.17). The other senses, sight, hearing, smell and taste have specialised receptors unique to that organ.

Speaking and the larynx

The quality of a person's voice communicates a great deal to listeners. A voice is often as unmistakable a signature as a face or laughter. Whether we intend to let people know what we are feeling or not, our voices often give us away. The larynx, or voice box, is an organ in the neck that plays a crucial role in speech and breathing (see Figs 4.18 and 4.19) and is the point at which the respiratory and digestive tract splits into two separate pathways. It is very sensitive to touch and foreign bodies such as crumbs, produce a protective cough, a response which can be damaged by brain injury or stroke.

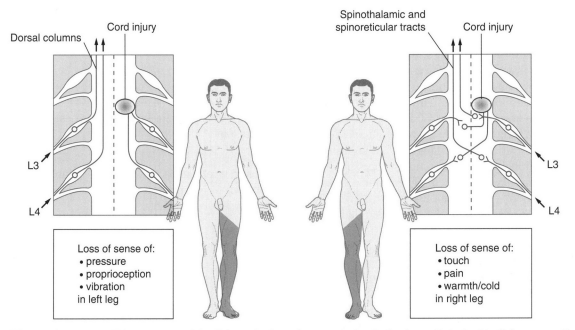

Fig. 4.17 Effects of an area of injury on one side of the spinal cord on sensation in the legs. Note that both legs are affected but in different ways (from Rutishauser 1994, with permission).

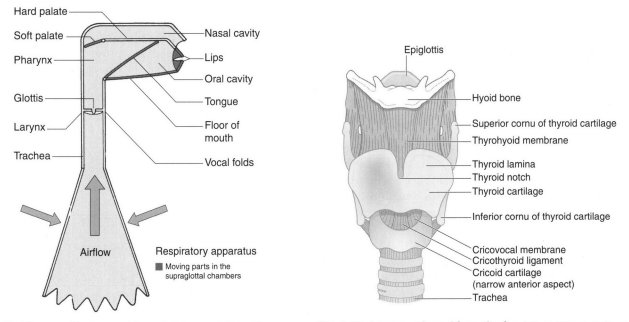

Fig. 4.18 The vocal instrument (from Rutishauser 1994, with permission).

Fig. 4.19 Larynx – viewed from the front (from Waugh & Grant 2001, with permission).

Exercise

Consider the structure and function of the larynx.

1. In what ways do you think the larynx might be affected in a person with a tracheostomy?

Psychological factors

Psychological factors in communication include both cognitive and emotional components. The cognitive rational mind works through words and the emotional mind generally works nonverbally. One rule of thumb used in communications is that probably as much as 90% of an emotional message is communicated through tone of voice, facial expression, gestures and subtle differences in body posture and movement. People receive and respond to these messages almost unconsciously. Good nurses are particularly skilled in noticing nonverbal signs of anxiety for example, and may give more weight to these if a person denies feeling anxious. Even if a patient's first language is English, the high level of emotional arousal can render processing information at a cognitive level inefficient. This happens because high arousal interferes with communication between the analytical and emotional parts of the brain. People in these situations may appear 'stupid' or irrational.

Most people have experienced this phenomenon when for example sitting an exam, going for a job interview or taking a driving test. Until the last decade, intelligence has been measured solely by cognitive outputs. Emotional intelligence as defined by Goleman (1996, p. 317) refers to 'the capacity for recognising our own feelings and those of others, for motivating ourselves and for managing emotions well in us and in our relationships'. He identifies five basic emotional and social competencies and argues that people with emotional intelligence demonstrate particular qualities to a high degree (see Box 4.1).

The more traditional meaning of intelligence, which used to be measured by IQ tests, is closely related to deductive reasoning based on symbolic knowledge such as numbers for numerical reasoning, words for verbal reasoning, and formal shapes and representational pictures for perceptual reasoning. These tests are also used to assess cognitive and perceptual states following a brain injury of some kind. There are dangers in relying solely on test batteries as indicators of cognitive intelligence. It is more common now to appraise how a person's mind processes information and handles data in a variety of real-life situations, looking for problem-solving abilities of different kinds. This type of intelligence is built up through experience as well as through formal education and a bright mind 'discovers' new associations and comes up with original ideas and hypotheses. Intelligence in this sense also implies a rich and complex network of neuronal pools and circuits, with new synapses being developed all the time rather than staying

Box 4.1 Five basic emotional and social competencies (adapted from Goleman 1996)

Self-awareness
Knowing what we are feeling in the moment, and using those preferences to guide our decision making having a realistic assessment of our own abilities and a well-grounded sense of self-confidence.

Self-regulation
Handling our emotions so that they facilitate rather than interfere with the task at hand; being conscientious and delaying gratification to pursue goals; recovering well from emotional distress.

Motivation
Using our deepest preferences to move and guide us toward our goals, to help us take the initiative and strive to improve, and to persevere in the face of setbacks and frustrations.

Empathy
Sensing what people are feeling, being able to take their perspective, and cultivating rapport and attunement with a broad diversity of people.

Social skill
Handling emotions in relationships well and accurately reading social situations and networks interacting smoothly; using these skills to persuade and lead, negotiate and settle disputes, for cooperation and teamwork.

static. There is, however, a strange exception to the idea of overall intelligence in a group of people rather insultingly called *idiots savants*. Defined as people with severe learning disabilities with a very low score in IQ tests, *idiots savants* have truly remarkable specific abilities such as in mental arithmetic, or in the ability to reproduce with startling accuracy ornate buildings seen only once, or a piece of music heard only once! Therefore, a single definition of 'intelligence' remains elusive and different kinds of intelligence need to be appreciated.

Exercise

1. Using the qualities adapted from Goleman in Box 4.1 and a scale of 1–10 (where 10 indicates very high), think of two very different people you know and score them on these qualities.
2. What sort of 'evidence' did you use to give them a score?
3. How can we incorporate these ideas in our nursing assessment of the communication needs of patients?

Sociocultural factors

Crystal (1992) states that:

> *There is considerable overlap between the psychological, social and cultural aspects of our existence. People indicate psychological identity such as personality, intelligence, emotional state, and attitude through communication and interpersonal relations. Geographical identity comes from language, accent, and dialect and national, ethnic and cultural identity through language, dress, customs, beliefs, and values. The dramatic increase in immigrant numbers in the 1960s has resulted in over 100 languages being used in Britain by ethnic minority communities. The most widely spoken immigrant languages appear to be Punjabi, Bengali, Urdu, Gujarati, German, Polish, Italian, Greek, Spanish, and Cantonese.* (Crystal 1992, p. 37)

In addition, social identity is indicated in terms of social stratification and social class, social role, and even gender through speech and language. From a growing body of sociolinguistic research, it is clear that we all make subtle, intricate and pervasive judgements about people based upon the way they speak.

The 'languages' of health care clearly differentiate between different professions involved in health care. Nurses, doctors, occupational therapists, physiotherapists, speech and language therapists and other specialists develop their own professional language or 'jargon', often incomprehensible to others outside the profession. Medical terms, for example, are not so much professional jargon as ancient Greek or Roman. Most anatomical terms are taken directly from Latin and Greek and when translated into English are not at all mysterious.

Exercise

Here is the English translation of several ancient Greek words: hyper = too much, poly = many, haem = blood, cyte = cell, lipos = fat, an = not, without, lacking, ology = study.

1. What do these medical terms mean: hyperlipidaemia, polycythaemia, cytology and haematology?
2. Find other words used in nursing and health care which are derived from Greek or Latin.
3. Listen to nurses talking to one another about patients in their care – as a nurse how easy was it for you to understand what they were talking about, and why?

Nurses need to be able to use their understanding of medical terminology to liaise with the medical team and to be able to communicate with patients in a language that patients understand. If nurses are not able to do this, the principles of informed consent and ethical practice are breached and patients cannot be truly involved in care planning.

Sociocultural differences also operate nonverbally in the form of gesture, eye contact, facial expression, body posture, proximity and dress. There are other nonverbal differences in greeting, in leave taking, and in expressions of emotions such as love, liking, disliking and disgust. Culture, socialisation and the brain equip individuals with a perceptual filter, which can lead to different interpretations of the same event. For example, in Taiwan, blinking while another person is talking is regarded as impolite, but to North Americans it is hardly noticeable (Adler & Rodman 1991). In addition, a beckoning finger in most Middle and Far Eastern countries is an insulting gesture, but not in the Western world. Eye contact also differs in traditional Afro-Caribbean and Caucasian cultures. Caucasians tend to look away from a conversational partner when speaking and at the other person when listening. Black culture does the reverse, and misinterpretation may well occur (Adler & Rodman 1991).

Exercise

1. Ask a colleague or friend from another culture or subculture what differences they find between communicating with a member of their own culture and a member of your culture.
2. How different is the nonverbal communication?

Environmental factors

Other environmental factors can influence communication. These include the auditory, visual and spatial features of the external physical environment as well as mental states of attention, concentration and distractibility. Health care settings have design difficulties in creating an environment that is public and private, sociable and peaceful and stimulating yet relaxed. The individual needs of patients with communication problems, and the different preferences people have in entertaining themselves have the potential to generate quite high noise pollution levels. Technology now makes the use of earphones, and networked radio and TV a welcome development in many hospitals. Different types of beds and equipment can also help. People can position themselves for conversation using four section-profiling beds or electronically operated beds. In the home people can operate doors, switch on a television, radio or lights using POSSUM (an electronic, environmental control system). The system also enables people with paralysis, or much reduced mobility to communicate with others via an intercom system. An adaptation of the security system in shops can help keep people with orientation problems more safe. An armband, which the patient has agreed to wear, activates an alarm to alert staff and the patient that he or she has left the building. Consider the following brief case study.

Ethical issues in electronically 'tagging' a person

Sam is a 23-year-old man in a neurohabilitation ward, who is recovering from an assault 8 weeks ago when he sustained a brain injury. He is making a good recovery, can mobilise very well, and is making good progress. He is unaware of danger and has lost his sense of direction. The nurses are concerned for his safety because several times he has wandered outside to smoke a cigarette and then got lost.

1. What ethical and practical issues might be discussed with him about the possibility of using a 'tagging' system?

Box 4.2 Communication behaviours

Confirming	Disconfirming
Sincere praise	Insults (even in fun)
Compliments	Humiliates
Acknowledging others, waving, smiling	Failing to return phone-call, letter, greeting
Listening attentively	Interrupting, irrelevant, or
Smiles	ambiguous responses
Laughter	Frowns and scowls
Humour	

Adapted from Adler & Rodman 1991.

High-tech environments, such as Intensive Care Units, or Accident and Emergency Units can also make difficult and awkward communication environments. They often have very little daylight, windows are high, there is little to connect patients with the outside world and high-tech equipment creates a disturbing background of hums, bleeps and sighs. This physical environment further compromises ease of conversation and the communication climate for example:

> *The term communication climate refers to the emotional tone of a relationship as it is expressed in the messages that the partners send and receive. Just as physical locations have characteristic weather patterns, interpersonal relationships have unique climates too.*
>
> *A climate does not involve specific activities as much as the way people feel about each other as they carry out those activities.* (Adler & Rodman 1991, p. 157)

Positive climates are characterised by value-affirming behaviour by the people in that environment such as praising and complimenting, showing appreciation, acknowledging by a wave or a smile, or listening attentively.

Exercise

1. Think back on some of your clinical experiences in different settings.
2. Would you say the communication climate was positive or negative?
3. What communication behaviours do you think contributed to this? Use Box 4.2 to help you identify the behaviours.

Politicoeconomic factors

Political and economic factors influence health care and the quality of health care. These include government health policy such as the NHS Plan 2000, pay and spending decisions, health care reforms and auditing frameworks such as the Commission for Health Improvement. The UK Department of Health website (http://www.doh.gov.uk) gives comprehensive information on all of these aspects.

However, health care is also influenced by nonspecific legislation relating to human rights. For examples see Box 4.3.

The Nursing and Midwifery Council (2002b) also produce guidelines for records and record keeping, based on the principle that good record keeping is a mark of the skilled and safe practitioner, and that there are important features of content and style as well as legal aspects.

Confidentiality This is a legal requirement embedded in the above acts. The Nursing and Midwifery Council in the Code of Professional Conduct (2002a) give clear guidelines on the nature of confidentiality and how nurses can protect confidential information.

Consent to treatment There is some discussion on this aspect of care in the second part of this chapter, particularly focusing on the capacity to consent. There are also some further reading suggestions at the end of this chapter and the website address of the Department of Health which gives government guidelines on informed consent.

Other politicoeconomic influences are revealed through literacy levels in the community. Under *Skills for Life*, the current government's strategy for improving adult literacy, the following issue is addressed:

> *Seven million people have poor literacy and numeracy skills, including half a million or more who struggle with English because it is not their first language. This has had disastrous consequences for the individuals concerned, weakens the country's ability to compete in the global economy, and places an enormous burden on society. People with poor literacy, numeracy and language skills tend to be on lower incomes or unemployed, and they are more prone to ill health and social exclusion.* (DfES 2001)

Exercise

1. Why do you think people with literacy problems are more prone to ill health?
2. Find out how health education and health promotion material is made user friendly for people of all ages who have literacy problems.

Box 4.3 Legislation relating to human rights

1976 Race Relations Act (amended 2000) which makes it unlawful to discriminate on racial grounds. The Act defines racial grounds as being colour, race, nationality, or ethnic or national origins. The act also makes victimisation and harassment illegal. This would include verbal or physical bullying, jokes, or excluding people because of race or sex.

1998 Human Rights Act which makes it unlawful for public bodies to act in a way that is incompatible with the Articles of the European Convention of Human Rights.

Article 2	Protection of life
Article 3	Freedom from inhuman treatment
Article 4	Freedom from servitude, slavery, or forced compulsory labour
Article 5	Right to liberty and security of person
Article 6	Right to a fair and public hearing
Article 7	Freedom from retrospective effects of penal legislation
Article 8	Right to respect for privacy
Article 9	Freedom of thought, conscience, and religion
Article 10	Freedom of expression
Article 11	Freedom of association and assembly
Article 12	Right to marry and found a family

Article 13	Right to an effective remedy before a national authority
Article 14	Prohibition of discrimination on the grounds of sex, race, colour, language, religion, political or other opinion, national or social origin, association with a national minority, property, birth or other status.

1998 Data Protection Act This Act declares that all records about clients which are filed will be seen as data, whether electronic or paper. Individuals are given rights, which include:

- The right to know what information is held about them and to see and correct the information if necessary.
- The right to refuse to provide information.
- The right that data should be accurate and up-to-date.
- The right that information should not be kept longer than is necessary.
- The right to confidentiality – that the information should not be accessible to unauthorised people.

The Department of Health (2002) has also produced guidelines for access to health records requests.

THE MODEL FOR NURSING

Using the model to individualize nursing for the Activity of Living: communicating

This section uses case studies that illustrate a range of communication problems that may arise in clinical practice. The discussion links the components of the model of living (lifespan, dependence/independence and factors affecting communication) with the nursing process.

Assessment and collection of data when taking a nursing history

Taking into account the issues discussed, assessment needs to include the person's physical, psychological and socio-cultural background, as well as the impact of environmental and politicoeconomic factors at work in the clinical setting, which affect communication. Nurses need to consider the relative advantages and disadvantages of the structured and unstructured means of gathering information and to differentiate between objectivity, subjectivity and interactivity in communication.

Assessment of AL of communicating

The following guideline questions can help structure assessment.

Lifespan

- Are there any potentially relevant factors in relation to the person's age, development, or life experiences that may affect communication style?

Independence/dependence

- Does the person normally need any kind of help to communicate and interact with others in either one-to-one or group situations?
- Does the person have a preferred means of communication?
- What means does the care setting have to meet this person's normal communication needs?
- What sort of family/friend support network does the person normally have?
- How might the current health breakdown affect the person's normal communication style and abilities?

Factors affecting the AL of communicating

- *Biological:* What is the specific health problem and does it present an actual or potential problem?
- *Psychological:* What does the person currently understand about their health problem? How has this affected confidence, self-image, mood, relationships and emotional wellbeing? Does or will the person need help from specialists or other members of the health care team to meet their information, learning or counselling needs?

- *Sociocultural:* what is the person's normal communication style and are there any specific social or cultural factors to be taken into account?
- *Environmental:* How does the care setting affect the person's ability to communicate effectively and meet the needs for company and privacy.
- *Politicoeconomic:* Is the current health problem likely to have a detrimental effect on income and occupation in either the long or the short term? What legal and ethical issues need to be considered?

Consider these guidelines in the assessment of the patients in the following case studies. The first case study explores communication concerning an unconscious patient; the second is complex and concerns a patient who has aphasia following a stroke and whose first language is not English. The third study discusses a patient who has a chronic and progressive health problem affecting all areas of physical, psychological and social life. As you read the case studies, reflect on patients you have nursed with similar problems and relate the discussion of some of the more general points to that patient. This will help to consolidate your knowledge base and develop your clinical reasoning in practice.

Reflect on the data collection tools you use such as structured and unstructured interview, structured observational assessment and include the less formal, conversational aspects of data collection. Finally, think about how you could use each of the tools to develop a care plan for the activity of communicating.

Case study 4.3

Paul

Paul is an 18-year-old young man who has just started at university. It is Freshers' Week and when his friends found him lying on the ground and 'very groggy' outside the Student Union bar they called an ambulance. He is semiconscious when the ambulance brings him to the Accident and Emergency Department. His friends arrive shortly after the ambulance.

Assessment of AL using guideline questions
Lifespan

Paul is in his late teens and in the first few weeks of a major life change in leaving home and attending university. However we cannot draw any conclusions from this or make any inferences, since this may lead to stereotyping. There may be relevant factors unknown to us. For example, he may have a health problem, which has made him very familiar with a hospital setting, or he may never have set foot inside a hospital since childhood. He may have relatives or friends involved in health care which make him more familiar with the environment or service.

Dependence/independence

We do not know whether Paul's first language is English, or whether he has a hearing problem, a speech impediment or a sight problem. We do not know whether he is usually quiet and withdrawn or outgoing and gregarious. Neither do we know anything of his family whereabouts or his social network. The only means people in the care setting have to communicate with Paul on his immediate arrival is to talk to him, hoping he can hear and understand, to move and handle him carefully so that he is not afraid and to try to elicit a response using a neurological assessment.

Biological factors

Unconsciousness may develop from neurological, metabolic or vascular causes. Brain injury may result from trauma or from spontaneous causes such as a cerebral bleed or infarction and lead to unconsciousness. Unconsciousness may also result from infections such as meningitis, the toxic effects of drugs and alcohol or from other metabolic causes such as hypoglycaemia, renal failure or liver failure. Whatever the reason, assessment of the conscious level is very important.

Neurological assessment

There are both structured tools and qualitative methods to help achieve a reasonable neurological assessment. This assessment can yield significant physical data about how the person's nervous system is functioning and what the level of consciousness is. From a nursing perspective it can:

- identify communication problems resulting from neurological damage
- detect life-threatening situations
- establish an initial database from which to develop a care plan, goal and nursing interventions
- compare data to previous assessments to determine change and trends, and to evaluate the effectiveness of the nursing interventions.

The Glasgow Coma Scale The initial tool to use in the emergency (after the Airway, Breathing and Circulatory protocol is carried out) in an unconscious patient is the Glasgow Coma Scale (GCS). This is a tool devised by two Glasgow neurosurgeons Jennet and Teasedale in 1974 (see Chapters 3 and 13). It is used all over the world and was welcomed because it is a reliable and valid objective measure of the level of consciousness, if carried out by those who are trained in its use. It allows nurses and medical staff to know over time whether the conscious level is lightening or worsening and whether further, possibly life-saving treatment needs to be initiated. The time factor is crucial and the GCS observations may need to be done several times in an hour if the situation is serious.

Using the Glasgow Coma Scale This scale is divided into three subscales, eye opening, best motor response and best verbal response (see Chapters 3 and 13). For simple and easy-to-follow guidelines on how to carry this out read Fuller (2000).

Other neurological assessment A full neurological assessment supplements the coma score. Careful neurological assessment indicates his cognitive function, his cranial nerve function, his motor function and sensation. The role of nurses is usually to focus on pupil size, which reveals if there is damage to the nerve that controls pupil reaction. Nursing assessment of limb power can also help assess damage to motor nerves. Nurses record these findings, and an overall trend can emerge as all these things are taken into account.

- Assessing the pupils of the eyes. The findings of one pupil are always compared to the findings in the other pupil and the differences, if any, between the two are noted.

For an assessment you need a pen torch but before beginning follow these instructions.

- Watch the person and see if they open their eyes spontaneously.
- Introduce yourself and ask the person to open his or her eyes, explaining that you need to assess their pupils using a light.
- If the eyelids do not open to speech, explain that you are going to raise the eyelids and shine a light into his eyes to assess the pupils and that this will not hurt.
- Raise the eyelids with the one hand holding the torch in the other.
- Look at the pupils.
- Are they equal in size?
- Are they regular in outline?
- Are their any holes in the iris or foreign bodies?
- Shine the light in one eye.
- Look at the reaction of that eye (this is called the direct reflex) and then repeat and look at the reaction in the other eye (this is called the consensual reflex).
- The person should be looking into the distance rather than at the light if possible.
- Repeat for the other eye.

Recording the findings This depends somewhat on the type of recording sheets used, but most will ask you to indicate the size of the pupil and the type of reaction of each pupil. Normally the pupils are equal in size (about 2–6 mm) and two methods are used to record pupil size: the millimetre scale, which is the most common, and verbal descriptors. These descriptors are:

- pinpoint
- small
- mid-sized
- large or dilated.

To record the information using the millimetre scale you need a diagrammatic gauge, usually illustrated on the recording sheet, which shows black circles ranging from 2 mm to 9 mm. Assessing and interpreting pupil size may take some experience before you feel confident. However, reliability always needs to be discussed as any changes can be very significant and must be the result of the change in the person rather than a change of observer. Most recording sheets will also ask you to record the rate of reaction to light in either words or symbols (see Glasgow Coma Scale, p. 77).

Assessing motor responses The next step in a neurological assessment is in evaluating motor function. Evans' (1995) explanation offers a good outline of what to look for (see Box 4.4).

Other data collection tools
Psychological/sociocultural factors
Other sources of information help identify actual, potential, temporary or long-standing problems with communication. Relatives and friends can give such information, and can tell the care team about people, places, activities and interests close to Paul's heart. These personal details can be used to stimulate a response at an emotional level, as these familiar things will have a more arousing effect. Nurses need to note and pass on to others anything which appears to elicit a response, even if this is as little as an eyebrow flare or eyelid flickering.

Environmental factors
Emergency admissions departments are often busy and noisy and people with brain injury often have impaired concentration. When carrying out observations there should be minimal distractions in the immediate environment. This may mean simply excluding visual distractions by drawing the curtains round the bed or trolley, and ensuring that people are not talking around the bed.

Politicoeconomic factors
In this case, where Paul is unconscious, application of the principle of informed consent needs to be discussed. English law and codes of professional conduct require a nurse to obtain consent from the patient before treatment is given. If consent is not obtained, either verbally or in writing, civil or criminal proceedings could be instituted. In advanced and specialist practice, where the scope is extended, nurses can be involved in invasive procedures and take on extra accountability as a result. In addition, although a doctor may have obtained a patient's consent, communication studies have shown (Dickson et al 1997) a patient may be confused or uncertain about their treatment choice and turn to the nurse for advice and clarification. This is linked with advocacy, where nurses act in the best interests of their clients (NMC 2002a) and explain, in words patients and families can understand, the issues involved. Advocacy is concerned with promoting and safeguarding the wellbeing and interests of patients and clients. The advocacy function is still being developed and discussed and its boundaries are uncertain.

However, in Paul's case it is an emergency. Emergency treatment in the best interests of the patient is lawful without

Box 4.4 Assessing limb power

Motor function

For a motor response to occur, nerve pathways from the brain to end organs and muscles must be intact. The upper motor neurones originate in the cerebral cortex and end at various levels in the spinal cord, where they synapse directly or via spinal neurones with lower motor neurones. Upper motor neurones are responsible for initiating voluntary movement. Lower motor neurones originate at various levels in the spinal cord and terminate on the muscle. They transmit upper motor neurone impulses or can be part of a motor reflex. Evaluate motor nerve function by assessing muscle movement and strength.

Start by having the patient simultaneously squeeze both of your hands with his hands. Evaluate the strength of the grip in both hands; document his grip as equal or unequal, strong or weak. Evaluate subtle extremity weakness and problems with proprioception by checking for arm drift. Have the patient stand with his hands extended outward (perpendicular with the body with palms up) and with his eyes closed. An affected arm slowly drifts down. In the comatose patient strength and grip cannot be tested voluntarily.

Ask the patient to move all his extremities. Record the presence or absence of movement or any unilateral or bilateral weakness. Determine whether movement is spontaneous or in response to command. Is spontaneous movement against gravity? Can the patient move an extremity against mild, moderate or forceful resistance? An entry might read 'Patient moves all Es in response to command, against gravity and against moderate resistance'.

Testing the patient's motor reflexes reveals the condition of sensory and motor pathways to and from muscle tendons and muscles to the spinal cord and brain. When the clinician taps on a muscle tendon (such as the one beneath the patella) with a reflex hammer, he is observing for an immediate, controlled jerk of the extremity in response to his action. A normal knee-jerk reflex indicates that the neural pathways to and from the spinal cord to the muscle and tendon are intact.

From: Evans (1995) Neurologic neurosurgical nursing, 2nd edn, p. 10. Springhouse Publications.

---

consent if the patient is unconscious or otherwise mentally incapable of valid consent. Emergency treatment may be taken to include all nursing care necessary to prevent significant deterioration.

Case study 4.4

Muhammed

Muhammed is a 72-year-old Asian man who has been admitted with a right-sided hemiplegia and aphasia. A CT scan shows that he has suffered a stroke and when his medical records arrive on the ward it becomes clear that he is also diabetic, and that this has unfortunately not been well controlled. He has lived in England since his early forties, working firstly in the local mill until it closed down 18 years ago, and then as a taxi driver. He speaks good English normally but his written skills in English are poor. His wife speaks very little English but his sons and two daughters are native English speakers. They also speak Urdu, which is Muhammed's first language.

Lifespan

Muhammed has learned to live his adult life using two languages and has been able to use English in his working and social life and Urdu with family and friends.

Dependence/independence

His spoken English is good in normal situations, but people who are suffering from illness or distress are more comfortable expressing themselves in their mother tongue (Robinson 1998).

His written English is less strong and his reading ability uncertain. We know so far that his sons and daughters can also speak both languages, but we do not yet know if the care setting has interpreters available.

Biological factors

A 'stroke' is a cerebrovascular accident (CVA). The injury to the brain can be caused by a ruptured blood vessel, which is called a haemorrhagic stroke, or by gradual or sudden ischaemic damage caused by a clot or embolus lodging in a blood vessel. In either case some areas of the brain are deprived of oxygen and may make only a partial recovery. The neurological deficit will depend on individuals and which area of the brain has been affected. There may be common deficits in people who have suffered either a right-sided or a left-sided stroke and these are summarised in Box 4.5 but each person is unique and will have a unique combination of care needs.

The World Health Organisation (2002) uses an international classification system of impairments, activities (disabilities) and handicap (participation). These are:

- **Impairment** Any loss or abnormality of psychological, physiological or anatomical structure or function.
- **Disability (activities)** Any restriction or lack of ability to perform an activity as a result of an impairment in a manner or within a range which is considered normal for a human being.

Box 4.5 Functional differences in right-sided and left-sided hemiplegia

Stroke syndrome on left side of brain (right-sided hemiplegia)	Stroke syndrome on right side of brain (left-sided hemiplegia)
Expressive aphasia or	Spatial–perceptual deficits
Receptive aphasia or	Denial and the deficits of the affected side require special safety considerations
Global aphasia	Tendency for distractability
Intellectual impairment	Impulsive behaviour; apparently unaware of deficits
Slow and cautious behaviour	Poor judgement
Defects in right visual fields	Deficits in left visual fields

From Hickey JV 1997 Neurological and neurosurgical nursing, 4th edn, p. 552.

- **Handicap (participation)** A disadvantage for a given individual resulting from an impairment or a disability that limits or prevents the fulfillment of a role which is normal for that individual.

The social model of disability, which goes far beyond the physical impairment is discussed under environmental aspects.

Assessing Muhammed's communication abilities

Goodwin (1995) points out that a language disorder strikes at a fundamental 'taken for granted' ability to communicate. In Muhammed's situation, there are three components of communication to consider:

1. the kind of aphasia he has
2. other perceptual and motor problems which may affect his ability to communicate. He may, for example, have visual problems because of either his stroke or his diabetes and his right-sided weakness may further impair his ability to use written or visual communication aids
3. his normal sociocultural and family life.

Aphasia is the overall term used for a language disorder. Dysphasia is a classification of a type of language disorder, which may be described as receptive dysphasia or expressive dysphasia. Receptively the problem may be auditory (unable to process verbal information) or visual (unable to interpret written information) or both of these. Expressively the problem may be seen as difficulty in expressing thoughts in speech or writing. The different categories are summarised in Table 4.1 but it is important to remember that this rough guide is in no way a substitute for thorough, interdisciplinary, individualised assessment.

Aphasia (or dysphasia) may be accompanied by a perceptual problem called agnosia that makes it difficult to

Table 4.1 Difficulties experienced in different aphasias

Disorder	Clinical findings	Location of lesion
Broca's aphasia (motor expressive nonfluent)	Patient knows what he wants to say but has motor impairment and can't articulate spontaneously. Also patient understands written or verbal requests but can't repeat words or phrases	Frontal (posterior)
Wernick's aphasia (sensory receptive/ expressive fluent)	Patient articulates spontaneously and well but uses words inappropriately or uses neologisms. Also patient has difficulty understanding written or verbal requests and can't repeat words or phrases	Temporoparietal (anterior)
Global aphasia	Patient has profound expressive and receptive deficits and can barely communicate	Temporoparietal
Anomia	When given an object, patient can describe its characteristics (colour, size, purpose) but cannot name it	Parietal, subcortical or temporal
Apraxia	When asked to speak, patient can't coordinate movement of lips and tongue. When left alone he may be able to do so	Frontal
Dysarthria	Patient knows what he wants to say but has motor impairment and fails to speak clearly. Also patient has difficulty swallowing and chewing	Cerebellar or frontal (posterior)
Perseveration	Patient continually repeats one idea or response	Throughout the cerebrum (primarily anterior)

Source: Evens MJ 1995.

recognise familiar objects, pictures or words. There may be some visual neglect, in which case the normal visual field is seriously distorted. There may also be apraxia, which means that the person has lost the ability to carry out planned purposeful movements. So for example, you may give Muhammed a pen to see if he is able to communicate that way. Inability to use the pen does not necessarily mean that the problem is with language. He may have other perceptual problems such as agnosia or apraxia that make it difficult for him to recognise or use the pen.

A Speech and Language Therapist will carry out diagnostic aphasia assessment, using a range of test batteries and techniques. Nursing assessment aims to establish a therapeutic relationship, over 24 hours, meeting both information giving and receiving needs. The overall purpose of a nursing assessment in this situation is achieved through a sequence of more short-term purposes:

- to build a trusting relationship
- to identify positive communication attributes
- to identify effective modes of communication and how and when to use them
- to generate information about communication abilities occurring naturally over the 24-hour period which may help the family and other members of the team
- to build a relationship with the family
- to incorporate the recommendations of the speech and language specialists into the care interventions (Iggulden 1994).

Benner (1984), through a series of patient vignettes identifies that at a very fundamental level people unable to communicate verbally have essential needs. These include:

- the need to understand
- the need to be reassured
- the need to learn trust
- the need to be involved.

Thus nurses are faced with situations in which the normal channels of communication are disrupted yet the nursing concern to meet the needs has to be resolved despite the inability to use language.

In Muhammed's case it might help to assess his needs when a family member or interpreter is available, making sure that:

- eye contact is made on the same level
- all are seated
- the curtains are drawn round the bed or the door to the room is closed to exclude visual and auditory distractions.

Explain to Muhammed, using facial expression, tone of voice and hand gestures where appropriate that his stroke has left him with some speaking problems and that it is important to establish a way of communicating with him. Note his nonverbal responses to you at this stage. It may be useful to ask a family member or interpreter to repeat your explanation and compare his responses. In order to establish an informal assessment of his verbal communication the next phase should be carried out using minimal nonverbal communication. The stages as outlined below can be helpful.

Assess understanding Ask him simple questions.
- What is your name?
- What is/was your job?
- Where do you come from?

If he does not appear to understand repeat louder and use the translator.

Test his understanding Ask questions with yes/no answers.
- Is this a pen? (showing something else such as a pair of scissors).

Check the consistency of yes/no responses as this is a vital and basic communication element.

- Give a one step command: 'Open your mouth please' or 'Please point to the floor'.
- Give a two step command such as: 'With your left hand touch your nose and with your right hand touch your tummy'.

If Muhammed appears to understand, but does not speak:

- Ask if he has difficulty finding the right word – this can elicit a good nonverbal response.
- Try to engage him in further, more natural conversation.
- Ask him about his job or his family using open questions so that he needs to reply in sentences and phrases.
- Take note of whether he speaks slowly, very indistinctly, or with difficulty or whether his voice lacks variable pitch and tone.

This may indicate that he has dysarthria rather than dysphasia. Dysarthria is a problem with the motor muscles of speech rather than a central problem of language in the cortex. This means that there is a strong possibility that other forms of graphical and symbolic language may be useful. For example, it may be possible to use eye pointing and gestures, as well as written communication and electronic communication aids.

If his speech is clear enough notice whether it is fluent, whether he uses words correctly, or whether he is unable to find just the word he is looking for. Asking him to name all the animals he can think of in a minute can further assess this word finding. The normal is 18–22 but Muhammed may not reach this anyway, as English is his second language. Then ask him to say all the words he can think of beginning with a particular letter, such as t or s. Word finding can also be assessed more practically by asking him to name objects in the room, items or components of clothing, or for washing or for eating.

Ability to repeat His ability to repeat can be assessed by:
- asking him to repeat a simple phrase, e.g. 'Today is Friday'

- asking him to repeat a more complicated phrase, e.g. 'There are 52 weeks in a calendar year'.

Reading and writing ability The final areas to check are his reading and writing ability, although in Muhammed's case his literacy skills were not good before his stroke.

- Use simple everyday tests such as a food menu or newspaper headline.
- Write down his name and ask him if that is his name.
- Ask him to write the names of the members of his family (be sure to repeat this in his native language).

Document the nursing assessment in the activity of communicating, the aims, interventions and evaluation. A sample of such an assessment is shown in Table 4.2.

Environmental factors

Pound et al (2000) suggest that a social model of disability shows that people are disabled not by their own disabilities, but by the socially constructed barriers which spring up around them. Oliver (1996) identifies that these are:

- Environmental barriers, which in aphasia or dysphasia would include background noise that can make it more difficult for the person to process what is being said.
- In addition, spoken and written language can have a disabling effect if it is too fast, too complex or too vague.
- Structural barriers arise when resources, services and opportunities are not available.
- Informational barriers arise when the information is unavailable, irrelevant or incomprehensible.
- Attitudinal barriers occur when people with a language disorder are deemed to be 'persona non grata' and unable to think or function in any way – the 'does he take sugar' syndrome. This was the title of a BBC programme, demonstrating society's and individuals' attitudes towards disabled people as if they were totally incapable. The attitude fosters unwarranted assumptions about dependencies. Such an attitude, although it may be unconscious, and may stem from pity, fails to take into account an individual's abilities set against the disabling effects of society and the environment. Neither is the situation helped by the medicalisation of disability, such as discussing 'the deaf', or talking about

Table 4.2 Suggested care plan for Muhammed

Assessment	Problem	Aim	Intervention	Evaluation
Muhammed attends to what is being said to him	Does not seem able to follow directions by language alone	Muhammed will understand and practise ways of overcoming language difficulty to make his needs known	Use gestures, clear simple speech, hand guided movements and aphasia boards	Record successful communication strategies in communication log-book
He is able to nod and shake his head appropriately and bows his head for thank you or waves his hand		Establish a consistent effective communication system with regard to meeting his elimination needs, nutritional needs and personal hygiene within the first 48 hours, negotiating with him and involving his family	Point to objects to increase his comprehension Ask closed questions with Yes/No response	
His family say that his facial expressions are very similar to those he used before he had a stroke and that he clearly expresses puzzlement, surprise, annoyance and pleasure			Respond to his facial expressions by asking for confirmation, e.g., 'Did I frighten you?'	Evaluate his mood through his facial expression
He is able to recognise familiar objects such as a cup and a bar of soap and uses them appropriately when handed to him	He does not yet recognise the male urinal or the call bell		Teach Muhammed how to use urinal and call bell Record effective teaching strategies	Check continence levels using urinal Evaluate perceptual function through his ability to recognise and use objects and equipment used in washing and dressing and eating and drinking
	He is not able to write his name or recognise his name written down		Refer to Speech and Language Therapist and liaise re interventions	

Table 4.3 A comparison of individual and social models of disability

Individual model	Social model
Personal tragedy	Social oppression
Personal problem	Social problem
Individual treatment	Social action
Medicalisation	Self-help
Professional dominance	Individual and collective responsibility
Expertise	Experience
Adjustment	Affirmation
Individual identity	Collective identity
Prejudice	Discrimination
Behaviour	Attitudes
Care	Rights
Control	Choice
Policy	Politics
Individual adaptation	Social change

From Oliver 1996 Understanding disability – from theory to practice, MacMillan, London, cited in Pound et al (2000) Beyond aphasia, Winslow Press, p. 9

Box 4.6 Research evidence and aphasia

The subjective experience of people with language impairments has been relatively little explored. Reasons for the exclusion of people who are 'inarticulate' from social research seem complex and are not yet fully understood. Certainly, in terms of aphasia, personal stories have largely been used as material for 'expert' commentary, although this is now starting to change. The research project by Parr et al (1997) explored the consequences and significance of acquired language impairment from the perspective of the people who have it. The study set out to examine the personal perspectives on aphasia within a social, economic and political context. Fifty people with long-term aphasia took part in in-depth interviews in which they described the onset of aphasia; its consequences for employment, education, leisure and social life and personal relationships; their access to information; their experience and evaluation of health, welfare and social care services; their perceptions and understanding of disability. The findings from this qualitative study indicated that aphasia is experienced as a complex, dynamic process which influences every domain of social functioning, and affects the individual at a number of different levels – as someone who interacts with others, as a member of groups and communities and as a citizen.

From: Pound et al (2000) Beyond aphasia. Winslow Press Ltd, pp. 11–12.

people as 'bound' to wheelchairs. The language reflects a patronising attitude, an attitude being seriouly challenged by social models of disability and disability rights activists. The emphasis of the social model of disability can be compared with the other main 'individual' model as shown by Oliver (1996) in Table 4.3. Pound et al (2000) also discuss research evidence from sufferers themselves to support this view (see Box 4.6).

It becomes much clearer in the light of how disabling aphasia can be that a social model of disability really gets to the heart of the impact of aphasia on an individual and the family.

Sociocultural factors

Gerrish (2001) points out that a recurrent concern arising from examining the provision of health care to ethnic minority persons relates to the problems that develop when the health care practitioner and the patient do not speak the same language. Whilst it is true that Muhammed does normally speak English, he does have literacy problems and as Robinson (1998) suggests, when ill, people will tend to revert to their first language. Of the 6% of the population in the UK who are from an ethnic minority background, people from South Asia and African-Caribbean backgrounds form the largest communities (Office of Population Censuses and Surveys 1991). The level of ability to speak, read and write English varies considerably, but what is of greater significance perhaps is the extent to which stereotyping can influence our relationships with patients and their families. Robinson (1998, p. 137) explains that:

> A number of stereotypes operate in the encounter between black people and the state welfare agencies. These are stereotypes of African Caribbeans as aggressive, excitable and defiant, and images of Asian people as meek, passive and docile. One common stereotype assigned to Asians by whites is that Asian culture is dominated exclusively by men, women playing a dependent, submissive role. … although the wife of a family patriarch pays a formal, and often perfunctory deference to her husband, especially in front of strangers, she may exercise considerable domestic power, not merely among the other women of the household, but with her husband, and she often makes many of the vital decisions affecting the family's interests.
>
> If a social or health worker expects Asian women to play a submissive role, then she/he will probably interpret the client's communication behaviour in that light. Social and health care workers must address themselves to the problem of overcoming the stifling effects of strong racial and ethnic stereotyping if multiracial and multi-ethnic communication is to occur.

One stereotyped image which exists about Asian people is that 'they do not speak English'. However, a large proportion of the Asian community speaks English as a second language and many people speak two or three languages as well as English. Asian women who do not work outside the home and older Asians who migrated to Britain in their later years are more likely not to speak English. Muhammed belongs to the latter yet he may still need the help of an interpreter at this vulnerable time. Robinson (1998) outlines some of the issues involved:

> *In another study of social and health authority services 38 social services departments (SSDs) and 39 health authorities (DHAs) for elderly people from black and minority ethnic communities, … half of both the SSDs and DHAs used no specifically funded interpreting services merely relying on families, phrase books or cards, or volunteers from their staff or community groups. All SSD respondents were aware of the inadequacy of interpreting services, and two thirds said they were reviewing or intending to review them. However, less than half the DHAs reported such intentions, and even these were mainly to do with improving leaflets rather than providing interpreters. The authors also interviewed 83 Caribbeans and 89 Asians. Two-thirds of the Asian sample said that communication was an issue for them. For example, 'more interpreters' was one of the two main answers given by Asians, the other being 'more Asian staff', to a question about how, if at all, people thought services could be improved. Ninety-eight per cent of service users said it was important to them that those looking after them spoke their first language. Yet only 5 per cent of Asians said they had ever made use of interpreters when consulting doctors etc.; only 40 per cent said they had ever been asked in hospital whether they needed help with interpreting, and only 34 per cent in outpatient clinics. In an earlier survey of health authorities, all the respondents mentioned language as a major obstacle to health care.*

(From Robinson 1998, p. 94)

There are however general difficulties in using trained interpreters, untrained interpreters, and family members including:

- the possibility of bias as communication is dependent on a third party
- meanings can be changed in the process of translation.

The messages that leave both the practitioner and patient have the potential to be modified and changed by the interpreter.

- Interpreters are sometimes unfamiliar with the terminology used.
- Interpreters might wrongly reinterpret the patient's ideas, or abbreviate responses.
- An interpreter's presence may embarrass the patient when the problem is perceived as a taboo subject.
- Breach of confidentiality is a serious issue – some Asians reject interpreters who belong to the same community.

Box 4.7 Family as interpreters

'Many Asian people frequently take their children to hospital to interpret. This brings its own problems. For example, in the gynaecological department, taking your children to interpret would seem utterly shameful to most parents. It cannot be assumed that people would wish to ask friends or acquaintances to interpret for them in highly personal and confidential situations. The disadvantages of using family members as interpreters should be recognised. … For example, social services tend to use children to translate for their elders. In sensitive situations, this can result in distress and humiliation and/or vital information not being elicited. Dominelli cites an example in which a child is used for interpreting for a Sikh woman who spoke Punjabi but virtually no English was referred by a health visitor to social services – because the woman was suffering post-natal depression. However, as there were no Punjabi-speaking social workers a white social worker visited the woman and used the woman's 9-year-old daughter as a translator. Rack argues under no circumstances should children be asked to interpret medical details for their parents'.

From Robinson (1998) Race, communication and the caring professions. Open University Press.

These last two will probably relate to Muhammed, particularly as it has been suggested that his family assist in helping to assess his communication needs (see Box 4.7).

Politicoeconomic factors

There are several issues here in relation to informed consent and privacy. Bergund (1998) suggests four main areas: competence, information, comprehension and voluntariness. The basic elements of consent are achieved when the person is:

- competent (has the ability to understand what he or she is being asked to consent to) *and*
- has the relevant information *and*
- comprehends the information *and*
- gives consent voluntarily (Bergund 1998, p. 104).

Also, in assessing competence there are seven main aspects to consider:

- Is the environment conducive to decision making?
- What is the person's cognitive function and is it stable over time?
- How does the person cope with activities of daily living?
- Has the person been adequately informed and has the information been understood?
- Is the person's frame of mind conducive to decision making?
- What is the health professional's frame of mind?
- What family and social factors are at work?

In considering these questions Muhammed's initial nursing assessment shows some situations in which he would be able to indicate his wishes by nonverbal means, using gesture and facial expression. However in other situations, particularly where there are no visual or concrete clues to offer him, such as when discussing his options for the future the situation is more complex. The role of the nurse here is to work with Muhammed, his relatives and other members of the multidisciplinary team in reaching decisions which are in his best interests, i.e. in maintaining and furthering his health and welfare.

Privacy is also an area to consider for Muhammed. By virtue of the fact that he has aphasia or may need interpreters and the family to support his communication, he loses control over what people can know about him. For this reason, if at all possible, it is better to limit the number of people involved in assisting his communication, and to discuss with those who do, the confidentiality clause under which health care professionals work.

Finally in respect of both politicoeconomic factors and sociocultural factors, it is a sad fact that racism is widespread in the UK (Archibald 2000) and that racism is a major problem in the health service as a whole. Institutional racism, as Macpherson (1999) sees it, is the collective failure of an organisation to provide an appropriate and professional service to people because of their colour, culture or ethnic origin. He warns that it can be seen or detected in processes, attitudes and behaviour through unwitting prejudice, ignorance, thoughtlessness or racial stereotyping which disadvantage ethnic minority people.

A study undertaken by Tod et al (2001), although limited, found that in cardiac rehabilitation services there was poor access and use of interpreting services and that use of written material did not take into account patient literacy skills and concludes that 'the low uptake of cardiac rehabilitation education group may well be exacerbated by these communication problems identified' (p. 1031).

Case study 4.5

Fiona

Fiona is a 38-year-old woman who developed multiple sclerosis (MS) 5 years ago. The progress of the disease has been very rapid in that time and she has needed help to support her in most of the Activities of Living. Every morning she has assistance from a carer to help her to wash, dress and prepare her and the children's breakfast. She is able to eat and drink independently as long as the shopping and food preparation is well thought out and of a suitable consistency and temperature. She is continent and uses self-catheterisation and a bowel management programme to maintain this. She can walk with the assistance of two sticks on good days, but can barely stand on bad days, on which occasions she uses a wheelchair.

Case study 4.5 (continued)

Her relapse this time has brought her into hospital for further therapy and a review of her situation. She works two mornings a week teaching in the school at which she used to work full time before her illness. However, this current relapse has meant she has not been able to do this for the last 3 weeks. She and her ex-husband separated 6 years ago and her husband has since remarried. Her two children are ten and eight; Fiona lives near her married sister and her mother who help her willingly. On this occasion Fiona is experiencing fatigue, she's very low in mood, tearful and feels that she is a nuisance to everyone. She fears that she won't be able to keep her job up much longer as the relapse has made it difficult to use the computer keyboard or control her handwriting. In addition, her speech is indistinct.

Lifespan

Up until 5 years ago Fiona had experienced a life of normal development of growth through babyhood, childhood, adolescence and young adulthood. She is well-educated and obviously intelligent and still works as a primary school teacher. However, Fiona has had very strong pressures on her coping mechanisms as she realises that her expectations and beliefs about her life and her future have been powerfully affected since the onset of her illness. As a mother she has not only the responsibilities of a single-parent family, she has the extra difficulties brought on by neurological diseases, which have affected her independence.

Dependence/independence

Although Fiona has lost absolute independence over the last 5 years, with suitable support and equipment she has been able to maintain her independence in her home and working life and in her activities of daily living. This is a very positive aspect of her character and can be built on during this time when she is feeling very low. Even so, the fact that she has lost some motor control which interferes with her writing may mean she has lost the motor control for other ALs such as self-catheterisation, which she used to maintain her independence in elimination. Also the speech problem is a development and it is not yet known whether this will resolve or become an ongoing problem for her. Fiona is facing the reality of less physical independence in the present, and fears that she is moving towards a more dependent and lonelier future, as she physically weakens and loses touch because of her reduced communicative ability. The Speech and Language Therapist needs to be involved. In the meantime, nurses caring for her need to understand the nature of dysarthria and the strategies that may be used to help her.

Biological factors

MS is believed to be an autoimmune disease affecting the brain and spinal cord. It is the most common neurological condition, affecting approximately 85 000 people in the UK (Layward 1998). Although the exact cause remains uncertain, the effects on a neurone are that it damages the myelin sheath in which many neurones are encased. This slows down the nerve transmission and makes it jerky, slowed and erratic. It affects both motor and sensory nerves in the central nervous system, but symptoms vary according to where the damaged nerve is situated. Common symptoms based on Graham (2001) include:

- blurring of vision, or double vision
- weakness or clumsiness or spasticity and lack of coordination of a limb
- altered feelings in the arms or legs such as tingling or numbness
- giddiness or lack of balance
- fatigue which is out of proportion to activity levels
- the need to pass water frequently and/or urgently.

Fiona is suffering from several of these symptoms and there is every possibility that they will resolve. There is a classification system, based on the course and duration of the symptoms, which shows that there is no one, inevitable pathway (Box 4.8). However each individual suffering from multiple sclerosis will experience it differently and each individual will have a unique experience, although often fellow sufferers can provide support and understanding for each other. In meeting Fiona's needs therefore what is important is how she is experiencing her illness at this time and supporting her emotionally as well as physically.

Multiple sclerosis can be difficult to diagnose as there is no foolproof diagnostic test, and once diagnosed no one can predict how mild or severe, relapsing or progressive the course might be. Diagnosis is usually made following thorough neurological examination by a neurologist and other radiological and physiological investigations such as visual and auditory evoked potentials, lumbar puncture, myelogram and magnetic resonance imagery. Careful attention must be paid to feelings of fatigue and vague sensory disturbances, as it is these that may cause subtle deterioration in overall ability to function. It is clear at the moment that Fiona is suffering from fatigue. Although there is no 'cure' for MS the symptoms can often be successfully managed using a combination of drug therapy, complementary therapy, the support of the multidisciplinary team and support groups. These are discussed below.

The commonest drugs used in the treatment of MS are:

- *Steroids*. These act by reducing the inflammation around the damaged nerve and are commonly used in relapse to assist recovery. They are usually given intravenously for a few days, when the effect is very rapid, or orally for a few weeks, with a gradually decreasing dose.
- *Baclofen*. This works in the central nervous system to calm down spasticity by reducing the neurotransmitters that cause such high tone in the muscles. Its use needs to be monitored carefully to ensure that weakness does not become a problem.
- *Oxybutinin*. This is commonly used because it relaxes smooth muscle and thus reduces the spasms that cause bladder difficulties. There may however also be troublesome side effects such as dry mouth, constipation, retention of urine and blurring of vision.
- *Amitriptyline*. This can be used in low doses to help alter the person's perception of pain. Pain may be a troublesome aspect of multiple sclerosis when sensory nerves are affected and cause neuropathic pain.
- *Carbamazepine*. This also helps to manage the neuropathic pain of MS and is thought to work by preventing excessive and spontaneous firing of sensory neurones.
- *Beta interferon*. There are two types of beta-interferon 1α and 1β. Interferons belong to a family of proteins that helps to regulate the body's immune system. It is effective because it regulates the body's immune system against myelin and stops it from being destroyed. It comes in a prefilled syringe and can be conveniently self-administered at home once a patient or family member is taught how to do so. Although not a cure beta interferon can reduce the number and severity of attacks, and slow the progression of disability. The side effects are mild to moderate and include flu-like symptoms such as fever, muscle aches and headache and there may be some irritation at the injection site.
- *Complementary therapies*. Complementary therapies treat 'the whole person' and for that reason have not been through the double-blind clinical trials used to assess the effectiveness of orthodox treatments. Also, what suits one person may not suit another, or it may take some time for the benefits or disadvantages

---

Box 4.8 The four main types of multiple sclerosis

Benign
With this type the person may experience one attack and then nothing further for ten or more years.

Relapsing–remitting
This type affects 25% of people suffering from MS and goes through cycles of relapse when new symptoms appear, but which then may disappear as remission is achieved.

Secondary progressive
This is the most common type and affects nearly half of all sufferers. It usually develops from the relapsing–remitting stage, and people begin to notice deterioration progressing over time.

Primary progressive
This develops in mid-life and generally follows a progressively deteriorating course from the onset.

of any treatment to become apparent. Acupuncture, acupressure, aromatherapy, cannabis (and the legal issues around this should make interesting reading over the next decade), chiropractic and osteopathy, herbalism and homeopathy all have reputable organisations which can be consulted to find practitioners.

The physiological processes may affect the cranial nerves, particularly the motor nerves needed to produce speech. Dysarthria is a disorder of speech, which includes difficulty in articulation due to the effect of damage to the motor nerves supplying the muscles of the lips, tongue, palate and throat. This means that pronouncing words is difficult, and sometimes the person may have slurred, drunken-sounding speech. In fact, the slurred speech of dysarthria is often mistaken for the speech of a person who is intoxicated. The rate of speech may be reduced and the slowed pace may lead listeners to infer that the thought processes are slow. This is by no means the case and can lead to deeper problems if the person is treated as if they have cognitive impairment. Sometimes the speech may lack melody and the result can be a flattened speech that can make the person sound bored or depressed and lacking in emotion. The communication problem is therefore not just one of verbal information exchange, it also affects the communication of emotion and the whole interpersonal experience unless other means are developed to convey feelings and interpersonal communication.

In order to help with speech production nurses can

- encourage Fiona to maintain a good posture whilst she speaks
- get her to use short sentences
- take appropriate breaths and break words up if necessary
- give her time
- phrasing questions that enable her to give short answers
- repeat what she has said to check your understanding
- use other assistive devices such as a lightwriter or communication board.

The important aim is to get the balance right between encouraging her to make herself understood verbally and yet not to allow this to make her feel fatigued.

Psychological factors

Fiona plays several roles in family, social and working life and in this respect it connects her with other women under the same stresses, strains and joys of these roles. However there are additional psychosocial factors to be found amongst MS sufferers. In a study of 110 people at the National Hospital for Neurology, Ron and Logsdail (1989) found that irritability, poor concentration, low mood anxiety and elation were all seen significantly more frequently in people with MS than in the control group who were people with other physical disabilities. Depression is however by far the most common, although this does not seem to be correlated with brain pathology. It relates more to environmental

factors such as social stress and lack of support (Ron & Logsdail 1989). Although cognitive impairment can be a feature of multiple sclerosis, it is by no means inevitable. Memory and attention impairments are usually the most commonly experienced problems, and these do tend to be correlated with brain pathology. We know that Fiona is tearful and low in mood, but it would be unreasonable to attribute this to a brain state caused by demyelination. Fiona needs immediate emotional support and it is important that nurses have the skills to offer that through what Burnard (1992) calls minimal counselling skills (see Box 4.9).

There are three main approaches to counselling, and some understanding of theoretical approaches is a valuable addition to basic skills.

- Freud and his followers developed complex psychoanalytical theories, which, although they had such a profound influence on Western thinking were based on only six published case histories that were, from the point of view of his patients, disasters (Dewdney 1997). Behaviour therapy approaches developed in complete contrast to this preoccupation with the unconscious workings of the mind.

Box 4.9 Counselling skills

Formal counselling requires lengthy training but, says Burnard (1992) all nurses should be taught 'minimal' counselling skills to enable them to help them to help clients with their problems in a positive, therapeutic way. He suggests:

- *Listening and attending:* giving the person one's full attention, and avoiding thinking about the 'rightness' or the 'wrongness'of what is being said – listening without being judgemental.
- *Using open-ended questions:* they usually begin with 'what', 'how' 'when' or 'where' enabling the person to expand on their problems, i.e. questions which avoid single word or yes, no answers.
- *Reflecting:* (a) reflection of thoughts, e.g. echoing the last few words the person has used; (b) reflection of feelings, i.e. echoing to the person, the feelings or unstated thoughts which underline a statement just made. Both need to be used judiciously, not over-used.
- *Summarizing:* (a) to pull together disparate strands of conversation and help the person to organise their thoughts; (b) to end a therapeutic conversation while still focusing on the other person's concerns.
- *Checking for understanding*: seeking clarification by asking, e.g. 'Can I just check what you are saying?' or 'You seem to be saying that...'.

From Roper et al 1996 Elements of Nursing, 4th edn, p. 125. Churchill Livingstone, Edinburgh.

- Behaviour therapists felt that there was more to be gained by concentrating on behaviour rather than analysing underlying causes of behaviour. Therapists work with the person in a trusting and supportive relationship focusing very much on the here and now. They work with people through a range of techniques to help overcome problems, including anxiety and depression. It is, however, considered as being generally unsuitable in psychotic conditions.
- Cognitive therapy on the other hand takes the view that behaviour is primarily determined by what a person thinks. This approach is particularly relevant in treating depression where thoughts of low self-worth and self-esteem are a common feature. Counselling challenges negative thoughts and explores the power of imagination, thought stopping and positive thinking to overcome problems.
- Another approach emphasises the power of active listening, where the role of the therapist allows the person to talk about their problems, their feelings about their problems and feeds back their understanding of that problem.

In practice all these theories contribute to the helper's approach in finding ways to help the person to find solutions to their distress. Whatever the theoretical stance, therapeutic nursing helps a person to:

- feel accepted and understood and therefore able to talk openly
- develop an increased understanding of their situation
- discuss alternative understandings of their situation
- make a decision about what to do
- develop specific action plans
- carry out those plans with support if necessary
- adjust to a situation if that situation is unlikely to change.

In Fiona's present situation, apart from the possibility of mood changes caused by demyelination, she is experiencing feelings of loss, apprehension about the future, which have at this time overwhelmed her coping strategies. Nurses can help in a number of different ways in developing a therapeutic relationship with her. Bowles et al (2001) found that this solution-focused brief therapy approach is relevant to nursing and offers a useful, cost-effective strategy towards training nurses in communication skills which is harmonious with nursing values. This approach may also be useful in determining whether Fiona may benefit from seeking the help of a qualified counsellor.

Sociocultural factors

Fiona has a supportive family and clearly has coped well with help from some of the community services. It is unusual for her to be admitted to hospital in an acute relapse such as this. Arrangements will need to be made for the care of her children while she is in hospital and the care team will need to anticipate and discuss with her the level of help she will need when she is discharged. It is the interface between the community and the interdisciplinary team and the effectiveness of the communication between them, which will go a long way towards helping Fiona. The people involved in the team may work in different care settings and different disciplines and because Fiona has an ongoing health problem that has made a big impact on her role and responsibilities her care network is wide. Wilson and McLelland (1997) highlight some of the problems of interdisciplinary working for both professional and patients:

> 66 *There are many potential problems in working with people trained in different disciplines. Each discipline or profession has its own theoretical framework, traditions, sense of mission, priorities and rules. They run the risk however of reinforcing a reluctance to look for ideas from elsewhere, and they can also run the risk of competition and friction between professional groups, as well as between professions and patients.* 99 (p. 8)

Fiona will probably come into contact with physicians, nurses, a specialist nurse, physiotherapists, occupational therapists, speech and language therapists, a social worker, and possibly a counsellor or clinical psychologist. Good teamwork not only across professions but also across care settings is essential if she is to experience continuity of care. Street and Blackford (2001) suggest a range of supporting strategies for effective formal modes of interdisciplinary communication across care settings in palliative care in Australia. Although on the other side of the world the communication problems they identify are universal:

- territoriality between professions
- lack of a common philosophy, language and style between professions and services
- restricted contact between busy professionals of one service and another.

Recent government initiatives in developing National Service Frameworks in the UK go some way towards helping to develop a framework which is more standardised, evidence-based and reliable in offering quality care. The framework for chronic health problems, including multiple sclerosis, is due for completion in 2004. In the meantime, nursing practices in Britain continue to explore collaborative working practices such as Collaborative Care Plans, Integrated Care Pathways and Patient-held records to try to improve continuity and communication in practice.

Environmental factors

Under this aspect for Fiona the social model of disability has a strong impact on her quality of life. Suitable adaptation of her home environment, provision of equipment and support to enable her to live as independently as possible, as well as help from a social worker can significantly improve her quality of life at home. Self-help organisations such as the Multiple Sclerosis Society can help Fiona overcome some of the wider environmental factors that may inhibit as full a social and communicative a life as possible. Wilson and McLelland (1997) explain that:

> *Sometimes the natural history of a condition such as multiple sclerosis, arthritis, glaucoma, deafness or Parkinson's disease is known to be one of steady or periodic deterioration, but the levels of severe incapacity may not be obvious until well into retirement age. This means that in the early stages the threat of disability can be an anxiety affecting the individual much more than the actual physical problems that present. Work potential is certainly often affected, but this can result far more from worry about things that could be adapted than from the actual inability to continue to work. People with these problems may welcome regular long-term support and a review of adaptive measures or equipment.* (Wilson & McLelland 1997, p. 126)

Politicoeconomic factors

For Fiona, a well-educated, professional, single parent with a chronic illness the economic implications are considerable because of her reduced ability to take on paid employment. Yet Wilson and McLelland (1997) point out that employment has significant wider functions (see Box 4.10).

The care team needs to be aware of these wider implications of the threat of the loss of the ability to work. Wilson and McLelland (1997) also warn that health care professionals may unwittingly make readjustment for

---

Box 4.10 Work occupation and disability

Work gives human beings the opportunity to have certain basic needs met, and although most people complain about how busy and stressful and tiring work is, they would probably be much worse if forced into inactivity. This is true of both paid work and volunteer work.

Work has these following functions

Income A job gives us the money to buy the goods and services others in society produce and provide. The 'poverty trap' is a term used to describe those who are not working (usually through disability) because its social benefits amount to more than could be earned.

Respect Social standards seem to favour those who are in work, and particularly those with high-status jobs. Individuals relying solely on benefits may feel low self-esteem and not respected by others.

Adapted from Wilson and McLelland 1997 Rehabilitation Studies Handbook, p. 115. Cambridge University Press.

---

patients more difficult by a preoccupation with clinical signs and pathologies (doctors), bowels and hygiene (nurses), painful physical jerks (physiotherapists) and the learning self-care tasks (occupational therapists). Patients with MS often find the service of an MS Nurse Specialist or the support of a self-help group such as the MS Society can help come to terms with the loss of social and economic status. The mission statement of the MS Society, founded in 1953 by Sir Richard Cave, indicates a clear concern with these issues:

> *Funds are also raised at branch and national level to provide welfare support for people with MS and their families. This includes producing information booklets and leaflets about MS, statutory services, and available and other sources of support. We also have a fund providing financial assistance to individuals and families for things not covered by state benefits. These include holidays, special equipment or mobility aids and respite care.*
>
> *As a national voluntary organisation, we also represent the concerns of people who have MS or are living with it, in all areas of government legislation and policy. Working to improve the things in everyday life which affect people's independence: for example working for the introduction of a comprehensive disability income through the social security system, access issues, seeking improved personal and social care facilities and the adequate provision of equipment for independent living.*

From: MS Society 'Perhaps We Can Help?'

Conclusion

It is cases such as Fiona's that show how the richness of a holistic model of nursing can accommodate the spectrum of issues that affect a person's wellbeing. The activity of communicating cuts through all these aspects, operating through biological, psychological, sociocultural, environmental and politicoeconomic modes to affect a person's wellbeing through all the Activities of Living.

Summary points

1. Communicating can take many forms, including verbal and written.
2. As an AL it is essential for effective assessment and care.
3. Nurses need to learn how to communicate with all age groups and take account of language differences in their care delivery.

References

Adler RB, Rodman G 1991 Understanding human communication, 4th edn. Holt, Rheinhart and Winston, Inc, London

Archibald G 2000 The needs of South Asians with a terminal illness. Professional Nurse 15(5): 316–319

Benner P 1984 From novice to expert. Addison-Wesley, London

Bergund CA 1998 Ethics for healthcare. Oxford University Press, Oxford

Bowles N, Mackintosh C, Tom A 2001 Nurse communication skills: an evaluation of the impact of solution focused communication training. Journal of Advanced Nursing 36(3): 347–354

Burnard P 1992 Counselling skills for health professionals, 2nd edn. Chapman and Hall, London

Crystal D 1992 The Cambridge encyclopaedia of language. Cambridge University Press, Cambridge

Department of Health 1998 Data Protection Act 1998: protection and use of patient information. DoH, HMSO, London

Department of Health 1998 Human Rights Act 1998. DoH, HMSO, London (http://www.hmso.gov.uk/acts/acts1998/19980042.htm)

Department of Health 2000 Race Relations Amendment Act. DoH, HMSO, London (http://www.homeoffice.gov.uk/raceact)

Department of Health 2002 Guidance for access to health records requests under the Data Protection Act 1998 (http://www.doh.gov.uk/ipu/ahr/dpa1998.pdf accessed Sept 30 2002)

Dewdney AK 1997 Yes we have no neutrons – a tour through the twists and turns of bad science. John Wiley and Sons, New York

DfES 2001 Skills for life: A strategy for adult literacy and numeracy skills improving. HMSO, London

Dickson D, Hargie O, Morrow N 1997 Communication skills training for health professionals, 2nd edn. Chapman and Hall, London

Evens MJ 1995 Neurologic neurosurgical nursing, 2nd edn. Springhouse Publications, Pennsylvania

Fromkin V, Rodman R 1983 An introduction to language, 3rd edn. CBS Publishing, London

Fuller G 2000 Neurological examination made easy, 2nd edn. Churchill Livingstone, Edinburgh

Gerrish K 2001 The nature and effect of communication difficulties arising from interactions between district nurse and South Asian patients. Journal of Advanced Nursing 33(5): 566–574

Goleman D 1996 Emotional intelligence. Bloomsbury, London

Goodwin C 1995 Co-constructing meaning in conversations with an aphasic man. In: Jacoby, S and Och E (eds) Research on language and social interaction (special issue on co-construction). Lawrence Erlbaum Assoc. Inc., NJ

Graham J 2001 What is MS? Multiple Sclerosis Society information booklet. Burnett Publications, London

Hickey JV 1997 Neurological and neurosurgical nursing, 4th edn. Lippincott, Philadelphia

Hunt M 1993 The story of psychology. Anchor Books, Doubleday, New York

Iggulden HM 1994 The nursing contribution in understanding and communicating with acute aphasia sufferers. Unpublished MSc Thesis, Manchester University

Layward L 1998 Understanding MS research. Multiple Sclerosis Society information booklet. Burnett Publications, London

Macpherson W 1999 The Stephen Lawrence Inquiry: report of an enquiry by Sir William Macpherson of Cluny. HMSO, London

Moonie N 2000 Advanced health and social care, 3rd edn. Heineman, Oxford

NMC 2002a Code of Professional Conduct. Nursing and Midwifery Council, London

NMC 2002b Guidelines for records and record keeping. London, NMC.

Office of Population Censuses and Surveys 1991 Census, local base statistics. HMSO, London

Oliver M 1996 Understanding disability: From theory to practice. Macmillan, London

Pound C, Parr S, Lindsay J, Woolf C 2000 Beyond aphasia. Winslow Press Ltd, Bicester

Robinson L 1998 'Race,' communication and the caring professions. Open University Press, Buckingham

Ron MA, Logsdail SJ 1989 Psychiatric morbidity in multiple sclerosis: A clinical and MRI study. Psychological Medicine 19: 887–895

Roper N, Logan WW, Tierney AJ 1996 The elements of nursing, 4th edn. Churchill Livingstone, Edinburgh

Rutishauser S 1994 Physiology and anatomy: A basis for nursing and health care. Churchill Livingstone, Edinburgh

Sharples N 2002 Communicating with patients who are pre-lingually profoundly deaf. Personal communication, University of Salford

Street A, Blackford J 2001 Communication issues for the interdisciplinary community palliative care team. Journal of Clinical Nursing 10: 643–650

Tod AM, Wadsworth E, Asif S, Gerrish K 2001 Cardiac rehabilitation: the needs of South Asian cardiac patients. British Journal of Nursing 10(16): 1028–1035

Waugh M, Grant A 2001 Ross and Wilson anatomy and physiology in health and illness, 9th edition. Churchill Livingstone, Edinburgh

WHO 2002 International Classifications of Functions, Disability and Health. (http://www3.who.int/icF; accessed 3.12.02)

Wilson BA, McLelland DL 1997 Rehabilitation studies handbook. Cambridge University Press, Cambridge

Further reading

Barnes MP, Ward AB 2000 Textbook of rehabilitation medicine. Oxford University Press, Oxford

Darley M 2002 Managing communication in health care. Baillière Tindall, London

Duck S 1998 Human relationships, 3rd edn. Sage Publications, London

Griffin J, Tyrell I 1999 Psychotherapy and the human givens. Monograph. The European Therapy Studies Institute, London

Parr S, Byng S, Gilpin S and Ireland C 1997 Talking about aphasia; living with loss of language after stroke. Open University Press, Buckingham

Piteroni M, Vaspe A 2000 Understanding counselling in primary care – voices from the inner city. Churchill Livingstone, Edinburgh

Thomas VN 1997 Pain: its nature and management. Baillière Tindall, London

Useful websites

http://www.aphasia.org (National Aphasia Association)
http://www.mssociety.org.uk (Multiple Sclerosis Society)
http://www.headway.org.uk (Brain Injury Association)
http://www.nmc-uk.org (Nursing and Midwifery Council – UK)
http://www.bac.co.uk (British Association of Counselling and Psychotherapy)
http://www.freedomtocare.org (Ethics in Health Care)
http://www.cultsock.ndirect.co.uk (Communication, cultural and media studies)
http://www.doh.gov.uk (Department of Health)

Breathing

Jane Jenkins

Introduction

Roper, Logan and Tierney (2000, p. 22) highlight the fact that breathing appears to be 'effortless and people are not usually consciously aware of the AL of breathing until some abnormal circumstances force it to their attention'. Being able to breathe normally ensures that we can attempt other activities without any difficulty, for example walking, running, swimming. However, breathing can be affected by health problems which relate to other Activities of Living, such as being overweight through unhealthy eating causing the individual breathing difficulties when running, walking or even talking. It is important to remember that we are all individuals with life activities that are inter-linked and when illness causes one or more activity to be affected then most of the activities can become compromised. This may then result in physical, emotional or social problems.

This chapter will focus on the following:

1. **The model of living**
   - Breathing activity in health and illness across the lifespan.
   - Dependence and independence in relation to the activity of breathing.
   - Factors which influence the activity of breathing.
2. **The model for nursing**
   - Nursing care of individuals with health problems which affect their activity of breathing.

THE MODEL OF LIVING

Initially, you will need to be able to answer the question: How do we breathe? It may be necessary for you to review your knowledge of the normal anatomy and physiology of the respiratory and circulatory systems before you continue with the chapter. (See further reading at the end of this chapter and the section entitled Biological Factors.)

Breathing activity in health and illness across the lifespan

At birth

Breathing is usually an independent activity immediately following birth. A mother's initial question, following the joys of labour, is to ask if the baby is alright. Whatever response is given, the first cry that is uttered from the baby signifies to the mother that all is well. From a health care professional's point of view that cry signifies that the baby is able to breathe on their own, albeit that suction may have been required to remove secretions from the upper respiratory tract which collect during the birth process. Observations of the baby's respiratory function will take place unobtrusively to ensure that this vital Activity of Living is not compromised in any way. It is important that the rate, depth and pattern of respiration is monitored along with the colour of the baby's skin.

Childhood

Children expend an enormous amount of energy and need a respiratory system that can meet these demands. The activity of breathing is performed effortlessly and children will be totally unaware of breathing unless they experience childhood illnesses, such as whooping cough and asthma.

Adulthood/older person

As in childhood, the activity of breathing continues to take place without conscious thought and is very much taken for granted. However, problems with the respiratory and cardiovascular system occur more commonly in adults and older people and breathing can then become a major factor in their lifestyle.

You may have noticed that the baby or child's rate of breathing was much faster than that of an adult and older person. The normal range for a baby is about 30 or more breaths per minute, 22–28 per minute for a child, 18–22 per minute for an adolescent and between 14–20 per minute for an adult and slightly higher in an older person. In healthy people, there is a relationship between their pulse rate and their respiratory rate. This is fairly constant and one breath occurs to every four or five heart beats. Where there are more than the usual number of respirations (above 24) then this is known as tachypnoea and bradypnoea if below 12. The depth of their respiration is again fairly constant and is often described as 'normal', 'shallow' or 'deep', but in an older person then the depth may become more shallow. Breathing patterns are usually regular and effortless, in all age groups (Jamieson et al 1992). If any of the people you observed had any health problems which affected breathing, such as the common cold, you may have noticed that their breathing rate was faster than normal and the pattern may have been altered and their breathing required effort and was possibly noisy.

Dependence and independence in relation to the activity of breathing

The degree of independence is closely related to the position on the lifespan with most of the activities. However, breathing is probably the exception to the rule, as already discussed, most individuals breathe unaided and independently from birth, throughout their lifespan until the moment of death. In fact, it is the cessation of breathing that signifies death to most people.

Roper et al (1996) identified that even in health, individuals can become dependent upon certain aspects in relation to breathing, such as, organising outdoor pursuits when the pollen count is low as they suffer from hayfever, or by ensuring that they take their respiratory or cardiovascular medications so that they can carry out their normal Activities of Living.

However, some individuals are not able to breathe on their own and are totally dependent upon specialised equipment and constant care. This may range from the need to have a constant supply of oxygen in their own home, to the person needing to be intubated and attached to mechanical ventilation. This latter level of dependency may be as a result of an accident which has caused paralysis of the nerves which affect breathing, infection such as poliomyelitis which causes paralysis of the muscles of the chest or a congenital problem. Although care for these patients requires specialist knowledge and skills, it is important that you have an awareness of mechanical ventilation as emergency situations may arise.

In relation to how mechanical ventilators work you may have discovered that there are different types of mechanical ventilators, e.g. the most common type being either positive pressure ventilators, or negative pressure ventilators which are used for patients with poliomyelitis. Walsh (2002) describes positive pressure ventilators as those which deliver gases directly into the lungs through a tube and an artificial airway, such as an endotracheal or tracheostomy tube, whereas negative pressure ventilators do not require an artificial airway as they work on the principle of removing air from within a closed container by generating negative pressure. This negative pressure causes the lungs to expand and air to flow into them as in the 'Iron Lungs' that were used for patients suffering from poliomyelitis.

Negative pressure ventilators may be used by individuals in their own homes but in Intensive Care Units it is usually the positive pressure ventilators that are used. There are also different modes of ventilating such as intermittent positive pressure ventilation (IPPV) and continuous positive airway pressure (CPAP).

Mechanical ventilation provides artificial support for breathing, maintains vital functions and optimum gaseous exchange and ensures adequate tissue perfusion, therefore allowing physiological functions to continue.

A bellows action within the ventilator acts as the diaphragm and the thoracic cage, thereby delivering oxygen to the lungs so that gaseous exchange can take place. The positive pressure ventilators allow oxygen to be delivered at a preset pressure at a concentration of 21–100%. This may be via either 'controlled ventilation' where the individual makes no respiratory effort and is totally dependent on the ventilator or via 'assisted ventilation' where the individual is able to make some respiratory effort but they are partially dependent on the ventilator to assist them to breathe adequately (Walsh 2002).

You may have watched medical programmes where patients are (or appear to be) ventilated or you may have been able to observe patients being nursed on a ventilator in an Intensive Care Unit or in an Operating Theatre. These patients are critically ill and require specialised care.

However, there are principles of care which you may be able to recognise, such as airway maintenance by appropriate endotracheal suctioning, delivery of warmed, humidified, filtered oxygen, observations of patient's vital signs (colour, oxygen saturation levels, consciousness, temperature, pulse, blood pressure, fluid balance), amount of sedation required and its effect on respiration, correct positioning for lung function, physiotherapy and whilst doing all of this technical activity it is vital to communicate with the patient. Care of the patient's skin is essential and the nurse must ensure that the patient is adequately hydrated and well nourished and that hygiene needs are maintained. Patients requiring this level of care are totally dependent on the health care professionals for the maintenance of all of their Activities of Living.

Specific monitoring devices for the measurement of arterial pressure, central venous pressure and pulmonary artery pressure will be utilised. Observation of the ventilator tubing, endotracheal cuff pressures will take place in addition to the other observations noted. (Further details of caring for the critically ill and ventilated patient can be found in Fulton 2000.)

Your response to how you may feel about being dependent on a ventilator will be affected by many aspects, e.g. 'Are you aware of the problem?', 'Is it long term?', 'Have you any previous knowledge of this type of care?'. However, you may well have thought that you would be frightened knowing that you could not breathe on your own, or angry at not being able to breathe or talk, or perhaps frustrated as you are not able to communicate with other people or become depressed and withdrawn because of lack of ability to communicate and worrying over the potential outcome. Responding to patient's mental, social and spiritual needs are as important as attending to their physical needs and technical equipment.

Another area of dependency to consider is in relation to smoking and this form of addiction. Because smoking is highly addictive, smokers find it difficult to give up smoking and therefore become dependent upon it for a variety of reasons. The World Health Organisation (1980) has defined three types of dependency:

1. *Social dependency* – the person depends on a chemical in order to conform to the behaviour patterns of his particular community.
2. *Psychological dependency* – the person depends on a chemical to provide enjoyment and/or suppress or come to terms with mental or emotional conflicts.
3. *Physical dependency* – the person depends on a chemical for normal functioning.

Exercise

1. Find out why people start smoking and try to find different age groups to see if reasons have changed.
2. Find out if any of them have tried to stop and if so how successful they have been.
3. Discuss with them how smoking affects their breathing and their day-to-day living activities.

You will probably have found many reasons why individuals start smoking. Children may start smoking to show their independence, because their friends or siblings do, because adults tell them not to, or to follow their role models. Advertising in sporting events or on billboards is also a reason why children start to smoke, as identified by the Department of Health (1998) in *Smoking Kills – White Paper on Tobacco*. This may initially start as an experiment but unfortunately they are unable to give up. Older people, especially men, may say they started smoking during the war periods where tobacco was given to troops. Now, older people may start smoking due to pressures at work or home and use it as a stress reliever (Department of Health 1998).

Social dependency may have been the originator of smoking for most people but this then slowly moves into psychological and physical dependency later on. At the physical dependency stage, it is more difficult to quit than at the previous levels of dependency. As the smoker has become dependent on the chemical, i.e. nicotine, unpleasant symptoms result from the withdrawal of this chemical, such as depression, irritability, anxiety, restlessness and lack of concentration as Roper et al (1996) identify.

You may have found out that smokers find it extremely difficult to stop, some may not wish to and some may have restarted after stopping smoking for a period of time. The statistics relating to smoking as found in *Smoking Kills* (Department of Health 1998) provide sober reading and demonstrate not only the dependency but also the cost in health.

Exercise

Read or show the statistics in Box 5.1 to:

1. Smokers – young and older persons.
2. A parent of a teenager.
3. Discuss with them their views on the facts raised by the DoH (1998).

You may find that a smoker may read them and pass no comment, or confirm that they already know the risks but still wish to smoke, or they may believe them and express a wish to quit. A parent who is a smoker or a nonsmoker may be horrified at these statistics and want to know how they can help to prevent their child from starting smoking.

Box 5.1 Statistics relating to smoking

- 120 000 people will die each year, in the UK, due to illnesses directly related to smoking.
- 13 people will die each hour, in the UK, due to illnesses directly related to smoking.
- 13 million adults smoke in UK.
- UK citizens smoke more cigarettes per person than in Europe.
- Principal avoidable cause of premature deaths in the UK.
- Smoking is the major cause of cancer (46 500 deaths per year in UK).
- Smoking is the major cause of heart disease (40 300 deaths per year in UK).
- Smoking is high in people with severe mental illness.
- Increasing numbers of young people smoke now.
- Smokers who take up the habit as teenagers generally go on to smoke all of their lives.
- Half of those (life-time smokers) die of the habit.
- A quarter die before the age of 69.
- Smokers lose 16 years from their life expectancy compared to nonsmokers.
- Someone starting smoking at 15 is three times more likely to die of cancer than someone who starts smoking at 25.
- UK death rates due to smoking are high compared to EU countries except Denmark.
- Higher rate of smoking in manual workers is matched with higher rates of disease.

(Department of Health 1998)

Factors influencing the activity of breathing

As identified by Roper et al (1996, 2000) speaking, laughing and eating alter breathing patterns even though individuals are rarely aware of this. Even in the healthy person a number of factors can and do influence the rate, depth and rhythm of breathing and other vital signs of pulse and blood pressure. These factors will be explored individually but include:

1. Anatomy and physiology related to breathing (biological factors).
2. Emotional issues related to breathing (psychological factors).
3. Practices, associated health beliefs and habits in different cultures related to breathing (sociocultural factors).
4. Pollutants in the air and how these are related to breathing (environmental factors).
5. Policies, laws and economics related to breathing (politicoeconomic factors).

Anatomy and physiology related to breathing (biological factors)

In order to promote health and be able to care for individuals who have breathing problems it is necessary for you to understand the normal structure and function of all systems in the body. In relation to breathing, the anatomy and physiology of the respiratory system and the cardiovascular system need to be considered.

The function of the respiratory system is twofold:

- to provide an adequate supply of oxygen to the cells, so that they can function properly
- to provide a means of removing the carbon dioxide, which is produced by the cells, as a waste product, following their activity.

The organs of the respiratory system allow the oxygen, present in the atmosphere, to enter the body and ultimately the cells, and for carbon dioxide to exit the body from the cells. It is vital that the cells receive this supply of oxygen as without it, even for a few minutes, major problems can result and death can occur. Breathing is effortless or laboured depending on how 'stiff' the respiratory system is and how narrow the airways are.

Respiration, according to Rutishauser (1994), is the term used to describe the processes which ensure that oxygen is transported to, and used by, the cells and that when carbon dioxide is produced it is taken away from the cells (see Fig. 5.1). For this process to work, it is necessary for the cardiovascular system to be utilised. The blood is the fluid medium used to transport oxygen and carbon dioxide, the blood vessels are the means by which the gases are transported to and from the cells in the blood and the heart provides the pump to ensure that the blood flows around the body in the blood vessels to deliver the oxygen and pick up the carbon dioxide.

These two systems (respiratory and cardiovascular) interlink to provide three processes, according to Rutishauser (1994): ventilation of the lungs with air, gaseous exchange between air and blood and perfusion of the lungs with blood. These processes will be briefly discussed in relation to the activity of breathing but you may need to refer to anatomy and physiology books noted in the Further Reading list at the end of this chapter for further details.

Ventilation process involving the respiratory system

Various organs make up the respiratory system (nose, pharynx, larynx, trachea, bronchi, bronchioles, lungs, alveoli, pleura and thoracic cage) and you need to be aware of the position, structure and function of each organ (Waugh & Grant 2001). The positions of these organs are shown in Figure 5.2.

The initial activity of the respiratory system is that of ventilation, moving air in and out of the lungs. Initially, air breathed in through the nose is warmed, moistened and filtered by the vascular, moist mucosal layer of the nose and the hairs in the nose. The mucus traps any inhaled particles

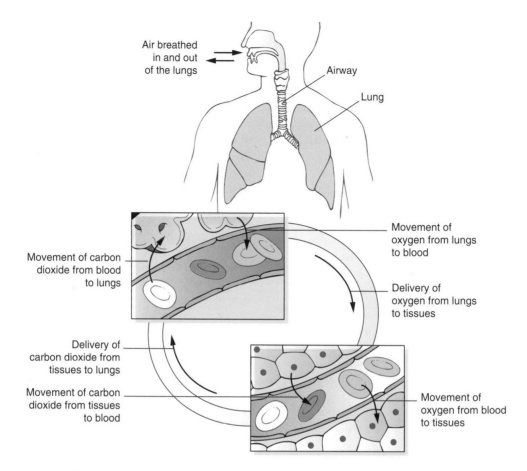

Fig. 5.1 Processes involved in the delivery of oxygen to the tissues and the elimination of carbon dioxide (from Rutishauser 1994, with permission).

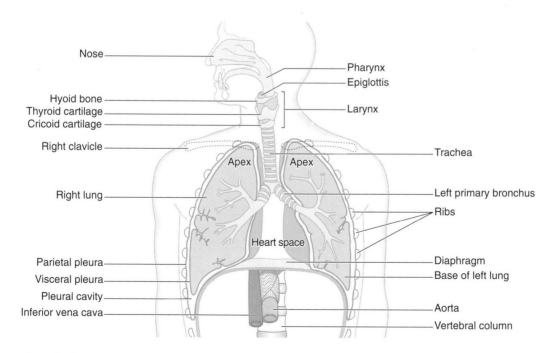

Fig. 5.2 Organs of respiration (from Waugh & Grant 2001, with permission).

and the cilia (hairs) help to drive this mucus with the particles up and out of the airway. As the air passes down the pharynx and larynx, the air continues to be warmed and moistened and is at body temperature when it reaches the trachea, although warming can still take place in the bronchi and bronchioles. The alveoli are at the end of the respiratory tract and it is here that gaseous exchange takes place between the air and the blood (Waugh & Grant 2001). The lower respiratory tract can be seen in Figure 5.3.

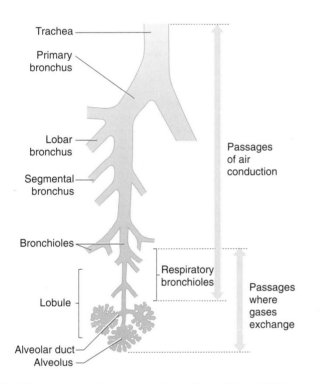

Fig. 5.3 Lower respiratory tract (from Waugh & Grant 2001, with permission).

For gaseous exchange to occur, the lungs need to inflate and this is achieved by increasing the size of the thoracic cavity due to the muscular activity of the external intercostal muscles (which are stimulated by the nervous system) and the diaphragm and this is known as inspiration. The diaphragm contracts and pushes the abdominal organs down, whilst the lower ribs swing outwards so increasing the size of the thoracic cavity to allow the air into the lungs. When the external intercostal muscles and the diaphragm relax air is pushed out of the lungs and this is known as expiration. No effort is normally needed for expiration to occur. The changes in the capacity of the thoracic cavity during ventilation are shown in Figure 5.4 (Waugh & Grant 2001).

You can also feel these changes if you place your hands on the sides of your rib cage and breathe in and breathe out. You will be able to realise that with extra effort (for example, lifting up shoulders) you can increase the size of the thoracic cavity and therefore breathe in more air, however breathing out just happens. These changes occur because of the links with the nervous system. The intercostal muscles are stimulated by the involuntary system which includes the respiratory centre in the brain stem. The respiratory centre receives information from the respiratory system itself on the state of the lungs and also from special receptors on the oxygen and carbon dioxide levels in the bloodstream as described by Rutishauser (1994) and is shown in Figure 5.5.

According to Rutishauser (1994), the amount of air breathed in and out varies between individuals, but in quiet breathing this should be about 500 ml and is known as the tidal volume (TV). However, the total lung capacity (TLC) is far greater than this and could be up to 6 litres of air. The total lung capacity includes the total amount of air that can be breathed in and out and also that which remains in the respiratory tract as not all air can be expelled. Extra air which can be breathed in, with maximum effort, could be

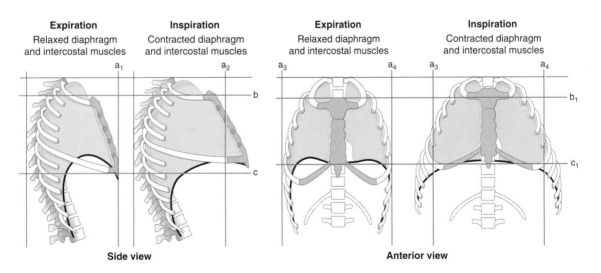

Fig. 5.4 Changes in the capacity of the thoracic cavity during breathing (from Waugh & Grant 2001, with permission).

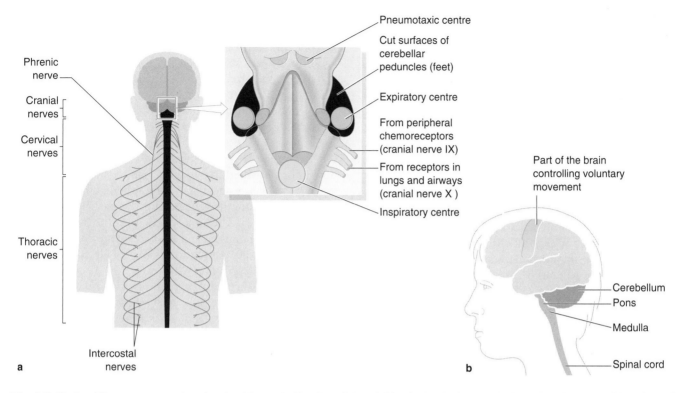

Fig. 5.5 Parts of the nervous system involved in controlling breathing, (a) brain, brainstem, spinal cord and nerves with enlarged inset showing respiratory centres in medulla and pons, (b) position of medulla and pons (from Rutishauser 1994, with permission).

up to 2 litres and is called the inspiratory reserve volume (IRV). The largest amount of air that can be breathed out, with maximum effort, is about 1 litre and is known as the expiratory reserve volume (ERV). The amount of air that cannot be expelled is known as the residual volume (RV) and is approximately 1500 ml. The last two volumes (ERV + RV) give the functional residual capacity (FRC), which is the amount of air left in the system at the end of normal expiration and should be between 2–3 litres. The maximum amount of air that can be moved in and out of the lungs (TV + IRV + ERV) is the vital capacity (VC) and is normally between 3500–4800 ml (Rutishauser 1994). The pattern of breathing and measurements of lung volumes can be recorded by spirometry as shown in Figure 5.6.

Respiratory function is assessed using these lung volumes and therefore it is important to be aware of their meanings in health and illness. Sayer (1999) comments on the increasing use of spirometers in GP surgeries which will provide a

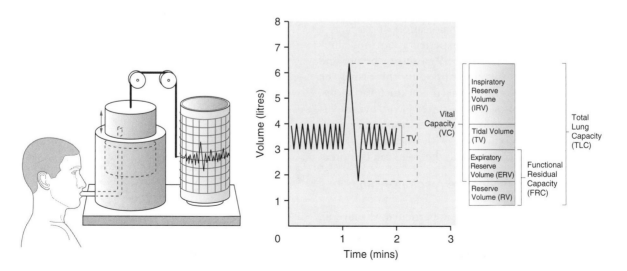

Fig. 5.6 The pattern of breathing and measurements of lung volumes by spirometry (from Rutishauser 1994, with permission).

reliable diagnostic tool for patients with chronic obstructive pulmonary disease.

Exercise

1. Investigate what alterations are found in lung volumes with individuals who have respiratory problems.

You may have been able to observe spirometry being carried out at the bedside, in a clinic, GP's surgery or at the patient's home. You may have visited a pulmonary function laboratory or discussed this with a Respiratory Specialist Nurse.

Patients who have obstructive airway disease (e.g. asthma) may have a normal or slightly reduced vital capacity (VC) as air is trapped in the lungs because individuals have difficulty in breathing out. Both the residual volume (RV) and functional residual capacity (FRC) are increased as more air remains in the lungs after each expiration.

You may have experienced difficulties in observing or finding out information in relation to lung volumes but you may have observed peak flow rate measurements (peak expiratory flow rate or PEFR). This can be undertaken at home, in a clinic, GP's surgery or at the bedside to assess respiratory function by an individual breathing in fully and then breathing out as fast and fully as possible into a peak flow meter. It, therefore, tests the maximum rate at which an individual can breathe out or exhale in litres per minute. As the rate at which the air flows through the airways is measured by the PEFR, it gives an indication of the size of the airways. If they are wider then the air flows easier through them and the PEFR will be higher but if the airways are narrowed then it will be harder for the air to flow through and the PEFR will be lower and problems will be experienced.

The normal range, in health, is 400–600 litres per minute but individuals with asthma, for example, will have a lower peak flow rate when their airway is narrowed. Many asthma sufferers monitor their own peak flow rate measurements to ascertain the effect of medication and act as a warning mechanism before they experience obvious alterations in their breathing. Sayer (1999) assesses the use and reliability of peak flow meters. Although there may be some discrepancies in readings due to product variations, user error or falsification of results, Sayer (1999) considers that the benefits are numerous as trends in respiratory function can be monitored, compliance with treatments may be improved and response to changes in therapies can be noted.

Gaseous exchange involving the respiratory and cardiovascular systems

Air has now reached the lungs and, in particular, the alveoli, and oxygen needs to be transferred from the air in the alveoli to the blood and carbon dioxide needs to be transferred from the blood to the alveoli (Waugh & Grant 2001). The oxygen moves from the alveolar air to the blood by diffusion and stops when the partial pressure of oxygen in the blood is the same as that in the alveoli. The carbon dioxide moves from the blood to the alveolar air again by diffusion and stops when the partial pressure of carbon dioxide in the alveoli is the same as that in the blood, as illustrated in Figure 5.7.

To understand how these gases exchange by diffusion, it is necessary to consider the differences in the partial pressures of the gases in the atmosphere and the alveolar air. According to Rutishauser (1994), the composition of air can be described in two ways, namely by the amount of each gas which is present in atmospheric air and alveolar air in terms of the percentage and the partial pressures of these gases (kPa). The atmospheric pressure, at sea level, is 100 kPa or 760 mmHg, and the percentage composition of oxygen is 21%, i.e. oxygen forms 21% of air. So the part of the atmospheric pressure, which is due to oxygen, is called the partial pressure of oxygen and is 21% × 100 kPa. This gives a partial pressure of oxygen which is 21 kPa. Carbon dioxide, on the other hand, is measured at only 0.04 as a percent in the atmospheric air, so the partial pressure of carbon dioxide is 0.04% × 100 kPa, giving a partial pressure of carbon dioxide of 0.04. In alveolar air, the percentage composition changes as the gases move through the respiratory tract to the alveoli. The percentage composition of oxygen, in the alveolar air, falls to 13.2%, so the partial pressure of oxygen is 13.2 kPa (as it is 13.2% × 100 kPa). The carbon dioxide level in the alveolar air is higher and the percentage composition is 5.3% giving a partial pressure of 5.3 kPa (as is it 5.3% × 100 kPa). The partial pressure of gases is denoted as pO_2 or pCO_2 kPa.

Oxygen moves from the alveolar air, which has a partial pressure of oxygen of pO_2 13.2 kPa, into the bloodstream, as the partial pressure of oxygen in the bloodstream only measures pO_2 5.3 kPa. This movement continues until the pO_2 is the same in the alveoli and the blood. Carbon dioxide leaves the alveolar air in the same way. The partial pressure of carbon dioxide (pCO_2) in the bloodstream is 6 kPa and

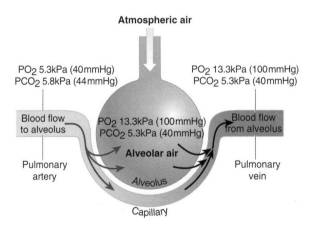

Fig. 5.7 Gaseous exchange of oxygen and carbon dioxide between alveolar air and blood (external respiration) (from Waugh & Grant 2001, with permission).

as this is higher than in the alveolar air (pCO$_2$ 5.3 kPa), the carbon dioxide moves from the blood into the alveoli and is eventually breathed out. Again the movement of the gases continue until the partial pressure of carbon dioxide is the same in the alveoli and the blood. Rutishauser (1994) explains that this process occurs very quickly.

It is useful to identify and differentiate between the terms external and internal respiration (Waugh & Grant 2001). External respiration is the term used to explain the process by which the blood is oxygenated and the subsequent elimination of carbon dioxide from the body, i.e. gaseous exchange as explained above. The use of the oxygen at cell level and the production of carbon dioxide is known as internal respiration and is illustrated in Figure 5.8.

Before birth, gaseous exchange is performed by the placenta and the exchange is between the mother's blood and that of the fetus. Immediately after birth, the gaseous exchange is taken over by the newborn baby's lungs.

Exercise

1. Identify what effects there may be on the fetus if the mother smokes and give the reasons why these problems may occur.
2. What information would you give a pregnant mother who smokes?

It is recognised that smoking is addictive and is therefore difficult to give up but there are serious health risks, not only to the mother, but to the unborn child and the baby as serious illnesses and cot deaths are more prevalent in houses where the mother smokes. There is evidence to support the fact that smoking during pregnancy harms the unborn child and leads to lower birth weights. These problems arise possibly because of a decrease in the blood flow to the placenta. There is also evidence that the mother can pass on harmful carcinogens to the baby. Some nicotine will also pass into the babies bloodstream if mothers smoke when they are breast feeding (Department of Health 1998).

The Department of Health (1998) state that 24% of women smoke during pregnancy and only 33% give up during pregnancy. Because of the problems noted it is vital that mothers quit smoking during pregnancy.

Helping mothers to give up smoking during pregnancy has many benefits. Not only should the health of the mother and baby be better but the NHS will save money also. This is because low-weight babies need intensive care which is extremely costly. Therefore, members of the primary health care team (midwives and health visitors in particular) have an important role to play in helping pregnant women to give up smoking.

Smoking cessation programmes are prominent at present as the risk of illness and death decrease with each year after stopping smoking. Therefore, it is vital that during pregnancy, health education is given, not only for the health of the fetus but for the pregnant mother's own health. Support groups, acupuncture and hypnosis are being used to assist smokers to quit (Department of Health 1998).

Nicotine replacement therapy (NRT) is not advocated in the UK at present for pregnant women. A pregnancy quitline was launched in 1997 and is run by the charity 'Quit'. In the first year, it answered 3000 calls and agreed individual smoking cessation programmes. There is evidence that prenatal counselling involving at least 10 minutes person-to-person contact and the use of written materials can double the quit rates (Department of Health 1998). Support needs to continue after the birth to ensure that the mother doesn't start smoking again.

Perfusion involving the respiratory and cardiovascular system

The amount of oxygen and carbon dioxide that can be diffused and therefore exchanged is dependent on the amount of blood passing through the lungs. For this to occur we must have a pulmonary circulation (Fig. 5.9).

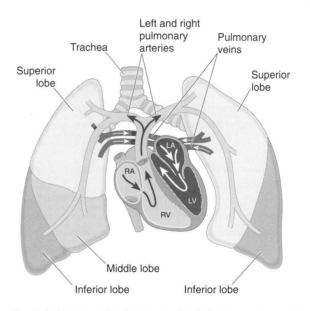

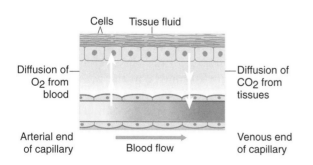

Fig. 5.8 Gaseous exchange of oxygen and carbon dioxide between capillaries and tissues (internal respiration) (from Waugh & Grant 2001, with permission).

Fig. 5.9 Heart and pulmonary circulation (from Waugh & Grant 2001, with permission).

You should have identified that the blood leaves the right side of the heart by the pulmonary artery (so named as, although carrying deoxygenated blood, it is taking blood to somewhere) to go to the lungs and then returns to the left side of the heart via four pulmonary veins (so called as taking blood away from somewhere, even though oxygenated now); check this in Figure 5.9. This results in a massive blood flow through the two systems at any time, as all the blood in the right ventricle goes to the lungs and all the blood in the lungs is returned to the left atrium. At rest, this is approximately 5 litres per minute and up to 25 litres per minute with maximum exertion (Waugh & Grant 2001).

Oxygen is transported mainly by the red blood cells and is linked to haemoglobin and is then called oxyhaemoglobin and gives blood its bright red colour when oxygen levels are high. However, when the oxygen leaves the red blood cell rendering the oxygen levels low, the deoxyhaemoglobin (deoxygenated haemoglobin) gives blood a purplish colour (Rutishauser 1994). Carbon dioxide is transported by reacting with several constituents of blood. At rest, the cells in the body use 250 ml of oxygen per minute and during exercise this can rise to 7500 ml. Two hundred ml of carbon dioxide are made when the body is at rest (Casey 2001).

1. Using your knowledge of the physiology of breathing, work out what happens to the breathing activities (short and long term) of the following individuals:

    a. A woman, aged 20, of average height, weighing 15 stones (95 kg), who decides to jog for 15 minutes a day as part of her new keep fit regime?
    b. A man, aged 50, who already undertakes regular aerobic exercise, three times a week by swimming, decides to start running 3 miles a day?

You may have decided that their breathing would be influenced by their age, weight and fitness levels. As muscles require more oxygen during physical exercise then, in a healthy adult, the respiratory rate will increase to provide this. Equally, as respiratory rates and pulse rates are linked then the pulse rate will also rise. The young woman is overweight and is new to exercise and therefore you would expect that her respiratory rate and pulse rate will increase quicker than the older man who is more used to exercise. When the body rests, then the respiratory and pulse rates will decrease. It may be that the older man's

respiratory and pulse rates return to normal quicker than the younger woman's.

Other factors need to be considered, such as the amount and effectiveness of the delivery of oxygen to the tissues, as this will also affect individuals' responses to lifestyle changes. Three factors determine the delivery of oxygen to the tissues: oxygen saturation, amount of haemoglobin in the bloodstream and how well it is transported around the body (Casey 2001).

Oxygen binds to haemoglobin molecules depending on the concentration of oxygen in the plasma and this is noted as PO_2. This figure is measured when taking arterial blood gases as a pressure in millimetres of mercury (mmHg). The amount of oxygen in the arterial blood depends on the amount entering the plasma as the blood passes through the lungs.

According to Casey (2001), at sea level, during inspiration, air is drawn in at a pressure of about 760 mmHg and this atmospheric air contains 21% oxygen. Through its passage to the alveoli, the air is warmed and humidified (water vapour pressure 47 mmHg) and this lowers the pressure of oxygen available to about 150 mmHg i.e. PO_2 of 150 mmHg (760 mmHg – 47 mmHg × 21%). This pressure is lowered further because of the dead space in the lungs where gaseous exchange doesn't take place (nose, trachea and bronchi). As blood entering the lungs has a PO_2 of 40 mmHg, diffusion occurs, thereby allowing oxygen to move from the air to the blood.

Changes occur when an individual experiences a change in altitude, for example athletes competing in other countries or climbers attempting to climb Mount Everest. For people who live in such places their breathing, lungs and red cells adapt to having less oxygen but for people who only visit for a short time problems can occur.

The inspired air pressure i.e. PO_2 at the top of Mount Everest is 42 mmHg (250 mmHg – 47 mmHg × 21%), with the PO_2 being 40 mmHg in the blood entering the lungs. Consequently, diffusion doesn't occur as the difference in the two pressures is not enough. The body would not be able to function properly as oxygen would not be entering the bloodstream and therefore would not be transported to the tissues. It is for this reason that individuals who climb at altitude may use oxygen (Casey 2001).

Oxygen can be used at different pressures: 24%, 28% or 40%. Using the same formula as above, it can be seen that any increase in oxygen pressures will increase the inspired air pressure i.e. PO_2 and therefore aid diffusion (Casey 2001). For 24% oxygen the inspired air pressure, i.e. PO_2 is 171 mmHg, for 28% it is 200 mmHg and for 40% it is 285 mmHg. As these are all considerably higher than the blood PO_2 of 40 mmHg then oxygen will be diffused into the bloodstream far more easily.

Arterial blood gas (ABG) samples are used to evaluate the partial pressures of oxygen and carbon dioxide in the blood and according to Coombs (2001), are commonly taken from acutely ill patients with respiratory and cardiac disease to assess their disorders. It is important to appreciate the physiological underpinnings of blood gas analysis and relate to changes that can occur in health as well as illness.

Normally the partial pressure of carbon dioxide (P_aCO_2) is 4.5–6 kPa (35–45 mmHg). Changes in people's breathing or ventilation affects the carbon dioxide levels, so by measuring the P_aCO_2 levels this will give an indication of the person's breathing and ventilation function. For example, in patients who are hyperventilating (breathing very fast and deep) large amounts of air are breathed in and out of the lungs. This lowers the amount of carbon dioxide and the P_aCO_2 level falls to below 4.5 kPa and causes respiratory alkalosis, which occurs when there is a fall in oxygen levels associated with high altitude (Coombs 2001). Anxiety may also cause people to hyperventilate and this can be treated by placing a paper bag over their nose and mouth and encouraging them to breathe in and out of the bag. This recycles the expired carbon dioxide so lowering the rate and depth of the respirations (Cornock 1996).

Respiratory acidosis arises when the person is hypoventilating (slow or shallow breathing) and so small amounts of air are breathed in and out of the lungs. This raises the amount of carbon dioxide and the P_aCO_2 level rises to above 6 kPa and causes respiratory acidosis, which can occur when there is an obstruction to the airways following inhalation of a foreign body (Coombs 2001). In this instance the obstruction needs to be removed to return respirations and blood gases to normal.

Normally, the partial pressure of oxygen (P_aO_2) is 8–12 kPa (60–90 mmHg) and measures the amount of oxygen dissolved in the blood. This level indicates the amount of oxygen which is potentially available to oxygenate the tissues. If the P_aO_2 levels fall below 8 kPa (hypoxaemia) then the cells are deprived of oxygen (hypoxia) and this can lead to cell damage and cell death. Hypoxaemia occurs following hypoventilation, obstructed airway and sometimes in older people.

Arterial blood gases can form part of an acutely ill patient's assessment alongside oxygen saturation levels. The oxygen saturation level (S_aO_2) can be measured by a pulse oximeter, using a finger probe, and is a useful monitoring device for evaluating the oxygen status of patients in a variety of clinical areas. It is important to remember that S_aO_2 measures the amount of oxygen being carried by haemoglobin in the arterial (oxygenated) blood but not the amount of oxygen that is delivered to the tissues. The oxygen saturation level should be 95% or more in a healthy adult (Casey 2001).

Other less invasive measurements can give useful information relating to respiratory function. Observing for cyanosis (blue–purple colour visible in nail beds, skin and mucous membranes, such as lips) is vital and this occurs when oxygen saturation levels fall below 70% and indicates that there is a large volume of haemoglobin which is poorly saturated and the oxygen levels are therefore low.

First aiders may be involved in situations where individuals have collapsed due to shock, circulatory and respiratory failure and as Roper et al (1996) point out they render help by using the mnemonic ABC: Airway (clear the airway), Breathing (give mouth-to-mouth resuscitation), and Circulation (carry out external cardiac compression). Finding individuals in a collapsed state, such as this, can be a frightening experience for onlookers, however there have been recent publicity and roadshows to teach the general public how to resuscitate people.

Another problem that individuals may experience in their everyday lives is that called the 'Flight or Fight' response which can help survival at times of extreme danger. The response to danger is to raise the respiration rate and depth, heart rate, blood pressure and blood flow to the muscles. This allows people to either run away from the danger or stand and fight off their attackers.

Emotional issues related to breathing (psychological factors)

Emotional events in life can affect breathing (Roper et al 1996). Consider the following exercise.

> **Exercise**
> 1. Observe individuals, when watching different programmes on TV, and identify the effect emotions have on their respirations, e.g. when happy, sad, grieving, anxious or frightened.
> 2. Ask a friend or colleague to observe your breathing whilst watching television programmes, a visit to the cinema or a sports event (making sure they do not make you aware of when they are doing this). Discuss your findings and theirs.

The actor's ability may have affected what you observed, but within your own family you may be able to confirm the associated changes in respiration. Roper et al (1996) identified that sadness and grieving can affect the rate and depth of breathing resulting in audible and visible activities such as sobbing and sighing. Also when individuals are frightened their respirations change and this can be noted by an initial indrawing and gasping respiration followed by an increase in breathing and pulse rates. Equally, pleasure and excitement result in raised breathing and respiratory rates. For some people, anxiety and panic attacks can result in marked changes in respiration.

West and Popkess-Vawter (1994) discuss classic literature from the 1960s which reports on the psychosocial aspects of breathlessness. For example, Dudley et al (1964), in West and Popkess-Vawter (1994), studied the effects of life stress, on pulmonary function, of individuals with normal and diseased lungs and concluded that psychological orientation was a major factor in the person's respiratory response to life events as changes in respiration rates during anger or anxiety were similar to respiratory changes during exercise.

Equally, Burns and Howell (1969), also cited in West and Popkess-Vawter (1994), studied chronic bronchitic patients who reported disproportionately severe breathlessness when compared with their lung function tests. Their level of breathlessness was found to be unrelated to the amount of exertion or their environment, but was related to their emotional status, where hyperventilation was associated with an emotionally distressing event.

West and Popkess-Vawter (1994) propose a holistic breathlessness model linking current life experiences (biological, psychological and social triggers) with antecedent conditions (perceived threat, past negative experiences, stress response, disease changes, fatigue and pulmonary congestion) which can then present with varying degrees of breathlessness, according to the individual's response.

Relaxation techniques and biofeedback can help individuals during periods of high anxiety or panic attacks and they should be encouraged to plan relaxation periods into their daily life. Biofeedback can also be used for individuals who suffer from migraine headaches, high or low blood pressure, epilepsy or even with paralysis. Biofeedback systems use electronic systems to measure stress and feed back the results in the form of a movement of a pen on graph paper or by the pitch of sound through earphones. Individuals can then practise using different techniques and compare the effects, such as being taught how to identify factors which trigger their problems, how to cope with these problems, how to change their lifestyles and how to gain self control. These techniques are a reminder that behaviour, thoughts and feelings can influence physical health and although they cannot cure disease they can help an individual. However for this to occur the individual must accept responsibility for their own health.

Practices, associated health beliefs and habits in different cultures related to breathing (sociocultural factors)

It is important that you consider the practices of individuals in relation to breathing. Most of the time, individuals are not aware of breathing until they have a problem, e.g. cough, choke, spit or sneeze. Coughing can be a sign of ill health (particularly cancer) if it is a nagging cough with hoarseness. The spread of disease through coughing, spitting and sneezing is well known, yet some individuals exhibit antisocial behaviour with regards to this, such as spitting on the pavement whilst walking along the street. It is obvious by observing onlookers, that this behaviour is perceived to be in poor taste. Tolerance to individuals polluting the air in social places warrants consideration, as does occupational practices and their effect on breathing and ill health.

Exercise
1. Identify links between various occupations and lung disease.
2. Tolerance of smoking in social places.
3. Differences in cultural attitudes to breathing habits.

There are numerous occupations linked to lung diseases. For example, long-term exposure to coal dust or cotton dust predisposes workers to lung disorders, such as pneumoconiosis and silicosis.

Another industrial disease, malignant mesothelioma, is linked to asbestos, which was used in the building industry in the 1960s and 1970s. Millar (2000) reports that experts estimate that over the next 35 years more than 250 000 people will die from this disease in Western Europe. The UK death rate is expected to be higher than any other European country, except The Netherlands with some 1750 dying from this disease. Men born between 1945 and 1950 and who worked as plumbers, gas fitters, carpenters and electricians, are at greatest risk. However, their family members are also at risk from secondary exposure via the asbestos fibres on their clothing. Millar (2000) reports on the recent development of a nurse-led project aimed at improving access to services and providing information on mesothelioma.

The general attitude to cigarette smoking in the early 20th century was that it relieved tension and produced no ill effects. However, it was noticed that lung cancer, rare before the 20th century, had dramatically increased and the link to lung cancer was made. Various measures have taken place since the 1960s in an attempt to limit smoking and the resultant diseases. Warnings on cigarette packets were introduced and all cigarette advertising was banned on television and radio.

The Hospital In-Patient Enquiry (OPCS 1985) reported that in a one in ten sample, 46 023 patients in England and Wales were suffering from respiratory illnesses and a further 5499 had lung cancer. The mortality rate, in 1986, for England and Wales for respiratory illness was found to be over 63 000 and a further 35 000 from lung cancer (OPCS 1986). Although the death rate in men from lung cancer was halved from 1971 to 1992, the death rate for women increased by 16% (Central Statistical Office 1995).

Smoking in public places has become less tolerated over the last few years and 'No smoking' sections in restaurants, theatres and on public transport have become commonplace. This is due to the risks to health, amongst nonsmokers, who are exposed to environmental tobacco smoke (Department of Health 1998), known as passive smoking, i.e. breathing in someone else's cigarette smoke. Statistics from the Department of Health (1998) show that passive smoking kills several hundreds of people every year in the UK from lung cancer and heart disease, could be responsible for a quarter of cot deaths every year in the UK and causes illness in several hundreds of people every year in the UK, such as asthma and glue ears in children.

Passive smoking has been linked to lung cancer for some time now. Roy Castle, an entertainer, is a classic example of a nonsmoking individual who died from lung cancer (Castle 1999). This may well have been because he breathed in cigarette smoke whilst entertaining in various clubs throughout the UK. Stanley (1999), one of five Roy Castle nurses in the UK, discusses the guilt, as relatives who smoke, express their possible role in lung cancer. He et al (1999) estimated that nonsmokers, exposed to passive smoking for a number of years, have a 25% increased risk of coronary heart disease and that exposure to smoke at home is more dangerous than exposure to smoke at work. Further details of the meta-analysis relating to this can be found on the Bandolier website http://www.jr2.ox.ac.uk/bandolier/booth/hliving/Passive.html

Nicotine is the chemical ingredient of tobacco, and smokers absorb small amounts of nicotine when they inhale. It is important to note that all forms of tobacco can cause cancer even though the effect of nicotine, on the nervous system, varies with individuals. It may serve as a stimulant by increasing the flow of adrenaline but in large doses may cause convulsions and death. Cigarette smoke causes constriction of the bronchus and eventually the airways become permanently narrowed and alveoli tissue is destroyed, which limits the lung area in which gaseous exchange can take place. Alveoli cannot be repaired once damaged but further damage can be prevented if the irritants are removed. Therefore, smoke and dust should be minimised at work and at home. Carbon monoxide in cigarette smoke binds with haemoglobin in the red blood cells and forms carboxyhaemoglobin and affects gaseous exchange resulting in lower oxygen levels throughout the body (Rutishauser 1994). It is estimated that individuals who are exposed to smoke have a 10–30% higher risk of developing lung cancer than nonsmokers who have not been exposed (Burgess 1994).

Cultural issues are linked to breathing habits in different ways. Deep breathing is a very effective method of relaxation and meditation is used by various cultures to enable individuals to experience total peace and self-empowerment. There are different forms of meditation which Buddhists use. However, all forms of meditation use concentration techniques, which allow thoughts to be slowed down and eventually stopped. When this occurs, the individual feels better and they are able to accomplish things in their daily life. Meditation may be achieved by concentrating on a picture or image or by using chanting or breathing control. Mindfulness is another form of meditation practised by Buddhists. It is based on their belief that whatever an individual focuses upon, they become. So, if they focus upon being happy then they become happy. Mindfulness and meditation are the two twin practices of Buddhist practice and involve controlling breathing.

Daily hygiene practices are fundamental to Japanese health beliefs and these relate to what is clean and dirty. According to Ohnuki-Tierney (1984), Japanese people use a face mask, similar to a surgical mask, when they go outside as this is classed as 'dirty' because this is where germs and pollution are located. Their rationale for this may be because the mask prevents the person from breathing in germs from the outside air or because it protects the sensitive membranes of the nose and throat from exposure to the cold air.

Japanese bathing is used as a means of cleansing the person before retiring to bed in the evening. However, this daily routine is discontinued once a person becomes ill, particularly with any of the respiratory illnesses. This is strictly enforced and a carer will decide when the person may resume bathing. Japanese consider that permission to resume bathing indicates recovery and they will bath themselves to cleanse themselves of the illness and mark a return to health.

Ohnuki-Tierney (1984), discusses the Japanese attitude to cancer which illustrates their philosophy in relation to life. They consider that the individual has no active role when they have cancer and the central role is that of fate and the person is totally passive, almost denying the existence of the disease rather than dealing with it. Family members will be informed of the disease but it may not be discussed with the sufferer. Cancer is the number one killer in Japan for people aged 30–69 and lung cancer accounts for 14.9% of these deaths. These cultural health beliefs will impact on a person's ability to deal with health and ill health.

Pollutants in the air and how these are related to breathing (environmental factors)

Atmospheric air is a mixture of gases (oxygen, nitrogen and carbon dioxide) and with each breath so much oxygen is inhaled and so much carbon dioxide is exhaled. Unfortunately, it also contains microorganisms and pollutants, such as sulphur dioxide, oxides of nitrogen and ozone. Microorganisms circulate in the atmosphere and can be inhaled into the respiratory tract giving, for example, the common cold. When a person sneezes, then these microorganisms can be recirculated and inhaled by another person. The same principle is involved in the spread of any infectious respiratory disease.

Exercise
1. Observe any public place where smoking is allowed.
2. Compare the atmosphere to an area where smoking is not allowed.
3. Consider the effect this would have on your lungs and your breathing.

You may have noticed that where smoking is allowed the air is not as clear and you may have difficulty seeing across the room. You may start to cough and notice your breathing. Long exposure in this type of environment may be harmful to you. Even in your own home there are dangers from other pollutants such as carbon monoxide poisoning. Carbon monoxide (CO) poisoning is, according to Thomson et al (1992) the commonest cause of fatal poisoning in the UK. Carbon monoxide binds to haemoglobin and forms carboxyhaemoglobin relatively easily, and prevents the oxygen from binding with the haemoglobin. If sufficient amounts of carbon monoxide are inhaled, the person will suffer from oxygen deficiency and yet maintain rosy features as carboxyhaemoglobin is bright red and therefore problems may be severe before treatment is commenced.

Carbon monoxide poisoning is due to either accidental poisoning from house fires, domestic appliances, central heating boilers or nonaccidental causes of self-poisoning and suicide attempts, usually involving car exhaust fumes which are diverted into the car. Durmaz et al (1999) identify that in the 82 patients, treated with hyperbaric oxygen therapy, in a 5-year period, 47 (57%) had suffered carbon monoxide poisoning as a result of self-poisoning with the remaining 35 (43%) mainly being poisoned through house fires and faulty gas appliances.

The Committee on the Medical Effects of Air Pollutants (COMEAP) concluded, after reading a report by the Institute for Environment and Health on the indoor air quality in the home with particular emphasis on carbon monoxide, that in homes where equipment malfunctions, there is a serious risk of severe illness and death may occur from carbon monoxide poisoning. Their advice is that all appliances capable of producing carbon monoxide must be installed properly and maintained regularly. The use of carbon monoxide monitors may have a useful role in identifying excess levels of carbon monoxide indoors, so that faults can be rectified before health is damaged, but their value is limited (Department of Health 1999a).

Smog is a major environmental problem facing the world today. It is a mixture of smoke particles and fog and it reduces natural visibility, irritates the respiratory tract and eyes. There are three types of air pollutants, according to the Advisory Group on the Medical Aspects of Air Pollution Episodes (Department of Health 1995a). These are summer smog (ozone mainly), vehicle smog (mainly oxides of nitrogen) and winter smog (mainly sulphur dioxide and some oxides of nitrogen).

There is some evidence that lung function is reduced in healthy individuals when smog pollutes the atmosphere. There is no evidence in the UK that smog causes ill health in well people, but researchers in the USA believe they have supportive findings to link the exposure of ozone to asthma in children (Miller 2001). However, there is some evidence that air pollution can produce adverse health problems in people with chronic respiratory and cardiac diseases. Air pollutants are not seen by COMEAP as responsible for the initiation and provocation of asthma and the increase in asthma is considered to be unlikely due to air pollution (Department of Health 1995b).

COMEAP note the findings of a UK study by Poloniecki et al (1997), which reports that there is a significant relationship between the incidence of myocardial infarction and air pollutants (Department of Health 1999b). This relationship was identified by analysing the number of hospital admissions with myocardial infarctions in London and the previous day's air pollution levels. Poloniecki et al (1997) suggest that 6000 patients, who suffer myocardial infarctions per year, may be related to exposure to air pollutants. This is seen as an important finding and further research is needed into this matter.

Department of Health (2001a), reported on the long-term effects of particles on mortality in the UK, after two studies in the United States had shown that those living in more polluted cities die sooner than those living in less polluted areas and that there was a positive association with death from lung cancer and cardiopulmonary diseases. It was concluded that, although there were many uncertainties, it was likely that there was an association between long-term exposure to particles and mortality in the UK.

To help reduce problems, smog levels, particularly ozone levels, are included in weather forecasts to alert the general public of this risk and individuals who are sensitive to ozone should limit outdoor exercise during the latter part of the day. Prevention of smog is also done by controlling smoke from chimneys, furnaces, industrial plants and noxious emissions from cars. Recent changes in the internal combustion engines and the use of catalytic converters have made these emissions lower in an attempt to lower the risk of smog (Department of Health 1991, 1998). Fine dust particles, suspended in the air, contain pollen, silica, animal fibres, bacteria and moulds. In cities these dust particles also contains smoke particles from industry and can cause a serious pollution problem and may cause silicosis. There is a need to use filters to obtain dust-free air.

A relatively new hazard is that of *Legionella pneumonophila,* a bacterium which causes infection and inflammation of the lung tissue. The bacteria are found in stagnant water in water tanks, shower heads and air conditioning systems so the source of the bacteria has often been linked to hotels and hospitals. It is known to transmit Legionnaires disease which produces symptoms of bronchopneumonia, complicated by gastrointestinal problems, headache, confusion and renal failure (Waugh & Grant 2001). The figures for 1999 identified 202 people had contracted Legionnaires disease, 151 men, 51 women, resulting in 30 deaths compared with 182 cases with 23 deaths in 1980 (http://www.phls.co.uk/topics).

Policies, laws and economics related to breathing (politicoeconomic factors)

Roper et al (2000, p. 119) clearly identify that political, economic and social issues are 'major determinants of health' and that health is not solely the concern of the National Health Service (NHS) but relates to public policies. The economic state of a country affects the living conditions, which in turn, affect the health and illness of that population.

The Public Health Act of 1875 heralded major reforms in the UK, with emphasis on sanitation and water supplies. Combined with this, as Roper et al (2000) discuss, there was a general improvement in the country's economy and as a result, living conditions improved. The general health of the population improved and diseases, which in those days were killers, were seen to decline prior to the implementation of preventative and curative care.

Today, preventative health measures are needed to promote health and prevent illness. As health care costs increase then the need for preventative health care is increased. For example, immunisation is now used to prevent respiratory diseases such as tuberculosis and influenza (flu). Every autumn, a national campaign is run, offering influenza (flu) vaccinations to protect people who are at risk of serious illness should they catch the flu. This includes everyone who is 65 years old and above and those who already suffer from chronic diseases, such as asthma, diabetes and heart disease. The vaccinations are given in GP's surgeries usually, but NHS Trusts also provide this service to their workers.

Environmental issues link to this factor also in relation to air pollutants as previously discussed, e.g. policies in relation to the purity of air, lessening the emissions from cars and industry and the banning of certain substances, e.g. asbestos. Poorer industrial towns have a higher than expected death rate compared to more affluent areas linking the effects of social factors and illness. For example, the Central Statistical Office (1994), found that mortality rates in 1992 in the north-west were 143 compared to 88 in East Anglia. It would appear that the poorer a person is, the more likely they are to die from respiratory disease (Walsh 1997).

> **Exercise**
> 1. Look on the Department of Health website
>   http://www.doh.gov.uk
> 2. Identify the current health policies relating to breathing and smoking up to 2002.

You should have found numerous links to breathing, smoking and related health problems on this website. Within the remit of public health and clinical quality, there are at least five areas that relate to breathing, e.g. air pollution, flu and pertussis (whooping cough) vaccines, smoking and tuberculosis. Information about various advisory committees is also included, such as SCOTH (Scientific Committee on Tobacco and Health) and COMEAP (Committee on the Medical Effects of Air Pollutants).

The NHS Plan published in 2000 by the Department of Health, identified the need for a major expansion in smoking cessation programmes. As a result, 26 Health Action Zones (HAZ) are to be established in England in areas of deprivation and poor health to tackle inequalities and provide services. Smoking cessation services were launched in 1999/2000, with £53 million being made available for these services plus extra for nicotine replacement therapy.

The results for 1999/2000 were published, as a Statistical Bulletin on 22nd February 2001 by the Department of Health (20001b) (http.//www.doh.gov.uk/public/sb0105.htm). This showed that 14 600 people had set a quit date through these services in HAZs and 5800 (39%) had successfully quit smoking at the 4-week follow up.

Silagy and Stead (2001) reviewed 34 trials, conducted between 1972 and 1999, involving 27 000 smokers and concluded that simple advice from physicians had a small effect on smoking cessation rates. Potential benefits were also found by Rice and Stead (2001), when 15 studies were reviewed to assess the effectiveness of nursing interventions in relation to smoking cessation. The odds of quitting were significantly increased when smoking cessation advice and counselling were given by nurses. Further research is needed to follow individuals who have ceased smoking and whether this has reduced their risk of developing lung cancer.

A significant White Paper on tobacco was published in 1998 entitled *Smoking Kills*. This was the first ever White Paper on smoking in the UK and it set out three targets in relation to smoking, as set out below.

Target 1. Reduce smoking amongst children from 13% to 11% or less by the year 2005 and to 9% by 2010.

Target 2. Reduce smoking amongst adults in all social classes from 28% to 26% or less by the year 2005 and to 24% by 2010.

Target 3. Reduce smoking amongst pregnant women from 23% to 18% or less by the year 2005 and to 15% by 2010.

> **Exercise**
> 1. Review these three targets and consider what action will be needed to meet these from the political perspective.
> 2. Discuss with colleagues the implications of these targets for health education initiatives.

You may have read the government's strategy in relation to these targets in which a need for a wide and integrated range of measures is identified (Department of Health 1998). A major issue is to help protect young people by helping them to quit and to prevent them from starting smoking. As a result, £60 million in England alone, will be invested to help smokers to quit, with a £50 million mass media publicity campaign planned to shift attitudes and change behaviour, over the next 3 years. Certainly this campaign will focus on priority groups, such as young people, adults and pregnant women.

One week's nicotine replacement therapy will be made available free to those who are less able to purchase these. A European ban on all tobacco advertising and sponsorship will be in place by July 2006 with earlier target dates for certain aspects. Smoking will be reduced in public places and a new Charter for Smoking in the licensed trade and a new Approved Code of Practice on smoking at work has been agreed. The tax increase on tobacco products will remain above inflation in an attempt to deter people from smoking due to the cost and stricter measures will be used to cut tobacco smuggling.

Health care professionals have an important role to play in ensuring that these targets are met in relation to health promotion activities, being nonsmoking role models and supporting individuals through smoking cessation programmes. It is recognised that some health care professionals smoke but these individuals can still play a role in ensuring that these targets are met and maybe take some personal responsibility in this and work with smokers through a smoking cessation programme.

An example of how legislation impacts upon health in breathing is in relation to the Health and Safety at Work Act (1974) which is directed at protecting the public. Within this Act the employer has a duty to provide a safe working environment and to inform and instruct employees about health risks and the precautions to be taken. Economic factors are a major influence in relation to breathing from the politicians and individual's perpective. Smoking costs the NHS £1.7 billion pounds per year. But how much does it cost the individual in monetary terms.

Exercise

1. Working on the basis of cigarettes costing £4 for a packet of 20, work out how much it will cost an individual who smokes:

   a. 10 cigarettes a day for 1 week, 1 month, 1 year, 15 years, 30 years and 50 years.

   b. 20 cigarettes a day for 1 week, 1 month, 1 year, 15 years, 30 years and 50 years.

You may be shocked at the cost of this activity. At 10 cigarettes a day, the cost in monetary terms is £14 a week, £56 a month, £728 a year, £10,920 for 15 years, £21,840 for 30 years and £36,400 for 50 years. For someone smoking 20 cigarettes a day, then these figures are obviously doubled, giving £28 a week, £112 a month, £1,344 a year, £20,160 in 15 years, £40,320 in 30 years and £67,200 in 50 years.

The cost of nicotine replacement therapy is between £10 to £20 a week and with a course lasting about 10 weeks, it amounts to costing between £100 and £200 to quit smoking. Surely an incentive of monetary gains is worthy of advertising.

Conclusion

The framework of the model of living has been used to demonstrate how the model can be used to guide your understanding of health and everyday life in relation to the activity of breathing (Fig. 5.10). From this it is hoped that you have been able to engage in the exercises and can appreciate the complexity of the model and the interrelativeness of the other Activities of Living. The final two exercises will concentrate on the interrelatedness with other activities and the factors which affect breathing specifically through the use of mini case studies to demonstrate how individuality in living occurs.

Exercise

1. Read through the family scenario in Case study 5.1 and consider how their activity of breathing may affect each other and the other Activities of Living.

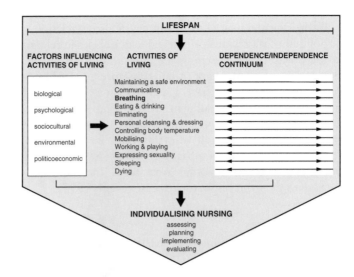

Fig. 5.10 Activity of breathing within the model for nursing (from Roper et al 1996, with permission).

Effect of smoking on ALs

John is 60 years old and has smoked 20 cigarettes for 40 years and has worked in the building trade for most of his life. His wife does not smoke now but she has done in the past. They have two children, aged 35 and 28. The elder son has two children and they visit their grandparents regularly, as well as going abroad on holiday as a family. Their youngest daughter, who also smokes, is expecting her first child.

You may have considered the following points:

- *Maintaining a safe environment* – safety issues relating to fire hazards in the home:
  - effects of stress in relation to smoking and quitting
  - air pollution and passive smoking
  - immunisation of grandchildren
- *Communicating* – smell of cigarettes on breath and teeth affected
- *Eating and drinking* – food and taste affected by smoking
- *Eliminating* – predisposition to cancers
- *Mobilising* – difficulty with walking, running etc., if suffer from shortness of breath
- *Expressing sexuality* – fetal damage possible
- *Maintaining body temperature* – predisposition to chest infections as noted by pyrexia
- *Working and playing* – social activities curtailed by nonsmoking areas:
  - cost of smoking
  - building work itself with dust and possible asbestos exposure
  - holidays abroad and risk of respiratory diseases
- *Sleep and rest* – coughing may affect sleep patterns
- *Dying* – predisposition to lung cancer for all the family.

Exercise

1. Read through the scenario in Case study 5.2 and consider how the activity of breathing is affected by biological, psychological, sociocultural, environmental and politicoeconomic factors.

Breathing and factors affecting health

A 20-year-old young man, who suffers from asthma, is taken ill at a disco. He takes his inhaler but unfortunately because he panics he is unable to control his breathing.

You may have considered the following:

- *Biological factors* – effect of asthma on lung tissue, effect on breathing, effects of smoke on lungs
- *Psychological factors* – anxiety, not using inhaler properly leading to panic state and hyperventilation
- *Sociocultural factors* – peer pressure to smoke and visit discos, macho male image
- *Environmental factors* – smoky environment
- *Politicoeconomic factors* – cost of smoking for a student.

Summary points

1. Breathing is affected by all the factors.
2. Breathing can affect all of the other Activities of Living.
3. Smoking is one of the major contributors to breathing problems.
4. Pollutants are a major problem worldwide which can cause respiratory problems.

THE MODEL FOR NURSING

Using the model for nursing to individualise nursing for the activity of breathing

Introduction

This part of the chapter will link the components of the model of living (lifespan, dependency/independency and factors affecting breathing) with the model for nursing in health and ill health states in relation to breathing. Exercises, mini case scenarios and one major case scenario will be used to allow you to apply the knowledge gained from the model of living section. The application of the model for nursing is based upon the integration of the model of living components and the four stages of the nursing process, according to Roper et al (1996), as shown in Figure 5.10. (See Chapter 1 for further details relating to the nursing process, i.e. assessing the individual, planning nursing activities, implementation of care and evaluation of care planned and given.) The initial stage of this process, i.e. assessment, begins with the point of contact of the nurse and the patient and is the start of the nurse–patient relationship. The aim of the assessment stage in relation to breathing is to collect information about how the individual relates to this Activity of Living when they are well and when they are ill.

Breathing in health

In order to do this assessment, all the other aspects of the model should be integrated into the breathing Activity of Living as shown in Box 5.2.

Box 5.2 Summary of the model for nursing with the activity of breathing – in health

Life span
- Consider effect of age on breathing, pulse rate, blood pressure.

Dependence
- Dependency is linked to lifespan and ill health, e.g. infection, congenital, trauma, paralysis.

Independence
- Independence linked to health.

Factors affecting breathing
Biological
- Degree of physical activity.
- Body's physiological responses to stressors.
- Intact respiratory system to enable effective internal and external respiration.
- Intact circulatory, lymphatic and nervous system to ensure that bodily systems benefit from the actions of the respiratory system.

- Noted by observations of normal breathing: rate, depth, rhythm, sound, patterns.
- Note any abnormal breathing: cough, wheeze, sputum produced, exposure to pollutants.

Psychological
- Effects of emotional state on breathing such as crying, laughing, anxiety, panic, fear.

Sociocultural
- Religious practices related to bathing/meditation/breathing control.
- Expectoration of sputum and coughing habits.

Environmental
- Exposure to microorganisms.
- Exposure to air pollutants at home, work, travelling.

Politicoeconomic
- Mechanisms to limit smoking related diseases and air pollutant diseases.

This Activity of Living in health is complex and the nurse needs to be aware of the normal health states of individuals before considering the activity of breathing in ill health. You will need to be able to integrate this information in each stage of the nursing process to identify individual patient needs and problems.

Breathing in ill health

The components of the model will be used to show you how a variety of ill health issues affect the activity of breathing.

Exercise
1. Using the components of the model (lifespan, dependency–independency continuum, factors affecting health – physical/biological, psychological, sociocultural, environmental, politicoeconomic) and your clinical experience to date, consider what illnesses patients may have in relation to breathing.
2. Check Box 5.3 for some examples.

Reflect on these conditions and identify your learning needs following this exercise. It may be useful for you to discuss your learning needs with a qualified nurse and formulate action plans to address them.

Assessing the individual

The aim of this section related to assessing an individual, in relation to breathing, is to demonstrate how you can utilise the components of the model of living to carry out the following three phases involved in assessment:

1. Collection of data when taking a nursing history in relation to the activity of breathing and other related activities.
2. Interpretation of data collected to assess the degree of alteration in the activity of breathing and the effect on other Activities of Living.
3. Identification of individuals' actual and potential problems related to the activity of breathing and other related activities.

It is noted that assessment is a continuous activity but a thorough initial assessment is vital and this chapter will describe how the components of the model can be integrated to support the assessment process. (For further details relating to assessment refer to Chapter 1.)

Collection of data when taking a nursing history in relation to the activity of breathing and other related activities

The assessment stage is vital, as all the other stages of individualising nursing are dependent upon it. Therefore, it is important to plan this activity and consider what may affect the collection of data, their interpretation and the identification of patients' problems.

Exercise
1. Consider that you have been asked to assess a patient who has been admitted to your clinical area with severe breathlessness.
2. Identify what physical, psychological, sociocultural, environmental and politicoeconomic factors may influence the collection of the data required.

Box 5.3 Summary of the model for nursing with the activity of breathing – ill health

Life span
- Congenital abnormalities
- Childhood, e.g. asthma, bronchiolitis
- Adult, e.g. chest trauma, tumours
- Older person, e.g. range of illnesses as below

Dependence/independence
- Breathing difficulties will affect many of the other Activities of Living and therefore the individual may become dependent on others, e.g. difficulties with mobilising due to dyspnoea

Factors affecting breathing

1. Biological
- a. Damage to respiratory tract
  - Airway obstruction e.g. chronic obstructive pulmonary/airways disease, emphysema, asthma, chronic bronchitis
  - Allergic reaction e.g. bronchial asthma
  - Infection e.g. pneumonia, pleurisy
  - Trauma e.g. chest injuries, flail chest, fractured ribs, haemothorax
  - Tumours e.g. benign, primary bronchogenic carcinomas, metastatic tumours
  - Blood flow obstruction e.g. pulmonary embolism in pulmonary capillaries

- b. Damage to cardiovascular tract
  - Congestion e.g. cor pulmonale, congestive cardiac failure, pulmonary oedema
  - Blood flow obstruction to myocardium e.g. myocardial infarction
  - Lack of oxygen in blood e.g. iron deficiency anaemia
- c. Damage to nervous tract
  - Respiratory muscle paralysis e.g. poliomyelitis, Guillain–Barré syndrome
  - Brain/spinal cord damage e.g. coma/head injuries

2. Psychological
  - Link with stress and anxiety e.g. asthma

3. Sociocultural
  - Cultural differences e.g. pulmonary tuberculosis
  - Smoking habits (active/passive) e.g. lung cancer

4. Environmental
  - Pollens/irritants e.g. hayfever, asthma
  - Smoking e.g. lung cancer
  - Inhalation of dust e.g. silicosis, asbestosis
  - Damp/overcrowding poor living conditions e.g. bronchial asthma, pulmonary tuberculosis

Box 5.4 Factors influencing activity of breathing

Physical
- Actual physical state of breathing as they may be unable to talk due to severe breathlessness, coughing or wheezing.
- May be in pain which will affect their ability to communicate.

Psychological
- Actual mental state due to oxygen transport being affected so may be hypoxic.
- Actual emotional state due to fear and anxiety relating to dying, may feel sense of shame.
- Actual knowledge of disease and past experiences.

Sociocultural
- Different social/cultural backgrounds of patient and nurse which may affect their ability to communicate.
- Level of interpersonal skills of the patient and the nurse.
- Presence, attitudes and reactions of others.

Environmental
- Ward environment noisy and not very private causing distractions and repetition of answers.

Politicoeconomic
- Time to conduct the interview.

You may wish to refer to Box 5.4 to check these factors and consider how you can minimise the influence these factors may have.

Reflect on how you can ensure that the collection of data is accurate and how these factors can be minimised so as not to influence the information collected. As noted, there are many factors that may affect the collection of the data and therefore you will need to use a variety of skills when collecting data. The following exercise will enable you to consider the skills needed.

Exercise
1. What skills will you need to develop to enable you to obtain a comprehensive nursing history from a breathless patient?
2. Check Box 5.5 with regards to these skills.
3. Reflect on your abilities in these skills. Consider which of these skills you believe you have mastered. Then identify the skills which you may need to improve upon and consider how you can do this.
4. Discuss this with your mentor or preceptor in practice and write an action plan for this learning need.

Box 5.5　Assessment skills – AL breathing

Interviewing skills
- Asking open and closed questions as appropriate so as not to tire the individual.
- Explain issues in lay terms and check understanding.
- Use of silence to allow individual to rest or think.
- Prioritise questions.
- Involve relatives.

Observation skills
- Verbal and nonverbal cues.
- Physical signs, e.g. pulse rate, respiratory rate, peak flow, pulse oximetry.
- Psychological cues, e.g. anxiety.

Listening skills
- Therapeutic relationship skills.
- Use own body language appropriately.

Having identified that various factors may affect your ability to collect information and that a variety of skills are equally required, it may be useful to consider what data you need to collect specifically and what purpose these data will be used for.

Exercise
1. Reflect upon a recent admission you have been involved with and identify potential questions that would help you collect specific data.
2. You may wish to check Box 5.6 for possible questions.

You may need to reflect on how you feel about asking these questions and how you would ask these questions in a conversational manner. You then need to consider specific questions which would be needed for patients with specific ill health issues related to breathing. The following exercise will allow you to consider additional questions relevant to three different ill health breathing problems. You are required to read the mini case studies in Box 5.7 to complete this exercise.

Box 5.7　Mini case studies

a. A 45-year-old builder, who has fallen at work, is complaining of severe right-sided chest pain. A fractured rib is suspected. The patient has been admitted to the Accident and Emergency Department.

b. A 70-year-old Asian man, with suspected pulmonary tuberculosis (TB), complains of feeling tired, night sweats, loss of weight and is coughing and expectorating sputum throughout the interview, following admission to a medical admissions unit.

c. An 18-year-old female, new university student, who has asthma is reporting to a practice nurse for a review of her medications and life style.

Exercise
1. Identify specific questions relating to the mini case studies in Box 5.7 with specific ill health breathing problems.

Box 5.6　Assessment questions – AL breathing

Life span and independence
- Does the individual breathe normally in relation to the expectations of the time of the life span?

Dependence
- Has the individual experienced any difficulties with breathing in the past or do they have a long-standing breathing difficulty?
- How has the individual coped with these difficulties experienced with breathing?
- How is the individual coping with these breathing difficulties?
- Could the individual experience difficulties with breathing in the future?

Factors affecting breathing
Physical
- What specific difficulties is the individual experiencing and what are the causes?
- What specific abnormalities are noted in the person's breathing pattern or habit?

- What other Activities of Living affect the individual's breathing difficulties?
- What effect does the individual's breathing difficulties have on the other Activities of Living?

Psychological
- What emotional responses affect breathing?
- What information or advice is required now or in the future to aid breathing and promote independence?

Sociocultural
- What are the individual's beliefs and attitudes to coughing, spitting and smoking?

Environmental
- What factors may alter/affect the individual's breathing at home, work and hospital?

Politicoeconomic
- What information and resources does the individual have or need, to assist in coping with any breathing difficulties to aid independence?

Here are some potential specific questions.

Scenario A questions

- When did the fall occur?
- Where is the pain specifically?
- What is the type of pain?
- When is the pain worse – on breathing in or out?
- What helps the pain?
- Have the problems/difficulties gotten worse?

Scenario B questions

- When did all the problems start?
- What type of cough does the individual have?
- Is there any sputum being expectorated?
- What colour and consistency is it?
- How difficult is it to expectorate?
- When is the cough the worst – day, night, with exercise?
- How long do you normally sleep for and how long do you sleep now?
- How much weight have you lost?
- What is your appetite like?
- Why are you not eating as well as before?
- What effect does coughing have on you?

Scenario C questions

- How effective is your present medication?
- When and how do you use your inhalers?
- Have you experienced any changes in breathing habits?
- Have you noticed any increase in wheezing, choking and coughing?
- How has your lifestyle changed now you are at university?
- Have you experienced problems with smoky atmospheres, stress, etc?
- How do you cope with your breathing problem in public?

It is impossible to cover all adult health problems and their associated breathing difficulties in this chapter but it is important for you to consider that the objective is to collect information to identify:

- the individual's normal habits when they are well
- whether there are any difficulties now in relation to their independence in breathing
- previous coping strategies with breathing and associated Activities of Living specific problems now.

However, there are common difficulties experienced by individuals with breathing problems such as:

- changes in rate, depth, rhythm of breathing
- marked changes in breathing habit (dyspnoea and wheezing)
- coughing
- production of abnormal secretions (sputum and haemoptysis)
- respiratory pain.

It is useful for you to consider how each of these difficulties can be assessed and what observations would be required.

Changes in rate, depth and rhythm of breathing

Mallik et al (1998, p. 199), state that it is 'relatively simple for a nurse to assess breathing by observing the rate, depth and rhythm of respiration' and these will give a basic indicator of respiratory function. Observations should be taken on admission, pre- and postoperatively, monitoring the patient's condition following invasive procedures and with patients who have respiratory, cardiovascular and neurological problems.

As noted previously the normal respiratory rate is 12–18 times per minute in usually fit adults and is called eupnoea. A rapid rate (tachypnoea) may indicate increased activity, anxiety, pain, pyrexia, shock or obstructed airway. Slow breathing (bradypnoea) may indicate sleep, head injury, brain tumours, hypothermia or depression of respiratory centre by drugs, e.g. opioids. Apnoea is the absence of breathing for at least 10 seconds and can occur in 'sleep apnoea' and causes snoring by a brief obstruction of the upper airways or can be the reason for 'cot deaths' (Walsh 1997).

The depth of respiration depends on the amount of air inhaled and can be observed by noting the movement of the chest wall during inspiration and is described as normal, shallow or deep. Observation of the chest movements is important as the thorax is usually symmetrical and breathing should be effortless. However, abnormal chest movements can be seen when an injury results in a flail chest. A flail chest occurs when several successive ribs are fractured and become dissociated from the rest of the rib cage which presents with breathing which is known as paradoxical. On inhalation, the rib cage expands and air is sucked in and the dissociated ribs are also drawn in. On exhalation, the rib cage contracts to expel the air and the dissociated ribs are also forced out (Edmond 2000). Peak flow meter or spirometer will give a more objective measurement of the depth of respirations.

Normally, adults have a regular breathing rhythm or pattern and their breathing is effortless, even, regular and automatic but it can become irregular when the respiratory centre is affected or the person has respiratory problems. Some of these are noted in the next section.

Marked changes in breathing habit (dyspnoea and wheezing)

It is, according to Walsh (1997), important to identify when the person becomes breathless and the effect this has on their normal activities including their sleep patterns. It is useful to listen to the person talking and assess whether it is jerky, with short phrases being used with an apparent effort or audible, effortless and clear. Another useful area to assess is the coping strategies they use to minimise their problems, such as pursed lips respirations.

Dyspnoea or shortness of breath or difficulty with breathing is accompanied by the use of accessory muscles of respiration, e.g. nostrils flaring and shoulder girdle raised, anxiety, restlessness and perspiring. This is a very distressing symptom but does indicate that the body is attempting to compensate by conveying more oxygen to the tissues. Orthopnoea is when the person experiences dyspnoea when lying down but is relieved when sitting up and is often found in patients who have heart failure. Another form of dyspnoea is that called paroxysmal nocturnal dyspnoea which occurs in patients with heart failure and pulmonary oedema and is characterised by sudden breathlessness at night.

Cheynes–Stokes respirations can occur as death approaches and are characterised by a cyclical pattern of a few seconds of apnoea (up to 20 seconds), followed by increase in rate and depth to a peak intensity followed by a period of apnoea again. Kussmaul's respirations, associated with pneumonia, involve an increase in the rate and depth with panting and grunting expirations (Jamieson et al 1992).

Breathing is usually silent so it is important to listen for breath sounds. Wheezing or rhonci occurs when whistling or musical sounds are heard which are associated with spasm of the bronchi and occur on expiration and are common in people with asthma and chronic bronchitis. Wheezing may also occur in response to exercise and inhalation of toxic substances. Severe bronchospasm is life threatening as the size of the bronchi is reduced and secretions are retained which become infected. Another distinctive noise is a harsh, high-pitched sound on inspiration, known as a stridor and is caused by an obstruction in the larynx, this again is life threatening.

Coughing

According to Walsh (1997), coughing is a frequently encountered problem and is when a sudden expulsive expiration is used to clear irritants from air passages. The nurse needs to note the presence, frequency, depth, nature and sound of a cough. Coughs may be described as hard, racking, croupy, hacking, shallow, deep, rattling, with a whooping sound. It may be worse in the morning or associated with exercise. It should be noted what effect the coughing has on the person, e.g. tired, not able to talk, sleepless nights or not able to carry out normal Activities of Living. It may be accompanied by sputum and this should be expectorated (coughed out) to prevent its accumulation within the lungs. A 'dry' cough has little sputum whereas a 'loose' cough is associated with sputum production.

Production of abnormal secretions (sputum and haemoptysis)

According to Walsh (1997), adults usually produce 100 ml of mucus a day. However, this is increased when the air passages are irritated and is then known as sputum and may result in a change of amount, colour, consistency and odour. The amount may need to be measured to show the effect of the disease or treatments. The colour must be noted as this may indicate an infection if purulent and green or if blood stained (called haemoptysis) which is found in inflammatory conditions (tuberculosis or pneumonia) that cause erosion of tissues and blood vessels, or lung cancer. Haemoptysis is very frightening for the patient and anyone else in the vicinity. It is also necessary to observe the consistency of the sputum as it may be watery or frothy (long-term respiratory conditions and/or cardiac problems as well), purulent (infections) or tenacious or thick (acute respiratory problems). Malodorous sputum, as noted by Roper et al (1996) is associated with infectious respiratory diseases and foul-smelling sputum can be expectorated in large quantities. Specimens of sputum can be collected and laboratory analysis of bacteriological culture of micro-organisms can aid the diagnosis of respiratory and cardio-vascular problems. As pathogens may be present in sputum, meticulous hand washing is needed to limit the cross-infection risk.

Respiratory pain

Pain in any part of the body can, as Roper et al (1996) point out, cause alterations in breathing. In relation to breathing difficulties, pain can be linked to poststernal pain and associated with coughing (usually inflamed trachea) or sharp, stabbing pain worsened by deep breathing and coughing (usually inflammation of the pleura or trauma). Therefore it is important to note if pain is associated with breathing activities or coughing, the nature, type, duration, severity of the pain and the strategies used to minimise the pain.

Interpretation of data collected

Once the data have been collected you need to utilise your knowledge and decision-making skills to interpret the information prior to the identification of the individual's actual and potential problems. Using the assessment questions outlined in Box 5.6 you need to consider the information that you may gather from Case study 5.3 by considering the components of the model.

Case study 5.3

Tom Jackson

Tom Jackson, a 78-year-old widower has been admitted to the elderly assessment ward following an episode of severe breathlessness. He is a retired mill worker and has been treated by his GP for a chronic chest condition with inhalers and tablets. He says that he is a bit confused with the inhalers and tablets. He lives alone in a terraced house since the death of his wife some 12 months ago. The house is rather damp and is in need of some repairs and modernisation as he only has coal fires in the downstairs rooms. His only daughter lives a few miles away and visits once or twice a week with his two grandchildren.

Case study 5.3 *(continued)*

He smokes some 10–15 cigarettes a day even though he is rather wheezy and his coughing keeps him awake at night. He used to enjoy a visit to the local pub but finds the walking too troublesome now as even going from room to room is difficult at times. He says that he has lost some weight since his wife died as he cannot shop or cook very well. His daughter does bring prepared meals with her when she visits but he prefers plain food so doesn't always eat them.

Over the last few days, he has felt too tired to shave himself or wash his hair. He has to stop many times during the interview to rest and cough. You note that his respirations are rapid and that he has a loose cough and is expectorating some sputum.

Exercise

1. Using the assessment questions found in Box 5.6 consider the possible responses in relation to Tom Jackson.
2. Consider the factors which may have led to Tom's health breakdown.
3. Identify the effect on other Activities of Living with the main case scenario.
4. Check your answers with those in Box 5.8.

From this exercise it can be seen that Mr Jackson has:

- an acute breathing problem affecting other Activities of Living
- a long-standing chronic breathing problem
- a knowledge deficit in relation to smoking
- an environmental problem regarding a damp and cold house
- alterations in social factors since bereavement and acute illness.

Following this interpretation of the data, it is then necessary to complete the final stage of the assessment process and identify actual and potential problems.

Identification of actual and potential problems

Actual breathing problems will be specific to the actual health problems but common problems have already been identified in relation to:

- changes in rate, depth, rhythm of breathing (see p. 141)
- marked changes in breathing habit – dyspnoea and wheezing (see pp. 141–142)
- coughing (see p. 142)
- production of abnormal secretions – sputum and haemoptysis (see p. 142)
- respiratory pain (see p. 142).

Box 5.8 Factors contributing to health breakdown

1. **Factors leading to this health breakdown**
   - Age possibly may be a factor
   - Dependency continuum altering now as dependent on daughter for some meals and company
   - Physical – long-standing chronic chest condition/smoking/mill worker
   - Psychological – bereavement
   - Sociocultural – losing social contact as not able to walk too far.
   - Environmental – damp terraced house, no heating in bedroom, fumes from coal fires, previous exposure to dust in mills.
   - Politicoeconomic – pension rates affected by death of wife, cost of food/heating

2. **Other activities being affected**
   - Maintaining safe environment – due to not taking his medication properly
   - Communicating – having to rest during interview as breathless, wheezing and tired
   - Eating and drinking – following bereavement and not being able to walk far, affecting shopping and cooking abilities which were already reducing
   - Mobilising – due to breathlessness and coughing.
   - Expressing sexuality – self-esteem affected by appearance
   - Working and playing – not able to walk to the pub. Lacks company since wife died
   - Sleep and rest – coughing during the night

Potential breathing problems

There are many potential problems which may be identified, some will relate to the individual's breathing condition, some specific to the factors which affect the individual. There are, however, two potential problems which may affect any individual with a breathing difficulty, namely being at risk of obstructed air passages and cardiac/respiratory arrest. It is important that you are able to recognise these potential problems so that prompt action can follow as both problems are potentially fatal. For example:

1. *At risk of obstructed air passages.* Airway obstruction may be due to a variety of causes, e.g. trauma, tumours, oedema, foreign bodies, blood, vomit or tongue falling backwards and occluding the airway. It may occur in the nasal passages, pharynx, larynx, trachea or bronchus. Hoarseness, dyspnoea, stridor, cyanosis and increased but ineffective respiratory effort can be seen (see pp. 151–152 for further care).

2. *At risk of cardiac/respiratory arrest.* Mallett & Dougherty (2000, p. 151) define cardiac arrest as the 'abrupt cessation of cardiac function which is potentially reversible'. Events leading up to an arrest may be

varied, e.g. surgery, asphyxia, accidents such as drowning, cardiac arrhythmias or respiratory failure. The diagnosis of an arrest is, according to Jamieson et al (2002), a sudden loss of consciousness, absence of respirations, absence of signs of circulating (including the carotid pulse and perfused skin). Although there are similarities in how you can recognise this event, there is one important difference between cardiac and respiratory arrest. In cardiac arrest there is an absence of an arterial pulse, whereas in a respiratory arrest the arterial pulses are present, although they may be difficult to locate and time should not be lost in trying to palpate these, just for a differential diagnosis. It is vitally important that these signs are noted early as cerebral damage can be caused by anoxia, i.e. no oxygen getting to the brain, if breathing and circulation is not restored effectively within 4 minutes. Basic life support measures are needed to restore breathing and circulation (see pp. 153–154 for further care).

Exercise

Re-read the case scenario in Case study 5.3 (Tom Jackson).

1. Using the 12 Activities of Living as a framework, identify Tom's actual and potential problems.
2. Check your identified actual and potential problems with those in Box 5.9.

Box 5.9 Actual and potential problems – Case study 5.3 Tom Jackson

Activity of Living	Actual problems	Potential problems
Maintaining safe environment	Tom has difficulty complying with the correct medication due to his stated confusion over his medication.	
Breathing	Tom has difficulty with breathing due to the exacerbation of his breathing disorder as shown by a loose cough, a raised respiratory rate and an audible wheeze.	
Communicating	Tom has difficulty communicating due to breathlessness and cough.	
Eating and drinking	Tom has difficulty cooking food so his dietary intake has decreased due to breathlessness affecting mobility and his ability to cook and shop.	
Eliminating		Tom may have difficulty getting to the toilet due to breathlessness.
Personal cleansing and dressing	Tom has difficulty maintaining his hygiene needs due to his breathless state.	
Mobilising	Tom has difficulty mobilising due to his breathlessness.	Tom may develop pressure sores, deep vein thrombosis, pulmonary embolism, and constipation due to limited activity.
Sleep and rest	Tom is experiencing difficulty sleeping due to coughing at night.	
Work and play	Tom is becoming isolated as he cannot socialise as he did previously due to breathlessness affecting his mobility.	
Expressing sexuality		Tom has difficulty maintaining his body image due to his breathing and mobility problems.
Maintaining body temperature	Tom may have difficulties maintaining body temperature due to his lack of mobility and because his house is in need of modernisation having only coal fires downstairs.	
Dying		Tom may be worried about the severity of his condition and he is still coming to terms with the death of his wife.

By working through this section you will have considered how to collect data when taking a nursing history in relation to the activity of breathing and other related activities; interpret the data collected to assess the degree of alteration in the activity of breathing and the effect on other Activities of Living and to identify individuals' actual and potential problems related to the activity of breathing and other related activities.

Planning nursing activities

Planning nursing activities involves the following:

- identifying priorities
- establishing short- and/or long-term goals
- determining nursing actions/interventions required
- documenting the plan (refer to Chapter 1 for further information).

To ensure that the nursing activities are planned appropriately, you must review the individual's actual and potential problems and then consider the level to which the activity of breathing can be helped. There are different levels of helping, such as:

1. to solve or alleviate actual problems
2. to prevent potential problems becoming actual ones
3. to prevent solved problems from re-occurring
4. to develop positive strategies for any problems which cannot be solved.

> **Exercise**
> 1. Re-read the three mini case studies in Box 5.7.
> 2. Consider these three case studies and identify the levels of helping within them.

You may have considered the following levels of care were appropriate.

Scenario A
- To alleviate severe right-sided chest pain.
- To prevent potential problems following rib fracture such as chest infection due to poor breathing and coughing habits.

Scenario B
- To alleviate congestion, tiredness, night sweats, weight loss and promote expectoration.
- To prevent possible spread of infection to others.

Scenario C
- To develop positive coping strategies for lifestyle changes so that potential problems don't become actual problems.

The focus must be on the individual's problems and what they want as opposed to the nurse's ideas. Therefore,

> **Box 5.10 Factors which influence planning care for a patient with breathing difficulties**
>
> **Nurse's perspective**
> - Knowledge of normal physiology and specific pathophysiological processes in relation to breathing disorders
> - Knowledge of normal living and dependency across the lifespan in various cultures in relation to breathing
> - Knowledge of breathing difficulties specific to the patient's problem
> - Knowledge of nursing interventions available and research-based evidence
> - Accuracy of assessment
> - Skills in relation to observing, assessment, interpreting and prioritising
> - Staffing levels and skill mix on individual shifts
>
> **Patient's perspective**
> - Ability and degree of involvement of patient in the decisions related to care to be planned
> - Knowledge of breathing difficulties specific to their problem
> - Personal beliefs, attitudes, experiences and coping strategies
> - Enactment of the sick role

involvement of the patient is crucial at this stage. However, this may be affected by the problems that the patient may have, e.g. pain, difficulty with communicating verbally as noted previously.

Many factors may influence the nurse and the patient in the planning stage of nursing activities with a patient with breathing difficulties. Consider this in relation to a patient you have nursed with breathing difficulties and check these in Box 5.10.

Identifying priorities

Following the assessment the next stage is to plan the care. You will need to determine priorities of care and this skill is a vital component of any nurse's repertoire. You need to be able to determine which problem is the most important and you could grade it as follows:

- life threatening – totally dependent
- urgent – mainly dependent but some ability to be independent
- semiurgent – some dependency but mainly independent
- nonurgent – totally independent.

This priority status may change day by day, shift by shift or hour by hour and therefore assessment must be a continuous activity to ensure that you remain alert to possible changes.

It can be seen that Tom's problems are varied in relation to their priorities and are complex in nature. A suggested priority order is:

1. has difficulty with breathing due to exacerbation of breathing disorder as shown by loose cough, raised respiratory rate and audible wheeze
2. has difficulty with mobilising because of breathlessness and may develop pressure sores, deep vein thrombosis, pulmonary embolism and constipation due to limited activity
3. has difficulty sleeping due to coughing at night.

The rationale for the priority order is that difficulties with breathing are the main problem that Tom has which is affecting many of his other Activities of Living. If nursing actions are not planned then the breathing difficulties will worsen. If, however, nursing actions are planned and implemented, then not only will the breathing difficulty be alleviated but also the difficulties with the other Activities of Living will be eased.

Mobilising difficulty will be eased once Tom's breathing difficulty is alleviated. In the meantime, however, potential problems which may become life threatening, e.g. deep vein thrombosis leading to pulmonary embolism could occur and therefore it is important to address this problem with preventative care.

Difficulty with sleeping is important to alleviate quickly as Tom's wellbeing is affected by lack of sleep.

Box 5.11 Priority status of actual problems – Case study 5.3 Tom Jackson

Activity of Living	Actual problems	Problem status
Maintaning safe environment	Tom has difficulty complying with the correct medication due to his stated confusion over his medication.	Urgent
Breathing	Tom has difficulty with breathing due to the exacerbation of his breathing disorder as shown by a loose cough, a raised respiratory rate and an audible wheeze.	Urgent
Communicating	Tom has difficulty communicating due to breathlessness and cough.	Semi-urgent
Eating and drinking	Tom has difficulty cooking food so his dietary intake has decreased due to breathlessness, affecting mobility and his ability to cook and shop.	Non-urgent
Personal cleansing and dressing	Tom has difficulty maintaining his hygiene needs due to his breathless state.	Semi-urgent
Mobilising	Tom has difficulty mobilising due to his breathlessness.	Urgent
Sleep and rest	Tom is experiencing difficulty sleeping due to coughing at night.	Semi-urgent
Work and play	Tom is becoming isolated as he cannot socialise as he did previously due to breathlessness affecting his mobility.	Non-urgent
Expressing sexuality	Tom has difficulty maintaining his body image due to his breathing and mobility problems.	Non-urgent
Eliminating	Tom may have difficulty getting to the toilet due to breathlessness.	Non-urgent
Mobilising	Tom may develop pressure sores, deep vein thrombosis, pulmonary embolism, and constipation due to limited activity.	Semi-urgent
Maintaining body temperature	Tom may have difficulties maintaining body temperature due to his lack of mobility and because his house is in need of modernisation having only coal fires downstairs.	Non-urgent
Dying	Tom may be worried about the severity of his condition and is still coming to terms with the death of his wife.	Semi-urgent

Goal setting

Goal setting is based upon sound assessment and the identification of problems and priorities. Goals can be short term (hourly to generally less than a week) or long term (for a longer period). Many short-term goals may be needed to achieve long-term goals.

The goal statement is essential so that the process of evaluation can take place. It is therefore important that the goal is written in the terms of what the patient ought to be able to, or has agreed to, achieve. The goals should be written in observable, realistic and measurable behavioural terms so that it is easier to monitor and evaluate the patient's progress. (Refer to Chapter 1 for further details on goal setting.) This may be a skill that you need to develop and practice. One example is shown in Box 5.12 for you to reflect upon.

> **Exercise**
> Re-read Tom Jackson's problems related to the main scenario, listed in Case study 5.3.
>
> 1. Choose three of these problems and set short- and long-term goals using one of the frameworks noted in Chapter 1.
> 2. Check the example given in Box 5.12.

Once the short-term and long-term goals have been set you will need to determine the appropriate nursing actions which will aid the alleviation of problems and the achievement of the short- and long-term goals.

Determining nursing actions

It is vital that the appropriate nursing actions are chosen to alleviate patient's problems. It is vital that each nurse constantly updates their knowledge and skills to ensure that care given is evidence based and delivered in a safe, competent and professional manner. Nursing actions will be considered in relation to dependency, comforting and preventative care with patients who have 'difficulty with breathing'.

Roper et al (1985) used these three aspects, in their second edition of *'Elements of Nursing'* to discuss care and it may be useful to consider their use in this activity.

Nursing actions associated with dependency care

The purpose of nursing actions associated with dependency care, related to breathing difficulties, is that you, the carer, provide specific care to the individual who is not able to provide care for themselves. The place on the lifespan, the level of dependency and biological factors identified in the model of living will need to be considered when the nursing actions are planned. There are many nursing actions, related to dependency care, which affect breathing but some of the main actions include:

- nursing observations of vital signs – TPR BP, peak flow, O_2 saturation levels, tissue perfusion
- administration of prescribed oxygen therapy
- administration of prescribed drug therapies/nebulisers
- localised airway passage obstruction
- postural drainage
- artificial airway maintenance
- cardiopulmonary resuscitation.

Let us consider these.

Nursing observations of vital signs

These actual observations have already been noted earlier in this chapter (see p. 141). However, it is important that you consider when these observations are done and how often. This will depend on the severity of the patient's condition and whether the problems are acute or chronic. The initial assessment of vital signs will be used as a baseline for future evaluations. It may be that these observations are carried out continuously as the patient is in a critical care environment and is monitored, or that they are carried out 4-hourly or daily. You may need to refer to Chapters 3 and 9 in relation to the activities of maintaining a safe environment and maintaining body temperature for further information.

It is the nurse who usually decides on the site for temperature recordings to be taken and the device to be used. Oral temperature recordings would be difficult for someone who is dyspnoeic and therefore the axilla or tympanic membrane would be the preferred site. Safety aspects, cost and ease of use may be the influencing factors and Tempadot and tympanic membrane thermometers could be used as opposed to glass or mercury thermometers.

The temperature observation could be completed when the pulse and respiration rates are being counted. The pulse

Box 5.12 Short- and long-term breathing goals set for Tom Jackson

Problem	Short-term goal	Long-term goal
Tom has difficulty with breathing due to exacerbation of his breathing disorder as shown by a loose cough, raised respiratory rate and audible wheeze.	Tom will be able to breathe easier and quieter with the aid of oxygen with a lower respiratory rate than on admission and is able to expectorate secretions.	Tom will be able to breathe normally, unaided before discharge, with no audible wheeze, no cough or sputum produced and have a respiratory rate of within 18–24 respirations per minute at rest for a minimum of 4 hours.

rate and respiratory rate need to be counted for a full minute each as sufficient time is needed to detect irregularities or abnormalities and these may not be identified if a full minute is not used (Mallett & Dougherty 2000). The blood pressure would normally be completed after the other vital signs have been recorded, as the patient will be at rest and factors which may affect their blood pressure, such as exercise, will have been minimised.

The use of automatic blood pressure machines, e.g. 'Dinamap' have speeded up the process of taking measurements of vital signs. These machines can also provide a recording of pulse rates and oxygen saturation levels. You must, however, remember to observe and touch the patient as pulse recordings and oxygen saturation levels on the 'Dinamap' machine only produce a reading, it does not give any indication to the fullness of the beat, the irregularity of the beat or the texture and colour of the skin. Peak flow recordings may be used as a general indicator of respiratory activity and are recorded 4-hourly or daily or they may be used to assess the effectiveness of medication and therefore the recordings may be done before and after medication has been taken.

As breathing is affected by mobilising, eating and communicating, then you would need to take these issues into account and record the vital signs prior to these activities. It is important for nurses to rationalise why such observations are being undertaken for each individual patient and in particular the frequency of these measurements. Ritualistic practices, particularly in relation to observations, have been identified and the recording of 4-hourly observations may well be an established practice but may not be necessary. As Walsh & Ford (1989, p. ix), identify 'Ritual action implies carrying out a task without thinking it through in a problem solving, logical way'.

When the observations have been taken, you must ensure that the recordings are accurately recorded on the appropriate chart and the significance of the observations identified and reported to senior members of the health care team. For example, if the recordings taken were as follows: pulse and blood pressure rising, pulse weaker, respirations initially increased, with sighing, yawning and dyspnoea being present, this combined with restlessness, confusion and decreasing conscious level may indicate hypoxia (insufficient oxygen for cells to work) and oxygen therapy may be required.

Administration of oxygen therapy

Oxygen therapy can be used for a variety of patients, e.g. acute and chronic respiratory problems, in an emergency situation, as a short- or long-term measure, but it must be remembered that it is a drug and therefore has regulations as to its administration. Serious consequences can develop if oxygen is administered inappropriately or incorrectly. Usually, as noted by Rutishauser (1994) and Hinchliff et al (1996), breathing is stimulated when the carbon dioxide levels are high. However, for people with chronic respiratory disease, their stimulus to breathe is due to an oxygen lack and not a build up of carbon dioxide. If these people are given above 24% of oxygen, then their stimulus to breathe is removed with potential fatal consequences. Oxygen should therefore, as noted by Jevon & Ewens (2001), always be prescribed and the flow rate, delivery system, duration and monitoring of treatment should be specified. This should be guided by arterial blood gas levels, for high concentrations of oxygen over a long period of time may cause severe lung damage, and so it is important that its use is monitored carefully. Local protocols, relating to its emergency use, should be available in every health care environment.

There are numerous delivery systems available and you need to be able to rationalise the choice to the patient and the other health care professionals. All of the systems include an oxygen supply (portable black cylinder with a white top clearly marked oxygen or piped oxygen), flow meter to regulate rate of oxygen per minute, oxygen tubing usually green and a delivery device with humidifier. The delivery device used may be low or high flow (nasal cannulae or masks) and depends on the amount and concentration of oxygen needed, compliance with the therapy and the condition.

Low-flow devices, e.g. nasal cannulae or simple face mask allow the patient to inhale room air and mix it with the oxygen being administered. Both nasal cannulae and face masks are for single patient use only and should be disposed of after use with one patient. Care must be taken when disposing of the devices if the patient is expectorating sputum because of any contamination. The respiratory rate and depth will affect the concentration of oxygen received. High-flow devices, usually Venturi masks or non-rebreathing masks, deliver a precise concentration of oxygen to the patient irrespective of their respiratory effort (Walsh 2002). See Figure 5.11 for these devices.

Nasal cannulae deliver oxygen via a length of tubing with two prongs which fit into the nostrils. They can deliver oxygen concentrations of 24–44% at a flow rate of 1–6 litres per minute, although patients may experience difficulties above 4 litres per minute. If a patient breathes through the mouth then the efficiency of this method is lessened and masks may be necessary.

Masks can be used to deliver various concentrations of oxygen and are designed to fit over the patient's nose and mouth or trachea. Simple low-flow masks can deliver oxygen concentrations of 21–60% but the amount of oxygen received will vary according to the patient's respirations as the patient rebreathes their own expired air, combined with air from outside the mask plus oxygen delivered through the system (Walsh 1997).

High-flow, fixed-performance or Venturi masks deliver accurate concentrations of oxygen as they are not affected by the patient's breathing pattern. The concentration of oxygen tends to be lower, but levels of 24–40% can be

You would need to ensure that the patient and their relatives received explanations, in relation to the need for oxygen therapy and the safety issues relating to this combustible gas, e.g. no smoking. A calm approach is needed and once the oxygen delivery system is in place the nurse needs to stay with them to ensure that the patient is able to tolerate the oxygen flow. They would need to be nursed in an observable position in the care environment and be nursed in an upright position in bed or a chair. Jamieson et al (2002) point out that the administration of oxygen does not require aseptic technique but that adequate cleanliness should be maintained to prevent crossinfection. The inside of the oxygen mask may become wet with condensation and can be dried to increase the patient's comfort and tolerance of the oxygen administration. Sheppard & Davis (2000) state that oxygen masks should be cleaned regularly, particularly if the patient has a productive cough and that the nurse must wash their hands after disposing of the oxygen equipment, to prevent cross-infection.

Administration of drug therapies/nebulisers

Moist inhalations may be used to loosen secretions in the upper respiratory tract and promote expectoration especially when infection is present. Tincture of benzoin or menthol crystals can be used with a jug and bowl or a Nelson's inhaler. Care must be taken to prevent scalding when handling the hot water and when in contact with the hot vapour. The vapour is breathed in through the mouth and out through the nose using a jug and bowl of hot water.

Bronchodilators are used to prevent or treat bronchoconstriction, e.g. salbutomol (Ventolin). Metered-dose inhalers are commonly used so that each time an inhaler is used the same amount of drug is delivered into the respiratory tract. The dose is usually two puffs three times a day. Corticosteroids, e.g. beclomethasone (Becotide), can be used with bronchodilators to reduce bronchial reactivity and broad-spectrum antibiotics, e.g. amoxycillin (Amoxil) may be used at the earliest signs of infection (Walsh 1997).

It is important for you to be aware of the effects and side effects of any drug therapy given. Teaching of inhaler techniques is vital and awareness of the different types of inhalers is needed so that patient's treatment can be tailored to their abilities. See Jordan & White (2001) for further information concerning bronchodilators and the implications for nursing practice.

Nebulisation is a method of converting a drug or liquid into an aerosol mist which can be used as a therapeutic inhalation, according to Jamieson et al (2002) (see Fig. 5.12). Nebulisers may be indicated when bronchodilators need to be administered or when mucolytic medication is required to lower the viscosity of sputum to aid expectoration. The medication and the air (oxygen is rarely used and only with selected clients because of the dangers) must be prescribed and the procedure should be coordinated with physiotherapy

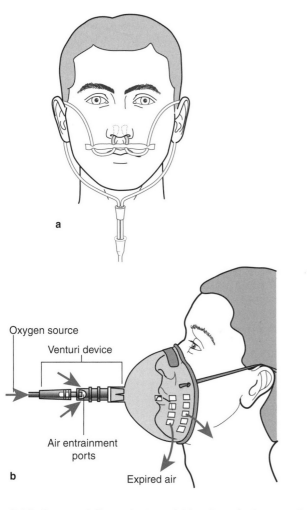

Fig. 5.11 Oxygen delivery devices, (a) low flow device, nasal cannula, (b) high flow device, Venturi mask (from Walsh 2002, with permission).

given. There are a number of holes in the side of the mask and this allows the expired air to escape and therefore eliminate the chance of rebreathing carbon dioxide. Hence, they can be used for people who retain carbon dioxide and use the lack of oxygen as their stimulus to breathe. Non-rebreathing masks can be used to deliver oxygen concentrations of 90–100%, at a flow rate of 12–15 litres per minute, as no outside air or expired air is allowed in through the mask (Walsh 1997).

Irrespective of the type of delivery device used, patients will require frequent mouth and nasal care because humidification of the inspired air will be lessened and breathing dry gas dries and irritates the mucous membranes. Specific measures to humidify the oxygen delivered may be necessary also, especially when oxygen concentration levels of 35% and above are prescribed, but not with nasal cannulae or Venturi masks. As all masks must fit closely over the nose and around the chin, then these areas must be inspected and pressure relieved on the underlying tissues.

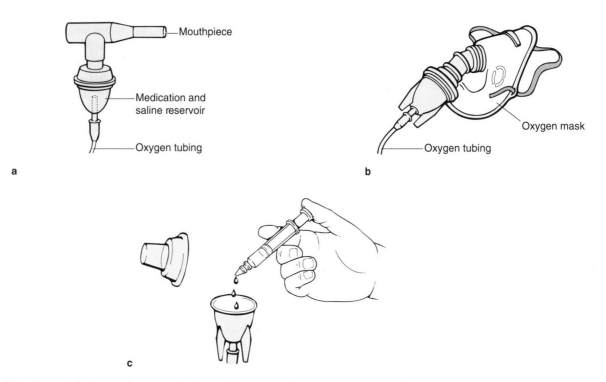

Fig. 5.12 Nebulisers, (a) attached to a mouthpiece, (b) attached to an oxygen mask, (c) taken apart to introduce a prepared medication (from Jamieson et al 2002, with permission).

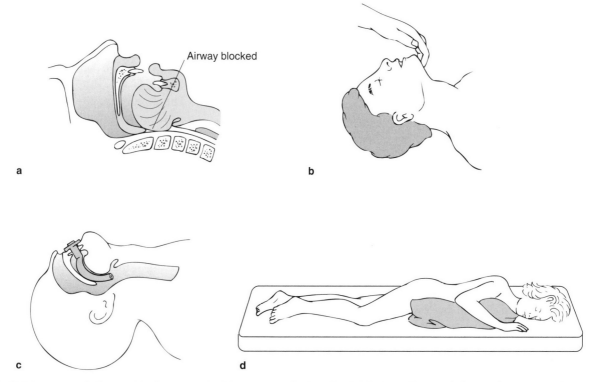

Fig. 5.13 Maintenance of airway, (a) airway blocked by tongue, (b) jaw lifted, (c) airway inserted, (d) semiprone position (from Roper et al 1996, with permission).

and peak flow readings taken before and afterwards to evaluate the prescribed therapy. Usually all the solution is administered in 10 minutes and it is important that you discourage the patient from speaking at this time and to breathe normally.

Nebulisers are for single patient use but must be cleaned after every use, and changed every 24 hours to prevent infection (Jamieson et al 2002). As the procedure doesn't sterilise the nebuliser, it must be discarded if the patient has an infectious illness. Guidelines for the cleansing of nebulisers will be found on the information leaflet that is provided with the equipment. However, it is usual that the residual drug is emptied from the nebuliser and water run through the nebuliser for 1 minute. The individual components of the nebuliser are washed in hot soapy water, rinsed in clean water to remove any residue and dried thoroughly. The nebuliser is reassembled, run on the compressor to remove any excess water and stored in a dry, clean place, ready for the next administration.

Localised airway passage obstruction

Where the airway is obstructed by a foreign body or the tongue, the positioning of the individual is important to ensure that the airway is patent and it may be necessary to insert an airway. This may be done by lying the patient flat on their back and then lifting up the jaw before inserting the airway, followed by placing them in the recovery position (see Fig. 5.13). Suction may be required to remove foreign material, blood or vomit. Prompt emergency measures are needed if the obstruction is at the larynx or trachea level as death may ensue as a result of asphyxia (Walsh 2002).

Sharp blows between the scapulae may move the obstruction or the Heimlich manoeuvre may be used. If the individual cannot stand, then the manoeuvre is performed by placing crossed hands just below the ribcage and exerting a firm thrust upwards. If they are able to stand then this manoeuvre is carried out differently. Someone stands behind the individual and places their arms around the individual's trunk, just below the diaphragm, clasping the hands in front. Pressure is then applied with the arms and the hands which forces air out through the airway and may dislodge the obstruction. If this is not successful, then an emergency tracheostomy may need to be performed to maintain the airway prior to the obstruction being cleared. See Figure 5.14 for the Heimlich manoeuvre.

Postural drainage

Roper et al (1996) identified that certain lung disorders produce an excessive amount of sputum which can obstruct the airways and must be removed or the oxygenation of the blood will be affected. Postural drainage can be used to remove these excessive secretions. According to Liddle (2000), postural drainage is where a person is placed in a variety of positions and treated by percussion. This repositioning allows gravity to assist in the clearance of each lung segment and is particularly used for patients with cystic

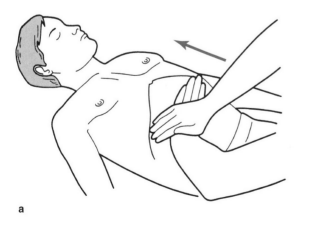

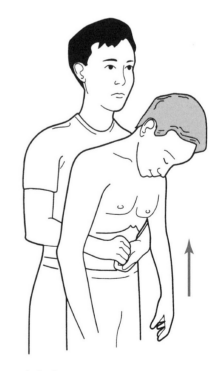

a

b

Fig. 5.14 Heimlich manoeuvre, (a) lying down, (b) standing up (from Walsh 2002, with permission).

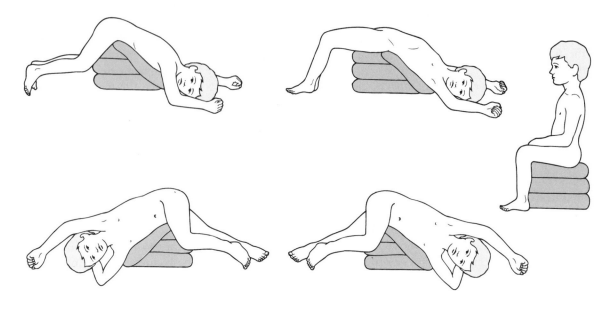

Fig. 5.15 Postural drainage positions (from Alexander et al 2000, with permission).

fibrosis, where they have persistent recurrent lower respiratory tract infections which result in lung damage. Figure 5.15 illustrates the positions used to enable postural drainage to take place.

Time needs to be spent teaching the patient and their relatives how to perform postural drainage along with specific breathing and coughing exercises. Patients may be exhausted following this exacting form of physiotherapy and the nurse may need to plan a rest period afterwards. Privacy is required as the expectoration of large volumes of sputum may be unpleasant for all concerned but the relief is great, especially in the morning after secretions have gathered overnight where movement is minimal.

Artificial airway maintenance

It may not be possible to clear the airway by physiotherapy, postural drainage, deep breathing and coughing exercises and suctioning, if there are excessive secretions and sputum retention. It is imperative that the airway is maintained and this may be achieved by the insertion of an endotracheal tube (through the mouth into the trachea) or by performing a tracheostomy (surgical opening in the trachea).

An endotracheal tube is held in situ by inflating a cuff with a specified volume of air (see Fig. 5.16), whereas the tracheostomy tube is inserted into the trachea and held in place by inflating a cuff and by tapes being tied at the back of the neck (see Fig. 5.17). These measures may be temporary or permanent and can be carried out as a planned or emergency procedure (Walsh 2002).

You would need to plan a variety of nursing actions once an endotracheal tube has been inserted or a tracheostomy has been performed. Humidified oxygen will be required to ensure that an adequate intake of moist oxygen is delivered.

Secretions will need to be removed by the use of sterile catheters and an appropriate suctioning technique which is not harmful to the sensitive mucosa. Explanations are needed prior to suction being used, as it can be a frightening procedure for the patient. Jamieson et al (2002) provide a description of the procedure for this. Figure 5.18 illustrates the position of a tracheostomy tube and aspiration of secretions from a tracheostomy tube.

Care of the skin around the tracheostomy tube needs to be considered as the secretions and the tape used to hold the tube in place can irritate the skin, so keyhole dressings can be placed underneath the tracheostomy tube and replaced twice a day. Mouth care and mouthwashes should be given with care. The tracheostomy tube does need changing at various intervals and the nurse needs the appropriate knowledge and skill to do this. There are many different types of tracheostomy tubes and Jamieson et al (2002) and Walsh (2002) discuss their specific care and the general care of patients requiring artificial airway maintenance. The patient will not be able to talk, initially, with an endotracheal or tracheostomy tube in position so the nurse must plan activities and use other communication methods such as a call bell and pen and paper to ensure that the patient can express their feelings and wishes to others. It may be useful for you to read the article by Serra (2000) for further information on tracheostomy care.

Mechanical ventilation will be required for patients who cannot breathe spontaneously and therefore maintain their own oxygen and carbon dioxide levels. Mechanical ventilators (negative or positive pressure) automatically expand the chest and oxygen is delivered into the lungs. Further details can be found earlier in this chapter and in Walsh (2002).

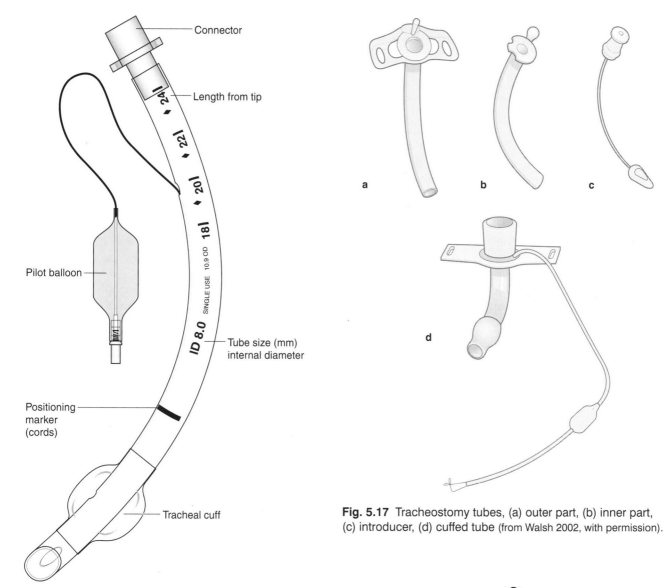

Fig. 5.16 Endotrachael tube with inflatable cuff (from Walsh 2002, with permission).

Fig. 5.17 Tracheostomy tubes, (a) outer part, (b) inner part, (c) introducer, (d) cuffed tube (from Walsh 2002, with permission).

Cardiopulmonary resuscitation in adults

Many writers discuss this action (Mallik et al 1998, Mallett & Dougherty 2000, Jamieson et al 2002) and there is consensus that it involves three procedures:

1. *Airway* – providing and maintaining a clear airway by removing any visible obstruction is the initial consideration. The head is then tilted backwards and the mandible pulled forward. This will open the airway and an oral airway may be inserted at this time. Care must be taken if a neck injury is suspected.

2. *Breathing* – supplying oxygen to the blood by means of artificial ventilation is the next consideration. Mouth-to-mouth ventilation can be used, with two initial ventilations then continue at a rate of 12 ventilations per minute. The rise and fall of the

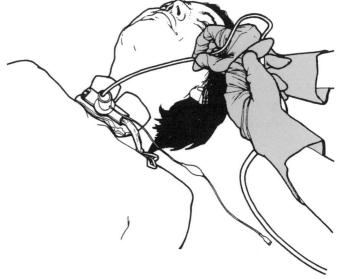

Fig. 5.18 Position and aspiration of secretions from a tracheostomy tube (from Chilman & Thomas 1987, with permission).

chest should be noted to confirm that air is entering the respiratory tract. However, this method can only deliver 16% oxygen to the individual and there may a risk from contact with body fluids. If at all possible, an airway should be used and ventilation continued with a Ambubag or a mask. Up to 90% oxygen can be delivered by this route but it needs practice to do this.

3. *Circulation* – forcing the blood out of the heart into the arterial system by means of cardiac compressions is needed if no carotid pulse can be found within 10 seconds. If the arrest is witnessed, then one precordial thump can be administered. This is achieved by a closed fist hitting the mid to lower third of the sternum. In some cases this one blow will restart the heart, if it does not then it is not repeated and external cardiac massage must be commenced. The heel of one hand is placed over the lower half of the sternum and the hand is placed on top. The arms are kept straight and the elbows locked and the sternum is then compressed by 4–5 cm towards the spine. The chest compression then needs to be repeated. The return of the pulse and breathing should be checked after 1 minute and every 3 minutes after that.

If two people are present then the compression to ventilation ratio is 5:1, i.e. five compressions to one breath, as there is no time lost in changing position. If there is only one person carrying out cardiopulmonary resuscitation then the compression to ventilation ratio is 15:2, i.e. 15 chest compressions followed by two breaths, as there is time lost in changing positions (see Fig. 5.19).

Training programmes for the general public have been promoted and well attended. However, it is essential that all health care professionals are trained in cardiopulmonary resuscitation techniques, as research by Wynne (1987) and Crouch (1993) did show that nurses have poor skills in

relation to resuscitation. The Resuscitation Council (UK) commenced Basic Life Support and Advanced Life Support courses in 1993 and there is some evidence that there has been an increase in the number of successful resuscitations since this time (Handley & Swain 1996).

There are legal, ethical and professional issues relating to resuscitation and you may need to consider these issues as well as the skills that are needed. According to Mallik et al (1998), there is no legal duty of care in the UK to a neighbour. So a nurse need not legally stop to give first aid to help someone in the streets but there is a moral issue of whether this is right. However, if the first aider has presented themselves as a nurse, then they do have a professional duty of care to help and would be responsible and liable for their acts and omissions in relation to the care given. It is, therefore, important that nurses have some form of personal indemnity insurance.

However, when the nurse is an employee and the arrest occurs in the context of employment, then the nurse would be classed as the designated first aider as defined in the Health and Safety at Work Act (1974). In this situation, it would probably be the employer who would be sued for negligence and not the individual nurse.

The Nursing and Midwifery Council (NMC) Code of Professional Conduct (2002a) however, complicates the matter as it states that 'As a registered nurse and midwife you must: protect and support the health of individuals and clients, protect and support the health of the wider community, act in such a way that justifies the trust and confidence the public have in you and uphold and enhance the good reputation of the professions'. This appears to override the legal issues and indicates that all nurses and midwives must render first aid to all people, whether they are in a health care setting or not.

Resuscitating individuals also raises ethical dilemmas and the issues of 'Do not resuscitate' policies and 'Living Wills' complicate this already 'grey area'. The Royal College of Nursing (1992) has produced guidelines to aid decisions into resuscitation practices. These decisions should be based on whether the action, i.e. resuscitation will bring about the best consequences and outcomes, whether it will respect the wishes of all concerned and whether human life will be respected and valued.

There are, therefore, many issues for you to consider when the decision to resuscitate someone is taken. Following a resuscitation event, debriefing is advocated by Gamble (2001) as the unpredictability of the event can result in unique feelings in the carer. The initial resuscitation call activates the stress response system known as the 'General Adaptation Syndrome'. If the effect of this stress response system is not discussed then the carer may be left with physical and psychological issues unresolved.

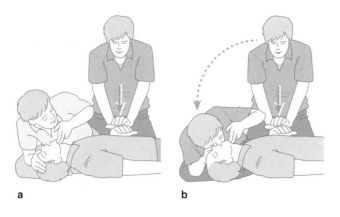

Fig. 5.19 Cardiopulmonary resuscitation, (a) two resuscitators – Ratio of 5:1, (b) one resuscitator – ratio of 15:2 (from Jamieson 2002, with permission).

Nursing actions associated with comforting care
You will need to consider what is the best position for the patient so that they can increase lung inflation, aid emptying

of the lungs and decrease respiratory effort. The patient may breathe easier sitting up and leaning forward, resting arms and shoulders on a bed table in a well ventilated area near a window. They may choose to sit in a chair as opposed to being in a bed. The nurse needs to adopt a calm approach to care, talking to the patient using closed questions and allaying their fears of dying. Deep breathing, coughing exercises and relaxation techniques need to be taught appropriately.

Nursing actions associated with preventative care

The nurse's role in health promotion and the prevention of disease is noted within the Department of Health's (1999c) document *'Saving Lives'* and within the activity of breathing there are many areas where this role is paramount to the patient's wellbeing. Their role in smoking cessation pro-grammes has already been discussed in this chapter.

Self-management is the mainstay of acute and chronic respiratory problems. So patients, and therefore nurses, need to have knowledge and skill in administering drugs via inhalers and/or nebulisers and need to be able to recognise when their regime may need altering and when medical assistance is needed. They need to know about the actions, side effects and method of administration of drug therapies. In particular, you will need to support patients with their inhaler technique as this is vital to the effectiveness of this therapy. Patients need to be able to identify allergens that precipitate an attack and consider what actions can be taken to try and minimise problems.

It can be seen that there are numerous nursing actions and these vary between emergency procedures and health promotion measures. You, therefore, may need to develop your knowledge and skills to ensure that you are able to give competent professional care to all patients alike.

Documenting the care plan

Once the nursing actions have been identified then the care plan needs to be written. Care plans should abide by the NMC (2002b) *'Guidelines for records and record keeping'* document and identify individualised actions and specify:

- who should be involved in the care planned
- what care should be given
- why that care should be given
- when the care should be given
- where the care should be given and
- how the care should be given.

> ### Exercise
> 1. Write the care plan for the three problems on p. 146 used in the previous exercise relating to Tom Jackson's main case scenario.
> 2. Check your answers with the following care plans in Box 5.13.

Box 5.13 Nursing care plan – Tom Jackson

PROBLEM 1

Tom has difficulty with breathing due to exacerbation of his breathing disorder as shown by a loose cough, raised respiratory rate and audible wheeze.

Short-term goal

Tom will be able to breathe easier and quieter with the aid of oxygen with a lower respiratory rate than on admission and is able to expectorate secretions.

Long-term goal

Tom will be able to breathe normally, unaided before discharge with no audible wheeze, no cough or sputum produced and have a respiratory rate of between 18–24 respirations per minute at rest for a minimum of 4 hours.

Nursing care plan

- Observe respiratory rate, rhythm and character of breathing 4-hourly.
- Observe sputum production for quantity, consistency and colour, ability to expectorate.
- Observe the duration and frequency of Tom's coughing and when his coughing is worse and the effect coughing has on Tom.
- Observe colour of skin, lips and nail beds.
- Observe temperature and peak flow recordings 4-hourly.
- Report changes in any of the observations immediately.
- Send a specimen of sputum for culture and sensitivity.
- Give oxygen, 2 litres per minute, via humidified MC mask as prescribed and note effect.
- Assist in the investigations ordered by the medical staff, e.g. chest X-ray, blood gases.
- Assist the physiotherapist in teaching and supervising deep breathing exercises and encourage Tom to expectorate sputum.
- Give oral care and nasal care 4-hourly.
- Ensure adequate hydration is maintained with 2 litres of oral fluids encouraged per day.
- Explain the need to expectorate sputum.
- Ensure a call bell is at hand and stay calm when with the patient.
- Ensure that Tom has a balance between company and rest.
- When talking to Tom allow him time to reply and if needed use closed questions so that Tom doesn't get overexerted trying to answer questions.
- Ensure the room is well ventilated and that Tom is sat up in bed or in an armchair, well supported by pillows.
- Ensure a bed table is at hand with pillows on it if this aids Tom's breathing.
- Ensure sputum pots are to hand and tissues available.

Box 5.13 Nursing care plan – Tom Jackson (*continued*)

PROBLEM 2 Tom has difficulty with mobilising because of his breathlessness and may develop pressure sores, deep vein thrombosis, pulmonary embolism, constipation due to limited activity. **Long-term goal** Tom will be able to mobilise unaided, without dyspnoea and will not experience complications of bed rest as shown by intact skin, calf soft, pain-free and normal size, no chest pain, bowels opened normally for him.	**Nursing care plan** • Observe Tom's ability to mobilise and his breathing rate. • Rest in bed initially, sitting up in bed supported well by pillows. • Ensure that Tom is comfortable. • When able to mobilise with minimal dyspnoea then encourage Tom to do so. • Complete risk assessments for pressure sores and plan accordingly. • Observe pressure areas 4-hourly, report redness and any breaks in the skin. • Re-position 2–4 hourly. • Move and handle appropriately. • Ensure skin is clean and dry. • Observe calf size for changes. • Report calf pain and pyrexia. • Note any sudden dyspnoea or chest pain. • Teach leg exercises (active and passive) and ensure Tom practices these in bed. • Explain why bed rest is needed initially. • Place bed cradle in situ. • Involve physiotherapist as required. • Record bowel patterns and actions daily. • High roughage diet as tolerated. • Oral fluids encouraged. • Allow to use the commode when on bed rest. • Ensure dignity and privacy is maintained.
PROBLEM 3 Has difficulty sleeping due to coughing at night. **Long-term goal** Tom will be able to rest in the day time and sleep undisturbed, by coughing, for at least 6 hours during the night.	**Nursing care plan** • Observe sleeping patterns and the effects coughing has on Tom's sleeping patterns. • Encourage Tom to expectorate sputum and carry out deep breathing exercises. • Assist physiotherapist with this. • Give medications as prescribed soothing cough syrup at night time and expectorants for the day time and monitor effect. • Ensure the environment is quiet and normal sleep routines are adhered to. • Sit and talk to Tom to ease anxieties that may affect sleep. • Educate Tom in how to rest during the day.

It may be useful for you to consider the five factors (physical, psychological, sociocultural, environmental and politicoeconomic) when writing the nursing care plan also. Re-read the nursing care plans and decide if all the factors are utilised.

Once the nursing care plan has been written then you must communicate this to other health care professionals by verbal handover ready for the next stage – implementation.

Implementing nursing activities

Implementation of nursing activities involves three stages:

1. Preparatory stage of reading the care plan, receiving handover report and ensuring that staff know what is required to accomplish the goals and decide on the skill mix needed.
2. Implementation where safe, competent practice is the key to successful care. The plan is then put into action and shows the artistic and scientific side of nursing.
3. Post-implementation stage when nursing activities are communicated to health care professionals (written and verbally) via progress notes.

Success of the implementation depends on the initial assessment, quality of the nursing care plan, organisation of care delivery and the competence of the care given. The written nursing care plan guides the implementation phase to help the patient achieve the goals set but the plan must be reviewed and updated according to changes in the patient's condition (see Chapter 1 for further information on implementation).

To ensure that this stage is both effective and efficient, there are numerous factors which can influence the care given. It is necessary for you to consider what influences care, what knowledge is needed and what skills are required by you to ensure that patients receive the best care that they can receive.

Exercise

Re-read the main case scenario in Case study 5.3 (Tom Jackson).

1. Consider what may influence the implementation of nursing activities planned.
2. Consider what knowledge you would need to implement this care.
3. Consider what skills you would need also.

English National Board (1999) and these can be linked to the implementation stage. The four domains are:

- professional and ethical practice
- care delivery
- care management
- personal and professional development (see Chapter 2 for further details).

These will now be explored in relation to breathing difficulties and the three scenarios used previously in this chapter.

You may have considered some of the factors in Box 5.14 and it would be useful for you to reflect upon your own level of knowledge and skills. The factors which influence care may differ in practice areas.

Four domains essential for professional practice have been identified in the 'Education for Focus' document by the

Exercise

1. Re-read the three mini case studies in Box 5.7.
2. Identify issues from these which relate to each of the four domains.
3. Check the answers in Box 5.15.

Box 5.14 Implementation of nursing activities

Factors influencing the implementation of nursing activities
- philosophy of care
- nursing model used
- assessment and planning stage
- care delivery system used
- resources available – skill mix, sufficient equipment and support services.

Knowledge required when implementing nursing activities
- normal and abnormal anatomy and physiology of respiratory and cardiovascular processes
- related psychological effects associated with breathing
- social and cultural issues relating to poor health or recovery

- environmental influences and concerns
- political and economic concerns.

Skills required when implementing nursing activities
- caring skills
- interpersonal skills
- clinical psycho-motor skills
- management skills – supervision, delegation, organising team/individuals
- counselling skills
- teaching skills
- research skills
- problem-solving skills
- leadership skills.

Box 5.15 Professional practice domains – mini case studies

Professional and ethical practice domain

Scenario A
- confidentiality
- information given to police relating to patients in A & E Dept.
- resuscitation orders
- equity and fairness in the A & E Dept.

Scenario B
- ethnicity and cultural differences
- antidiscriminatory policies

Scenario C
- patient's role in decision making
- links of smoking to ill health/ health promotion and ethics.

Care delivery domain

Scenario A
- communicating with patients who are in pain, shocked and stressed
- different ways of assessing patients in an A & E Dept., e.g. Fancap
- pain relief required
- first aid activities required
- health promotion relating to the prevention of falls.

Scenario B
- communicating with patients with whom English is not their first language
- health promotion for family members
- drug therapy required.

Scenario C
- health promotion activities
- drug therapies required.

Box 5.15 Professional practice domains – mini case studies *(continued)*

Care management domain

Scenario A
- triage system of care in A & E Dept.
- Nurse Practitioner role
- liaison with X-ray Dept., Occupational Nurse, fracture clinics
- ROSSPA
- pain services.

Scenario B
- barrier nursing
- role of TB Liaison Nurse.

Scenario C
- asthma clinics
- role of Practice Nurse
- stepwise care approach for asthma.

Personal and professional development domain
Portfolio of knowledge and skills to include:

Scenario A
- triage
- first aid
- pain management
- industrial injuries
- Health and Safety at Work Act.

Scenario B
- specimens of sputum for culture and sensitivity or TB culture
- barrier nursing
- communication skills
- cultural issues
- social effects on health.

Scenario C
- peak flow observations
- nebuliser care
- teaching skills
- nurse prescribing and protocols.

Having identified the potential aspects within these domains, it may be necessary for you to increase your knowledge and skills relating to the aspects identified.

Evaluation of nursing activities

Evaluation of care is integral to the professional accountability of nurses to their clients and is an essential stage of the process yet, according to Clothier et al (1994) in the Allitt Report, it is unfortunately a neglected part. Evaluation involves the degree of goal achievement so that feedback on care can be gained. Evaluation should be ongoing to gain an insight into the patient's progress and effectiveness of nursing activities. Evaluation can be continuous, hourly, daily, on a shift basis or longer depending on the individual patient's problem and the goals set. (For further information on evaluation see Chapter 1.) Again various factors can influence this evaluation stage and a number of skills are required and you need to recognise these factors and skills.

Exercise

Re-read the main case scenario found in Case study 5.3.

1. Consider the influencing factors which may affect the evaluation of nursing activities.
2. Consider the skills needed to evaluate nursing activities.
3. Check your answers in Box 5.16.

You may have considered some of these influencing factors and skills and it may be useful for you to reflect upon your own level of knowledge and skills but remember that the factors which influence care may differ in different practice areas. There are various steps which need to be followed when evaluating care:

Box 5.16 Evaluation of care

Factors which influence the evaluation stage
- abilities of nurse and patient
- standards and quality assurance mechanisms
- assessment, planning and implementation stages
- goals set
- timing of evaluation.

Skills required in the evaluation stage
- re-assessment to include:
  - observation
  - interviewing
  - listening
  - identification of plan
  - time scale
  - plan of action
- analysis of patient's response to care
- auditing.

---

1. Check goals against the patient's progress (discuss with patient if possible):
   - Have the goals been completely or partially met?
   - Have they been met at all?
2. Is the timescale realistic?
3. Record the findings and plan accordingly:
   - goal completely met – state evidence for this and discontinue the problem
   - goal partially met – decide if need to extend the evaluation time or modify the plan
   - goal not met at all – decide if need to extend the evaluation time, modify the plan or reassess the problem.

Exercise

1. Read the information in Box 5.17 and review the goals set for Tom's problems and evaluate his progress.
2. Consider what needs to be done in the next few days and write a revised plan of action if needed.

You may have considered that some of the long-term goals had been completely met, i.e. Tom was able to breathe normally, unaided and has no audible wheeze. However, some of the long-term goals had not been met, i.e. Tom still has a cough and is now expectorating thick, green tenacious sputum with a respiratory rate of 18 breaths per minute. Where goals have not been met then the following questions may be asked:

- Is more information required?
- Should the plan be modified?
- Has the problem changed?
- Has the problem worsened?
- Should the goals be reviewed?
- Were the goals appropriate?
- Does the plan need interventions from other health care professionals?

Therefore, the plan of action needs to be modified as the problem has changed, i.e. Tom has probably developed a chest infection. A modified plan may be:

- increase physiotherapy
- send further sputum specimen for culture and sensitivity immediately
- monitor 4-hourly temperature, pulse and respiration rate
- report changes in vital signs
- encourage Tom to increase his fluid intake to liquefy sputum

Box 5.17 Long-term goal review

Long-term goal previously set

Tom will be able to breathe normally, unaided before discharge with no audible wheeze, no cough or sputum and have a respiratory rate of 18–24 respirations per minute at rest for a minimum of 4 hours.

Evidence available

- Tom is breathing unaided now and no oxygen is required now
- Tom is able to walk around the bed now with minimal difficulty
- Tom has no audible wheeze
- Tom's respiratory rate is now 18 breaths per minute
- Tom still has a cough and sputum is now green, thick and tenacious.

- observe Tom's smoking habits and discuss with Tom the need to limit or discontinue smoking, if he has recommenced smoking
- if results of sputum specimen indicates a chest infection then administer the appropriate antibiotics and monitor effect on breathing, coughing and sputum production.

Summary points

1. An underpinning knowledge of the physiology of breathing is essential in order to deliver care to patients with breathing difficulties.
2. There are many ill health problems related to breathing and many of these can be linked to smoking.
3. Breathing as an activity is vital to life.

References

Burgess L 1994 An epidemic of massive proportions. Smoking and the health of the nation. Professional Nurse 9(8): 566, 568, 570, 572

Burns BH, Howell J 1969 Disproportionately severe breathlessness in chronic bronchitis. Quarterly Journal of Medicine 38: 277–294.

Casey G 2001 Oxygen transport and the use of pulse oximetry. Nursing Standard 15(47): 46–53

Castle F 1999 The breath of life. Nursing Standard 13(33): 20

Central Statistical Office 1994 Regional trends. HMSO, London

Central Statistical Office 1995 Annual abstract of statistics. HMSO, London

Chilman A, Thomas M 1987 Understanding nursing care, 3rd edn. Churchill Livingstone, Edinburgh

Clothier C, MacDonald C, Shaw D 1994 Independent enquiry into deaths and injuries on the Children's ward at Grantham and Kestevan General Hospital during the period February to April 1991 (Allitt Inquiry). HMSO, London

Coombs M 2001 Making sense of arterial blood gases. Nursing Times 97(27): 36–38

Cornock MA 1996 Making sense of arterial blood gases and their interpretation. Nursing Times 92(6): 30–31

Crouch R 1993 Nurses' skills in basic life support: A survey. Nursing Standard 7(20): 28–31

Department of Health 1974 Health and Safety at Work Act. HMSO, London

Department of Health 1991 Advisory group on the medical aspects of air pollution episodes first report: ozone. HMSO, London

Department of Health 1995a Advisory group on the medical aspects of air pollution episodes. Report: health effects of exposure to mixtures of air pollutants: fourth report of the advisory group on the medical aspects of air pollution Episodes. HMSO, London

Department of Health 1995b Committee on the medical effects of air pollutants. Asthma and outdoor air pollution. HMSO, London

Department of Health 1998 Smoking kills. A white paper on tobacco. HMSO, London

Department of Health 1999a Committee on the medical effects of air pollutants. Statement on the health effects of indoor exposure to carbon monoxide in the UK. HMSO, London

Department of Health 1999b COMEAP statement on the study by Poloniecki et al: Daily time-series for cardiovascular hospital admissions and previous day's air pollution in UK. HMSO, London

Department of Health 1999c Saving lives. HMSO, London

Department of Health 2000 NHS plan. HMSO, London

Department of Health 2001a Committee on the medical effects of air pollutants report on long-term effects of particles on mortality. HMSO, London

Department of Health 2001b Statistical bulletin. HMSO, London (http://www.doh.gov.uk/public/sb0105.htm)

Dudley DL, Martin CJ, Holmes TH 1964 Psychophysiologic studies of pulmonary ventilation. Psychosomatic Medicine 26: 645–659

Durmaz E, Laurence S, Roden P, Carruthers S 1999 Carbon monoxide poisoning and hyperbaric oxygen therapy. British Journal of Nursing 8(16): 1067–1072

Edmond CB 2000 The respiratory system, Chapter 3. In: Alexander MF, Fawcett JN, Runciman PJ (eds) Nursing practice hospital and home, 2nd edn. Churchill Livingstone, Edinburgh

English National Board 1999 Education for focus. ENB, London

Fulton CE 2000 The critically ill patient, Chapter 29. In: Alexander MF, Fawcett JN, Runciman PJ (eds) Nursing practice hospital and home, 2nd edn. Churchill Livingstone, Edinburgh

Gamble M 2001 A debriefing approach to dealing with the stress of CPR attempts. Professional Nurse 17(3): 157–160

Handley AJ, Swain A (eds) 1996 Ethics and legal aspects. In: Advanced life support manual. Resuscitation Council, London

Hinchliff SM, Montague SE, Watson R 1996 Physiology for nurses, 2nd edn. Baillière Tindall, Edinburgh

He J, Vupputuri S, Allen K, et al 1999 Passive smoking and the risk of coronary heart disease – a meta analysis of epidemiologic studies. The New England Journal of Medicine 340: 920–926 (http://www.jr2.ox.ac.uk/bandolier/booth/hliving/Passive.htlm)

Jamieson EM, McCall JM, Blythe R 1992 Guidelines for clinical nursing practices related to a nursing model, 2nd edn. Churchill Livingstone, Edinburgh

Jamieson EM, McCall JM, Whyte LA 2002 Guidelines for clinical nursing practices, 4th edn. Churchill Livingstone, Edinburgh

Jevon P, Ewens B 2001 Assessment of a breathless patient. Nursing Standard 15(16): 48–53

Jordan S, White J 2001 Bronchodilators: implications for nursing practice. Nursing Standard 15(27): 45–52

Liddle K 2000 Cystic fibrosis. In: Alexander MF, Fawcett JN, Runciman PJ (eds) Nursing practice hospital and home, 2nd edn. Churchill Livingstone, Edinburgh

Mallett J, Dougherty L 2000 The Royal Marsden Hospital manual of clinical nursing procedures, 5th edn. Blackwell Science, Oxford

Mallik M, Hall C, Howard D 1998 Nursing knowledge and practice: A decision making approach. Baillière Tindall, London

Millar B 2000 'A cruel and nasty disease'. Nursing Times 96(21): 32–33.

Miller G 2001 Tainted air. New Scientist 169(2272): 7

Nursing and Midwifery Council 2002a Code of professional conduct. Nursing and Midwifery Council, London

Nursing and Midwifery Council 2002b Guidelines for records and record keeping. Nursing and Midwifery Council, London

Ohnuki-Tierney E 1984 Illness and culture in contemporary Japan. Cambridge University Press, Cambridge

OPCS 1985 Hospital in-patient enquiry. HMSO, London

OPCS 1986 Mortality Statistics England and Wales: Cause. HMSO, London

Poloniecki JD, Atkinson RW, de Leon AP, Anderson HR 1997 Daily time series for cardiovascular hospital admissions and previous day's air pollution in London, UK. Occupational and Environmental Medicine 54(8): 535–540

Public Health Laboratory Service 2002 Legionnaires' disease cases and deaths. England and Wales residents, by sex 1980–2002. (http://www.phls.co.uk/topics-az/legionella/data_deathsex.htm)

Resuscitation Council UK 1997 The 1997 resuscitation guidelines for use in the United Kingdom. Resuscitation Council UK, London

Rice VH, Stead LF 2001 Nursing interventions for smoking cessation (Cochrane Review). In: The Cochrane Library, 2. Oxford, Update Software

Roper N, Logan W, Tierney AJ 1985 The elements of nursing: A model for nursing based on a model of living, 2nd edn. Churchill Livingstone, Edinburgh

Roper N, Logan W, Tierney AJ 1996 The elements of nursing: A model for nursing based on a model of living, 4th edn. Churchill Livingstone, Edinburgh

Roper N, Logan W, Tierney AJ 2000 The Roper–Logan–Tierney model of nursing based on activities of living. Churchill Livingstone, Edinburgh

Royal College of Nursing 1992 Resuscitation: right or wrong? The moral and legal issues faced by health care professional. Royal College of Nursing, London

Rutishauser S 1994 Physiology and anatomy: A basis for nursing and health care. Churchill Livingstone, Edinburgh

Sayer Q 1999 Put to the test. Nursing Times 95(29): 55–56

Serra A 2000 Tracheostomy care. Nursing Standard 14(42): 45–52

Sheppard M, Davis S 2000 Oxygen therapy – 2. Nursing Times 96(30): 43–44

Silagy C, Stead LF 2001 Physician advice for smoking cessation (Cochrane Review). In: The Cochrane Library, 2. Oxford, Update Software

Stanley H 1999 Facing cancer hand-in-hand. Nursing Times 96(9): 59

Thomson L, Mardel SN, Jack A, Shields TG 1992 Management of the moribund carbon monoxide victim. Archives of Emergency Medicine 334: 1642–1647

Walsh M (ed) 1997, 2002 Watson's clinical nursing and related sciences, 5th edn, 6th edn. Baillière Tindall, London

Walsh M, Ford P 1989 Nursing rituals: research and rational actions. Heinemann, Oxford

Waugh A, Grant A 2001 Ross and Wilson anatomy and physiology in health and illness, 9th edn. Churchill Livingstone, Edinburgh

West N, Popkess-Vawter S 1994 The subjective and psychosocial nature of breathlessness. Journal of Advanced Nursing 20: 622–626

World Health Organisation 1980 International classification of impairments, disabilities and handicaps: a manual classification relating to the consequence of disease. WHO, Geneva

Wynne G 1987 Inability of trained nurses to perform basic life support. British Medical Journal 294(6581): 1198

Further Reading

Department of Health 1998 Smoking kills. A white paper on tobacco. HMSO, London

Department of Health 2000 Smoking, drinking and drug use among young people in England in 2000. HMSO, London

Edmond CB 2000 Chapter 3 In: Alexander MF, Fawcett JN, Runciman PJ (eds) Nursing practice hospital and home, 2nd edn. Churchill Livingstone, Edinburgh

Jordan S, White J 2001 Bronchodilators: implications for nursing practice. Nursing Standard 15(27): 45–52

Rutishauser S 1994 Physiology and anatomy: A basis for nursing and health care, Chapter 7. Churchill Livingstone, Edinburgh

Serra A 2000 Tracheostomy care. Nursing Standard 14(42): 45–52

Sinclair J 1999 Environmental effects on health. Nursing Standard 13(26): 42–46

Stocks J 2000 Chapter 5.3. In: Hinchliff SM, Montague SE, Watson R (eds) Physiology for nurses, 2nd edn. Baillière Tindall, Edinburgh

Walsh M (ed) 2002 Caring for patients with respiratory problems (Chapter 13). In: Watson's clinical nursing and related sciences, 6th edn. Baillière Tindall, London

Useful websites

http://www.cochrane.org (Cochrane Library – Cochrane Databases of Systematic Reviews (CDSR) and the Database of Abstracts of Reviews of Effectiveness (DARE))

http://www.europa.eu.int (European Union website)

http://www.nelh.shef.ac.uk (protocols and care pathways library)

http://www.jr2.ox.ac.uk/bandolier

http://www.clinicalevidence.com

http://www.sign.ac.uk (new asthma guidelines January 2003)

http://www.brit-thoracic.org.uk

Eating and drinking

Jackie Solomon

Introduction

Eating and drinking are essential to existence (Roper et al 1996, 2000) and nutritional status is influenced by general health, chronic disorders, mobility and psychological or socioeconomic factors as well as age (McLaren et al 1997). The ability or inability to eat and drink can impact on many of the other ALs, if not all, for example overeating resulting in obesity may impact on the ability to mobilise or lack of adequate fluids may lead to dehydration and imbalance of homeostasis thus impacting on the activity of maintaining a safe environment. It is important to remember that ALs are closely related to each other and when illness compromises one activity then this will undoubtedly impact on the other ALs. The Roper, Logan and Tierney model for nursing provides nurses with a framework through which they are able to recognise and take account of the interrelatedness of the Activities of Living when assessing, planning, implementing and evaluating patient care. The nurse has a primary role, within the multidisciplinary team, in ensuring that patients receive food, fluids and adequate nutrition whilst they are in their care and health education regarding a healthy diet. Unfortunately, several reports have highlighted the poor nutritional status of patients in acute care, the lack of nurses' knowledge of nutrition and involvement in the nutritional care of patients, and the need for medical and nursing staff to assess patient's nutritional status (Lennard-Jones 1992, McWhirter & Pennington 1994, Kowanko et al 1999). To maintain a healthy diet we all need to ensure that we have an adequate supply of nutrients and in the right proportions for our need. Throughout this chapter the term malnutrition is used to include undernutrition due to inadequate food intake, overnutrition due to over consumption of food, deficiencies in nutrients, or dietary imbalance (Bond 1997).

This chapter will focus on the following:

1. **The model of living**
   - eating and drinking in health and illness (across the lifespan)
   - dependence/independence in eating and drinking
   - factors influencing the AL of eating and drinking.
2. **The model for nursing**
   - nursing care of individuals with health problems affecting the AL of eating and drinking.

THE MODEL OF LIVING

Eating and drinking are essential to our survival as human beings (Roper et al 1996, 2000). Food, water and essential nutrients are necessary to provide energy, growth, repair of body tissue and to maintain physiological functioning (Gobbi & Torrance 2000). Eating and drinking form part of our social activities and psychological wellbeing and a certain level of intelligence is required to understand the requirements of a well-balanced diet. The availability of food and drink is subject to social, economic and political influences and within well-developed countries is often taken for granted; unlike in less-developed countries where the access to food and drink is a daily struggle. Food safety and access to uncontaminated water sources is of vital importance. Eating and drinking are also central to cultural and religious rituals and ceremonies, for example the service of communion within a Christian community.

The nurse has a key role within the multidisciplinary team for assessing the nutritional needs of patients and ensuring that patients receive the right food, encouraging patients to eat and drink or managing artificial feeding regimes. They are also ideally placed to ensure a pleasant environment at mealtimes and minimise interruptions.

Eating and drinking in health and illness (across the lifespan)

Before birth

Before birth the fetus obtains its essential nutrients for growth and development from the mother via the placenta and amniotic fluid. Therefore it is important that the mother during her pregnancy maintains a healthy diet to provide nourishment for the growing fetus and successful lactation, and if she drinks alcohol that she reduces her intake to avoid the risk of birth defects (Roper et al 1996).

After birth

The first few days after birth the mother produces a substance known as colostrum from her breasts. The baby sucking the nipple stimulates the production of colostrum in the first instance followed by breast milk, which begins to flow on or around the third day after delivery (Hinchliff et al 1996). Colostrum and breast milk contain all the nutrients that a baby needs in the right proportions (National Child Birth Trust 1999). The 'fore milk' which is full of lactose quenches the baby's thirst is followed by a richer food known as the 'hind milk' that contains the calories that the baby requires. It is easily digested and absorbed and contains antibodies that help to protect the baby against infection and disease (Rutishauser 1994).

> **Exercise**
> 1. Discuss with your colleagues or family your views (and theirs) about breastfeeding.
> 2. Access the MIDIRs website (www.nelh.nhs.uk/maternity) for information about breastfeeding and find out what advantages breastfeeding has for the mother and the baby.

Breastfeeding has been shown to be advantageous for both the baby and the mother in preventing certain diseases. You may have found that there is some evidence to indicate that breastfeeding can protect the baby against gastroenteritis, otitis media, respiratory infections, urinary infections and diabetes mellitus. Breast milk also provides the baby with added immunity and enhances the benefits from immunisation (Effective Health Care Bulletin 2000). There is a belief that there are some situations in which breastfeeding might not be in the best interest of the baby including some maternal medications and specific viral infections such as HIV, hepatitis and T-cell leukaemia. Despite the risk Dobson (2002) points out that an overwhelming majority of babies will benefit from breastfeeding, even those born to HIV-infected women and that babies who receive formula milk or feed are six times more likely to die before they are 3 months old than breast-fed babies (Box 6.1).

> **Box 6.1 Health problems associated with bottle-fed babies**
>
> - gastroenteritis
> - respiratory infection
> - otitis media
> - urinary tract infection
> - necrotizing enterocolitis
> - atopic disease.
>
> From: MIDIRS Informed Choice (www.nelh.nhs.uk/maternity).

> **Exercise**
> 1. Find out it if there is any information available on the number of women who started to breast feed within your local area over a period of time.
> 2. What initiatives are available to support and encourage mothers to breastfeed their babies?
> 3. What advice is given to expectant and breastfeeding mothers about their own nutrition?

An infant feeding survey conducted by the Department of Health (2000b) has shown that breastfeeding rates within the UK have increased since 1990 and are associated with social demographic characteristics for example social class, age and education. Factors that also influence uptake include an acceptance that artificial feeding is the cultural norm. Other factors include the father or partner's commitment to breastfeeding, cultural norms and the provision of facilities in public places where women can breastfeed their baby. Breastfeeding a baby can be difficult for some women and it is important that they receive instruction and support in how to breastfeed successfully. In some areas mothers who have breastfed act as peers to help and support new mothers to breastfeed (Effective Healthcare Bulletin 2000).

You may have also found out about a number of initiatives designed to increase the prevalence of breastfeeding within your area. These may include the following:

- media campaigns
- health education activities
- support groups
- peer support
- training for both mothers and health professionals.

> **Exercise**
> 1. If you have had children, how did you feed your baby? If you breastfed your baby reflect on why you chose to do so and who or what helped you.
> 2. If you have not had children, discuss with a relative or colleague who has breastfed their child or children. Why did they chose to do so and who or what helped them?

Some mothers will not want to breastfeed their baby for many different reasons, some of these personal, such as needing to go back to work soon after the baby is born, flexibility, and confidence in the ability to breastfeed. You may have found that others' previous experience of breast-feeding and their support or otherwise may have influenced a decision to breastfeed or not.

Formula milk provides the necessary nutrients and is easy for the baby to digest. All formulas marketed in the UK must meet rigorous legislation and contain certain levels of protein, carbohydrates, fats, vitamins and minerals. Feeding a baby formula milk requires a supply of bottles and teats and an environment where these can be washed and sterilised by either boiling, steaming or chemical sterilisation. It is very important to make a formula feed up according to the instructions to ensure correct strength and dilution, there-fore the mother must be able to read and understand the instructions otherwise the baby may not receive adequate nutrition. The cost of buying formula milk can put pressure on the household budget. Recognising this some health clinics in the UK sell formula food cheaper than in local supermarkets or local shops.

Formula milk marketed in the UK has to meet strict regulations and standards regarding the levels of protein, carbohydrates, fats and vitamins. Preparing formula milk for a baby's feed requires strict hygiene and equipment. If there is any history of allergies in the family this should be taken into account when making a decision on whether to feed a baby formula milk. Mothers are advised to discuss this with a health professional who will advise on the brands of milk available.

Infants

When a baby is between 4 and 6 months old it is ready to begin taking solid food. The baby is introduced to these gradually by introducing solids on a spoon. The solids that might be tried include pureed fruit, vegetables and baby rice made up with breast or formula milk. It is important that these are introduced gradually and certain foods avoided before the baby is 6 months old.

Foods that should be avoided include: wheat-based products; nuts and seeds; eggs; fish and shellfish; citrus fruits and juices; cow's milk and milk products; salt; sugar; honey and spiced foods. Many of these foods are known to cause allergies, for example allergic reactions to peanuts can cause anaphylactic shock and be fatal. It is therefore necessary to pay careful attention to food labels when purchasing proprietary products. Some children are thought to be sensitive to additives in processed foods. Within the European Community only additives that have been passed as safe and given an E number are recommended for use, however, in the UK and other countries additives without E numbers are used. Processed foods contain a higher amount of salt, fat and sugar than homemade foods. Drinks that contain sugar should be avoided as they can cause tooth decay and fruit juices should be diluted with

water. Infants should be encouraged to drink from a cup rather than a feeding cup or bottle.

Children

Children rely on adequate nutritional intake for growth and energy and need regular nutritious meals. The amount of food will depend on their age, gender, weight, height and physical activity. Sometimes children will refuse to eat. Unless the child is showing signs of malnutrition this should not be a cause for concern, as children have a ten-dency to eat when they are hungry. It is more concerning when the child refuses to eat nourishing food for example fruit and vegetables in favour of high-energy snacks. The National Fruit Scheme and increasing access to healthy foods in schools are examples of how the UK Government is trying to improve nutrition in children (DoH 2001g). An example of this is setting up a breakfast club for local school children. The children who attended the breakfast club per-formed better in the classroom. Parents and their teachers have an important role in ensuring that children and young adults understand what a well-balanced diet is and that they lead by example. Nevertheless obesity in children is on the increase and this may continue into adulthood. Indeed according to the Third National Health and Nutrition Survey (NHANES 111) nearly 14% of children age 6–11 years were overweight and at risk of developing asthma, type 2 diabetes mellitus and orthopaedic conditions (Covington et al 2001). Research undertaken in the North of England found that whilst most 11–12 year olds under-stood what they should eat for a healthy diet they had little knowledge of fats, carbohydrates, and dietary fibre (Frobisher & Maxwell 2001).

Adolescents

During adolescence young people begin to become more independent, perhaps leaving home for the first time and beginning relationships. They will choose to try out new foods perhaps adopting a vegetarian dietary regime and be willing to experiment with alcohol. Young people are also conscious of their body image and can be susceptible to eating disorders such as anorexia nervosa in their mid-teens (Cremin & Halek 1997) (see further information on anorexia nervosa and bulimia at the Royal College of Psychiatrists website www.rcpsych.ac.uk).

Adulthood

Within the Western world the choice of food has increased with globalisation and access to foreign travel. Eating and drinking has become a major social pastime and over recent years there has been an increase in the number of fast food outlets and restaurants, which together with more sedentary lifestyles are contributing to the rise in the incidence of obesity. Adults should try to eat a healthy diet as described by the Department of Health COMA (DoH 1991) recommendations and in enough amounts to maintain an optimal weight for their height. This is a model that helps people to understand what healthy eating means in terms of food choice. Adults also need to keep their intake of alcohol within 'safe' limits and take sufficient exercise to prevent coronary heart disease and other diet related diseases (Roper et al 1996). A diet that is rich in oily fish, such as salmon, sardines and tuna contains a fatty acid (Omega-3) and appears to have an effect on the heart rhythm, as well as a reduction in the incidence of stroke and a positive effect on rheumatoid arthritis and asthma. Increasing the intake of fruit and vegetables and reducing the amount of saturated fat in the diet can protect against cardiovascular disease (see Box 6.2).

The decline of oestrogen levels in women approaching the menopause and increased bone reabsorption can lead to osteoporosis. Whilst osteoporosis is usually seen in the older person, increasing the level of calcium and vitamin D supplements in the diet alongside medication can help to slow down the disease in those at risk of other calcium-deficient diseases in adulthood, including osteomalacia and Paget's disease. Calcium also has a role in controlling blood pressure and reducing the likelihood of kidney stones. Some foods which contain phyto-oestrogens, are thought to be especially beneficial to menopausal women (Sutcliffe 2001). These are believed to control excess oestrogens in the body and prevent excess excretion of calcium from our bones. Phyto-oestrogens are found in fruit and vegetables and the soya bean. Soya contains more protein than cow's milk, it is high in fatty acids and also contributes to reducing cholesterol levels. Some women prefer to use phyto-oestrogens as an alternative to hormone replacement therapy.

Box 6.2 Summary of food groups

Bread, other cereals and potatoes
Recommendations: eat lots.

Milk and dairy foods
Recommendations: eat and drink moderate amounts and choose lower-fat versions whenever you can.

Fruit and vegetables
Recommendations: eat lots (at least five portions a day, excluding potatoes).

Meat, fish and alternatives
Recommendations: eat moderate amounts and choose lower-fat versions whenever you can.

Foods containing fat, foods containing sugar
Recommendations: eat foods containing fat sparingly and look out for the low-fat alternatives.

Foods containing sugar should not be eaten too often as they can contribute to tooth decay.

Adapted from Roper et al (1996).

Older people

Around 18% of the UK population is over 65 years of age and it is estimated that by 2030 this will rise to 23%. Older people are more likely to suffer from debilitating factors associated with ill health, psychological, physiological and biological changes, social isolation, reduced income and environmental issues that impact on their ability to take an adequate diet and maintain an appropriate nutritional status (Bond 1997). The older person is likely to have lower activity levels and lead a more sedentary lifestyle than younger people. They are also likely to be receiving medication that may cause side effects (e.g. nausea, constipation) alter their appetite, absorption of nutrients, their sense of taste and/or influence their nutritional status.

A decrease in the ability to handle food and cutlery perhaps due to arthritic hands or mental capacity, difficulty with shopping and cooking, declining oral health and ill-fitting dentures, as well as loss of senses such as taste and smell, can contribute to malnutrition in the older person. However, due to improved oral health and dental care older people are now retaining their teeth. Fitzpatrick (2000) points out the need for improved attention to oral hygiene to improve patient comfort and maintenance of nutritional status (Holmes & Mountain 1993).

Malnutrition in the older person is a frequent and serious problem (Chen et al 2001) and often goes unnoticed, mistaken instead for signs of ageing or symptoms of underlying disease (McLaren et al 1997). Untreated it will lead to increased mortality, morbidity and influence the length of admission to hospital (Lennard-Jones 1992). A study in Sweden (Elmståhl et al 1997) found that a high proportion of older people in long-term care were reported as having lower energy and nutrient levels than was recommended and that they also had a higher mortality rate. In the UK between 10% and 40% of older people admitted to hospital are thought to be undernourished. With a rapidly increasing elderly population the issue of malnutrition is gaining the interest of policymakers and professional bodies (DoH, 2001a, 2001b, 2001c, 2001d, 2001f).

Exercise

1. Talk to a teenager, an adult and an older person and find out:

   - What they eat and drink and when?
   - Are there any foods that they avoid and if so why?
   - Do they shop for their food?
   - Do they cook for themselves or others?

You may have discovered differences in their responses to your questions. A teenager living at home will more likely still be reliant on their parents to provide their food. Their lifestyle may mean that they rely on convenience or fast foods. Because they are still growing and need high energy levels, they are likely to eat bigger portions and have snacks between meals. There may be some foods that they dislike and therefore avoid.

The adult's choice and variety of food may be constrained or enabled by their socioeconomic status and access to healthy foods. The times and frequency with which they eat may depend on working patterns, and if a parent, children's routines and choice of food. Their view of what constitutes a healthy diet may be influenced by their knowledge and health beliefs and this in conjunction with their financial circumstances will have a bearing on their purchase of food. Environmental factors relating to facilities for the safe storage and cooking food may also be a factor.

The older person is more likely to suffer from health problems, live alone and have a reduced income. Cooking for one person and eating alone reduces the pleasure associated with mealtimes and perhaps after a lifetime of preparing food for others they see no purpose in the preparation of food (Gustafsson & Sidenvall 2002). They may find it hard to adapt recipes for one person and choose ready-prepared meals instead. If the older person is housebound they are reliant on others to shop and make choices for them. They may also avoid certain foods because of health conditions such as citrus fruits in arthritic conditions. The older person is likely to have lower activity levels and a more sedentary lifestyle than younger people and therefore may believe that they do not need to eat as much as a younger person. A study by McKie et al (2000) of older people living in Scotland showed dietary beliefs are based on childhood and lifetime experiences and that access to food, the cost and quality of the food influenced what people ate.

Exercise

1. Compare what people eat with what they said they ate against the five-food group plan below (see Boxes 6.3 and 6.4).
2. How do they compare?
3. Monitor your diet for a week. How does your diet compare with the five-food group plan?

Box 6.3 Five-food group plan for adult's daily requirements

Cereals/bread/potatoes
Make these the main part of every meal. Whole grain products are preferred. This group provides carbohydrates (starch), fibre (nonstarch polysaccharides), some calcium, iron and B vitamins.

Fruit and vegetables
Aim to eat at least five portions a day. Eat a wide variety of fresh, frozen, canned or juiced fruit and vegetables. This group provides vitamins C and A, folates and some carbohydrates.

Meat, fish and alternatives
Eat moderate amounts of these foods. Lower fat alternatives are preferred. Include two portions of fish each week, one of which should be oily fish. This group provides protein, iron, zinc, magnesium and B vitamins.

Fats and sugars
Eat fatty foods as sparingly as possible. Some fats contain vitamin A, D and E and essential fatty acids. Eat sugary foods infrequently and in small amounts as sugar contributes to tooth decay and contains no other nutrients.

From Gobbi & Torrance 2000.

Box 6.4 Five-food group plan for vegetarian adults' daily requirements

Cereals/bread/potatoes
Make these the main part of every meal. Whole grain products are preferred. This group provides carbohydrates (starch), fibre (nonstarch polysaccharide), some calcium, iron and B vitamins.

Fruit and vegetables
Aim to eat at least five portions a day. Eat a wide variety of fresh, frozen, canned or juiced fruit and vegetables. This group provides vitamins C and A, folates and some carbohydrate.

Milk and milk alternatives
Eat moderate amounts of these foods. Lower fat alternatives are preferred. This group provides protein, calcium and vitamins A, B_{12} and D. Alternatives include vitamin B_{12} soya milk and vegetarian cheese.

Alternatives to meat and fish
In vegetarian diets, it is not sufficient just to avoid meat. Such food must be replaced by other foods from the same food group. Choose protein-rich plant foods such as pulses, soya bean, quorn, nuts and seeds. Eat moderate amounts of these foods. Lower-fat alternatives preferred. This group provides protein, iron, zinc, magnesium and B vitamins.

Fats and sugars
Eat fatty food sparingly and choose low-fat alternatives if possible. Fats contain vitamins A, D and E and essential fatty acids. Eat sugary foods infrequently and small amounts as sugar contributes to tooth decay and contains no other nutrients.

From Gobbi & Torrance 2000.

Healthy eating

Gobbi and Torrance (2000) identify a five-food plan for an adult's daily nutritional requirements, including those of adults who are vegetarian (see Boxes 6.3 and 6.4).

Reflect on the outcome of the exercise on p. 167. Do you need to change your dietary intake and if so in what way?

Dependence/independence

Dependence/independence in the ALs is closely related to an individual's lifespan and the other Activities of Living (Roper et al 1996, 2000). Viewed as a continuum it is central to the concept of the model (see Fig 6.1).

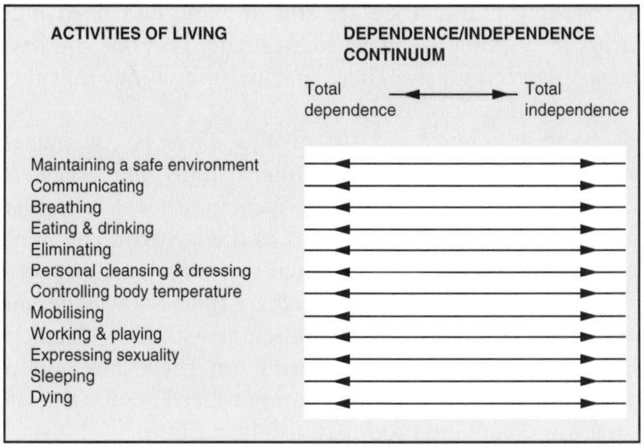

Whilst in the uterus the fetus is dependent on the mother for its nutrients via the umbilical cord. After birth babies and young children are very dependent on adults to provide them with food and drink. By the age of 18 months a baby will be making attempts to feed itself and by the age of two most children are able to undertake this activity independently. However, children will continue to depend on adults to make informed choices about the purchase, provision and safe preparation of food and drink for some considerable time and those who are physically disabled or suffer from learning difficulties may be dependent on others to assist them to eat and drink for even longer. Ill health, physical or psychological disability in all ages may impact on an individual's ability to be independent in the activity of eating and drinking (Roper et al 1996).

> **Exercise**
>
> Consider the following brief case studies.

> **Case study 6.1**
>
> **Temporary disability**
>
> Mark is a 22-year-old university student. He has recently been involved in a road traffic accident and injured both his arms. He lives in student accommodation with two other students. He is reluctant to move back home as he needs to attend lectures in preparation for his exams later in the year.

> **Exercise**
>
> 1. How will Mark's temporary disability impact on his independence in the activity of eating and drinking?

Mark will need help from his friends and colleagues, if they are willing, to buy in and prepare the food. He may require help to feed himself and to attend to his personal

Fig. 6.1 Dependence/independence continuum (from Roper et al 1996, with permission).

hygiene, washing and dressing and elimination. He may be unable to clean his teeth resulting in altered sense of taste and lack of appetite. However his dependence is temporary and he should return to independence within a short timescale.

> **Case study 6.2**
>
> **Dependence on others**
>
> Agnes is a 48-year-old lady who suffers from multiple sclerosis. She lives with her husband, who is the main wage earner, and two teenage children. She is wheelchair-dependent and needs assistance with most ALs.

> **Exercise**
>
> 1. In what way is Agnes dependent on others in relation to the activity of eating and drinking?

Multiple sclerosis is a chronic degenerative disease, the incidence of which is higher in women than men (Walsh 2002). The effects of the disease vary from person to person and recurring relapses will increase dependency on others for assistance with many of the Activities of Living. Whether or not she is in remission, Agnes will be dependent to a lesser or greater degree on her family for support and to provide food and drink. It may also be necessary to provide resources from the community and social services such as specialist devices to assist in feeding. Occupational Therapists and Speech Therapists can provide help with assessment of swallowing problems and specialist interventions. Agnes is also dependent on her husband to ensure that finances are available to purchase food and drink.

Exercise
If you are a student nurse on clinical placement arrange to spend some time with the following health care professionals. Find out what support they provide for patients who are dependent on others to ensure they receive food and drink. You may like to use Case studies 6.1 and 6.2 as a focus for your discussions.

- Speech and Language Therapist
- Occupational Therapist
- Dietitian
- Social Worker.

Exercise
Reflect on your own circumstances.

1. Have you ever been in a situation in which you have been dependent on others to provide your food and drink or feed you?
2. How did you feel?
3. To illustrate dependence undertake this exercise with a colleague.

At a mealtime take turns in feeding each other a meal and a drink. Do this under the following conditions, firstly in silence, then blindfolded and finally normally. Discuss how you felt in each situation. What did you learn from this exercise?

How did you manage to communicate with the person you were feeding? While you were blindfolded what was it like not to be able to see the food? Did this make any difference to your enjoyment of the food?

You may have experienced a loss of self-esteem, felt out of control and reliant on the person feeding you to anticipate your needs.

Assisting patients to eat and drink

Sometimes patients require assistance to eat and drink. Being fed by others can be quite threatening and demoralising. A full assessment of the patient's ability should be undertaken and interventions designed to promote independence agreed. When feeding patients the nurse should attempt to make the experience as normal as possible by using normal crockery and tableware. The patient should be made comfortable and encouraged to contribute in whichever way he or she is able and care should be taken not to rush the meal.

In some situations patients may be unable to eat enough solid food to meet their nutritional needs and require nutritional supplements or sip feeds. These are prescribed by the dietitian following a nutritional assessment or given according to protocol or guidelines. Where this is necessary it is useful to monitor the patient's intake of food to ensure the patient is receiving enough nutrition.

Enteral and parenteral feeding

In other situations patients are fed directly into the stomach or enterally. Enteral feeding involves passing a fine-bore tube into the stomach either via the nasal route, orally or directly into the gut (usually stomach or small intestine) through the abdomen (gastrostomy) usually reserved for longer-term feeding. Specialised feeds are passed through the tube either intermittently or by bolus and absorbed by the gut. If patients are unable to meet their nutritional needs orally or enterally it is possible to provide nutrients directly into a vein bypassing the gut and the need for ingestion, digestion and absorption of food and is known as parenteral nutrition. This route should only used if the gut cannot be used. The general rule is if the gut can be used use it as this helps to maintain gut integrity. Patients receiving enteral or parenteral nutrition are dependent on the nurse and members of the multidisciplinary team to provide their nutritional and physical needs and psychological support. It is outside the scope of this chapter to provide a complete synopsis of the indications, administration and monitoring of patient care associated with enteral and parenteral nutrition (Jamieson et al 2002).

Exercise
1. If you are a student nurse undertaking a clinical placement seek the opportunity to assist in the care of a patient who is receiving enteral or parenteral nutrition.
2. Identify the knowledge and skills you need to develop to ensure safe and accountable practice.
3. Discuss how you will develop these with your mentor and personal tutor.

Dependency on food and drink

Some individuals can become dependent on certain foods and drink for example caffeine (chocolate, Coca Cola® and coffee) and alcohol. Caffeine has a stimulating effect on the central nervous system. A study by Silverman et al (1992) found that participants who were on a caffeine free diet suffered more headaches, required more analgesia, suffered tiredness and showed a higher level of depression than those who included caffeine in their diet.

Alcohol

With the exception of some cultures (e.g Islam), alcohol is widely used by adults in social situations to facilitate interaction with others and remove inhibitions. The availability of alcohol and its inclusion in everyday life means that children are exposed to alcohol at an early age. In the UK it is against the law to serve alcohol to a person under the age of 18. There is no law that prohibits children under the age of 18 from drinking alcohol in the home.

Alcohol misuse may result in long-term disability or in some cases death. Regular heavy alcohol use can increase the

Box 6.5 Alcohol use: associated harm

Consequences of intoxication
- accidents
- acute poisoning
- acute gastritis
- drug overdose
- epileptic-type seizures
- head injury
- suicidal behaviour.

Consequences of excessive regular use
- anxiety
- cancer of the mouth/throat
- depression
- fatty liver
- liver cancer
- liver cirrhosis
- pancreatitis
- peripheral neuritis
- phobic illness
- sexual impotence
- stomach haemorrhage.

Consequence of dependence
- alcoholic psychosis
- anxiety
- delirium tremens
- depression
- hallucination
- paranoid states
- polydrug abuse
- withdrawal: epileptic seizures.

From: Cooper 2000.

risk of various diseases (see Box 6.5). A person who over-indulges in alcohol may become malnourished due to the toxic effect of alcohol on the intestine, which can impair the absorption of nutrients and impaired metabolism leading to loss of weight. If alcohol is replacing food in the diet, the effects on malnutrition are accelerated. Alcohol can also interact with or reduce the effectiveness of medicines.

An online Report by the Royal College of Physicians (2001) highlights the increasing burden on the National Health Service due to alcohol misuse. The report suggests the need to consider strategies to reduce the hazardous drinking in the population, assume more responsibility for health promotion and tackle the underlying problems of alcohol rather than just treating the physical disease.

Factors influencing the AL of eating and drinking

This next section will help you to understand the factors influencing the activity of eating and drinking. Each of these will now be explored.

Biological factors

All living organisms must have some form of nutrition to sustain life. In order for you to care for people who have problems with the activity of eating and drinking it is necessary for you to understand the anatomy and physiology related to the gastrointestinal system. These will be briefly discussed in relation to the activity of eating and drinking, however you may need to refer to the Further Reading list for further information.

Under normal circumstances a person will consume approximately 1 kg of solids and 1.2 kg of fluid each day (Hinchliff et al 1996). However, most of what we eat is unsuitable for immediate use by the body to provide energy and for growth and repair. As food passes through the gastrointestinal tract it undergoes three main processes: ingestion, digestion and absorption. In their model of living, Roper et al (1996) link these processes alongside that of the AL of eating and drinking. However the interrelatedness of the AL means that it is also necessary to consider the biological factors associated with movement, for example, to be able to transport the food or drink from the plate or cup into mouth (Roper et al 1996) (see Fig. 6.2 for anatomy of the digestive system).

Ingestion

Food is ingested through the mouth. As well as being necessary for communication the lips are necessary to help to take hold of food when eating and fluids when drinking.

Exercise
1. Think about a time when you have had a local anaesthetic at the dentist.
2. Before the local anaesthetic wore off, did you have any problems eating and drinking?
3. Talk to others who have had similar treatments. What were their experiences?

Discomfort or impairment of the lips will impact on an individual's ability to eat and drink normally. Such problems might include:

- neurological problems, e.g. stroke
- infections of the lips, e.g. herpes simplex
- trauma of the face or lips, e.g. assault or RTA
- environmental, e.g. chapped lips due to wind or sunburn.

Once food is taken into the mouth it is chopped up into little pieces by the teeth, mixed with saliva and passed down the oesophagus by the tongue.

Swallowing

Roper et al (1996) describe swallowing in three stages.

Preparatory stage During this stage an individual will transfer the food or drink from a receptacle (cup, plate, package, etc.) to the mouth. This usually involves a functioning

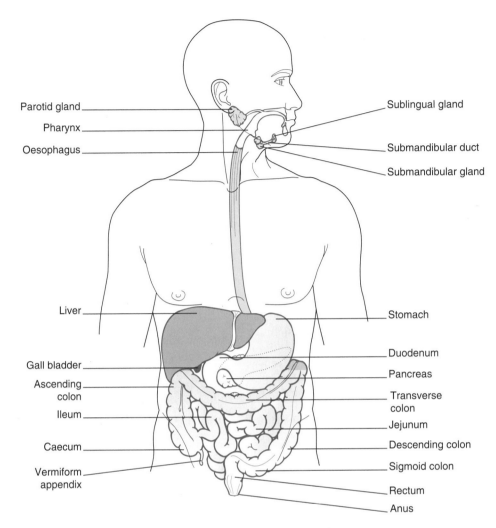

Fig. 6.2 Anatomy of the digestive system (from Hinchliff et al 2000, with permission).

upper limb or assistance from another individual. The normal mouth, gums, tongue and mucosa should be pink and moist. Small papillae should be visible on the surface of the tongue and the teeth should be free from caries and the breath free from odour. Any changes in the appearance of a person's mouth may indicate a digestive or general disorder and can assist in diagnosis.

Exercise

To illustrate how inspection of the mouth can assist in diagnosing nutritional deficiencies or gastrointestinal problems, consider the following case studies.

1. Ellen is an 82-year-old lady admitted to hospital following a fall. On assessment you find her lips are dry, her tongue is dry and furred.
2. Mary is a 36-year-old lady who is complaining of recurrent oral ulceration.

In each of these cases how might oral assessment help in diagnosis?

In Ellen's case you might suspect that she is suffering from dehydration or lack of fluids. However, you might also enquire about her medication, as some medicines, for example some antispasmodics or antidepressive drugs cause dry mouths. In Mary's case recurrent oral ulceration may be a sign of a deficiency of folic acid.

Exercise

1. Find out what other information you can obtain by inspecting a patient's mouth and how this might link to the activity of eating and drinking (see Alexander et al 2000 Chapter 15 for further reading).

The tongue is a vascular organ, extremely sensitive and plays an important part in speech. Its function within the AL of eating and drinking is not only to move the food around the mouth but also to allow us to taste and enjoy our food. On the surface of the tongue are many papillae, which contain taste buds. These taste buds with the aid of stimuli from the olfactory nerve enable us to differentiate between sweet, sour, salt and bitter tastes. In Ellen's case her taste may be altered due to her dry mouth and furred tongue.

An adult has 32 permanent teeth, canine teeth for tearing food, incisors for cutting and the molars and premolars for grinding food. Each tooth is covered in enamel and protects the underlying dentine, a substance similar to that of bone. Underneath the dentine is the pulp cavity that contains the nerve fibres. If there is a break in the enamel then acid formed from sugars in the diet can attack the dentine, cause intense pain and lead to tooth decay. Fluoride added to toothpaste is effective in helping to control dental decay (Anderson & Nathan 1991). Regular oral hygiene and dental care are essential to prevent dental disease and aid taste, eating and communication.

The voluntary/preswallowing/oral stage This is when the tongue moves about the food in the mouth. The action of the tongue enables mastication by the teeth and mixes the food with saliva. The parotid, the submaxillary and the sublingual glands produce saliva. The thought, sight or smell of food or the presence of food in the mouth stimulates the production of saliva in the mouth. As well as helping to soften the food and bind it into a bolus, saliva contains a digestive enzyme, which acts on cooked starches and changes polysaccharide into disaccharides.

Involuntary/swallow/pharyngeal stage This is when the bolus of food is pressed against the hard palate by the tongue and using an arching movement thrusts the bolus of food towards the oropharynx (Hinchliff et al 1996). So that food is not inhaled into the trachea breathing is inhibited during this time (see Fig. 6.4). The oesophagus is a

Box 6.6 Health problems associated with ingestion of food and drink
Disorders of the mouth
• dry mouth (xerostomia)
• dental caries
• peridontal disease
• acute tooth infection
• stomatitis
• thrush (oral candidiasis)
• gingivitis
• leucoplakia
• cancer
• inflammation of the parotid gland
• obstruction of the flow of saliva
• trauma (fracture of the jaw).
Adapted from Finlay 2002.

hollow muscular tube and has no role in digestion or absorption; its sole purpose is to connect the pharynx to the stomach. Once in the oesophagus the bolus of food is propelled by the action of peristalsis into the stomach and small intestine (see Fig. 6.3). This movement is under involuntary neural control and hormonal factors. The parasympathetic supply is via the vagus nerve and leads to an increase in the motility and secretion and relaxation of the sphincters whereas the action of the sympathetic supply serves to decrease the blood supply to the gut and reduce motility and secretions (see Hinchliff et al 1996, p. 466 for further reading).

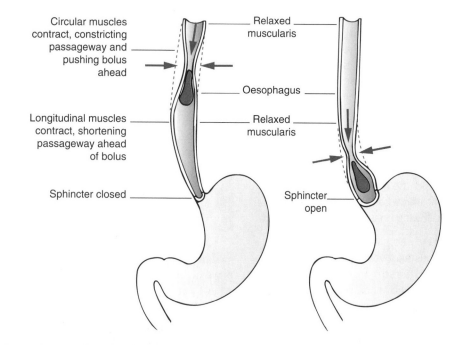

Fig. 6.3 The oesophageal stage of swallowing showing peristalsis (from Hinchliff et al 1996, with permission).

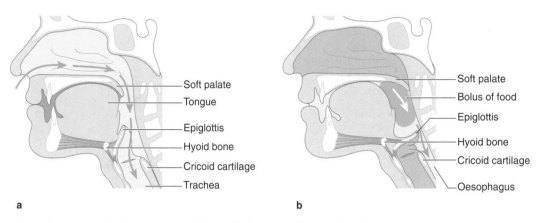

Soft palate
Tongue
Epiglottis
Hyoid bone
Cricoid cartilage
Trachea

a

Soft palate
Bolus of food
Epiglottis
Hyoid bone
Cricoid cartilage
Oesophagus

b

Fig. 6.4 The position of structures in the mouth and throat during breathing and swallowing (from Rogers 1993, with permission).

Patients who have suffered a stroke may experience swallowing difficulties known as dysphagia due to neurological impairment. Up to 45% of patients admitted to hospitals following a stroke may have dysphagia (SIGN 1997).

> **Exercise**
> 1. Look up the Scottish Intercollegiate Guidelines Network site on the web.
> 2. Find out about the management of patients with stroke, identification and management of dysphagia.

You will have discovered that it is extremely important for the nurse to be able to assess a stroke patient's ability to swallow, as there is a possibility that if swallowing is impaired they may inhale food or fluid into the bronchial tree. This is referred to as aspiration and can be life-threatening. If a patient displays any difficulty in swallowing they should be referred to a Speech and Language Therapist for full assessment. It may be necessary to feed the patient through a nasogastric tube until the swallowing reflex returns when foods of different consistencies may be introduced (see Box 6.7 for a list of other health problems associated with swallowing difficulties).

> **Exercise**
> Reflect on the knowledge and skills you need to develop to enable you to undertake a swallowing assessment. Include these in your personal development plan and discuss these with your mentor and personal tutor.

Digestion

Digestion begins in the stomach, where food is mixed with gastric juices (mucus, hydrochloric acid and pepsinogen) to produce chyme. As the food enters the stomach via the lower oesophageal sphincter the stomach wall stretches and in doing so stimulates receptors to release the gastric juices. The release of gastric juices is also stimulated by the

> **Box 6.7 Health problems associated with ingestion of food and drink**
>
> **Disorders of the oesophagus**
> * neurological disorders
> * congenital disorders
> * reflux oesophagitis
> * oesophageal achalasia
> * trauma
> * benign neoplasm
> * cancer
> * oesophageal varices
> * hiatus hernia.
>
> Adopted from Finlay 2002.

thought, sight and smell of food and certain foods such as protein and caffeine (see Fig. 6.5).

The stomach acts as a reservoir for food and allows us to eat enough food at widely spread intervals. The stomach can hold up to 1.5 litres of food and fluids and up to 4 litres in extreme conditions. Patients who have had a portion of their stomach removed should be advised to take small frequent meals to avoid unpleasant symptoms, for example, dumping syndrome or hypoglycaemia.

It usually takes 4–5 hours for the contents of the stomach to empty. Meals that contain a high fatty content take longer to leave the stomach and will leave a person feeling more satisfied. This is important to consider when advising a patient to fast before surgery. It is not just sufficient to ask the patient to fast without providing advice on which foods they should avoid.

> **Exercise**
> 1. Find out what information is given to patients preoperatively.
> 2. How long are patients advised to fast for?
> 3. Are they given any information on what foods to avoid prior to fasting?

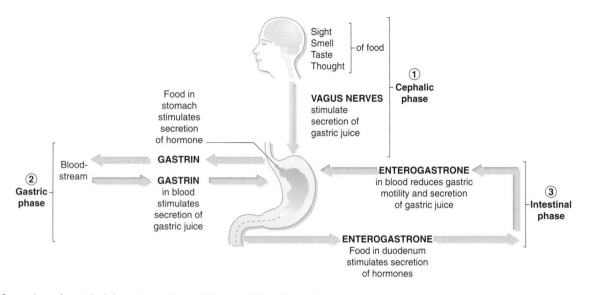

Fig. 6.5 Secretion of gastric juices (from Wilson & Waugh 1996, with permission).

Patients are advised to fast before surgery because anaesthesia can cause vomiting, aspiration of acid secretions and lung damage. Traditionally patients have been fasted from solids and fluids for up to 12 hours prior to surgery (Hamilton-Smith 1972, Butterworth 1974) and in some cases longer (Thomas 1987). This practice can lead to dehydration and nutritional deficit postoperatively especially in patients who have a reduced intake of protein (protein energy malnutrition) resulting in loss of weight and muscle wastage and loss of subcutaneous fat predisposing to pressure sore development (Shireff 1990). The practice of starving people for long periods of time has been challenged recently with most anaesthetists agreeing that, in the absence of any condition or disease that delays gastric emptying, a fast of 6 hours for solids and 3 hours for clear fluids for both inpatients and day patients is good practice (Ogg & Hitchcock 1993, Maltby 1993).

To prevent overloading the small intestine, the pyloric sphincter controls the passage of chyme into the duodenum where it is mixed with the secretions of the gall bladder (bile) and pancreas, which enter through the ampulla of Vater. Chyme has low pH due to the hydrochloric acid and as it enters the duodenum it is neutralised by the pancreatic juices. The hormones cholecystokinin and secretin control the secretion of pancreatic juices and bile. Bile consisting of bile salts and bile pigments is manufactured in the liver and stored in the gall bladder. The action of bile is to emulsify fats into smaller particles so that they can be broken down further and digested. Disorders of the stomach include:

- gastritis
- peptic ulcer
- haemorrhage (perforation)
- cancer
- pyloric stenosis.

Absorption

Once the food is broken down into a form that can be absorbed digestion is complete and the nutrients are ready to pass into the bloodstream. The chyme is moved along the small intestine by a series of movements known as peristalsis and segmentation. In addition to digestive enzymes present in the pancreatic juice, enzymes are secreted through the walls of the small intestine, which consists of finger-like projections known as villi and which serve to increase the surface area of the intestine. Each villi contains an arteriole and a venule. As the nutrients are absorbed through the villi they pass into the lymphatic system (fats) and bloodstream (other nutrients).

Failure to absorb nutrients is known as malabsorption syndrome. Adults with malabsorption syndrome will present with loss of weight, abdominal distension, anaemia and diarrhoea. In children, parents will have noticed that they are failing to thrive. Howie et al (2000) suggest several reasons for malabsorption, including pancreatic dysfunction, liver disease, extensive bowel resection, coeliac disease, and impaired enzyme activity. Crohn's disease is a chronic inflammatory disease of the gastrointestinal tract that is common in young adults in the West. Damage to the mucosal lining because of inflammation reduces the ability to absorb nutrients and protein can be lost through gastrointestinal bleeding (Metcalf 2002). Patients with Crohn's disease will need to ensure that they have a balanced diet and during an active phase of the disease that they increase their intake of protein and calories. Metcalf (2002) suggests that whilst there is no validated dietary advice available on what should be avoided there are some foods, for example milk, that might make patients feel better. Patients who have coeliac disease are unable to tolerate gluten, found in wheat, rye and barley in their diet. Classically, they present with loss of weight and fat in their faeces, but in many cases the symptoms are more vague, e.g. lethargy, anaemia.

Metabolism

Eveyone needs food for energy and the cellular activity of major organs even at rest. The amount needed to maintain these functions at rest is known as the basal metabolic rate or BMR. The BMR is at its highest during childhood and declines with age, it is also influenced by the sex and size of the body. As digestive processes break down the food the cells take it up and it undergoes further physical and chemical metabolism.

The amount of energy produced by foods is measured by calories or joules (SI units). A calorie is the amount of energy that is needed to raise the temperature of water by 1°C. Different foods produce different levels of energy with fats providing the highest level (see Table 6.1 and Fig. 6.6 and Table 6.2 for further information on metabolism and energy).

Exercise

1. Think about a hot summer's day. How active were you?
2. What types of food did you eat?
3. Now think about a cold winter's day. How active were you?
4. What types of food did you eat?
5. Consider the effects on eating when living in either a cold climate or a hot climate on a permanent basis.

The level of activity determines how much energy is required from food. On a hot summer's day you may have reduced your activity and ate small light meals, such as salads whereas in winter it is likely that you have been more active and eaten larger meals with more carbohydrates. This is because in the cold more energy is required to keep warm.

Table 6.1 Energy yielded by different foods and drinks*

Food/drink	kcal/100 g[†]	kJ/100 g[†]
Tea (no milk or sugar)	< 1	2
Coffee (no milk or sugar)	2	8
Beer	25–39	104–163
Milk (whole)	66	275
Wine (dry–sweet)	66–94	275–394
Vegetables (mushrooms–potatoes)	13–75	55–318
Fruit (melon–bananas)	19–95	81–403
Fish (cod)	76	322
Lean meat (chicken–lamb)	121–162	508–679
Eggs	147	612
Fish (mackerel)	223	926
Bread (Hovis–naan)	212–336	899–1415
Nuts (peanuts–macadamia)	564–748	2341–3082
Butter	737	3031
Vegetable oil	899	3696

* Representative values compiled from Holland et al 1991 McCance and Widdowson's The composition of foods, fifth revised and extended edition, by permission of HMSO, London.

[†] Applies to the edible part of each food. Energy depends largely on the relative proportions of fat (9 kcal/g), carbohydrate (4 kcal/g) and water (0 kcal/g) in each food and drink. Thus, tea and coffee (mostly water) yield few calories whereas butter and vegetable oil (mostly fat) yield a lot. Bread (mostly carbohydrate plus water) and potatoes (mostly water plus some carbohydrate) are intermediate.

Table 6.2 Predicted basal metabolic rates of adult men and women of different ages, each weighing 65 kg*

Sex	Age range (years)	BMR		
		mJ/day	kcal/day	kcal/min
Male	18–30	7.07	1690	1.17
	30–60	6.82	1630	1.13
	>60	5.73	1370	0.95
Female	18–30	6.11	1460	1.01
	30–60	5.86	1400	0.97
	>60	5.32	1270	0.88

* Compiled from the report of a Joint FAO/WHO/UNU Expert Consultation 1985.

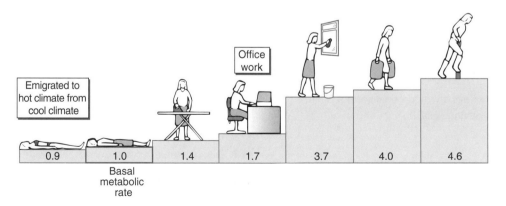

Fig. 6.6 The relative energy costs of different activities undertaken by a woman, as compared with her metabolic rate (from Rutishauser 1994, with permission).

Diabetes mellitus

The number of people suffering from diabetes mellitus is increasing worldwide. It is estimated that there are around 1 million people in England suffering from diabetes mellitus. Diabetes is a serious and major health concern for which there is no known cure. Around 5% of the NHS budget is spent on treating people with diabetes and accounts for up to 10% of hospital resources. People suffering from diabetes mellitus have a high level of glucose (hyperglycaemia) in their bodies and because they are unable to use it properly it accumulates in the blood. Diabetes is more likely to occur in people of South-Asian descent, older people, those in deprived areas and is more common in males than females (DoH 2001d).

Insulin is a hormone produced by the pancreas that plays an important role in regulating blood glucose. A low level of blood glucose is known as hypoglycaemia. Diabetes mellitus is a major health concern as people with this condition are more likely to go on to develop a number of chronic complications as a result of vascular degenerative changes including, e.g., diabetic retinopathy, arteriosclerosis, peripheral neuropathy and cardiovascular or cerebrovascular disease.

There are two main classifications of diabetes mellitus, insulin-dependent diabetes mellitus (IDDM) and noninsulin-dependent diabetes mellitus (NIDDM).

Exercise
Find out what the difference is between NIDDM and IDDM.

People with insulin-dependent diabetes mellitus are also know as Type 1 diabetes. This type of diabetes usually presents before the age of 40 and because the body is unable to produce insulin regular injections of insulin and modification to the person's diet is required. Patients with non-insulin-dependent diabetes, or Type 2 diabetes, still produce insulin but in this case it does not work properly. This type of diabetes is usually found in people over the age of 40 who are likely to be overweight and can be treated with diet and exercise. Many patients with noninsulin-dependent diabetes go on to require insulin injections. Once diagnosed a person can live a healthy life with help and support of health care professionals. It is important that the nurse understands the role of diet in diabetes.

Exercise
Find out what dietary advice would be given to a patient newly diagnosed as having NIDDM.

A newly diagnosed diabetic will be referred to a dietitian for dietary advice. Diet is an important factor in maintaining a normal blood sugar and patients should be advised to follow a healthy diet. The management of diabetes requires input from the members of a multidisciplinary team.

The healthy diet

A healthy diet should consist of an adequate supply of nutrients to ensure survival. There are several main food groups: carbohydrates, proteins, fats, vitamins and minerals and water. Each of these must be in the correct proportion and quantity according to a person's size, gender, age, health and level of activity. Other nutrients such as fibre are also needed whilst others, such as amino acids, are synthesised by the body.

Exercise
1. Look up the nutrition information on an item of prepacked food.
2. What information does it contain?
3. How will it help you to maintain a well-balanced diet?

The nutritional information on food labels will include the fat content and may provide information on the different types of fat, saturates, polyunsaturates and monosaturates as well as protein, carbohydrates, sugar and starches. The labels sometimes contain a useful guide on the recommended daily amount of calories and fat that adults should be eating each day and indicate the amount of salt. For further information access the British Dietetic Association website http://www.bda.uk.com.

Water Approximately 60% of the body comprises of water. Approximately 2/3 of water is contained within the intracellular fluids and the remaining 1/3 within the extracellular fluid (blood plasma, synovial fluid, lymph, etc) and interstitial fluid. The recommended daily intake of water is 2500 ml, however, this might vary according to environmental issues and the amount of water lost through expiration and excretion of bodily fluids such as urine and sweat. If there is an increase in the amount of sodium in the blood through sweating this stimulates receptors located in the hypothalamus and a feeling of thirst. The need for water is controlled by osmoreceptors located in the digestive tract and stretch receptors in the circulatory system. Information is passed to the hypothalamus, which influences the need to drink, and controls the excretion of urine. The importance of hydration is not always recognised by the nurse and Madden (2000) provides a helpful review of the types of fluids that nurses might promote to reduce the risk of dehydration (see Fig. 6.7 for regulation of water intake and loss).

Exercise
1. Find out how you would know that a person is dehydrated.
2. Discuss the effects of dehydration with your mentor and other colleagues.
3. How many patients with dehydration have you cared for? Consider their symptoms and compare to the theoretical knowledge discovered in question 1.

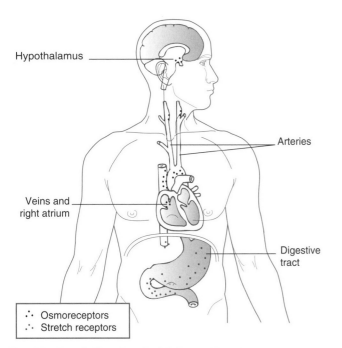

Hypothalamus

Arteries

Veins and
right atrium

Digestive
tract

∴ Osmoreceptors
∴ Stretch receptors

Fig. 6.7 Regulation of water intake and loss (from Rutishauser 1994, with permission).

Dehydration occurs when water loss exceeds intake, for example through sweating, vomiting, diarrhoea, polyuria, fever and loss of appetite. On examination the person will have sunken eyes, dry mouth, dry skin with loss of elasticity and be constipated. They may also have a low blood pressure, a tachycardia or be in a state of shock. In cases of mild dehydration it may be possible to replace fluids orally but in more severe cases intravenous fluids may be needed. The administration and monitoring of intravenous fluids is an important task that the nurse working in acute care will undertake regularly. Gobbi (2000) stresses the importance of the nurse understanding the physiology of fluid replacement when administering and monitoring fluid intake and output and managing complex fluid regimes. Safe administration of intravenous fluids also requires knowledge of professional and legal responsibilities, an understanding of the fluids being administered and the reasons why they are being administered (Hand 2001).

Exercise

1. Access a physiology textbook and update your knowledge of fluid and electrolyte balance.
2. What skills and knowledge do you need to be a safe and competent practitioner when administering an intravenous infusion to a patient?
3. If you are a student nurse on a clinical placement find out how fluid balance is documented.
4. Are there any factors that limit the accuracy of this process?

Include these responses in your development plan and arrange to discuss these with your mentor and personal tutor.

Carbohydrates Carbohydrates are the main source of heat and energy for the body and should supply the majority of calories needed. There are three main groups of carbohydrates: sugars, starches and complex polysaccharides. These can be found in bread, potatoes, cereals, fruit and vegetables. During digestion carbohydrates are broken down into glucose before being absorbed.

Proteins Protein is required for repair and growth. Whilst protein is found in most foods, the extent to which the body can absorb proteins, in the form of amino acids, from some foods differs considerably. Protein from animal products, for example meat, fish and eggs, and from legumes, has a higher absorption rate than that of plants or cereals.

Fats Fats also provide a source of energy and insulation. It is an essential component of the body composition and of the diet but taken in excess it can contribute to a number of health problems including obesity. Saturated fats found in foods from animals may contribute to an increase in blood cholesterol levels and likelihood of coronary heart disease. However not all fat is unhealthy and polyunsaturated fatty acids, like those found in oily fish, have been shown to reduce the likelihood of coronary thrombosis (Daniels 2002).

Vitamins There are two main types of vitamins, fat-soluble (A, D, E, K) which we can store in our body and water-soluble (B, C) which we need to get from our daily food but are easily lost. Vitamins are found in fruit and vegetables, dairy products and meat and oily fish. A deficiency in one or more of the vitamins may result in specific diseases such as scurvy (vitamin C).

Minerals These are found in many different foods and are essential for health. They have many different roles including hormonal, enzymatic, transportation of molecules and electrolyte balance. A major trace element, iron, is necessary for the transportation of haemoglobin around the body, whereas sodium, a mineral, is essential in maintaining the electrolyte balance within the cell. Other minerals include calcium, phosphorus, potassium, chlorine, magnesium and sulphur.

Sociocultural factors

The AL of eating and drinking extends to more than just providing nutrients for the body, it forms an important part of our personal, religious, sociocultural and ethical aspects of living (Roper et al 1996, 2000). In many cultures eating and drinking is given a great deal of attention and provides much pleasure. For example, Henley and Schott (1999) state that:

> ❝ *Food is not simply a matter of nutrition; it often has deep personal significance, symbolising, for example, security, love, moral and religious values and identity* ❞ (Henley & Scott 1999, p. 104).

Some families make a point of sitting down at a table as a family for a meal at least once a day, others may never eat at a table. Others may only eat as a family at special occasions, family birthdays or holidays and have special foods. In some cases adults may eat separately from the children. Some people may pray before a meal. Other rituals may be considered to be polite or respectful, like waiting until everyone has sat down and has been served food before eating. Some cultures and religions observe different rituals.

In some family structures the male and female roles are clearly distinguished. For example in the Jewish orthodox faith the mother is responsible for the home and children and the father for religious education. Only food that is kosher (permitted by the Torah) is allowed and dairy products are not eaten at the same time or following a meal containing meat unless several hours have elapsed (Collins 2002). On the Sabbath (Saturday) Jewish families celebrate with a special family supper and lighting of candles. There are many religious groups that follow dietary restrictions and observe rituals. There are also strong beliefs in some cultures about what one should eat to keep healthy and what to avoid.

Chan (1995) discusses the influence of the Chinese philosophy of yin and yang on dietary beliefs and customs. The Chinese believe that harmony and health can only exist when these two competing forces are balanced. Yin is linked to cold energy and to infections, gastric upsets and anxiety. Foods, which are said to be yin, are vegetables, milk, water and dairy products. Yang on the other hand is related to hot energy and dehydration, fever, and irritability, these are foods such are red meat, alcohol, wheat and fatty foods. Dietary remedies are an important part of the Chinese culture and relatives may bring in food and herbal remedies to redress the balance of yin and yang.

Not all people use a knife and fork to eat a meal. The Chinese use chopsticks and people living in South Asia and Muslim countries use only their right hand and often their fingers to eat their food. Their left hand is reserved for washing and using the lavatory (Henley & Schott 1999, Akhtar 2002).

Fasting from food and drink is expected in some religions. Fasting is one of the five pillars of Islam and it teaches Muslins self-discipline and self-restraint and reminds Muslims of those in poverty and hunger. During the month of Ramadan Muslims will avoid food and drink from sunrise to sunset. Strict Buddhists may decline food after midday (Northcot 2002).

When visiting the sick, relatives and carers will often bring food. Taking time to provide food for a person who is ill is a sign of caring or love (Henley & Schott 1999). If a patient is unable to eat or drink this can be very stressful for the relatives or carers. The wish to preserve life at all costs is, in some cultures, very intense. Some people will insist on artificial feeding, even in patients in the final stages of death. They may see the reluctance of medical and nursing staff to feed a patient artificially as failing in their duty of care. The British Medical Association's guidance for decision-making *'Withholding and Withdrawing Life: Prolonging Medical Treatment'* recognises ethical dilemmas and the emotional and psychological burden on staff involved with withdrawing or withholding treatment (BMA 1999). There is often a misconception that when a patient is receiving hydration via an intravenous infusion that this is nutrition. McAulay (2001) identified the need to raise awareness of the effects of dehydration in terminally ill patients so that they are able to comfort relatives who are concerned about the withdrawal of hydration in patients who are terminally ill and would no longer benefit.

Environmental factors

Environmental factors have an important role to play in the AL of eating and drinking. The quality and availability of food and water depends on a stable and safe environment. Many people in the world depend on local produce and on access to good soil and amenable weather conditions (Roper et al 1996). Climate changes can mean the difference between a good harvest and starvation for many thousands of people in some countries. The World Health Organisation website (www.who.int) has up-to-date information on the number of people affected by famine in the world. In countries with access to good road and rail networks, people have access to a wide variety of foods, which are imported and exported, from many different parts of the world. Easier access to package holidays and foreign travel has also increased the demand for different foods.

Access to a safe supply of drinking water is a fundamental health requirement. Approximately 20% of the population of the Earth lack access to safe drinking water. Contamination of the water supplies is of grave concern to the more affluent countries of the world. Within the UK the Department for

Environment, Food and Rural Affairs is responsible for all aspects of water policy, supply and research.

> **Exercise**
> Access the Department for Environment, Food and Rural Affairs website www.defra.gov.uk. Increase your knowledge about maintaining safe water supplies.

Where, when and with whom we eat and drink can determine how we enjoy our food. Roper et al (1996) suggest that an environment that promotes a relaxing atmosphere contributes to both the physiological and psychological enjoyment of eating and drinking. If we are rushed we are less likely to enjoy our food.

> **Exercise**
> 1. Think about a meal you have enjoyed in the restaurant with friends or family.
> 2. Now think about a meal you have taken whilst at work or in a snack bar.
> 3. Did the environments differ and how did they contribute to your enjoyment?

You may have enjoyed the ambience of the restaurant, being able to choose your food from a menu and being served your food by others. The comfort of the restaurant and company of others may have added to your enjoyment of your meal. However, if the restaurant was dirty, noisy or the service slow and the food poor quality then this may have affected your enjoyment of your meal. On the other hand your may have found that the meal at work was rushed because of lack of time and you did not have time to enjoy your food and the choice of food on offer may be limited and of poor quality. Once again this may not always be the case and a chance to sit down with colleagues and enjoy a meal may prove an enjoyable experience. Ensuring a pleasant environment and patient experience at mealtimes is an important role of the nurse.

> **Exercise**
> 1. If you are a student nurse on a clinical placement, observe the patient environment at mealtimes.
> 2. Speak to patients and ask them how they enjoyed their meal.
> 3. How did the environment contribute to the patient's experience?
> 4. Compare this to your own experiences.
> 5. Are there any changes you would make to improve the patient's experience?

Food hygiene and the provision of a safe and clean environment for food storage, preparation and cooking are essential to health and wellbeing. Hospitals, restaurants, cafes, bars, in fact anywhere food is sold, prepared, cooked and served to the public are required to comply with stringent standards to ensure the general public is not put at risk.

> **Exercise**
> 1. Increase your knowledge about food hygiene and food safety.
> 2. Access the Food Standards website at www.foodstandards.gov.uk
> 3. Look in your own refrigerator. How do you store your foods?
> 4. Find out about any guidelines within the clinical area regarding the serving of food and storage of food within the clinical area.

You will have found out about the importance of strict hand washing and the separation of cooked meats from uncooked meats both within the refrigerator and in retail outlets, ensuring foods are cooked thoroughly and at the correct temperature, and ensuring food is not used after its sell-by date.

Psychological factors

As Roper et al (1996) point out individuals need to have a certain level of intelligence to be able to select, prepare and cook a healthy diet. They need to understand the role of the major nutrients and to be able to prepare foods safely.

The amount of food one eats depends on a number of factors not only on the degree of hunger but also on appetite and the function of the hypothalamus. Appetite can be affected by emotional state, mood and behaviour, for example, overeating or undereating due to stress or loss of self-esteem.

> **Exercise**
> 1. Think about a time when you have felt stressed. This may have been before an examination or interview for a new job.
> 2. How did you feel?
> 3. Did you use food to help you cope with the stress?
> 4. If so what foods did you eat?
> 5. Did you increase your intake of alcohol?

Some people when stressed might eat more cakes, sweets and chocolates than when less stressed. Research has shown that some people crave carbohydrates when depressed (Rinomhota & Rollins 2001). A study by Lieberman et al (1986) found that people who snacked on carbohydrates in between meals reported a more positive mood.

Eating disorders

People who experience symptoms of depression are likely to report loss of appetite and eating disorders. A number of well-known people have admitted to suffering from eating disorders. Most notably Princess Diana who admitted that she had suffered from bulimia, as did the actors Jane Fonda and Joan Rivers.

Eating disorders, whilst usually associated with young women, can affect both men and women of any age and background (Cremin & Halek 1997). Anorexia nervosa usually presents during adolescence and can persist throughout life. Individuals present with severe loss of weight due to strict dieting, they are preoccupied with their weight and have a distorted image of their body. Bulimia on the other hand usually manifests itself in later life. Those who suffer bulimia crave food and binge on food before vomiting the food up. They are reluctant to seek help as they see this as giving up the control they have over their food intake. Depression and suicidal thoughts and behaviours are not uncommon and require psychological treatment.

Obesity

Within the Western culture a slim body shape is preferred. People who are overweight are often stigmatised and suffer discrimination. If intake of food exceeds activity levels over a period of time then there is a risk that this will result in weight gain. Obesity is defined as where someone puts on weight to the point that it damages health. In the UK the number of people who are obese or overweight continues to grow. An estimated 20% of males and 25% of females are likely to be overweight by 2004 (NAO 2002). The reasons for this are believed to be a gradually more sedentary lifestyle, a change in eating patterns and genetic factors (Various 1998, NAO 2002).

In 1998, the direct costs of obesity to the NHS were estimated to be in the region of half a billion pounds and indirectly around £2 billion. Obesity increases the risk of many common diseases (see Fig. 6.8) and is an important public health problem (Effective Health Care Bulletin 1997).

An epidemiological study carried out over a period of 50 years in the USA (Framington Heart Study) has revealed an association between obesity and heart failure (Kenchaiach et al 2002).

The recent National Service Framework for Coronary Heart Disease (DoH 2001c) and Diabetes (DoH 2001d) have highlighted the need for health promotion, promotion of a healthy diet and weight reduction. A body mass index of >30 kg/m^2 increases the risk of cardiovascular disease. Any approach to reducing weight needs to induce a negative energy balance, by reducing calorie intake and/or increasing energy expenditure. Whilst there are several diets and weight-loss products on the market there is no evidence to demonstrate their effectiveness and indeed some products may be deficient in essential nutrients. Dietary and behavioural interventions combined with exercise have been found to be more successful (Effective Health Care Bulletin 1997, Milne 2001). Ekpe (2001) suggests that nurses can help patients with chronic mental health problems to take control of their obesity by encouraging user-empowerment

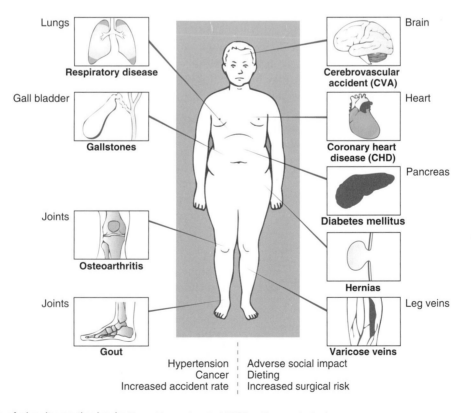

Fig. 6.8 The effects of obesity on the body (from Alexander et al 2000, with permission).

Box 6.8 Body mass index

The BMI is calculated by dividing a person's weight (in kilograms) by the square of their height (in metres). For example someone with a body weight of 57 kg and a height of 1.62 m has a BMI of $57/1.62^2 = 22.3$ kg/m^2. The BMI tends to vary between 20 and 30. The ideal range is 20–25; 25–30 indicates overweight and a ratio of over 30 indicates obesity.

From Gobbi & Torrance 2000.

strategies that consider the wider psychosocial and environmental factors. Weight alone is not an accurate indicator of whether a person is over- or underweight. The body mass index (BMI) is a much more reliable indicator and estimation of total body fat (see Box 6.8).

The body mass index (BMI) provides a more accurate reflection of whether a person is obese or underweight than just weight alone. However, this is a general guide as very muscular people may have a high BMI without being overweight and some people may be underweight without being thin.

Exercise

Using the calculations outlined in Box 6.8 calculate your BMI.

The shape of a person's body is also an important indicator of risk of heart disease and diabetes. A person who carries a lot of weight around the middle of his or her body 'apple shaped' has a greater health risk than someone who is 'pear shaped' (see Box 6.9 for impact of being overweight).

Politicoeconomic factors

Malnutrition is a global problem and contributes to nearly 5.25 million deaths each year. The World Health Organisation

Box 6.9 Impact of being overweight on the body

Being overweight can affect most parts of the body:

- coronary heart disease
- breathlessness
- cancer
- osteoarthritis
- back pain
- sleep difficulties
- infertility
- sweating
- difficulties in walking
- low self-esteem, poor body image.

(From British Dietetic Association Fact Sheet 1)

has sought the help of all sectors of society to help to tackle malnutrition in infants and young children that is causing grave concern. As a result of global communications, the recent crop failures in Africa have been once again brought into our homes. These pictures serve to remind us of the plight and fight for human survival of these people who are undernourished and live in extreme poverty. Roper et al (1996) highlight the complex reasons for the misdistribution of food throughout the world including poor soil and crop rotation, lack of irrigation, social unrest, natural disasters, lack of funding, poor education and food regulation.

A study by Mahasneh (2001) of the health perceptions and health behaviours of poor urban Jordanian women found that a fifth of Jordanian households, mostly in urban areas, live below the poverty line. Many of the women in the study were illiterate, did not work and had little or no income. The Jordanian government control food prices to ensure access to basic food at affordable prices, nevertheless despite this Mahasneh (2001) found that Jordanian women were now consuming a less well-balanced diet. Their diet consisted of bread, vegetables, rice and dairy products, whilst chicken and meat were eaten less frequently. Many of the women reported an increase in weight, which they believed to be a result of pregnancy and lack of exercise.

Over recent years the UK Government has set targets in line with its health policy to place emphasis on the contribution of diet to health (DoH 1992). Coronary heart disease is the main cause of premature death in the UK and costs the NHS around £1 billion and results in around 53 million lost working days each year. As the risk of coronary heart disease is linked to the amount of saturated fats in the diet, the UK government has introduced targets and a range of initiatives to reduce the amount of fats in our diets by 12% by 2005.

There are also economic reasons why it is important that people eat healthily. The costs of treating patients with malnutrition is higher than in patients who are not malnourished as they require more tests, take longer to recover resulting in a longer stay in hospital (Royal College of Physicians 2002).

Exercise

1. Visit the Health Development Agency website www.hda-online.org.uk.
2. Find out about initiatives and interventions aimed at encouraging people to adopt a healthier diet.

You may have found out that the UK government is working with industry to increase the provision of fruit and vegetables by encouraging the establishment of food cooperatives that allow people to increase the availability of fresh fruit and vegetables at affordable prices. Other interventions may be aimed at increasing the knowledge of a healthy diet within schools for example the 'Cooking for Kids' initiative, which reinforces food hygiene and nutrition.

Initiatives such as breakfast clubs are aimed at encouraging children to have a breakfast and those from low-income families to have at least one nutritious meal a day. Food suppliers, supermarkets and retailers also support healthy eating campaigns by providing nutritional information on foods and food packaging. Unfortunately, there is a lack of research evidence to demonstrate the effectiveness of these interventions.

On an individual basis there are resource implications in ensuring a healthy diet, including enough money to buy or grow food, access to the right sort of food, access to food storage facilities, cooking utensils and equipment, and access to health and social services support if necessary.

Meeting the nutritional needs of patients in hospital

In 1992 the King's Fund Centre published a report 'A Positive Approach to Nutrition as Treatment' by Professor JE Lennard-Jones concerned with the recognition of nutritional status of patients admitted to hospital as a consequence of illness. The report indicated that as many as half of certain patient groups (surgical and medical) were malnourished on admission to hospital and during prolonged hospital stay malnutrition often becomes worse or develops for the first time (Table 6.3).

The Report recommended a multidisciplinary team approach to recognising and dealing with malnutrition and acknowledged the nurse's role as essential within that team. McWhirter and Pennington (1994) undertook a prospective study of the nutritional status of patients admitted to a Scottish hospital and found that 40% (200) of patients were undernourished and had a body mass index of less than 20, of these only 96 patients had any information on nutrition documented in their case notes. This problem is not unique to the UK. Kowanko et al (2001) undertook a similar study in Australia and found that the nutritional intake of many patients was poor. Lennard-Jones et al (1995) found that most nurses and doctors in 70 hospitals failed to recognise the importance of asking patients questions about nutrition and height and weight. Attempting to raise awareness of the importance of assessing nutritional needs Reilly et al (1995) developed a simple assessment tool to be used on admission to encourage staff to assess nutritional needs.

As a result of the recommendations of the Kings Fund Report (Lennard-Jones 1992), the British Association for Parenteral and Enteral Nutrition (BAPEN) was formed. BAPEN subsequently published two reports: the first 'Organisation of Nutritional Support in Hospitals' (Silk 1994) recommended that nutrition support teams responsible for organising the diagnosis, treatment should be established; the second report set standards of clinical practice in nutritional support (Sizer 1996). Both reports highlighted the general lack of awareness of both medical and nursing staff of nutrition and the importance of nutritional assessment.

In response to a report 'Hungry in Hospitals' by the Association of Community Health Councils (1997) and

Table 6.3 Malnutrition

Causes	Effects
Reduced dietary intake	• impaired growth and development of children
• reduced appetite	• weight loss
• difficulties with eating	• loss of muscle strength
• nausea and vomiting	• delayed wound healing
• depression/anxiety	• increased risk of pressure ulcer development
• environment	• impaired immune response leading to increased risk of infection
• pain	
• starving for tests	
• difficulties with shopping and cooking	• impaired psychological well being
• side effects of medication	• depression of appetite
Increased nutritional requirements	• prolonged recovery and rehabilitation
• liver disease	• increased morbidity and mortality
• renal disease	• increased dependence
• respiratory disease	
• abdominal losses (e.g. through stoma)	
• major surgery/trauma	
• increase in involuntary movements secondary to neurological condition	
Impaired ability to utilise, absorb metabolic nutrients	
• Crohn's disease	
• untreated coeliac disease	
• untreated diabetes	
• laxative abuse	

Kings Fund Centre Report 1992.

concern about the dietary care in hospitals in the UK, the Department of Health through the Chief Nursing Officer supported the development of a resource pack 'Eating Matters' (Bond 1997). The pack was designed to assist nurses and organisations to improve the nutritional needs of patients.

More recently, the UK government through the NHS Plan (DoH 2000a) sought to redress the unacceptable variations in standards of catering and nutrition in hospitals across the country. Initiatives such as the Department of Health 'Better Food for Hospitals' scheme have resulted in nurses, Modern Matrons, dietitians, hospital managers and catering staff looking at ways in which the patient's experience of food by introducing new menus and ward housekeepers or ward hostesses could be improved. The NHS Plan (2000a) also identified the need for nationally agreed standards for the fundamental aspects of nursing care. Working with patients, user groups and practitioners a number of essential aspects of care were identified and benchmarks of best practice agreed. Food and nutrition is one of those eight essential aspects of care. Benchmarking is seen as a process through which best practice is identified and continuous improvement pursued through comparison and sharing. In Scotland the Nursing and Midwifery Practice Development Unit (NMPDU) has published best practice statements available on their website, which describe best and achievable practice for Nutritional Assessment and Referral in the Care of Adults in Hospital (www.nmpdu.org).

Nutrition and hydration are important aspects of nursing care and are just as important as monitoring vital signs. Assessing and meeting the needs of patients at risk is a fundamental part of a nursing assessment and planning care to ensure that 'patients get the right sort of food and drink, in the right place at the right time, with the right help' (Mullally 2000). However, nurses do not work in isolation and meeting the nutritional needs of patients requires a multidisciplinary approach.

Exercise

1. If you are a student nurse on a clinical placement in a hospital find out which health professionals have a role in ensuring that patients' nutritional and hydration needs are met.
2. Arrange to meet with one or two of these professionals and find out more about their role and how you can refer for specialist advice and support.
3. Consider what happens to patients being cared for in the community.

During your allocation you may have met with the following health care professionals:

- *Ward Nurse* – who has overall responsibility for ensuring that the patient's nutrition and hydration needs are identified, that there is a plan of care designed to meet individual needs and subject to ongoing evaluation. The ward nurse will work in collaboration with other health care professionals and co-ordinate their input.
- *Health Care Assistant* – who is responsible for ensuring that patients receive the right food at the right time and receive any assistance that they need. Some hospitals may have introduced ward housekeepers whose role is to support ward staff by serving meals and preparing snacks.
- *Occupational Therapist* – who will assess the patient's ability to feed themself and provide specialised equipment where necessary.
- *Dietitian* – who will assess nutritional status, calculate dietary requirements, monitor patients on nutritional support and provide specialist dietary advice and support to patients.
- *Catering Manager* – who is responsible for the catering arrangements, menus and nutritional content of meals.
- *Doctor* – who has overall responsibility for the nutritional regimes and the suitable route of nutritional support.

- *Pharmacist* – who will supply intravenous foods and advise on how drug regimes may impact on nutrition, parenteral, enteral and intravenous regimes.
- *Gastroenterologist* – who is increasingly becoming involved in artificial nutrition support.
- *Chemical Pathologist* – who will monitor the biochemical activity.
- *Microbiologist and Infection Control Nurse* – who together will provide support and monitoring of possible catheter-related sepsis.
- *Speech and Language Therapist* – who will assess the patient's muscular control and swallowing reflex and work with patients to improve swallowing.

Summary points

---

1. Food and water are essential for our survival.
2. Access to sufficient food and water for survival however is affected by many different politicoeconomic as well as sociocultural factors.
3. What we eat and drink is very much affected by the culture we live in as well as our health status, e.g whether we are ill or not.

THE MODEL FOR NURSING

Introduction

Within this chapter, in addition to the following main case study, you will be encouraged to transfer your understanding of eating and drinking to other individual patients and consider its relationship to other ALs. Using the model for nursing you will consider what information you would obtain from a main case scenario, identify patient problems and develop a plan of care. You may choose to record the information on the Patient Assessment Sheets provided in Appendix 2.

Assessing individual needs and problems

If patients' expectations are to be understood and their problems (whether actual or potential) with this AL are to be addressed then an assessment must be undertaken. Assessment involves the following three phases:

- collecting information from the patient and nursing history
- interpreting the information collected
- identifying the patient's actual and potential health problems.

However, if the nurse is to undertake a comprehensive and holistic nursing history it is essential that all the Activities of Living as seen in Chapter 1 and taken into account. This is not only undertaken at the beginning of the patient's episode of care or admission to hospital but is an ongoing and dynamic process. Before assessing the AL of eating and drinking in ill health the nurse must first of all understand and have knowledge of the AL of eating and drinking in health.

Assessing the individual

Assessment is the cornerstone on which the patient's care is planned, implemented and evaluated. In most cases the nurse undertakes an initial nursing assessment within the first few hours of admission to hospital by gathering information that informs the nursing assessment without overburdening the patient and duplicating assessments. However, we must remember that nursing assessment is continuous and patients must be reassessed as their condition changes or in response to the outcome of evaluation.

Using the model of living as a framework to collect information on the patient's normal habits and routines and any factors that might cause the activity to be altered is the first step in applying the Roper et al (1996, 2000) model of nursing in practice. Box 6.10 provides a summary of the key factors, which you may consider assessing the activity of eating and drinking.

When assessing the patient you will need to use interviewing, observational and listening skills (see Chapter 4). In addition you will also need to understand the biological, sociological, psychological and environmental issues associated with eating and drinking. Poor or incomplete assessment subsequently leads to poor care planning and implementation of the care plan (Sutcliffe 1990). The care plan should identify the nursing interventions required to meet patient needs related to eating and drinking. These interventions may include promoting health, preventing ill health, providing nutritional support, helping patients to eat and drink and maintaining a safe environment.

Exercise

1. Consider the activities in Box 6.11 and identify which skills you have already and the ones you need to develop when undertaking an assessment of eating and drinking.

A thorough patient assessment is the basis on which a relevant and realistic individualised nursing care plan is founded. The nursing care plan should aim to:

- solve actual problems
- prevent potential problems becoming actual problems
- prevent solved problems from recurring
- alleviate problems which cannot be solved
- help the person cope with temporary or permanent altered states
- provide information to others to enable the delivery of individualised care
- provide information on the effectiveness of nursing care through evaluation.

Box 6.10 Assessment framework for the activity of eating and drinking

Life span
- Consider the effect of age on the activity of eating and drinking.

Dependence/independence
- Dependence is linked to lifespan and age, e.g. childhood/old age.
- Dependence is linked to specific needs, e.g. disability, communication, certain foods and drink.
- Ill health affects the dependence–independence balance, e.g. dehydration, neurological problems.

Factors affecting eating and drinking
Biological
- ingestion
- digestion
- absorption
- neurological impairment
- metabolism
- nutrients
- exercise.

Psychological
- attitudes to eating and drinking, health behaviour and beliefs
- intellectual capacity
- emotional state
- cognitive state
- social class
- body image.

Sociocultural
- recognition of individual attitudes, beliefs and values
- sociocultural similarities/differences
- religion.

Environmental
- access to food and drink
- food storage and food hygiene
- cooking facilities
- environment.

Politicoeconomic
- finance
- access to feeding aids
- access to health and social services support.

Box 6.11 Skills and behaviours necessary for undertaking assessment

Interviewing
- asking open and closed questions relevant to the health status of the patient
- use of appropriate language
- determining the priority of the questions to be asked
- giving information, relating and checking understanding
- involving relatives and carers.

Observation
- verbal and nonverbal responses
- body language
- appearance
- vital signs
- height and weight
- skin condition
- oral health and dentures
- dexterity
- swallowing reflex
- anxiety and stress.

Listening
- verbal and nonverbal cues
- checking out understanding and giving explanation.

Patient assessment

When assessing the Activities of Living you may consider the following questions.

Lifespan
- How old is the person?
- Do they have a life history of health problems?
- Is there anything in their life history that may affect the way in which they view their present health problems?

Dependence/independence
- Has the individual experienced any difficulties in relation to independent living?
- Are they able to prepare food and drink or are they dependent on others?
- Are they able to shop for food and drink or are they dependent on others?
- Will they experience difficulties in the future as a result of their current health problems?
- Do they have any dependence on food or drink?

Factors affecting health
Biological
- What specific health problem are they suffering from?
- What do they understand about their present health status?
- Are there any disabilities?
- What is their BMI?

- Is there evidence of loss of weight recently?
- Are there any allergies to food and/or drink?
- What is their nutritional status? You may choose to use one of the recognised nutritional assessment tools to assess their nutritional status as discussed previously in this chapter.
- Is there any pain?

Psychological
- Is there any intellectual deficit?
- What effect is their health problem having on their emotional wellbeing?
- Are there any emotional problems?
- Is the patient suffering from stress?
- Are there any memory problems?
- What is their motivation?

Socioeconomic
- Are there any specific spiritual or religious practices or needs?
- Do they have any beliefs about food and diet?
- What support do they have in the home?
- Do they have any contact with others?

Environmental
- What type of housing does the individual live in?
- What facilities for preparing food are there?
- Does the individual have any environmental needs which affect nutritional care?
- Are they exposed to any environmental hazards or risks of infection?

Politicoeconomic
- What resources could be required to help the individual manage their health problems both in hospital and at home?
- Is the patient aware of the resources that are available?
- Are there any financial constraints compromising recovery or maintenance.
- What effect is this having on their nutritional status?

Case study 6.3

Admission to hospital

Mavis, an 83-year-old woman, is admitted to your ward after being found on the floor at home by a neighbour. She has a history of arthritis and hypertension. She lives alone in her own home. Her husband died 4 years ago and she has a son and a daughter and three grandchildren. Her daughter lives 50 miles away and visits at weekends. Until recently she has been fiercely independent and refused any form of support other than help with her cleaning and assistance with shopping from her son. On admission she is dehydrated and disorientated and her son has noticed that she has lost weight recently.

Whilst helping patients maintain an adequate nutritional intake is everyone's responsibility, as a nurse you will have the most contact with patients. Working in partnership with other health professionals, you are in a unique position to ensure that that patient's nutritional needs are met and not compromised (Bond 1997, Norton 1996, Roper et al 1996, Wood & Creamer 1996).

> **Exercise**
> 1. Using your knowledge of the Roper et al model for nursing and the questions on p. 185, reflect on how you will include these in your assessment of the patient in Case study 6.3.

Using the Roper et al model for nursing (1996), you may have decided to devise a number of questions that will enable you to identify the patient's normal habits and routines in relation to the ALs, dependency, and identify actual and potential problems associated with the AL of eating and drinking and how this might impact on the other ALs. Even if the patient is able to communicate effectively, it is usually helpful with the permission of the patient to make arrangements to speak to the patient's relatives or carers to elicit any extra information and opinions.

Having considered your questions and likely responses check these out against the following.

Lifespan

In later life nutritional status is influenced by physiological changes as a result of normal ageing, disease, chronic disorders and reduced mobility. Mavis, an 83-year-old widow, may not fully understand the importance of nutrition in later life. Her medical records reveal that she has a history of osteoarthritis in her knees and hip and hypertension. Osteoarthritis is more likely to occur in older women and is a noninflammatory degenerative condition which affects the hyaline cartilage of the synovial joints (Jamieson et al 2000).

Physically frail older patients are more likely to have problems associated with eating and drinking and suffer from malnutrition. This should alert you to the importance of ensuring adequate nutrition whilst in hospital and also when she returns home, thus highlighting the nurse's role and responsibility for health education.

Dependence/independence

Mavis has been fiercely independent and has refused any help other than help from her son with shopping and her neighbour's help to do the cleaning. You may have questioned Mavis about how she manages to do the cooking, who helps her with the cooking and are there any constraints. You will need to consider how her chronic health problems in particular her osteoarthritis is affecting her independence. The answers to these questions will provide information on Mavis's normal functioning. Admission to hospital and a change in health status will impact on Mavis's current level of dependence/independence. Therefore you will need to assess any change from the normal functioning.

An older person can find admission to a hospital ward disorientating. You will need to take account of whether the patient has been in hospital before and how they coped. You will need to assess what the impact of hospital admission will have on Mavis's independence and if necessary what help she will need to regain her independence. Taking account of her current situation is she able to eat herself? Does she need help to feed and if so what help does she need? How will she respond to changes to her independence as a result of her admission?

You will have also considered the impact of dehydration and that Mavis will be dependent on the medical and nursing staff to restore hydration and rectify her electrolyte balance by intravenous fluid replacement.

> **Exercise**
> 1. Reflect back on your discussions with your mentor and tutor following the previous exercise (p. 186).
> 2. Is there anything else you need to know, see and do in relation to meeting the hydration needs of patients?

Biological

It is important to understand Mavis's normal health situation. When was she diagnosed with osteoarthritis and hypertension and how did this impact on her ALs? You would want to understand what Mavis could remember about the incident and any symptoms or events leading up to her fall. You would need to know if she had any physical difficulties or disabilities, including any sensory loss (sight, hearing, smell, taste) or pain. Whilst people don't normally feel ill with osteoarthritis they are likely to suffer dull nagging pain or periods of acute pain, which will require medication for pain relief. You will need to know if the presence of pain has had any effect on Mavis's appetite.

You would want to understand how her raised blood pressure is affecting her health status. Hypertension can be defined as primary, where no cause is found, or secondary, due to underlying medical conditions for example renal disease. If the rise in blood pressure is only moderate and occurs over a long period of time it is said to be mild, whereas a sudden increase in blood pressure is referred to as malignant (Thompson & Webster 2000). A number of dietary factors are associated with hypertension including obesity, sodium intake and alcohol and so you would need to take these factors into account when assessing Mavis's normal Activities of Living.

To understand Mavis's current health status you would monitor her vital signs and in discussion with medical staff determine the frequency of future monitoring. You would record her temperature, pulse, respiration and blood pressure. Mavis's son thinks she has lost weight over the last 6 months. You would also need to record her weight and height and calculate her BMI (see Box 6.10). A patient with a BMI of less than 19 is said to be 'at risk' and associated with higher mortality (Bond et al 1997). It is important to record this in her medical and nursing notes against which any future weight gain or loss can be monitored.

Observation of Mavis's physical condition will also aid your assessment in relation to the activity of eating and drinking. You would want to observe whether there is evidence of recent loss of weight. Do her clothes or rings look too big? Is there any evidence of oedema in her lower limbs? Can she grip your hands? Is there any evidence of loss of muscle power?

Psychological

As psychological factors can affect people's attitude to food and drink, you would need to understand Mavis's attitude towards her diet and if this has changed recently. You questions and observations would be aimed at establishing her understanding and knowledge of her current situation. Does she give any indication that she might be suffering from depression? Does she understand the importance of a healthy diet? Has she any problems with her memory? Does she have any abnormal attitudes about her weight or body image?

Sociocultural

We know that Mavis was bereaved 4 years ago and that her son and a neighbour support her. Her daughter lives some 50 miles away and visits whenever she can. You would need to determine her normal social situation and how her current health problems impact, or have the potential to impact, on this. You might have considered the following questions:

- What social contacts and support does she have?
- Does she get out of the house?
- Does she meet up with friends?
- Is she isolated?

The older person living alone can become isolated and this can influence their motivation and interest in eating and drinking. Gathering this information will assist you to discuss with Mavis any support she might wish to access on her discharge from hospital to help her maintain a healthy living style.

Whilst in hospital you would also need to understand any food preferences that Mavis has in relation to any religious beliefs or cultural upbringing. Does Mavis avoid any foods, e.g. spicy foods? Does she have any beliefs about particular foods? What time of day does she have her main meal? Does she eat breakfast? Beginning to understand our patient's food habits will enable us to know if a patient is eating appropriately or not and inform future health education needs and any support the patient needs to maintain the AL.

Environmental

When taking environmental factors into account you would need to consider both the home and hospital environment.

In the home you would need to understand the design of the home and facilities. Does she have hot and cold running water? What cooking and food storage facilities does she have? Can she use these safely? What about toilet facilities? If Mavis's only toilet facilities are upstairs, and she is unable to negotiate the stairs without feeling pain, she might be reluctant to drink. Have there been any adaptations made to her accommodation?

As previously discussed there have been several studies that have highlighted the prevalence of malnutrition in patients in hospital (Lennard-Jones 1992, McWhirter & Pennington 1994). You will also need to consider the impact being in the hospital environment might have on Mavis's nutritional status. She is unlikely to be able to find her way around the ward or understand the routines. Depending on the type of ward she has been admitted into, she will be in contact with other ill patients who might have feeding difficulties, and exposed to different sights and smells that might affect her appetite and ability to eat and drink. She might not be familiar with the type and standard of food served in hospital. You should also have taken into account the impact the environment has on her ability to reach her food and drink.

Politicoeconomic

Sensitive questioning and observation may reveal any concerns or issues relating to lack of financial support that may influence Mavis's access to adequate nutrition. You may enquire if she is accessing any resources to which she is entitled and if she requires any advice or support from a social worker.

By using the components of the model we are able to identify how lifespan, dependency, psychological, sociocultural and economic factors have contributed to health breakdown. We are also able to discover normal coping mechanisms and identify which of the other ALs may also be affected. In addition we are able to begin to recognise actual and potential problems associated with the activity of eating and drinking.

However, Roper et al (2000) point out that each Activity of Living does not stand alone and it is the interaction of each of these that contributes to the individualisation of nursing. Hence we need to assess the patient's other Activities of Living to obtain a holistic view.

Exercise

1. Consider how you might assess each of the other ALs in order to provide a holistic assessment of the patient.

You may have considered and observed the following:

1. *Breathing*
   - Does she have any problems breathing?
   - Does she smoke and if so how many and how often?

2. *Eating and drinking*
   - How much fluid is she drinking?
   - Is her appetite affected? If yes, in what way?
   - Is she able to eat and drink? If not, why not?
   - Does she need help to eat and drink?
   - When does she eat and drink?
   - What does she eat and drink?
   - Does she take any food supplements?
   - Is she taking any medication that may affect her appetite?
   - Does she avoid or have allergies to any foods or drink?
   - Does she have any problems with oral hygiene, e.g. dentures, crowns, gum disease?
   - Is there any nausea or vomiting?

3. *Eliminating*
   - Is she continent?
   - How often does she have her bowels opened?
   - Has she any gut problems?
   - What does her urinalysis tell you?

4. *Mobilising*
   - Has she any disability that restricts her mobility or ability to eat and drink?
   - If so how does this impact on her ability to eat and drink, obtain and/or prepare food?

5. *Expressing sexuality*
   - What is her appearance?
   - What does she like to wear?
   - Is she in a relationship?

6. *Personal cleansing and dressing*
   - Is she able to shower or bathe?
   - How frequently does she bathe or shower?
   - Does she require any assistance to get dressed?

7. *Working and playing*
   - How does she spend her day?
   - Does she have any visitors?
   - Is she able to get out of the house?
   - Does her health problem impact on her home and social life?

8. *Communicating*
   - Is she able to express her needs?
   - Does she require glasses or hearing aid?

9. *Maintaining a safe environment*
   - Does she have any pain?
   - Does she have any visual or auditory impairment?
   - Are there any risks, e.g. infection, pressure sore development, falls, and moving and handling?
   - Does she understand her medication regime?

10. *Sleeping*
    - How does she sleep?
    - Does anything disturb her sleep?
    - What helps her to sleep?

11. *Controlling body temperature*
    - Does she feel cold?
    - How does her diet influence her body temperature?
    - How does she keep warm at home?
    - What heating system does she have?
    - Is she able to maintain this?

12. *Dying*
    - Does she express any beliefs about dying?
    - Does she have any spiritual or religious beliefs?

Exercise

Using the information presented so far in this chapter, consider the following brief case studies and plan your assessment of the activity of eating and drinking. You may use the Nursing Care Plan template found in Appendix 2.

1. John is a 52-year-old joiner who has noninsulin-dependent diabetes mellitus (NIDDM), is overweight and has a chest infection. He is married and is the sole wage earner in the family.
2. A 65-year-old patient who is admitted with a stroke and is unable to swallow.

Compare your responses in each scenario and discuss your questions with your mentor or personal tutor.

Planning nursing activities and care

Within the UK nursing records may be used in evidence in a court of law, by the Health Service Commissioner or in order to investigate a local complaint (NMC 2002a,b). The Nursing and Midwifery Council Professional Conduct Committee may also use them when investigating complaints about professional conduct. The NMC (2002a) have published a number of key principles that underpin good nursing documentation including:

- a full account of your assessment and the care you have planned and provided
- relevant information about the condition of the patient or client at any given time and the measures you have taken to respond to their needs
- evidence that you have understood and honoured your duty of care for the patient and that any acts or omissions on your part have not compromised their safety in any way
- a record of any arrangements you have made for the continuing care of a patient or client.

By using the Roper et al (1996) model for nursing to assess, plan and implement care we will be able to demonstrate a holistic patient assessment, develop an individualised plan of care and take account of the input of other health care professionals in the patient's care. This involves the following activities:

- identifying the problems or needs
- identifying priorities
- establishing short- and long-term goals
- determining the nursing actions and interventions required
- documenting the care plan.

Identifying problems or needs

Roper et al (2000) state that:

> ❝ *the nurse's role is to enable the patient/client to prevent, alleviate or solve, or cope positively with problems (actual or potential) related to the ALs.* ❞

Whilst undertaking the nursing assessment the nurse should be able to detect potential problems, which the patient may not be aware of. This is where the nurse's knowledge of the factors relating to ill health, socio-economic, biological, psychological and environmental is important.

During the initial nursing assessment the nurse may obtain a considerable amount of information from the patient, their relatives or carers, other health care professionals and the patient's medical records. Roper et al (2000) seek to clarify the use of the word assessment in relation to their model for nursing as follows:

- collecting information from or about the person
- reviewing the collected information
- identifying a person's problems with Activities of Living
- identifying priorities amongst the problems.

It must be remembered that assessment is an ongoing and interactive process. Having undertaken a thorough assessment you should be able to identify any problems or patient needs and determine the nursing interventions required in order to meet those needs. It is important to stress that such problems and needs must be patient-focused, relate to the nursing assessment and what is needed to aid recovery in the immediate, short and long term. They may be actual or potential problems or needs and should be prioritised to take account of life-threatening situations.

Prioritising problems

Prioritising problems is an important component of care planning. By using the independence/dependence continuum of the model of living it is possible to identify and prioritise those problems that patients require nursing care and assistance to regain or maintain their independence, or where the patient is totally dependent on the nurse (Roper et al 2000).

There are different ways by which dependency scoring can be used and you should discuss with your mentor or preceptor local systems of prioritisation or dependency scoring systems. Alternatively you may wish to use the following example as suggested by Whittam in Chapters 3 and 11.

Dependency/independency priority criteria

Priority 1   Completely independent in the AL/independency maintained.

Priority 2   Potential problems in the AL/remains mostly independent.

Priority 3   Actual problems identified within more than one AL/some dependency noted but remains mainly independent.

Priority 4   Existence of actual and potential problems in a number of other ALs with associated increasing dependency.

Priority 5   Life-threatening actual and potential problems/total dependency.

Once the patient problems or needs have been identified and prioritised the nurse can review these and plan the nursing interventions required to:

- solve actual problems
- prevent potential problems occurring
- prevent solved problems from re-occurring
- develop positive coping strategies for any problem that cannot be solved.

Exercise

1. Reflect on what skills and knowledge you consider a nurse will need to plan care for a patient?
2. Check your knowledge and skills against your list and those listed below.
3. Identify any areas for further learning and/or skills development.
4. Discuss these with your personal tutor and mentor.

List of knowledge and skills required to plan care:

- analytical skills
- problem-solving skills
- knowledge of the illness
- knowledge of anatomy and physiology
- decision-making skills
- negotiating skills
- priority setting.

Identifying actual and potential problems

Having undertaken a nursing assessment let us consider what actual and potential problems have been identified and how these might be prioritised. Within the context of this chapter we will focus on those problems, actual and potential in relation to the activity of eating and drinking that might be relevant to Mavis's admission to hospital. We will also demonstrate how using the Roper et al (1996, 2000) model for nursing can contribute to provide a holistic nutritional assessment and inform care planning and nursing interventions.

Nutritional risk assessment screening

There are a number of nutritional assessment tools available that are designed to help nurses to identify patients who may be malnourished or at risk of malnutrition. Reilly et al (1995) developed a quick and simple tool that nurses could use on every patient admitted to hospital. Some tools include guidelines on when to refer to dietitians and advice on nutritional interventions according to a score. However, nurses need to ensure that assessment tools are based on evidence rather than rhetoric and validated in practice. The British Association for Parenteral and Enteral Nutrition Report (Allison, 1999) recommend that nutritional screening should be an integral part of the medical and nursing admission process and suggest that patients should be asked:

- Have you intentionally lost weight recently?
- Have you been eating less than normal?
- What is your normal weight?
- How tall are you?

The Department of Health (2001b) in the Essence of Care – Clinical Practice Benchmarking Report and the Nursing and Midwifery Practice Development Unit in Scotland Best Practice Statement – Nutritional Assessment and Referral in the Care of Adults in Hospital (NHS Scotland 2002) both recommend nutritional screening and assessment as best practice and identify the need to incorporate this into the nursing assessment and nursing care planning process.

Exercise

1. Locate literature on a nutritional risk assessment tool and the evidence to support its use in practice. Discuss the value and/or limitations of the tool with your personal tutor and mentor.
2. If you are a student nurse undertaking a clinical placement, find out if a nutritional risk assessment tool is used.
3. If so, establish how this is used, what information is collected and what guidelines are in place to support its use.
4. What evidence base is there to support its use?
5. If a tool is not used find out why and if any plans are underway to introduce one.
6. You may wish to discuss your findings with your mentor or personal tutor.

The Nursing and Practice Development Unit in Scotland (NHS Scotland 2002) have suggested that the following criteria should be included in any screening tool used:

- weight loss in the last 3 months
- body mass index (BMI)
- ability to eat and drink/absorb food
- appetite
- stress factors
- physical condition
- mental condition.

Having undertaken a thorough nursing assessment using the Roper et al (1996, 2000) model for nursing you should have sufficient information to complete a nutritional screening tool, identify actual and potential problems associated with the activity of eating and drinking and maintaining adequate nutrition.

Now let us return to the main case study. Using the Roper et al (1996, 2000) model for nursing has enabled us to undertake a thorough nursing assessment, which may look something like the following hypothetical example for Mavis.

1. *Breathing*
   - Mavis has never smoked and has no problems with her breathing.

2. *Eating and drinking*
   - She has reduced her fluid intake because her toilet is upstairs and she is unable to negotiate the stairs without pain in her hip.
   - Her appetite has been poor and she has not felt like cooking for herself 'What's the use of cooking for one?'.
   - Mavis is able to feed herself but with IV therapy in place she finds this difficult.
   - She has toast for breakfast, a sandwich at lunchtime and soup for her evening meal. She used to like to cook for her husband. Her BMI is 16.
   - She doesn't like fish or tomatoes.
   - She likes a small whisky at night before going to bed.
   - Her mouth is dry and her dentures are too big.
   - She has a sore mouth.

3. *Eliminating*
   - She has recently had some incontinence of urine and is complaining of constipation.

4. *Mobilising*
   - She is experiencing pain in her hip and has found it increasingly difficult to move around recently. There is one step down into her kitchen. She used to like to go out to Age Concern to meet up with her friends for lunch but her mobility problems have made this increasingly difficult recently.

5. *Expressing sexuality*
   - Mavis was always very proud about her appearance but her recent weight loss has made her clothes look untidy and she feels she is not smart. She likes to wear smart clothes and used to visit the hairdresser each week.

6. *Personal cleansing and dressing*
   - Until recently she has been able to get into her shower but because of mobility problems she is finding it increasingly difficult. Under normal circumstances she does not need any assistance to dress herself.

7. *Working and playing*
   - Before she retired she was a schoolteacher. Until recently she was able to do most of her own

housework, shopping and cleaning. She had a circle of friends whom she would meet in Age Concern and at church social events. Since she has been unable to get out of the house her friends have been visiting her at home. She is a Christian and regularly attended church on a Sunday. She spends most of her day watching the television or listening to the radio.

8. *Communicating*
   - Mavis is able to communicate; she wears a hearing aid and glasses. She has a telephone and frequently phones her daughter and speaks to her grandchildren. Her eyesight has begun to deteriorate recently and she is unable to read the newspaper.

9. *Maintaining a safe environment*
   - Mavis has pain in her hip when mobilising. She has had a couple of falls at home and walks with a stick. Her eyesight is poor and there is a risk of further falls.
   - Because she is undernourished she is at risk of developing pressure ulcers.
   - She understands her medication although she does not understand that because she is hypertensive she needs to reduce her salt intake.

10. *Sleeping*
   - Normally she sleeps well for 7½ hours but recently she has had difficulty in getting off to sleep.

   - She likes to have a small drink of whisky before retiring.

11. *Controlling body temperature*
   - Her house is centrally heated but she is unwilling to keep it on because of the high cost of fuel bills.

12. *Dying*
   - She does not express any beliefs about dying openly but she was very upset when her husband died. Her Christian beliefs have helped her to cope.

Exercise

1. Having undertaken a thorough nursing assessment you will have already begun to identify a number of potential and actual problems in relation to the activity of eating and drinking.
2. Make a list of what you think these might be and check your list against those identified below. This list might not be exhaustive but will give some indication to those that you might consider in relation to eating and drinking. You should remember to take account of the factors which influence the Activities of Living, i.e. physical, psychological, sociocultural, environmental and politicoeconomic.

Whilst undertaking this exercise you will begin to appreciate the interrelatedness of the actual and potential problems relating to the other Activities of Living. For further

---

Table 6.4 Potential problems – Case study 6.3 Mavis

Activity of Living	Actual problem	Potential problem
Eating and drinking	Mavis is dehydrated and reluctant to drink IVI in place, which may hamper her ability to reach her food and to feed herself	Fluid and electrolyte imbalance Mavis may not eat her meals and receive adequate nutrition
	Her BMI is 16	Further weight loss and protein energy malnutrition whilst in hospital
	Her appetite has been poor and she has not felt like cooking for herself	Mavis may not receive adequate nutrition
	Mavis is disorientated due to dehydration and hospital admission	Mavis may not understand how to choose her meals from the menu or how to call for help
Eliminating	Occasionally incontinent of urine	Reluctance to drink fluids thus increasing symptoms and effects of dehydration
	Constipation due to reduced fluid intake	Impacted faeces
Mobilising	Pain on mobilising	Depression due to pain and inability to get out and socialise
Personal cleansing and dressing	Unable to wash and dress due to IVI in situ	
Communicating		Inability to see menus due to poor eyesight Inability to hear dietary instructions and advice
Maintaining a safe environment	Risk of further falls Risk of pressure ulcer development due to loss of subcutaneous fat	Risk of fractured femur due to falls

information and reading on these Activities of Living you are referred to the relevant chapters in this book. You may like to return to the brief case studies and consider the actual and potential problems that might arise and discuss these with your personal tutor.

Setting goals

Having identified the actual and potential problems, it is now necessary to agree, ideally with the patient, short- and long-term goals or outcomes for nursing care and nursing interventions. This will enable you to evaluate whether the expected outcome has been achieved.

Goals should be realistic, achievable and measurable. It is advisable to include dates and times to indicate when the goal is to be achieved. This enables the nurse to evaluate progress and achievement and demonstrate how nursing has benefited the patient (Roper et al 1996). In some cases it may be necessary to agree long-term goals, i.e. those goals that might take longer to achieve than those that can be achieved within a shorter timescale. Roper et al (1996, 2000) liken goals to signposts on a journey indicating when you have arrived at your destination.

Table 6.5 shows examples of how goals might be set in the case of Mavis in relation to her activity of eating and drinking.

You may have considered other goals in relation to her psychological, sociocultural and environmental needs that have been identified in the case study. For example you may have considered the need for a home assessment in relation to her ability to negotiate the kitchen and prepare meals

or referral to a social worker to assess if she is eligible for financial support and how she might access services to enable her to get out more. You may wish to include these in your nursing care plan.

Determining nursing actions and interventions

Having undertaken a nursing assessment and identified actual and potential problems, the nurse is now ready to develop the nursing care plan. Roper et al (1996) point out that 'the nursing care plan is just that – a plan'. The nursing care plan, in addition to the direct observation of the patient, monitoring of vital signs and verbal report, should guide professional and ethical practice, care delivery, care management and personal and professional development (NMC 2002a, b) (see Box 6.12).

Box 6.12 Objective of the plan (Roper et al 1996, p. 57)

- to prevent identified problems with any of the ALs from becoming actual ones
- to solve actual problems
- where possible to alleviate those that cannot be solved
- to help the person cope positively with those problems that cannot be alleviated or solved
- to solve identified actual problems
- to prevent recurrence of a treated problem
- to help the person to be as comfortable and pain free as possible when death is inevitable.

Table 6.5 Eating and drinking goals

Actual problem	Potential problem	Goal
1. Mavis is dehydrated and reluctant to drink	Fluid and electrolyte imbalance	Mavis will receive IV fluids as prescribed Mavis will drink 1.5 litres of water a day
2. IVI in place, which may hamper her ability to reach her food and to feed herself	Mavis may not eat her meals and receive adequate nutrition	Mavis will receive assistance to reach her food and drink
3. Mavis' BMI is 16	Further weight loss and protein energy malnutrition whilst in hospital	Further weight loss whilst in hospital will be prevented
4. Mavis's appetite has been poor	Mavis may not receive adequate nutrition	Mavis's dietary intake will be monitored. Mavis will state that her appetite has improved
5. Mavis is disorientated due to dehydration and hospital admission She also has poor sight and hearing	Mavis may not understand how to choose her meals from the menu or how to call for help	Mavis will receive assistance and explanation on how to choose nourishing meals
6. Sore mouth due to loose dentures	Mavis may be reluctant to eat because of pain	Mavis's painful mouth will be relieved
7. Mavis is constipated	Faecal impaction	Mavis will receive dietary advice and increase amount of fibre in her diet and fluid intake Mavis will report normal bowel movements

Availability of resources

When planning the care and determining nursing actions and interventions the nurse must take account of the resources available to her, including staffing levels, knowledge and skills available, the environment and equipment and any evidence-based guidelines, protocols or policies. They will also need to take account of any interventions and care prescribed by other members of the health care team and incorporate these in to the nursing care plan where necessary.

Care pathways

The introduction of clinical governance into the NHS in the UK (DoH 1998) has placed greater emphasis on ensuring quality care to patients and effective outcomes. A care pathway is a tool that sets out the evidence-based care a patient should receive for an episode of care (Ellis & Johnson 1999). When planning the nursing care of a patient it is necessary to consider where care pathways have been developed and take account of these when determining the nursing interventions and individualising care.

Collaboration

As we have already discussed nurses do not work in isolation; they work in teams and in collaboration with others. In hospital nurses are with the patients for 24 hours a day and in many cases they may take the lead role in coordinating the care of the patient referring if necessary to specialist nurses and health care professionals.

Exercise

1. Revisit Mavis's assessment and identify other health care professionals who may be involved in her care.
2. What would be their role?

You may have considered the following:

- Dietitian
- medical staff
- junior medical staff
- Physiotherapist
- Health Care Assistant
- Ward hostess.

Other professionals who may input indirectly or at a later date include:

- Social Worker
- Dentist
- Occupational Therapist
- Discharge Liaison Coordinator.

When preparing a nursing care plan you will need to take account of the input and assessments undertaken by these professionals.

Return to the brief case studies and consider which other professionals are likely to be involved.

Exercise

1. Review Mavis's assessment and nursing care plan.

- Reflect on your experience to date; what knowledge and skills do you already possess to enable you to plan her nursing care?
- What knowledge and skills do you need to develop?
- What do you need to see and do to gain the knowledge and skills?
- What resources do you need to access care for this patient?

Nursing interventions

The nursing care plan details the nursing interventions required to achieve the stated goals. The plan should enable other staff including other health care professionals to provide continuity of care for the patient (Roper et al 2000). The nursing care plan may be paper-based or computerised.

When determining the nursing interventions you will need to consider where the patient is on the independency/dependency continuum as identified in the model of living (Roper et al 1996). The nurse provides nursing interventions for a dependent patient whereas nursing interventions in an independent patient aim to encourage and maintain independence. As discussed in the first part of this chapter dependency may be influenced by the factors associated with living across the lifespan.

Exercise

1. Review Mavis's assessment, actual and potential problems and goals and identify the nursing actions and interventions required.
2. Consider your knowledge and skills to undertake or supervise these. Identify those that you need to develop further and discuss these with your mentor or personal tutor.
3. Consider your suggested nursing actions and interventions in relation to the activity of eating and drinking against those listed below. These are by no means exhaustive.

Problem 1 *Mavis is dehydrated and is reluctant to drink*

The nurse has an important role in ensuring that the patient's hydration needs are met. In Mavis's case the nursing actions would involve ensuring that the intravenous fluids are administered safely and according to the medical prescription. You would need to ensure the integrity and patency of the cannula site and that it does not pose a problem with washing, dressing or feeding. The nurse must observe the cannula site for any signs of phlebitis or extravasation, the most common complications of intravenous therapy (Gobbi 2000). The intake and output of fluids must be accurately monitored, measured and charted. The reasons for intravenous therapy should be explained to Mavis.

You would need to agree with Mavis how often she would take oral fluids and what she preferred to drink. It is sometimes useful to agree with the patient that they would keep a record of what they drink and when. You would ensure that fluids are made available and within reach or that Mavis understands how to call for assistance to drink if necessary.

Problem 2 *Mavis has an IVI in place, which may hamper her ability to reach her food, and feed herself, she may therefore not eat her meals or receive adequate nutrition*

Intravenous access is more likely to be made through one of the lower extremities, such as the arm or hand. When determining which arm or hand, consideration should be given to using the arm other than the one she uses to feed herself. Consideration should be given to her positioning for meals and whether she can reach her food. Whilst wishing to promote independence, Mavis may require nursing assistance according to her dependency to drink or feed herself. Food should never be left out of the reach of the patient.

Problem 3 *Mavis is underweight with a BMI of 16*

A person with a BMI of 16 is regarded as underweight. Mavis should be referred to the dietitian who will undertake a detailed nutritional history and determine if Mavis requires a therapeutic diet. In some hospitals there are guidelines on when to refer to a dietitian and providing nutritional food supplements based on a nutritional assessment score for patients. Nutritional food supplements contain nutrients and are used in the short term to complement the normal hospital diet (Bond 1997). A doctor or dietitian must prescribe some food supplements unless there is a locally agreed protocol.

You may consider recording Mavis's food intake for a period of 3 days to enable a more detailed assessment of Mavis's nutritional intake whilst in hospital. Nurses, health care assistants and ward hostesses should be alerted to the need to monitor and observe Mavis's dietary intake, especially any food supplements. Mavis will also need assistance with choosing food from the menu.

In order to monitor any improvement you would need to check Mavis's weight at least once a week. You should try to do this using the same machine each time and ensuring that Mavis wears the same clothes each time.

Problem 4 *Mavis's appetite is poor*

As in the previous problems you would discuss Mavis's likes and dislikes and help her to choose nourishing meals from the hospital menu. The hospital environment including smells and other patients' behaviours can have an influence on a person's appetite. You should attempt to ensure the environment is as conducive as possible at mealtimes so that

they are as pleasurable as possible (Tolson et al 2002). Attention to the presentation, amount and serving of meals can help to encourage patients to eat. You will need to discuss with Mavis reasons why she believes her appetite is poor and try to identify any underlying reasons for this. You should aim to discuss strategies for improving her appetite and monitor and record her food intake especially when removing her food tray at the end of a meal.

Problem 5 *Mavis is disorientated due to hospital admission. She also has poor eyesight and hearing*

It is not uncommon for older patients to be disorientated on admission to hospital. Mental state is affected by malnutrition and Mavis may well have little motivation, energy or will to help herself. Mavis will need to be orientated to her surroundings and any procedures and routines explained. It should be explained to her that by eating a better diet she might begin to feel better. She will need instructions and assistance in completing any relevant forms for her menus. She might be unused to the type of food on the menu and will need to be helped to choose nourishing high calorie food. This may provide an opportunity to promote healthy eating and offer patient information leaflets to support your advice in readiness for her discharge.

Problem 6 *Mavis has a sore mouth due to loose dentures*

Because Mavis is dehydrated her mouth is dry and as she has also lost weight her dentures are too big resulting in a sore mouth and a reluctance to eat and drink. Older people have specific oral care needs and it is essential that nurses understand and are able to meet these needs (Fitzpatrick 2000). You may choose to use one of a number of oral hygiene assessment tools developed to assist nurses in assessing patient's needs to identify any nursing actions or interventions. Nursing interventions should include inspection of her oral cavity noting any ulceration or abnormality. The plan should include the frequency of oral hygiene, cleansing of dentures, advice on removal of debris and any prescribed use of topical anaesthetic mouthwash or lozenges and possible referral for dental advice. It is important to consider Mavis's dignity and self-esteem when attending to her oral hygiene.

Problem 7 *Mavis is constipated*

Constipation may be caused by low fluid intake therefore an increase in fluid intake should assist in a returning to normal defecation. Mavis's problems with mouth pain and her inability to cope with foods that need to be chewed can also contribute to constipation. In addition, unfamiliarity with her surroundings and access to toilet facilities will also compound the problem. Therefore nursing interventions and actions should aim to increase fluid intake, administer any prescribed medication or laxatives, reduce mouth pain and familiarise Mavis with her surroundings. Her bowel movements should be monitored and recorded daily.

Implementing the plan

When implementing the plan of care nurses need to take account of the resources available, including staff and skill mix, knowledge, the skills required to deliver care and systems of organising nursing care delivery.

> **Exercise**
> 1. If you are a student nurse undertaking a clinical placement observe how nursing care is organised.
> 2. How does the system of organising care delivery contribute to individualising patient care?

You may have observed one of the following methods.

Task allocation where the nurses are assigned to tasks such as taking temperatures for a group of patients or a whole ward. This method leads to fragmentation of care and lack of continuity. Patient care is not individualised and no one nurse will have an overall view of an individual patient.

Team nursing where nurses work in teams to deliver the care to a group of patients sometimes in a defined area of the ward. Sometimes the nurses are allocated to a team for a whole shift or allocated to a team permanently. This system of care delivery can provide continuity of patient care but there is always a danger that the team can revert to task-centred nursing within a team.

In primary nursing a nurse is responsible for the care of a patient for the whole period of care from admission to discharge. Because they are unable to be present 24 hours a day they work with an associate nurse who will assume delegated responsibility in his or her absence. This method provides continuity for the patient and the nurse.

Alternatively, you may have observed hybrid systems of care delivery being used depending on the number of nurses and their level knowledge and skills available to meet the individual needs of patients.

> **Exercise**
> 1. What factors would you need to take into account when implementing the plan of nursing care for Mavis?

You may have considered the following factors might influence implementation:

- the philosophy of care on the ward or department (beliefs and values, advocacy)
- the nursing model used
- the care delivery system (primary nursing, team nursing, case management or task allocation)
- resources available (skill mix of staff available, equipment, support staff and other health care professionals).

You may have considered that the following knowledge is required when implementing nursing activities:

- anatomy and physiology of digestive system and nutrition
- psychological effects associated with eating and drinking
- sociocultural issues relating to eating and drinking
- environmental issues and concerns
- political and economic concerns.

You may have considered that the following skills are required when implementing nursing activities:

- caring skills (listening, comforting, reassuring, helping)
- clinical psychomotor skills (catheterisation, intravenous infusions)
- management skills (organisational, supervision, delegation skills)
- counselling skills (listening, problem solving, advising)
- teaching skills
- research skills (literature searching, critical appraisal, synthesis)
- problem-solving skills (problem identification, goal setting, priority setting)
- leadership skills (advocacy, teamwork, transformational leadership skills, networking).

> **Exercise**
> 1. Reflect on these and assess your current knowledge and skills in relation to the activity of eating and drinking.
> 2. Record your reflections in your diary.
> 3. Identify those areas in which you need further development.
> 4. Take these to your next tutorial or clinical supervision session. Discuss with your mentor or preceptor how you plan to develop these further.

Evaluation of nursing actions and interventions

Evaluation of nursing care is an important part of professional practice and provides feedback on the patient's progress (NMC 2002a). Evaluation is an ongoing process, which should be undertaken by the nurse in conjunction with the patient and his or her relatives or carers and other health care professionals (for further information refer to Chapter 1).

Evaluating care consists of checking the patient's progress against the identified goals and timescales to determine whether these have been fully or partially met or indeed not been met at all.

When evaluating the care plan you will need to establish if the goals have been completely met, partially met or not met at all. If the goal has not been met or partially met then the nurse must consider if the agreed timescale was realistic. If not then you may decide to extend the timescale. Alternatively you may need to reassess the problem and modify the plan. In some cases the problem may have changed or the goal may have been inappropriate. Not all goals will be achievable during a hospital stay. In which case you might need more information on the problem, is it worse or has it changed?

You might also reconsider the appropriateness of the prescribed nursing actions and interventions – do these need to be changed or modified? By involving patients in their nursing care planning it is possible to identify and agree realistic goals and meaningful evaluation of outcomes.

Discharge planning

The nursing care plan should include a plan for discharge or transfer of care between secondary, tertiary and primary care. It is advisable to begin planning discharge when a patient is first admitted to hospital. By using the Roper et al (1996, 2000) model for nursing based on a model of living will also provide the basis of a well-developed discharge plan and facilitate safe and effective discharge back into the community.

Summary points

> 1. This chapter introduced the fourth Activity of Living, eating and drinking as described by Roper, Logan and Tierney in their model of nursing (Roper et al 1996, 2000).

> It systematically explored the framework of the model and its application in clinical practice, the use of a case scenario, exercises, and reflection and directed reading. It has been impossible within this chapter to cover every aspect in relation to the activity of eating and drinking and it is important that you keep up-to-date with new information and evidence-based practice in order to be able to meet the changing needs of patients and health care delivery.
>
> 2. The activity of eating and drinking is essential to existence and nurses have a very important role in ensuring the quality of the patient experience that patient needs are met. There is a significant amount of evidence that patient's nutritional needs in hospital are not being met. Throughout this chapter it has been shown how the ability or inability to eat and drink can impact on many of the other Activities of Living and how by using the Roper, Logan and Tierney model for nursing as a framework, nurses are able to recognise and take account of the patient's nutritional needs when assessing, planning, implementing and evaluating holistic patient care.

References

Akhtar S 2002 Nursing with Dignity: Part 8: Islam. Nursing Times 98(16): 40–42

Allison SP (ed.) 1999 'Hospital Food as Treatment' a report by the Working Party of the British Association for Parental and Enteral Nutrition. Maidenhead

Alexander MF, Fawcett JN, Runciman PJ 2000 Nursing practice for hospital and home (the adult), 2nd edn. Churchill Livingstone, Edinburgh

Anderson C, Nathan A 1991 Promoting oral health (3). The Pharmaceutical Journal 15: 734–736

Association of Community Health Councils 1997 Hungry in hospital. ACHEW, London

Bond S (ed.) 1997 Eating matters: A resource for improving dietary care in hospitals. Centre for Health Services Research, University of Newcastle, Newcastle

British Medical Association 1999 Withholding and withdrawing life prolonging medical treatment. Guidance for decision making. BMJ, Buckingham

Butterworth ACE 1974 The skeleton in the hospital closet. Nutrition Today March/April: 4–5

Chan JYK 1995 Dietary beliefs of Chinese patients. Nursing Standard 9(27): 30–34

Chen CG, Schilling LS, Lyder CH 2001 A concept analysis of malnutrition in the elderly. Journal of Advanced Nursing 36(1): 131–142

Collins A 2002 Nursing with dignity. Nursing Times Series Part 1 Judaism. Nursing Times 98(9): 33–35

Cooper DB 2000 People who use and abuse substances. In: Alexander MF, Fawcett JN, Runciman PJ (eds) Nursing practice for hospital and home (the adult), 2nd edn. Churchill Livingstone, Edinburgh

Covington CY, Cybulski MJ, Davis TL et al 2001 Kids on the move: Preventing obesity of urban children. American Journal of Nursing 101(3): 73–75, 77, 79, 81–82

Cremin D, Halek C 1997 Eating disorders: Knowledge for practice. Nursing Times Learning Curve Volume Unit 451(5): 5–8

Daniels L 2002 Diet and coronary heart disease. Nursing Standard 16(43): 47–52, 54–55

Dobson R 2002 Breast is still best even when HIV prevalence is high, experts say. British Medical Journal 324: 1474

DoH 1991 Dietary reference values for food energy and nutrients for the United Kingdom. Report of the Panel on Dietary Reference Values. Report on health and social subjects No 41. HMSO, London

DoH 1992 Health of the Nation Report. HMSO, London

DoH 1998 A first class service: Quality in the New NHS. The Stationery Office, London

DoH 2000a The NHS plan: a plan for investment – a plan for reform. The Stationery Office, London

DoH 2000b (2001a) Infant feeding survey in 2000. The Stationery Office, London

DoH 2001b The essence of care: patient-focused benchmarking for health care professionals. The Stationery Office, London.

DoH 2001c National service framework for coronary heart disease. The Stationery Office, London

DoH 2001d National service framework for diabetes. The Stationery Office, London

DoH 2001e Modern standards and service models of older people: National Service framework for older people. The Stationery Office, London

DoH 2001f Caring for older people: Nursing priority integrating knowledge, practice and values. Report by the Nursing & Midwifery Advisory Committee, HMSO, London

DoH 2001g Tackling health inequalities: Consultation on a plan for delivery. The Stationery Office, London

Effective Healthcare Bulletin 1997 The prevention and treatment of obesity. NHS Centre for Reviews and Dissemination, University of York, 1(2)

Effective Healthcare Bulletin 2000 Promoting the initiation of breast feeding. NHS Centre for Reviews and Dissemination, University of York, 6(2)

Ekpe HI 2001 Empowerment for adults with chronic mental health problems and obesity. Nursing Standard 15(39): 37–42

Ellis BW, Johnson S 1999 The care pathway: a tool to enhance clinical governance. British Journal of Clinical Governance 4(2): 61–71

Elmståhl S, Person M, Andren V, Blabolil V 1997 Malnutrition in geriatric patients: a neglected problem? Journal of Advanced Nursing 26: 851–855

Finlay T 2002 Caring for the patient with a disorder of the gastrointestinal system. In: Walsh M (ed) Watson's clinical nursing and related sciences, pp. 435–506. Baillière Tindall, Edinburgh

Fitzpatrick J 2000 Oral health care needs of dependent older people: responsibilities of nurses and care staff. Journal of Advanced Nursing 32(6): 1325–1332

Frobisher C, Maxwell SM 2001 The attitudes and nutritional knowledge of a group of 11–12 year olds in Merseyside. International Journal of Health Promotion and Education 39(4): 121–127

Gobbi M 2000 Fluid & Electrolyte Balance. In: Alexander MF, Fawcett JN, Runciman PJ (eds) Nursing practice for hospital and home (the adult), 2nd edn. Churchill Livingstone, Edinburgh

Gobbi M, Torrance C 2000 Nutrition. In: Alexander MF, Fawcett JN, Runciman PJ (eds) Nursing practice for hospital and home (the adult), 2nd edn, pp. 697–718. Churchill Livingstone, Edinburgh

Gustafsson K, Sidenvall B 2002 Food-related health perceptions and food habits among older women. Journal of Advanced Nursing 39(2): 164–173

Hamilton Smith S 1972 Nil by mouth. Royal College of Nursing, London

Hand H 2001 The use of intravenous therapy. Nursing Standard 15(43): 47–55

Henley A, Schott J 1999 Culture, religion & patient care in a multi-ethnic society. A handbook for professionals. Age Concern Books, Glasgow

Hinchliff S, Montague SE, Watson R 1996 Physiology for nursing practice, 2nd edn. Harcourt Publishers Ltd, Edinburgh

Holland B, Welch AA, Unwin ID, Buss DH, Paul AA, Southgate DAT 1991 McCance and Widdowson's The composition of foods, 5th revised and extended edn. The Royal Society of Chemistry & Ministry of Agriculture, Fisheries and Food, London

Holmes S, Mountain E 1993 Assessment of oral status: Evaluation of three oral assessment guides. Journal of Clinical Nursing 2: 35–40

Howie E, Miller MEA, Murchie MB 2000 The gastro-intestinal system, liver and biliary tract. In: Alexander M, Fawcett JN, Runciman PJ (eds) Nursing practice – hospital and home (the adult). Churchill Livingstone, Edinburgh

Jamieson L, McFarlane CM, Brown JM 2000 The musculoskeletal system. In: Alexander M, Fawcett JN, Runciman PJ (eds) Nursing practice – hospital and home (the adult). Churchill Livingstone, Edinburgh

Jamieson EM, McCall JM, Whyte LA 2002 Clinical nursing practices. Churchill Livingstone, Edinburgh

Joint FAO/WHO/UNU Expert Consultation 1985 Energy and protein requirements. WHO Technical Report Series 724. WHO, Geneva

Kenchaiach SK, Evans JC, Levy O et al 2002 Obesity and the risk of heart failure. The New England Journal of Medicine 347(5): 305–313

Kowanko I, Simon S, Wood J 1999 Nutritional care of the patient: nurses knowledge and attitudes in an acute setting. Journal of Clinical Nursing 8: 217–224

Kowanko I, Simon S, Wood J 2001 Energy and nutrient intake of patients in acute care. Journal of Clinical Nursing 10: 51–57

Lennard-Jones J 1992 A Positive Approach to Nutrition as Treatment. The Kings Fund Centre, London

Lennard-Jones J, Arrowsmith H, Davison C, Denham AF, Micklewright A 1995 Screening by nurses and junior doctors to detect malnutrition when patients are first assessed in hospital. Clinical Nutrition 14: 336–340

Lieberman HR, Wurtman JJ, Chew B 1986 Changes in mood after carbohydrate consumption among obese individuals. American Journal of Clinical Nutrition 44(6): 772–778

McAulay D 2001 Dehydration in the terminally ill patient. Nursing Standard 16(4): 33–37

McKie L, MacInnes A, Hendry J, Donald S, Peace H 2000 The food consumption patterns and perceptions of dietary advice of older people. Journal of Human Nutrition and Dietetics 13(3): 173–183

McLaren S, Holmes S, Green S, Bond S 1997 An overview of nutritional issues relating to the care of older people. In: Bond S (ed) Eating matters: A resource for improving dietary care in hospitals, pp. 15–21. Centre for Health Services Research, University of Newcastle, Newcastle

McWhirter JP, Pennington CR 1994 Incidence and recognition of malnutrition in hospital. British Medical Journal 308: 945–948

Madden C 2000 Nutritional benefits of drinks. Nursing Standard 15(13–15/2000): 47–52

Mahasneh SM 2001 Health perceptions and health behaviours of poor urban Jordanian women. Journal of Advanced Nursing 36(1): 58–68

Maltby JR 1993 New guidelines for pre-operative fasting. Canadian Journal and Anesthesiology 40: 5/BPR113–R117

Metcalf C 2002 Crohn's disease: an overview. Nursing Standard 16(31): 45–52

Milne L 2001 Do diets work? Nursing Times 97(44): 46–48

Mullaly S 2000 The Chief Nurse's view. Nursing Times Plus 96(8): 1

NAO 2002 National audit report: Tackling obesity in England report by the Comptroller and Auditor General. The Stationery Office, London

National Child Birth Trust 1999 Complete baby care from birth to 3 years for parents. National Child Birth Trust, Harper Collins, London

NHS Scotland 2002 Best practice statements – Nutritional assessment and referral in the care of adults in hospital. The Nursing and Midwifery Practice Development Unit (NMPDU), Edinburgh (www.nmpdu.org)

Northcot N 2002 Nursing with dignity. Part 2: Buddhism. Nursing Times 98(10): 36–38

Norton B 1996 Malnutrition in hospitals: The nurses role and prevention. Nursing Times 92(26) (Supplement in Association with British Association for Parenteral and Enteral Nutrition) 1(1): June 26

Nursing and Midwifery Council 2002a Guidelines for records and record keeping. NMC, London

Nursing and Midwifery Council 2002b Code of professional practice. NMC, London

Ogg TW, Hitchcock N 1993 What is the optimum NPO time prior to day surgery. Journal of One Day Surgery Summer: 4–5

Reilly HM, Martineau JK, Moran A, Kennedy H 1995 Nutritional screening – Evaluation and implementation of a simple nutrition risk score. Clinical Nutrition 14: 269–273

Rinomhota S, Rollins H 2001 Energy, mood and behaviour: part 2. NT Plus Nursing Times 97(44): 50, 52

Rogers AW 1992 Textbook of anatomy. Churchill Livingstone, Edinburgh

Roper N, Logan WW, Tierney AJ 1996 The elements of nursing: A model for nursing based on a model for living, 4th edn. Churchill Livingstone, London

Roper N, Logan WW, Tierney AJ 2000 The Roper Logan Tierney model of nursing based on activities of living. Churchill Livingstone, Edinburgh

Royal College of Physicians 2001 Alcohol can the NHS afford it? Online publication. RCP (http://www.rcplondon.ac.uk/pubs/wp-actnhsai-summary.htm)

Royal College of Physicians 2002 Nutrition and patients: A doctors responsibility. Online publication. RCP (http://www.rcplondon.ac.uk/pubs/wp-np-summary.htm)

Rutishauser S 1994 Physiology and anatomy. A basis for nursing and health care. Churchill Livingstone, London

Scottish Intercollegiate Guidelines Network 1997 Management of patients with stroke. Identification and management of dysphagia. Publication no 20. SIGN, Edinburgh

Shireff A 1990 Pre-operative nutritional assessment. Nursing Times 86(8): 68–72

Silk D (ed) 1994 Organisation of nutritional support in hospitals: A report by a working party of BAPEN. The British Association for Parenteral and Enteral Nutrition, Maidenhead, Berks

Silverman K, Evans SM, Stragin EC et al 1992 Withdrawal syndrome after the double-blind cessation of caffeine consumption. New England Journal of Medicine 327(16): 1109–1114

Sizer T (ed) 1996 Working Party of the British Association for Parenteral and Enteral Nutrition. Standards and guidelines for nutritional support of patients in hospital. BAPEN, Maidenhead

Sutcliffe A 2001 Osteoporosis: prevention and treatment. Nursing Times 97(3): 53–55

Sutcliffe E 1990 Reviewing the process progress. A critical review of the literature on the nursing process. Senior Nurse 10(a): 9–13

Tolson DT, Schofield J, Booth R, Ramsey R 2002 Best practice statements Part 2: Nutrition for the physically frail older people. Nursing Times 98(28): 38–40

Thomas AE 1987 Pre-operative fasting, a question of routine. Nursing Times 83(49): 46, 47

Thompson DR, Webster RA 2000 The cardiovascular system. In: Alexander MF, Fawcett JN, Runciman PJ (eds) Nursing practice – hospital and home (the adult), pp. 7–58. Churchill Livingstone, Edinburgh

Walsh M (ed) 2000 Watson's clinical nursing and related sciences, 6th edn. Baillière Tindall, in association with the RCN

Wood S, Creamer M 1996 Malnutrition in hospitals. Nursing Times 92(26): 67–68

Further reading

Hinchliff SM, Montague SE, Watson R Physiology for nursing practice, 2nd edn. Baillière Tindall, London

Holland K, Hogg C 2001 Cultural awareness in nursing and health care. Arnold, London

Useful websites

British Dietetic Association www.bda.uk.com

Committee on Medical Aspects of Food and Nutrition www.doh.gov.uk/coma/about.htm

Department for Environment, Food and Rural Affairs www.defra.gov.uk

Department of Health Essence of Care www.doh.gov.uk/essenceofcare/index

Department of Health – Health Inequalities www.doh.gov.uk/healthinequalities

Department of Health National Service Framework for Diabetes www.doh.gov.uk/nsf/diabetes

Department of Health National Service Framework for Coronary Heart Disease www.doh.gov.uk/nsf/coronary

Department of Health National Service Framework for Older People www.doh.gov.uk/nsf/olderpeople.htm

Food Standards Agency www.foodstandards.gov.uk/older

Health Development Agency www.hda-online.org.uk

MIDIRS informed choice www.nelh.nhs.uk/maternity

National Centre for Health Statistics (NHANES III) http://www.cde.gov/nchs

National Heart, Lung and Blood Institute www.nhlbi.nih.gov/aboutframington

Nursing and Midwifery Council www.nmc-uk.org

Nursing and Midwifery Practice Development Unit (NMPDU) http://www.nmpdu.org

Royal College of Psychiatrists www.rcpsych.ac.uk/

Royal College of Physicians http://www.rcplondon.ac.uk

Scottish Intercollegiate Clinical Guidelines www.sign.ac.uk/guidelines

Various 1998 Why and how should adults lose weight. Drugs and Therapeutics Bulletin 36(12): 89–92

World Health Organisation www.who.int

Eliminating

Jackie Solomon

Introduction

Elimination is an activity that individuals, undertake several times throughout each day and is necessary to rid the body of the waste products (urine and faeces) associated with metabolism. It is an activity that is undertaken in private. Influenced by societal and cultural norms, the inability of individuals to control elimination is often frowned upon in all but the very young child. The ability to control elimination is referred to as being 'continent' and relies on mature physiological systems. Illness or disability may impact on the ability to remain continent. Problems associated with elimination may impact and compromise many of the other Activities of Living, such as mobilising, eating and drinking, expressing sexuality, personal cleansing and dressing, working and playing, and maintaining a safe environment. Each AL is closely related to each other (Roper et al 2000) and it is important that the nurse takes these into consideration when assessing, planning, implementing and evaluating care of patients with such problems.

This chapter will therefore focus on the following:

- elimination in health and illness
- dependence/independence in the AL of elimination
- factors influencing the AL of elimination
- nursing care of individuals with health problems affecting the Activity of Living: elimination.

THE MODEL OF LIVING

Elimination in health and illness (across the lifespan)

Childhood and adolescence

At birth babies have no control of their bladder or bowels and depend solely on their parents to keep them dry and clean. Most children will gain control around the age of 18 months and many children will be dry during the daytime by the time they reach 3 years with boys taking longer than girls to do so. As soon as the child is able to recognise the need to pass urine or faeces ('wee' (urine) or 'poo' (faeces) are frequently used words used by British children to describe these activities) and is able to understand simple instructions and pull his/her clothes up and down, parents will begin potty training. Later when the child progresses to using the toilet they may require a low stool and toddler seat to make it less daunting and easier to sit on. A boy will need to learn that it is acceptable to stand to pass urine and in front of other children. In the early days there are likely to be 'accidents' when they lose control and are incontinent, especially if they are upset, excited, distracted or engrossed in something.

Exercise

1. Reflect on your own childhood. Can you recall an event or situation in which you were unable to control your bladder or bowel? What were you doing at the time? How did you feel?
2. How does society view the young child who is unable to control his bladder? Would this attitude change if this were an older person?

Environmental and psychological factors can influence a child's toileting regime. During a period of excitement, activity or fear, a child may become incontinent. Some children may suppress the need to go to the toilet in a different environment, for example at school, preferring instead to use their own toilet at home. It is important to be sympathetic and understanding about any accidents. If the child gets worried then the problem may become worse.

Whilst society is understanding of the young child who is unable to control their bladder, it is much less tolerant of the older child or adult who is incontinent.

Enuresis

If a child is unable to control his or her bladder either during the day or night this is known as enuresis. Daytime wetting can be either due to delaying the need to go to the toilet, giggling, or urge incontinence due to detrusor instability (Rogers 2002). Being dry at night takes a little longer and there are the inevitable bedwetting accidents. Most children grow out of this by the age of five; however, boys tend to take a little longer. If a child continues to wet the bed and has no other urinary symptoms or disease this is known as nocturnal enuresis (Evans 2001). Some children who have been dry for some time may begin to wet the bed again. This is known as secondary enuresis. This may happen if they are upset or are feeling insecure, for example if a new baby has arrived in the family. The number of children living in Cumbria suffering from secondary enuresis rose during the foot and mouth outbreak in 2001 (Beaton 2001). It is important to give encouragement and support and identify those children who require physiological and psychological help at an early stage. A child who has never been dry at night is said to have primary nocturnal enuresis.

There are approximately 500 000 children in the UK suffering from nocturnal enuresis or persistent bedwetting (DoH, 2000). Whilst the prevalence of enuresis decreases with age surveys have shown that it affects;

- one in six of children aged five
- one in seven children aged seven
- one in 11 children aged nine
- one in 50 teenagers.

Exercise

1. Find out what support is available for parents of children who persistently wet the bed at night.
2. What do you think are the consequences of bedwetting, a) for the child, b) for the parents?

You may have found out about local and national support groups and organisations that provide written information to parents such as the Enuresis Resource and Information Centre (ERIC). These organisations provide information and practical help to parents. They may be able to put parents in contact with other parents with children with similar problems. The General Practitioner will be able to undertake a physical examination to determine if there are any physical or congenital abnormalities and to exclude a urinary infection. Local health services may have a team of health professionals including specialist nurses, physiotherapists and psychologists to provide expert advice and therapy.

There are a number of treatments or interventions for children of school age with nocturnal enuresis. These include: enuresis alarms, dry bed training, the use of star charts, and medication, e.g. antimuscarinic medicines, tricyclic antidepressants or hormones. Enuresis alarms are pads with sensors, which are placed on the bed or worn on the body and an alarm sounds when the child begins to pass water. Alternatively parents may choose to wake their child every 2 hours to go to the toilet. They may do this without the help of an enuresis alarm. There are two types of nocturnal incontinence. The first is where the child produces

excessive urine thought to be as a result of hormonal insufficiency, and has an impaired arousal mechanism. This type of enuresis is usually treated with antidiuretic hormones. The second is due to hyperactivity of the detrusor and failure of the arousal mechanisms (Neveus et al 2000). This type is treated with anticholinergic drugs. Star charts and dry bed training involve systems of rewards or incentives to encourage the child to become dry at night. A systematic review of the research undertaken by Glazener and Evans (2001) found that the use of alarms for nocturnal enuresis is an effective treatment for nocturnal bedwetting in children. The effect of hormonal or tricyclic antidepressant treatment was effective but was not sustained in the long term.

It may be difficult for parents to cope with continual wet beds and they may become stressed and impatient due to lack of sleep. They may also suffer a financial burden if they need to buy pads and extra bed linen to cope with the wet beds. The child who wets the bed may get teased or bullied at school and their siblings may also ridicule them. Waking up in a cold wet bed is unpleasant and interrupts the child's sleep. As a result they may be unable to concentrate and this could affect their progress in school. Socially, they may be unable to sleep over with friends due to the embarrassment of being woken frequently during the night.

Some parents may find if extremely difficult to cope with a child who is incontinent. Amanda Page writing under a pseudonym shared her experience of bringing up a daughter with urinary incontinence and how the stigma of incontinence impacted on their relationship to the extent that at the age of 16 her daughter chose to go into the care of the local authority. Reflecting on her experiences Amanda felt the need to be better informed about urinary incontinence to have been able to support her daughter. She also recognised that she herself needed support and the opportunity to speak to other parents in similar situations (Page 1999).

Physical and mental disabilities

Some males may suffer from a condition know as phimosis. Phimosis is a situation where the foreskin or prepuce of the penis is too tight to be retracted over the glans penis. Natural separation of the two layers of the skin occurs around the age of 2 years. If this is attempted before the two layers have naturally separated then scar tissue will form which can lead to urinary retention, pain and discharge. Circumcision may also contribute to phimosis if it is incorrectly performed.

There are some children who are born with neurological lesions such as spina bifida. The location of the lesion will depend on the extent to which the child's ability to pass water is affected. High lesions will result in detrusor and sphincter overactivity and the inability to recognise when they have a full bladder. Many of these children may be wheelchair dependent and may have difficulty accessing toilets as well as managing their clothes without help (McMonnies 2002). For some of these children intermittent catheterisation is usually considered the best option (McMonnies 2002). Children with learning difficulties such as Down syndrome and cerebral palsy may suffer from incontinence; however they respond well to behavioural toilet training sessions (Rogers 2001).

Encopresis

Faecal incontinence or soiling in children is known as encopresis and is defined as the passage of a normal consistency stool or an incomplete or loose stool in a socially inappropriate place. Faecal incontinence in children is also common with best estimates suggesting that 1.5% of children still lack bowel control by their 7th birthday (see Box 7.1) (Royal College of Physicians 1995).

The Royal College of Physicians (1995) identified a number of factors and health problems why children may not achieve continence of faeces including failure or delay in normal development, neurological deficiency, and abnormality of the anal sphincter muscles, faecal retention, incorrect laxative treatment and psychological and emotional problems. Children may suffer from one or more of these health problems and both they and their parents will require input and support from a multidisciplinary team. The possibility of invasive procedures and investigations can be very distressing and add to the psychological and emotional turmoil for both the child and their parents.

Adulthood

In adulthood we are expected to have full control of our bladder and bowels. Incontinence is the inability to maintain voluntary control resulting in excretion of urine and/or faeces in inappropriate places or at inappropriate times (Royal College of Physicians 1995). Often associated with old age, incontinence is a taboo subject and has a significant impact on an individual's social and occupational activity, psychological functioning, and physical and sexual relations.

A postal survey within two health authorities in the UK revealed that a large number of adults (23%) had experienced urinary incontinence at some time during their adult years (Roe & Doll 2000). Roe and Doll (2000) also found that people who were incontinent had a lower health status than those who were continent. Whilst it is difficult to measure accurately the prevalence because of the subjective nature of the problem and associated embarrassment, it is estimated that six million people within the UK have continence problems (Willis 1999).

A Royal College of Physicians report on Incontinence – Causes, management and provision of services (1995) reviewed the current knowledge about continence and the management of incontinence. They suggested that the prevalence of urinary incontinence is widespread. More recently this has been confirmed by the Department of Health (2000) that published the following statistics for people living at home and those in institutions (see Box 7.2).

Common symptoms of urinary incontinence include frequency of micturition, needing to go to the toilet in the

---

Box 7.1 Prevalence rates of children incontinent of faeces

- one in 30 of children aged four to five
- one in 50 of children aged five to six
- one in 75 of children aged seven to ten
- one in 100 of children aged 11 to 12.

Source: Good practice in continence services (DOH 2000).

Box 7.2 Statistics for the incidence of urinary incontinence

For people living at home:
- between 1 in 20 and 1 in 14 women aged 15–44;
- between 1 in 13 and 1 in 7 women aged 45–64;
- between 1 in 10 and 1 in 5 women aged 65 and over;
- over 1 in 33 men aged 15–64;
- between 1 in 14 and 1 in 10 men aged 65 and over are incontinent.

For people living in institutions:
- one in three in residential homes
- nearly two in every three in nursing homes
- half to two-thirds in wards for elderly and elderly mentally infirm are incontinent.

Source: Good practice in continence services (DoH 2000).

---

night, a sense of urgency or need to void urine urgently, leakage of urine when trying not to void and sneezing or coughing, and being incontinent during sleep. Childbirth, obesity, chronic constipation, chronic chest problems and weak pelvic floor muscles are common causes of urinary incontinence in adults. Physical exercise, coughing or sneezing may exacerbate the problem. The menopause in women is thought to increase the risk of urinary symptoms as a result of hormonal changes and reduction in oestrogen levels. In males, diseases of the prostate may lead to obstruction of the flow of urine. In both males and females retention of urine due to an obstruction can lead to incontinence. Males may also suffer from postmicturition dribble, this is when leakage of urine occurs as the penis is placed back in underclothes. A summary of the age-related disorders associated with incontinence in males is provided in Box 7.3.

Faecal incontinence affects both males and females of all ages. Whilst less prevalent than urinary incontinence it is reported to affect about 2% of the adult population and 7% of healthy independent adults over the age of 65 (Nelson et al 1995, Johanson et al 1996). It is the cause of a great deal of embarrassment for people who suffer from faecal incontinence (Herbert 1999).

Around 30% of women suffer damage to one or both anal sphincter muscles during their first vaginal delivery

---

Box 7.3 Age-related disorders of the lower urinary tract associated with incontinence in males

Childhood/youth
- Anatomical abnormalities
- Detrusor instability
- Neuropathic bladder
- Bladder neck weakness

Middle age
- Detrusor instability
- Neuropathic bladder
- Bladder neck obstruction
- Underactive bladder disorders

Older men
- Outflow tract obstruction:
  - uncomplicated
  - associated with instability
- Neuropathic bladder
- Detrusor instability
- Underactive bladder states
- Extraurological causes:
  - constipation
  - pharmacological agents
  - environmental difficulties

From RCP report 1995

Box 7.5 Causes of faecal incontinence in later life

1. Constipation/faecal impaction with overflow incontinence.

2. Neurogenic incontinence – due to loss of cortical inhibition in dementia.

3. Colorectal disease
   - colorectal cancer
   - diverticular disease
   - inflammatory bowel disease.

4. Causes of diarrhoea
   - drug-induced (e.g. laxatives, magnesium-containing antacids, iron preparations)
   - gastric and small bowel disorders
   - irritable bowel disease.

5. Anal sphincter defects, rectal prolapse.

6. Factors relating to access to toilets and handling clothing, in association with impaired mobility.

From RCP report 1995

Box 7.4 Causes of faecal incontinence (Norton 1996)

Sphincter or pelvic floor damage
- Obstetric trauma
- Direct trauma or injury

Diarrhoea/intestinal hurry
- Inflammatory bowel disease
- Irritable bowel disease

Iatrogenic/postsurgery
- Post haemorrhoidectomy
- Sphincterotomy for fissure
- Anal stretch

Anorectal pathology
- Rectal prolapse
- Anal or rectal–vaginal fistula
- Congenital abnormalities

Neurological disease
- Spinal cord injury
- Multiple sclerosis
- Spina bifida/sacral agenesis
- Parkinson's disease (often secondary to constipation)
- Secondary to degenerative disease, neurological disease, e.g Alzheimer's, environmental

Impaction with overflow
- Institutionalised or immobility
- Elderly
- Severe constipation in children

Environmental
- Poor toilet facilities
- Inadequate care

Idiopathic
- Unknown causes
- Psychological factors

(Kamm 1998). Forceps delivery, large baby, a long second stage of labour and occipitoposterior presentation of the fetus are all common risk factors. Of the women who have a third-degree tear during delivery, despite repair, a significant number develop anal incontinence (gas) or urgency (Sultan et al 1993). Anal surgery, structural damage to the internal sphincter, neurological disease and congenital anorectal malformations may lead also to faecal incontinence. Faecal incontinence occurs in 50% of people who have multiple sclerosis and is the cause of significant distress (Hinds et al 1990). Norton (1996) provides a useful summary (Box 7.4) of the causes of faecal incontinence.

Older people

Whilst people at all ages may be affected by inability to remain in control of bladder and bowel functions it is more prevalent in the older person and in particular the frail elderly due to the loss of muscular control, changes to the central nervous system, atrophic vaginitis, cerebrovascular disease, constipation, immobility and drug usage (see Box 7.5). Older people also tend to pass more during the night due to changes in homeostatic mechanisms controlling the production of urine. The prevalence of incontinence is higher in older people living in institutions than those living in their own homes (see Box 7.2).

The care of the older person is one of the key priorities for the NHS in England and in order to reduce inequalities the Government has published a National Service Framework for Older People (DoH 2001d). The framework sets out the standards for services for the older person and aims to ensure these are delivered to the same standard irrespective of geographical location. The framework identifies the need for integrated continence services (Box 7.6) to be in place by April 2003.

The influence of faecal and urinary incontinence on the individual's health, their quality of life and self-respect is enormous. The health and social care issues and impact on the individual are summarised in Box 7.7.

Box 7.6 Integrated continence services

Integrated continence services should:

- be in line with published guidance on good practice
- link identification, assessment and treatment across primary, acute and specialist care

and should include:

- primary and community staff giving general advice to older people and their carers about healthy living (in particular diet, and drinking appropriate fluids)
- staff in nursing and residential care homes to identify, assess, treat and review the needs of residents within agreed protocols
- hospital nurses to identify people with incontinence, and to ensure that treatment is provided and that continence needs are assessed and a plan agreed before discharge from hospital
- specialist continence services to provide expert advice and be available to people whose condition does not respond to initial treatment and care
- links to designated medical specialties such as urology and geriatrics
- links to regional and national units for specialist surgery to form part of the care pathway for continence services
- availability and provision of continence aids/equipment
- access to bathing and laundry services
- patients and carers in developing local services.

Source: Integrated Continence Services (NSF for Older People, DoH 2001d)

Box 7.7 Impact on the individual

As a health issue incontinence can:

- cause skin breakdown which may lead to pressure sores
- be indicative of other problems in children, such as emotional problems rather than physical discorders.

As a social issue, faecal and urinary incontinence can:

- lead to bullying of children at school, adults in the workplace and older people in residential care and nursing homes
- in children, cause emotional and behavioural problems
- restrict employment, educational and leisure opportunities
- result in people moving to residential and nursing homes – incontinence is only second to dementia as an initiating factor for such moves
- cause conflict between the individual and their carer
- cause soiling and ruin clothes and bedding leading to extra laundry costs and increased expense for those items.

Impact on the individual (taken from the Good Practice in Continence Services, DoH 2000).

Dependence/independence in the AL of eliminating

Dependence/independence in the ALs is closely related to a person's lifespan (Roper et al 1996, 2000). Viewed as a continuum it is central to the concept of the model (see Chapter 1).

Babies and young children rely on adults to keep them clean and dry. From the age of five most children are able to undertake this activity independently during the daytime. However, in some cases it may take longer at night. Children who are physically disabled or suffer from learning difficulties may be dependent on others to assist them in elimination.

Likewise most adults remain independent in this activity for the most part of their life unless illness, injury or disability occurs.

If physically or mentally disabled, individuals are likely to require help in the form of aids and adaptations to their accommodation to help them to be independent in the activity of elimination. In Mary's case you may have considered asking an occupational therapist, physiotherapist or social worker to visit her in her own home to assess how she might be helped to maintain her independence in the activity of elimination. Vickerman and Whitehead (2001) outline the benefits to patient care of adopting a multidisciplinary approach. Mary may benefit from adaptations to her home to enable her to maintain her independence, for example, a stair lift may help Mary to get upstairs to the toilet. She may also require grab rails to assist her getting on and off the toilet. In addition she may also be eligible for financial support to enable her to fund extra help or to access other resources.

Other patients may be unable to pass urine without the aid of a catheter or evacuate their bowels without the assistance of a nurse or carer. Within the Western culture elimination is a very private activity. Dependence on others to assist in this private and personal Activity of Living can be very humiliating. Nurses must ensure privacy and dignity and take account of the patient's self-esteem when assisting with elimination.

Diseases of the intestinal tract and urinary tract may require surgical intervention or a temporary or permanent diversion on to the abdomen to enable passage of waste products from the body. In these cases patients are dependent on stoma appliances and the assistance from others, e.g. stoma nurses to maintain elimination and teach them how to become independent in managing their stoma care, emptying their stoma bags and coping with the change in body image and functions.

Exercise

1. Find out what services exist in your area for patients who have had an ileostomy or colostomy.
2. What advice is given to patients on how to manage their stoma?
3. When is this advice given?

You may have found out about a specialist nursing service within your local area. These nurses work as part of a multidisciplinary team including medical staff, clinical psychologists, surgical appliance officers and community nurses to provide a comprehensive service. Advice and counselling is provided prior to surgery and the patient is encouraged to be involved in their care as soon as they are able following surgery. A stepwise approach managing their stoma is taken until the patient is able to become independent (Walsh 2002).

Factors influencing the AL of eliminating

This next section will help you to understand the factors influencing the activity of elimination. Each of these will now be explored.

Biological factors

Any living organism must eliminate waste products. In human beings this is achieved through the renal system and urinary tract as urine and the intestinal tract as faeces.

Renal system

Normally each individual has two kidneys that lie on the dorsal wall of the abdomen. Each kidney consists of a million nephrons and collecting tubules and receives a supply of blood from the renal artery and a capillary network of arterioles (see Fig. 7.1). A good blood supply to the kidneys is crucial in maintaining their functioning (Walsh 2002) (see Fig. 7.2). The kidneys also play an important part in maintaining homeostasis by regulating the water and electrolyte content and acid–base of the body (see Box 7.8).

The removal of the waste products of metabolism is achieved through a process of ultrafiltration and reabsorption in the nephrons and passed via the ureter into the bladder, before being excreted as urine. Urine consists of urea, creatinine, uric acid, sulphates and nitrates (Box 7.9).

Each day an average healthy adult will excrete in the region of 1–1.5 litres of urine. The exact amount will depend on a number of factors such as how much fluid has been taken in, diet, the amount of water lost in sweat and expired air.

Exercise

1. Monitor your fluid intake and your urine output for 24 hours.
2. Is there any difference in volume in your intake and your output?
3. How many times did you pass urine?

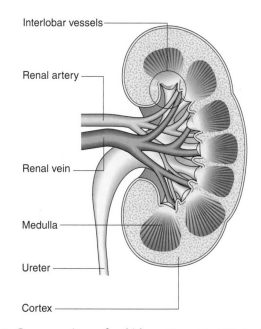

Interlobar vessels
Renal artery
Renal vein
Medulla
Ureter
Cortex

Fig. 7.1 Cross section of a kidney (from Hinchliff et al 1996, with permission).

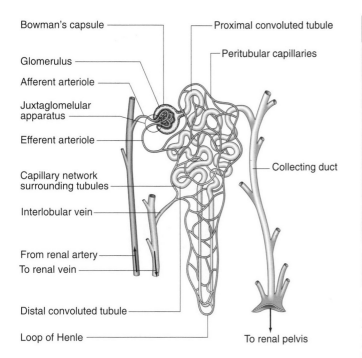

Bowman's capsule
Glomerulus
Afferent arteriole
Juxtaglomelular apparatus
Efferent arteriole
Capillary network surrounding tubules
Interlobular vein
From renal artery
To renal vein
Distal convoluted tubule
Loop of Henle

Proximal convoluted tubule
Peritubular capillaries
Collecting duct
To renal pelvis

Fig. 7.2 Anatomy of a nephron with associated blood supply (from Hinchliff et al 1996, with permission).

Box 7.8 Principle function of the kidney

To regulate the volume and composition of the extracellular fluid

The kidney maintains homeostasis by performing the following roles:

1. *Production:*
   - Vitamin D metabolite (calcitriol)
   - Erythropoietin
   - Renin

2. *Regulation:*
   - Volume of water in extracellular fluid
   - Concentration of electrolytes in extracellular fluid
   - Osmolality of extracellular fluid
   - Concentration of hydrogen ions in the extracellular fluid

3. *Excretion:*
   - Endogenous – end products of protein catabolism
   - Exogenous – medications

Source: Walsh M (ed.) 2002 Watson's Clinical Nursing and Related Sciences, p. 613. Baillière Tindall, Edinburgh.

You will have found that intake roughly matches output. However this can depend on your activities during the day and the type of fluid that you drank. For example, if you are exercising your may lose more water in sweat and expired air. Some substances such as alcohol and caffeine act as diuretics and increase the urine flow. Recording a patient's

Box 7.9 The composition of urine in an adult

pH	5.0–6.0
Osmolality	500–800 mosmol
Specific gravity	1.003–1.030
Urea	200–500 mmol/l
Creatinine	9–17 mmol/l
Sodium ions	50–130 mmol/l
Potassium ions	20–70 mmol/l
Organic acids	10–25 mmol/l
Protein	0–50 mg/24 h
Urochrome	Traces
Glucose	0–11 mmol/l
Cellular components (epithelial cells, leucocytes)	<2000/l

Source: Hinchliff et al 1996.

intake and output of urine is an important responsibility for the nurse and will aid diagnosis and treatment. For instance patients with heart failure may be unable to excrete fluid and because of this may develop dyspnoea and peripheral oedema. Recognising this early will enable timely medical intervention.

Urine

Observing and reporting the colour and odour of urine can inform diagnosis. For example cloudy urine may indicate infection whereas dark urine may indicate a patient is dehydrated or the presence of bilirubin. Undertaking urinalysis on the ward or in a clinic allows the nurse to measure the Ph and test for the presence of protein, glucose, ketones, blood and bilirubin. Urine that smells offensive can often suggest the presence of an infection. Accurate recording of the results in the nursing care plan or patient record is essential. Often the nurse will be expected to obtain a specimen for laboratory testing. In which case this is best obtained first thing in the morning before being diluted by fluid intake later in the day.

Exercise
1. If you are a student nurse undertaking a clinical placement test a patient's urine, observe and report your findings to your mentor and discuss the significance of your results. Find out where the results should be recorded in the patient's nursing care plan or medical notes.
2. Find out what the presence of glucose in the urine (glycosuria) would indicate.

The presence of glucose in the urine (glycosuria) may suggest that the patient has diabetes mellitus. A patient with diabetes may also pass large volumes of urine (polyuria), in severe cases the patient may become dehydrated. It may also indicate an acute response to stress.

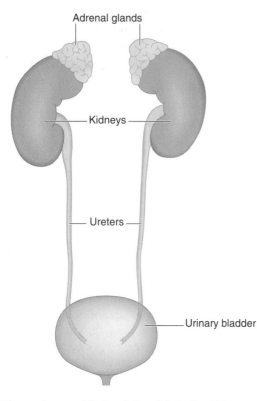

Fig. 7.3 The ureters and their relationship to the kidneys and bladder (from Waugh & Grant 2001, with permission).

Micturition

Urine is propelled down the ureters by peristaltic action into the bladder, which is a hollow highly muscular organ lined by epithelial cells (see Fig. 7.3). The bladder holds about 0.5 litres. The detrusor muscle is a layer of smooth muscle, which lies beneath the lining of the bladder (Fig. 7.4). As the bladder fills the lining stretches and the detrusor muscle

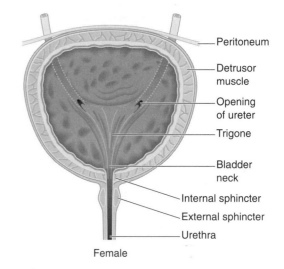

Fig. 7.4 Structure of the bladder (from Rutishauser 1994, with permission).

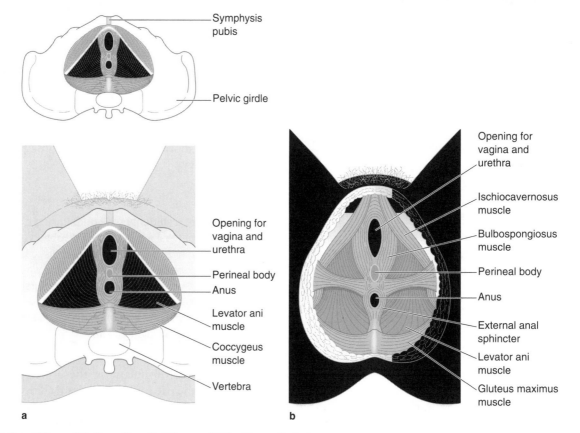

Fig. 7.5 Muscles of the pelvic floor (from Rutishauser 1994, with permission).

contracts, the internal sphincter also contracts. As the urethra widens the muscles of the pelvic floor relax (Fig. 7.5). This allows the urine to flow into the urethra. For micturition to take place normally the bladder must be healthy and its neural supply intact. Evacuation of urine from the bladder is controlled by both voluntary and involuntary systems. As the pressure in the bladder increases the bladder wall distends and stimulates the stretch receptors in the wall of the bladder. The external sphincter opens and urine passes into the urethra. As it is not always convenient to pass urine, the voluntary control mechanism via the pudendal nerve will prevent contraction of the external sphincter (see Fig. 7.6).

When it is convenient to pass urine contraction of the bladder is aided by contraction of the abdominal muscles. This effect of the contraction of the abdominal muscles can be seen when coughing or sneezing. This may result in a leakage, known as stress incontinence it is usually found in females. The bladder may develop spontaneous contractions, which results in the intravesical pressure exceeding the intraurethral pressure and leads to involuntary leakage of urine. This is known as detrusor instability or in cases where there is known neurological disease, detrusor hyperreflexia.

Urinary retention

In some cases a patient may be unable to empty their bladder or they might be passing frequent small amounts of urine or dribbling. On examination the abdomen might be distended and the bladder palpable, the patient might also be complaining of pain and be distressed. Retention of urine is usually due to an obstruction, e.g. prostatic disease or neurological disease and interruption of the nerve supply. Other reasons include patients who have undergone surgery, lack of privacy, pain and discomfort.

One of the commonest causes of urinary retention is seen in males over the age of 50 who suffer from benign prostatic disease (Walsh 2002). The prostate gland is enlarged and obstructs the normal flow of urine from the bladder (Fig. 7.7). Unable to empty their bladder completely they frequently experience dribbling and frequency. On examination of the abdomen the bladder may be distended. A comprehensive and sensitive nursing assessment is required when dealing with these patients.

Patients who have atonic bladders or dysynergia, where the bladder contraction does not synchronise with opening of the urethral sphincter, intermittent self-catheterisation may be an option. These patients may be constantly wet or suffer pain from retention of urine that requires urgent medical treatment. The bladder is allowed to fill and a clean catheter is passed into the bladder and the urine drained away. Patients are taught to pass the catheter several times a day thus putting the patient in control of emptying their bladder and improving their quality of life (Hunt et al 1996). However, not all patients are able to self-catheterise

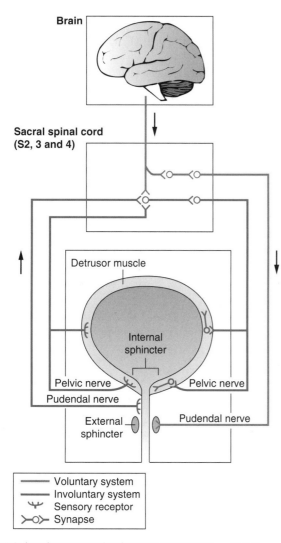

Fig. 7.6 Involuntary and voluntary systems (from Rutishauser 1994, with permission).

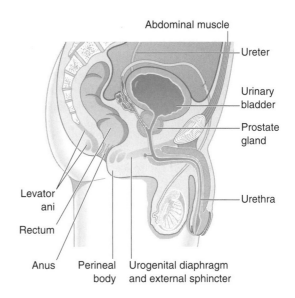

Fig. 7.7 The male urinary system (from Rutishauser 1994, with permission).

and a thorough assessment of their manual dexterity, motivation and mental capacity is required before introducing intermittent self-catheterisation. If a patient is not able to self-catheterise then with the patient's agreement a relative or carer may be trained to undertake the procedure.

Urinary catheterisation

In some situations, following a full assessment and informed consent of the patient the bladder may be emptied by insertion of a urethral catheter on a continuous or intermittent basis. However, catheterisation should not be performed routinely as it increases the risk of infection. Insertion of a catheter must be undertaken under strict aseptic technique and with care to lessen the risk of trauma. Depending on the reason for catheterisation, the catheter may be left in place or removed and inserted intermittently if necessary. If the catheter is left in place, the urine can be collected in a urine bag which is attached to the catheter and to the patient's leg or alternatively on a stand under the bed. It is important that urine bags are kept below the height of the bladder to encourage drainage and that catheters are observed for kinking so that the risk of retention is reduced. It is also important not to disconnect the catheter from the drainage bag unnecessarily so that the risk of infection is reduced. This is known as maintaining a closed system.

Long-term catheterisation in the management of incontinence should only be undertaken after all other options have been explored. The nurse must consider the patient's wishes, lifestyle and likelihood of compliance. In the event of a patient having an abnormality or injury to the urethra it may be necessary to insert a suprapubic catheter into the bladder via the abdomen.

Exercise

1. If you are a student nurse undertaking a clinical placement find out about the infection control guidelines for catheter care and how you would care for a patient with a catheter.
2. Discuss with your mentor and personal tutor the knowledge and skills you need to care for a patient with a catheter and undertake catheterisation safely and competently.

You may have discussed the following:

- principles of asepsis
- indications for catheterisation
- anatomy and physiology of both the female and male urethra and bladder
- counselling skills and gaining informed consent
- knowledge of the different types of catheters available, indications for use and product liability
- procedure for catheterisation
- recording observations.

Urinary tract infections

Infection of the urinary tract is common in women (Selfe 2000). The close proximity of the vagina to the urethra allows the passage of organisms normally found in the bowel and perineum, into the urinary tract more easily than in males (Fig. 7.8).

Normally the route of the infection is through the bladder but in some cases the infection may enter through the bloodstream. Pyelonephritis is an infection of the renal pelvis. Patients may present with a sudden onset of pain in the loin radiating to the iliac fossa. They may also have pyrexia, rigors, nausea and vomiting. A midstream specimen of urine should be collected and sent for bacteriological examination. Once the bacterial organism is identified then the doctor will prescribe the appropriate antibiotic. However, it is important that further diagnostic investigations are undertaken to understand the underlying cause of the infection.

Exercise

1. Find out which organisms are likely to cause a urinary tract infection.
2. What are the predisposing factors for urinary tract infection?
3. What other investigations would be undertaken to assist diagnosis?
4. What advice would you give to a patient to prevent recurrence of a urinary tract infection?

Organisms likely to be involved are *Escherichia coli, Klebsiella,* proteus, pseudomonas, *Streptococcus faecalis* and *Staphylococcus albus.* Some of the factors which predispose urinary infection are listed in Box 7.10.

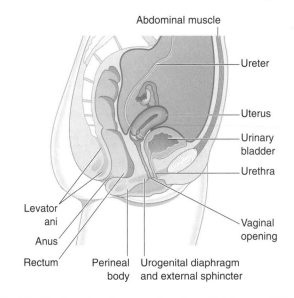

Fig. 7.8 The female urinary system (from Rutishauser 1994, with permission).

Box 7.10 Urinary infection: predisposing factors

Vesico-ureteric reflux
This may be congenital or acquired.

Obstruction such as stricture, tumours of the bladder, prostate or kidneys
The inability to empty the bladder (urinary retention) due to stricture or abnormality of neighbouring organs may result in a build up of pressure and backflow on the kidneys. This predisposes the individual to urinary tract infection, formation of stones and possible renal impairment.

Fistula
An abnormal opening between the bowel and the bladder will allow organisms to pass into the urinary tract.

Sexual trauma
The female ureter may suffer trauma during sexual intercourse and allow the passage of organisms.

Personal hygiene
Lack of attention to personal hygiene, contamination from the rectal area or inadequate hygiene facilities may also predispose to urinary tract infection.

Surgical and diagnostic procedures
Unless strict asepsis is maintained medical and nursing interventions such as catheterisation can introduce organisms or indeed exacerbate an existing infection.

Adapted from Selfe 2000.

Urinary investigations for urinary tract infections
Investigations may include:

- routine ward testing using a dipstick
- collection of a midstream specimen of urine (MSU), which is sent to the laboratory for culture and sensitivity. The MSU should be collected under clean conditions to reduce the risk of contaminants
- a full blood count, urea and electrolytes
- an ultrasound scan to identify any obstruction.

The nurse has an important role in health promotion and the prevention of recurrence of urinary tract infections by providing advice to patients on handwashing and personal hygiene in particular after defecation.

Pelvic floor muscles
The pelvic floor muscles support the bowel, the bladder and in women the uterus (see Fig. 7.5). The muscles are attached to the inner surface of the pelvic girdle. The urethra, anus and the vagina in women pass through openings in these muscles. Weak pelvic floor muscles due to repeated heavy lifting, surgery, obesity, constipation, chronic cough and lack of general fitness both in men and women can lead to incontinence. In women childbirth and the menopause are also major factors. Pelvic floor exercises can help

to increase the power of the pelvic floor muscles to aid urinary continence.

Exercise
1. If you are female, find your pelvic floor muscles by placing the tip of your finger in or against your vagina. Try to contract the muscle against your finger.
2. If you are male, find your pelvic floor muscles by placing your finger just behind your scrotum. When you try to contract your muscles you will feel them tighten away from your fingers. This should give you some idea of the strength of your pelvic floor muscles.
3. Now find out how to do pelvic floor exercises and how often they need to be done.

You will have discovered that pelvic floor exercises need to work against gravity and so they should be done either standing or sitting upright. Sitting on a chair you should concentrate on lifting your perineum off the chair by tightening the muscle inwards and lifting up at the same time. Make sure you are not moving your leg or thigh muscles and buttocks or pulling in your abdominal muscles. Pelvic floor exercises should be done regularly. The pelvic floor muscles consist of different muscle fibres, which need to be exercised differently. You should aim to do at least 10 slow contractions and 10 fast contractions four times a day over several weeks in order to gain any benefit.

The intestinal system
The digestive system consists of the mouth, oesophagus, stomach and intestines (Fig. 7.9). Food is consumed and during its passage through the digestive system undergoes a number of digestive processes to enable absorption of nutrients into the body's cells. Food residue is propelled along the digestive system by peristaltic action and segmentation brought about by the contraction of smooth muscle. The substances which are not of use to the body are eliminated as faeces at the final stage (see Rutishauser 1994 and Hinchliff et al 1996).

A large number of bacteria colonise the large intestine and their function is to break down food residue. These bacteria live in harmony with each other within the gut and are known as commensals (Box 7.11). However, if they are introduced to another part of the body they become pathogenic. So attention to personal hygiene after going to the toilet and/or before undertaking patient care is extremely important.

Box 7.11 Commensal bacteria

- *Bacteroides fragilis*
- *Clostridium perfringens (welchii)*
- *Enterobacter aerogenes*
- *Escherichia coli.*

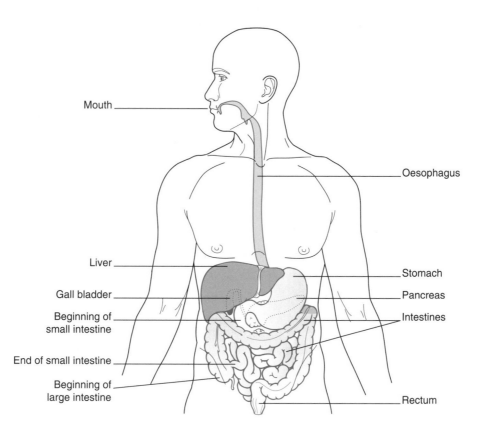

Fig. 7.9 The digestive system (from Rutishauser 1994, with permission).

Exercise
1. Find out what happens to patients on long-term antibiotic therapy.
2. What effect does this have on the bacteria in the gut?

Exercise
1. Visit the PHLS site on the internet (www.phls.co.uk) or speak to your local infection control nurse or public health department.
2. Find out the incidence of gastrointestinal infection in the UK and other countries.
3. What other bacteria cause these infections?
4. Which people are at most risk from these infections?
5. Find out what reporting systems are in place within your clinical area for patients who display symptoms of gastrointestinal infection.

You will have discovered that the commensal bacteria are destroyed in patients on long-term antibiotic therapy and that the first sign of this is usually diarrhoea.

Gastrointestinal infections

Gastrointestinal infection is an important cause of morbidity in England and Wales (PHLS Review of Communicable Diseases 1999/2000). *E. coli* is a Gram-negative bacillus. It is normally present in the gut and is probably the commonest cause of bacterial diarrhoeal disease. *E-coli* (VETC) produces potent cytotoxins and is commonly responsible for human infection in the UK. Food handlers who fail to maintain high standards of hygiene are likely to spread the bacteria. Outbreaks have been associated with uncooked cold meats contaminated by butchers handling raw meat. However the largest outbreak in 1999 was the result of improperly pasteurised milk. People most at risk are the elderly in hospitals and nursing homes, and young children in schools and day nurseries (PHLS Advisory Committee on Gastrointestinal Infections 2000).

You will have discovered that not all people who are infected with a pathogen display symptoms, therefore it is possible that the incidence of gastrointestinal infection is underreported. Despite a greater awareness of the need for hygiene and public health initiatives trends remained stable during the 1990s.

Other bacterial organisms include:

- Campylobacter, usually acquired from poultry, unpasteurised milk and contaminated water.
- Salmonella has been associated with eggs and poultry. Since improvements and control measures

in the poultry industry have been introduced the incidence of Salmonella has reduced. More recently however the infection has been associated with imported lettuce.

- Small round-structured virus (SRSV) is predominately spread from person to person, particularly in hospitals and nursing and residential homes.
- Cryptosporidiosis is a bacteria associated with contaminated water supplies. The source of an outbreak in the north-west of England during 1999 was found to originate from the Thirlmere reservoir and infected 347 north-west residents.

Infection control issues are paramount in today's health care. Each hospital in England is required to have in place a multidisciplinary Infection Control Team and policies and guidelines on the management of patients with gastro-intestinal infections including procedures for dealing with outbreaks within hospitals. Make yourself familiar with the contents of these documents, procedures and contact numbers of the members of the Infection Control Team. Reducing the risk of gastrointestinal infection and ensuring adequate hygiene requires access to adequate toilet facilities, toilet paper, hot running water, soap and hand-drying facilities.

Faeces

Faeces consist of 30–50 g of solids (cellulose, epithelial cells, bacteria, salts and a brown pigment stericobilin) and 70–100 g of water. The characteristic odour is due to bacterial decomposition. The amount of faeces passed each day by an individual will vary according to their diet, lifestyle and mental state.

Defecation

Normally the rectum, a muscular tube, is empty. Defecation is under the control of both the parasympathetic and sympathetic nervous system (see Hinchliff et al 1996, p. 496). As faeces pass from the colon into the rectum, the walls of the rectum distend. This action stimulates sensory receptors in the walls of the rectum and raises awareness of the need to defecate. This is known as 'call to stool'. The rectum has both internal and external anal sphincters. As the internal sphincter relaxes, the faeces pass into the rectum, the external anal sphincter contracts. This enables faeces to be contained until such time as it is convenient to defecate. Abdominal muscles contracting and increasing the intra-abdominal pressure assist evacuation of the rectum (see Fig 7.10 for structures involved in defecation).

Exercise

Find out why people who have had a stroke are likely to suffer from faecal incontinence.

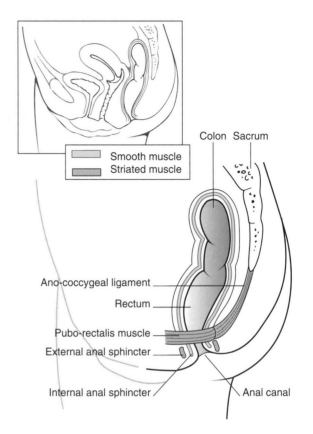

Fig. 7.10 Structures involved in the storage and evacuation of faeces (from Rutishauser 1994, with permission).

You will have found out that patients who have damage to their pudendal nerve or spinal cord because of a stroke, due to loss of voluntary sphincter control, may not be able to inhibit defecation until a time when it is convenient. This may result in faecal incontinence whilst in some cases patients may need to evacuate their rectum manually in order to eliminate faeces.

Kamm (1998) suggest that faecal incontinence affects 2% of all adults and 7% of all adults over the age of 65 years and is more prevalent in patients with multiple sclerosis, spinal injuries and congenital disorders. A summary of the causes of faecal incontinence can be found in Box 7.12.

Stool assessment

The colour and consistency of faeces and any alteration in a person's pattern of defecation may indicate a potential health problem. Hence, the importance of assessing the patient's normal bowel habits and reporting any abnormal findings to the doctor. Careful assessment and recording of the frequency and appearance of stools in the patient's nursing care plan or health record is an important part of nursing care. The Bristol Stool Chart devised by Dr KW Heaton is a tool used in some areas to aid accurate and descriptive recording (Heaton 1999).

Box 7.12 Causes of faecal incontinence in adults

Causes of faecal incontinence in adults	Common examples
Sphincter or pelvic floor damage	Obstetric trauma Direct trauma or injury
Diarrhoea	Inflammatory bowel disease Irritable bowel syndrome
Iatrogenic/post surgical	Post haemorrhoidectomy sphincterotomy for fissure or anal stretch
Anorectal pathology	Spinal cord injury Multiple sclerosis Spina bifida Parkinson's disease (usually secondary to constipation) Secondary to degenerative neurological disease, e.g. Alzheimer's disease, dementia (environmental see below)
Impaction with overflow 'spurious diarrhoea'	Institutionalised or immobile elderly
Environmental	Poor toilet facilities Inadequate care
Idiopathic	Unknown cause Possible psychological factors

From (Norton C 1996 Faecal incontinence in adults 1: prevalence and causes. British Journal of Nursing)

Exercise

The following are abnormal types of stools that you may come across. Find out what each indicates:

- black and tarry (malaena)
- maroon
- bright red (blood)
- putty coloured
- black stool
- diarrhoea.

You may have found out that the first three types of stools indicate some form of bleeding in the gastrointestinal tract. A malaena stool is an indication of bleeding from the upper gastrointestinal tract caused by oesophageal varices, bleeding duodenal ulcer or peptic ulcer. Malaena has a characteristic smell of altered blood due to the action of digestive enzymes. The maroon stool indicates bleeding from the lower gastrointestinal tract, possible causes include inflammatory bowel disease and malignancy. The presence of fresh blood is usually due to haemorrhoids but could also indicate malignancy or inflammatory bowel disease.

A bulky, pale foul-smelling coloured stool is indicative of an obstruction to the flow of bile into the duodenum.

Diarrhoea

Diarrhoea, a loose watery stool, may be the result of an infection, medication, e.g. antibiotics, laxative abuse, inflammatory conditions such as ulcerative colitis or irritable bowel syndrome, malabsorption syndrome, stress, tumours or thyrotoxicosis. Diarrhoea is a distressing and embarrassing condition for patients, who will require reassurance and support from nursing staff to help relieve the problems (see Hinchliff et al 1996, p. 497). Strict attention of the nurse and the patient to hand-washing and personal hygiene is essential to reduce the risk of crossinfection. Diarrhoea can also be present in patients who are constipated as a result of faecal overloading and irritation of the lining of the intestine.

Constipation

The food residue can remain in the colon for 2–3 days as water and salts are gradually reabsorbed. The longer the residue remains the more water is absorbed and the faeces will become compact and hard, possibly leading to constipation.

Everyone has an individual pattern of defecation. Constipation is when that pattern is less frequent than normal and stools are hard and difficult to pass. A frequency of less than three times a week has been used as an objective measure to define constipation (Effective Health Care Bulletin 2001). Symptoms associated with constipation include flatulence, bloating, abdominal pain and a feeling of incomplete evacuation. Factors which may increase the likelihood of constipation include diet, fluid intake, mobility, drug regimes and psychological factors such as impaired cognitive function and anxiety. Again an accurate nursing assessment should be made including questions about frequency and consistency of stools, access to a toilet or commode, mobility and dexterity. The nurse should be aware that the patient may feel embarrassed to talk about their bowel and therefore should ensure privacy when undertaking a nursing assessment.

Constipation is one of the most common reasons for people visiting their General Practitioner in the UK especially the very young and the older person (Effective Health Care Bulletin 2001). Treatment for constipation may include reviewing the patient's dietary habits and increasing the fibre content in the diet such as wholemeal bread, bran and fruit and intake of fluids. It may be necessary to review any medication especially analgesics such as opiates as a common side effect is constipation (British National Formulary 2002). However, laxatives remain the most common choice of treatment. Laxatives work by (a) increasing the bulk of the stool, (b) stimulating the intestinal motility, (c) softening the stool by increasing water absorption by osmosis. In England £46 million per year is spent on laxatives (Effective Health Care Bulletin 2001).

In some instances it may be necessary for a nurse to undertake a rectal examination to examine for faecal loading. Whilst every attempt should be made to avoid manual evacuation Powell & Rigby (2000) point out that it may be the only viable method of evacuating the bowel in some cases. This should only be undertaken by a nurse who is professionally competent to do so, following individual assessment and with the informed consent of the patient (NMC 2002a, RCN 2000, DoH 2001a, 2001c). The nurse should also take account of the cultural and religious beliefs of the patient.

> **Exercise**
> 1. Familiarise yourself with the local procedures for administration of an enema, insertion of a suppository and rectal examination.
> 2. Do you possess the knowledge and skills to undertake these procedures?
> 3. If not, find out how you can develop these skills. Discuss with your mentor and personal tutor the knowledge and skills you need to undertake these procedures safely and record this in your personal development plan.
>
> Useful resources to guide you in your exercise are The Royal Marsden Manual of Nursing Procedures (2000) and the RCN Digital rectal examination and manual removal of faeces (RCN 2000).

Psychological factors

Psychology is concerned with explaining the way people think, behave and experience the world. Roper et al (1996) state that 'psychological factors cannot be considered in isolation; they are related to biological and also sociocultural, environmental and politicoeconomic factors'. Psychological factors and perspectives influence individuality and the way a person undertakes each AL across the lifespan.

Kenworthy et al (2002) outline four main psychological theories or perspectives, which seek to explain human psychological development:

- the psychodynamic perspective
- the behaviourist perspective
- the cognitive perspective
- the humanist perspective.

Nurses will need to draw on these perspectives and psychological theories when assessing planning, implementing and evaluating care. (For further information on each of these see Kenworthy et al 2002, p. 203–210.)

Eliminating is a personal Activity of Living and patients may be too embarrassed to talk about their urinary and bowel functions. Incontinence has an impact on the quality of life and psychological wellbeing of individuals (Shaw 2001). The extent to which people with incontinence seek help depends on their knowledge of the problem and treatment options, how severe they believe the symptoms to be and the resources they have available to deal with the problem (Shaw 2001). As a result they may delay seeking help until they feel more able to do so or they feel unable to cope by which time the problem will have been present for a few days if not longer.

Health beliefs

Each of us may hold a different view or belief of what is health and what is illness. A patient's health beliefs will guide how they access health services and take responsibility for their own health. For example, an older person who believes that problems with eliminating are part of the natural process of ageing may not seek the help of professionals believing that nothing can be done or the problem is outside their control. Equally people may associate old age with incontinence and accept it as the norm.

> **Exercise**
> 1. Reflect on your own health beliefs.
> 2. How will these beliefs influence how you assess patients' Activities of Living?

Health locus of control

The extent to which individuals will take responsibility for their own health is dependent on what they regard as controllable by themselves or others (Ogden 1996). The extent to which a person will take responsibility for their own health will depend upon their locus of control (Wilkinson 2002). Consequently a person who has a problem with incontinence may decide to seek out the help of a health professional to assist in making a decision about how they can take responsibility for managing or taking ownership of the problem (internal locus of control) alternatively if they believe that their situation is outside their control, they may hand over the responsibility for making decisions for their health to the health professional (external locus of control). A literature review by Shaw (2001) found that evidence to suggest that different personality types might also influence the outcome of treatment for incontinence, with introverted patients responding better to bladder training than extroverts. Consider the following exercise.

> **Exercise**
> Mrs Smith is a 50-year-old lady who suffers stress incontinence when she sneezes or coughs. She has sought the advice of her GP who has referred her to the specialist physiotherapist for advice and treatment.
>
> How might she respond to:
>
> (a) adopting an internal locus of control?
> (b) adopting an external locus of control?

Firstly, by adopting an internal locus of control she would want to begin to understand her problem and question how she might work with the physiotherapist to manage the problem. She would seek out other sources of information and would possibly join self-help groups.

In the second scenario, she would adopt a more passive role and expect the physiotherapist and GP to provide information and take ownership of her problem. She may also fail to comply with the instructions and exercises provided by the physiotherapist. Understanding a patient's health belief will assist the nurse when planning care and providing health education.

The concept of classical conditioning developed by Pavlov in the late 19th century and operant conditioning by BF Skinner in the mid 1900s underpins the behaviourist perspective (Wilkinson 2002). Nurses may choose to use these theories by positively reinforcing activities that contribute to achieving continence, for example, giving rewards and praise for remaining dry or prompts to confused patients to visit the toilet at regular intervals. Research undertaken by McDowell et al (1999) showed that behaviour therapies could reduce incontinence in older people who were cognitively intact. Using a randomised crossover trial the intervention group received behaviour therapies, e.g. pelvic floor exercises, bladder retraining and urge and stress strategies. Nurses also visited them at regular intervals and spent much more time with them than those patients in the control group. The control group of patients received the information on the exercises without the behaviour therapy interventions. Patients who received behaviour therapies and increased input from nursing staff had fewer incidences of incontinence than those who were in the control group.

Stress

Problems associated with the activity of elimination can be a source of shame and stigma and a source of stress. People experience stress in many different ways (Ogden 1996). Requiring help with the activity of elimination can result in loss of a person's sense of dignity and a feeling of 'being like a child', which may lead to anxiety and/or depression. Caring for an incontinent person can be a major source of stress for carers who are required to help with toileting, faced with constant laundry and lack of personal time.

There is a relationship between stress and disease (Wilkinson 2002). As well as certain types of food stress is thought to exacerbate the condition irritable bowel disease which occurs in people aged between 15–40 years. It is reported to affect around one in five women and one in ten men and little is known about effective treatment (Bandolier Library 2000). Symptoms include pain, fullness, bloating and flatulence. Stress management and counselling and dietary advice are helpful. In some cases where the patient is anxious or depressed psychotherapy may be helpful; although in all cases investigations should be undertaken to exclude more sinister bowel disease.

Exercise

1. Think about a stressful situation you may have experienced.
2. What impact did the stressful situation have on your urinary and intestinal systems?

You may have thought about an exam situation, an interview for a new post or a presentation to a group of people. Prior to the event or situation you may have visited the toilet frequently or experienced loose stools.

Sociocultural factors

Elimination is undertaken in private and in some cultures separate facilities are provided for males and females. The facilities provided can however differ depending on the country. Facilities also differ according to economic, religious and cultural needs, for example, in many places in Europe and in Asia the toilet facility is a hole in the ground.

Exercise

Think about a country that you may have visited.

1. What toilet facilities were there?
2. Did they differ from what you were normally used to and if so how?
3. How did you feel about this?

You may have visited a country where men and women share the same toilet facilities and felt embarrassed. In some countries you may have experienced urinating or defecating into a hole in the ground. If you are used to sitting on a toilet you may have found the experience uncomfortable or difficult. Likewise a person who is used to this way of life will find sitting on a toilet uncomfortable.

Attitudes to continence are influenced by several factors, including the ability to access appropriate medical help, expectations and education. Country of origin is also thought to influence the attitude of women to their incontinence. A study of migrant women in Australia revealed that Vietnamese and Chinese women were reluctant to discuss their incontinence problems with their families (Burton 1996). It is important to remember that in any community discussing continence is a very sensitive topic and consideration must be given to those people whose first language is not English. Many Muslim women will not discuss their continence problems in the presence of their husbands or a male interpreter (Haggar 1997). They will also refuse to be examined by a male doctor.

People who suffer from incontinence problems or who require assistance from another to enable them to pass urine or faeces can experience social isolation, embarrassment and may isolate themselves from their family and friends. It can also impact on their quality of life including sleep disturbance, mobility problems and discomfort.

Environmental factors

What is acceptable in one culture and/or religion may not be acceptable in another. Some cultures place emphasis on respecting a person's modesty and segregation. Within England in recent years many wards were designated mixed-sex wards in an attempt to maximise the use of beds. However for many patients, irrespective of their religious beliefs, being nursed in mixed sex accommodation caused anxiety and distress. More recently attempts have been made to eradicate mixed-sex accommodation and improve single-sex accommodation, including separate washing facilities and lavatories in hospitals.

Patients whose cultures require strict modesty will find the collection of bodily fluids and substances (e.g. faeces and urine) and investigations involving the rectum or urethra very distressing (Henley & Schott 1999). Facilities that do not afford patients privacy or dignity (e.g. using a bedpan in hospital or in the presence of another person) may lead to constipation and stress. Access to washing facilities is required for South Asians and Muslims who using their left hand wash their perineal area with running water after going to the lavatory. The right hand is reserved for handling food and clean things. These patients need access to a bidet, basin or a jug to be able to pour running water over them.

> ### Exercise
> 1. Undertake an assessment of the toilet facilities in your practice setting.
> 2. Does the environment afford your patients privacy and dignity?
> 3. What facilities are there for patients who are Muslim or have other religious beliefs about elimination activity?

Individuals need access to suitable toilet facilities. In the event of disability toilet facilities will need to be adapted. For example, a person suffering a stroke will need assistance to go to the toilet until such time as he or she is able to function independently. Adaptations may include raised toilet seats, grab rails and easy access to a suitably placed call bell. Toilets will need to be of sufficient width to allow the carer and person enough space to manoeuvre, including if needing wheelchair access. They should be warm and private. Adequate washing facilities are also required either within the person's own home or within an institution in order to reduce any risk of infection.

Patients who have continence problems should be positioned within easy access of a toilet and assessed regarding their dexterity and ability to mobilise with or without assistance. Assessment and input from physiotherapy and occupational therapy may be helpful here. Adaptations to the environment may be needed to enable the patient to function independently within their own home.

Politicoeconomic factors

Incontinence affects large numbers of people in the UK yet it remains a hidden problem by comparison with other conditions. Despite incontinence being underreported because of embarrassment, stigma and lack of understanding and awareness of treatment available the Continence Foundation (2000) estimated 5 million people over the age of 30 have experienced urinary incontinence and 0.6 million have experienced faecal incontinence. The risk of hospitalisation is greater in people who are aged 65 and over and who suffer from incontinence (RCP 1995). In 1991 the NHS was reported to spend £56 million per year on continence products and £20 million on continence devices (RCP 1995). A survey undertaken by Clayton et al (1998) found that the costs incurred by incontinent women ranged from £0.27 to £237 in a 3-month period.

The cost of providing incontinence aids on low-income families can be very high. It is essential that they be advised on the correct supplies and how to access advice and support. A review of continence services within the UK during 1997 undertaken by Incontact highlighted a number of problems with continence services (DoH 2000). These included a variation in type and access to NHS services and the number of staff trained to provide specialist care, lack of involvement of users in determining how services should be provided and variation in the range of treatments provided and time spent waiting. In some areas because of lack of access to the continence advisor incontinence pads were offered without assessment and attempting curative treatment.

> ### Exercise
> 1. Visit your local pharmacy and make a note of the products on sale for people who are incontinent.
> 2. Consider what might be the cost to a person suffering from an incontinence problem.
> 3. What information is available?
> 4. Find out what services are available for people with incontinence problems within your local area.
> 5. Whilst on a clinical placement find out if there are any standards or benchmarking activities being undertaken for continence.

The Department of Health Good Practice in Continence Services (2000) sets out a model of practice for health services involving various professionals working at different levels. In addition a number of professional organisations and charities have produced a continence charter designed to meet the needs and rights of people with continence problems (see Swaffield 2000, p. 766). You may have found out that there is a specialist team involving specialist continence nurses and specialist continence physiotherapists working to common policies, procedures and guidelines. They also have a role in supporting and working alongside other practitioners providing expert advice and raising awareness. There may also be a continence service supplying continence aids and providing education and training to both patients and professionals.

You may also have discovered that some clinical areas are undertaking benchmarking activities (DoH 2001b) to ensure that patients'/clients' bladder and bowel needs are met. More information on this initiative can be found at www.doh.gov.uk/essenceofcare.

Within the first part of this chapter the factors influencing the Activities of Living within the model of living and lifespan have been used to illustrate the activity of eliminating in health and everyday life. By engaging in the exercises and reflective activities it is hoped that the reader has begun to appreciate the complexity of the model and its interrelatedness of the AL of eliminating to the other 11 ALs.

Summary points

1. The ability to eliminate relies on mature physiological systems.
2. Illness or disability can have an impact on elimination.
3. The activity of eliminating is influenced by societal and cultural norms.
4. The prevalence of urinary and faecal incontinence is high.

THE MODEL FOR NURSING

Introduction

Within this part of the chapter, you will be encouraged to transfer your understanding of eliminating and consider its relationship to other AL. Using the model for nursing and a main case scenario you will consider what information you will need to develop an assessment framework, identify patient problems and develop a plan of care. If you wish you may choose to record the information on the Patient Assessment Sheets provided in Appendix 2.

Assessing individual needs and problems

If patients' expectations are to be understood and their problems (whether actual or potential) with this AL are to be addressed then an assessment must be undertaken. Assessment involves the following three phases:

- collecting information from the patient and nursing history
- interpreting the information collected

- identifying the patient's actual and potential health problems.

However to undertake a comprehensive and holistic nursing history it is essential to take account of all the Activities of Living as seen in Chapter 1. This is not only undertaken at the beginning of the patient's episode of care or admission to hospital but is an ongoing and dynamic process. However, before assessing the AL of elimination in ill health the nurse must first of all understand and have knowledge of the AL of elimination in health.

Roper et al (1996) provide us with an aide memoir of areas which may be considered in relation to each of the components of the model of living, these will serve as a reminder of the many dimensions and components of the model which underpin a nursing assessment.

Assessing the individual

Assessment is the cornerstone on which the patient's care is planned, implemented and evaluated. In most cases the nurse undertakes an initial nursing assessment within the first few hours of admission to hospital by gathering information that informs the nursing assessment without overburdening the patient and duplicating assessments. However, it must be remembered that nursing assessment is continuous and patients must be reassessed as their condition changes or in response to the outcome of evaluation.

Using the model of living as a framework to collect information on the patient's normal habits and routines and any factors that might cause the activity to be altered is the first step in applying the Roper et al (1996) model for nursing in practice. Box 7.13 provides a summary of the key factors, which may be considered when assessing the activity of eating and drinking.

In most cases the nurse undertakes an initial nursing assessment within the first few hours of admission to hospital. Assessment is the cornerstone on which the patient's care is planned, implemented and evaluated. As already stated in Chapter 2 nurses work in partnership with other professionals to deliver an integrated and collaborative approach to care delivery. The introduction of nurse-led preassessment clinics within the UK and NHS Direct provide a unique opportunity for early holistic assessment of a patient being admitted to hospital for elective surgery. Working in collaboration with other health care professionals, nurses are able to gather information that informs the nursing assessment without overburdening the patient and duplicating assessments.

When assessing the patient the nurse will need to use interviewing, observational and listening skills. In addition she will also need to understand the anatomy and physiology associated with eliminating. Poor or incomplete assessment subsequently leads to poor care planning and implementation of the care plan (Sutcliffe 1990).

Box 7.13 Assessment framework for the activity of elimination

Lifespan
- consider the effect of age on the activity of eliminating.

Dependence/independence
- dependence is linked to lifespan and age, e.g. childhood/old age
- dependence is linked to specific needs, e.g. disability
- ill health affects the dependence–independence balance, e.g. trauma, paralysis.

Factors affecting eliminating
Biological
- muscle tone
- neurological impairment
- muscular damage, e.g. child birth.

Psychological
- attitudes to elimination
- emotional state
- cognitive state.

Sociocultural
- sociocultural similarities/differences
- religion.

Environmental
- access to toilets
- privacy
- home circumstances.

Politicoeconomic
- diet
- access to aids
- finance
- access to health services.

Exercise

Consider the following activities and identify which skills you have already and the ones you need to develop when undertaking an assessment of eliminating. In your personal development plan identify how you plan to further develop these skills.

1. **Interviewing**
   - asking open and closed questions relevant to the health status of the patient
   - use of appropriate language
   - determining the priority of the questions to be asked
   - giving information relating and checking understanding
   - involving relatives and carers.

Exercise *(continued)*

2. **Observation**
   - verbal and nonverbal responses
   - body language
   - appearance
   - vital signs and urinalysis
   - skin condition
   - pain
   - anxiety and stress.
3. **Listening**
   - verbal and nonverbal cues
   - checking out understanding and giving explanation.

Patient assessment

A relevant and realistic individualised nursing care plan is founded on a thorough patient assessment. The nursing care plan should aim to:

- solve actual problems
- prevent potential problems becoming actual problems
- prevent solved problems from recurring
- alleviate problems which cannot be solved
- help the person cope with temporary or permanent altered states.

Within this chapter, in addition to the main case scenario, you will be encouraged to transfer your understanding of eliminating to other individual patients and consider its relationship to other ALs. Using the assessment guide consider what information you would obtain from Case study 7.1 (p. 218). You can record the information on the Patient Assessment Sheets provided in Appendix 2.

Using the Activities of Living as a framework for assessment you may consider the questions in Box 7.14.

Box 7.14 Using the assessment framework in practice

Lifespan
- How old is the person?
- Do they have a life history of health problems?
- Is there anything in their life history that may affect the way in which they view their present health problems?

Independence/dependence
- Has the individual experienced any difficulties in relation to independent living?
- Are they able to go out and meet other people or are they dependent on others to transport them?
- Will they experience difficulties in the future as a result of their current health problems?

Box 7.14 (continued)

Factors affecting health

Biological
- From what specific health problem are they suffering?
- What do they understand about their present health status?
- Are there any disabilities?

Psychological
- What effect is their health problem having on their emotional wellbeing?
- Is the patient suffering from stress?

Socioeconomic
- How might cultural needs be taken into account?
- Are there any specific spiritual or religious needs that the patient may have?
- How does the health problem impact on working and playing?

Environmental
- Does the individual have any environmental needs that will affect future care?
- Are there any environmental hazards or risks of infection?
- Is there a need for adaptations or resources?

Politicoeconomic
- What resources could be required to help the individual manage their health problems both in hospital and at home?
- Is the patient aware of the resources that are available?
- Are there any financial constraints compromising recovery or maintenance?
- What effect is this having on their other Activities of Living?

Case study 7.1

Cyril

Cyril, a 63-year-old man with a history of recurrent urinary tract infections and an enlarged prostate is admitted to your ward for a transurethral resection of the prostate (TURP).

Exercise
1. Consider the questions in Box 7.14 and reflect on how you might use this framework as a basis for your assessment of this patient in your care.
2. Make a list of the questions you might ask and check your answers against those listed below.

You may have decided to ask the following questions to identify what the patient's needs are in relation to the ALs, taking account of the lifespan, dependency and factors which contribute to health.

Lifespan
- Benign prostatic hyperplasia is a condition associated with ageing in males.
- Urinary tract infections in men from the age of 60 are associated with tumours of the prostate, bladder and kidney (Selfe 2000, p. 329).
- There is an increase in prostatic cancer in the older male in the West.

Dependency
- Does he require help to get to the toilet?
- How does he manage at home?

Physical
- How long has the problem existed?
- When did the problem start?
- Does he have any pain?
- Does he have any problems starting to micturate?
- Does he have any difficulty stopping micturition?
- Does he have any frequency or urgency?
- Does he have dribbling or incontinence?
- Does he have any nocturia?
- Does he have any haematuria?
- What do his urinalysis and vital signs tell you?
- What medication is he taking?

Psychological
- What does he think the problem is?
- Is the problem worrying him?
- Has he had any information?
- How does he feel about being in hospital?
- Is he anxious?
- Is he embarrassed?
- How is he coping with the situation?

Sociological
- How has his problem impacted on his everyday activities?
- Does it affect his ability to interact with other people?
- Has the problem impacted on his family and social life?
- How has he managed at home?
- Does he have any cultural or religious needs?

Environmental
- What toilet facilities are there at home?
- What are the risks of further infections?

Politicoeconomic
- Does the health problem impact on the patient's ability to work?
- Does the patient require access to resources in the community to enable independent living?

Roper et al (2000) point out that each Activity of Living is interrelated and it is the interaction of each of these that contributes to the individualisation of nursing. Hence it is necessary to assess the patient's other Activities of Living to obtain a holistic view.

You may have considered and observed the following.

1. *Breathing*
   - Does he have any problems breathing?
   - Does he smoke and if so how many and how often?

2. *Eating and drinking*
   - How much fluid is he drinking?
   - What does his intake and output chart tell us?
   - Is his appetite affected?
   - What is his weight?
   - Has he suffered any weight loss?
   - Does he have any problems with oral hygiene, e.g. dentures, crowns, gum disease?

3. *Eliminating*
   - Does he need to use a urinal?
   - What does his urinalysis tell you?
   - What are his urinary symptoms?
   - Is he able to recognise when he needs to void urine?
   - How often does he have his bowels opened?
   - Does he have any diarrhoea?
   - Does he have any pain?

4. *Mobilising*
   - Has he any disability that restricts his mobility?
   - If so how does this impact on his ability to mobilise to the toilet?

5. *Expressing sexuality*
   - What has been the nature of the problem on his relationship with his partner?

6. *Personal cleansing and dressing*
   - Is he able to shower or bathe?
   - How frequently does he bathe or shower?
   - Does he require any assistance to dress/undress?

7. *Working and playing*
   - Does the health problem impact on his work, home and social life?

8. *Maintaining a safe environment*
   - Does he have any pain?
   - Does he have any visual or auditory impairment?
   - Are there any risks, e.g. infection, pressure sore development, falls, and moving and handling?
   - Does he understand his medication regime?

9. *Sleeping*
   - Does he get up to go to the toilet or have any episodes of incontinence at night?
   - Does this disturb his sleep?
   - Does this affect his performance at work or leisure?

10. *Controlling body temperature*
    - Does he have a temperature because of the infection?

11. *Dying*
    - What does he understand the prognosis to be?
    - Does he have any religious and cultural beliefs?

Using the information presented so far in this chapter, think about the following short case studies and plan your assessment of the activity of eliminating. You may use the template in Appendix 2.

Case study 7.2

A patient with inflammatory bowel disease

Mary is a 30-year-old secretary who has inflammatory bowel disease.

Irritable bowel disease or inflammatory bowel disease (IBD) is a term used to describe ulcerative colitis or Crohn's disease that usually affects younger adults in the Western world (Walsh 2002).

1. *Biological*
   - How long has she suffered from IBD?
   - What are her symptoms?
   - Does she suffer from any pain?
   - What treatment does she take?
   - Does she suffer from incontinence?
   - If so how does she manage her incontinence?
   - What is her weight?
   - How is she sleeping?

2. *Psychological*
   - Is she suffering from stress or anxiety?
   - What is her mood?
   - Is she depressed?
   - How is she coping with the situation?
   - What does she understand about her illness?
   - Does the problem impact on her sexual relationships?

3. *Sociological*
   - How does the problem impact on her social life?
   - What support does she have?
   - How does she cope with everyday living?
   - How does her problem impact on her family and relationships?

4. *Environmental*
   - What facilities are at home?
   - How does she cope with the problem in the community and at work?

5. *Politicoeconomic*
   - How does the problem impact on her working life?
   - Are there any economic factors that may be causing stress and anxiety?

Case study 7.3

A patient with urinary incontinence

Ellen is an 82-year-old lady with congestive cardiac failure who has recently become incontinent of urine. She is slightly deaf and has poor eyesight.

Within the UK heart failure is reported to be responsible for 5% of all hospital admissions (Clarke et al 1994, p. 323). One of the symptoms of heart failure is generalised oedema. One objective is to reduce fluid excess by prescribing diuretics (see Walsh 2002)

1. *Biological*
   - How long has she suffered from urinary incontinence?
   - What are her symptoms?
   - How does she manage her incontinence?
   - Does she suffer from any pain?
   - What treatment does she take?
   - When does she take her treatment?
   - Is she constipated?

2. *Psychological*
   - Is she suffering from stress or anxiety?
   - What is her mood?
   - Is she depressed?
   - How is she coping with the situation?

3. *Sociological*
   - Does she live alone?
   - What support does she have at home?
   - How does she cope with everyday living?
   - Does she manage to do her shopping?
   - Does she go out?
   - How does her problem impact on her family?

4. *Environmental*
   - What facilities are at home?
   - What type of accommodation?
   - Does she have an upstairs toilet?
   - Can she climb the stairs?
   - Does she have a commode downstairs?
   - Does she have any adaptations to her house?

5. *Politicoeconomic*
   - Does she have access to resources to help her cope with her incontinence?
   - Are there any economic factors that may be causing stress and anxiety?

Planning nursing activities and care

Planning nursing activities and care involves the following:

- identifying the problems or needs
- identifying priorities
- establishing short- and long-term goals
- determining the nursing actions and interventions required
- documenting the care plan.

Having undertaken a thorough assessment the nurse is now able to identify any problems or patient needs and determine the nursing interventions required in order to meet those needs. It is important to stress that such problems and needs must be patient-focused, relate to the nursing assessment and what is needed to aid recovery in the immediate, short and long term. They may be actual or potential problems or needs and should be prioritised to take account of life-threatening situations.

Whilst undertaking the initial nursing assessment the nurse may obtain a considerable amount of information, it must be remembered that assessment is an ongoing and interactive process. Roper et al (2000) seek to clarify the use of the word assessment in relation to their model for nursing as follows:

- collecting information from or about the person
- reviewing the collected information
- identifying a person's problems with Activities of Living
- identifying priorities amongst the problems.

Once the patient's problems or needs have been identified the nurse can review these and plan the nursing interventions required to:

- solve actual problems
- prevent potential problems occurring
- prevent solved problems from reoccurring
- develop positive coping strategies for any problem that cannot be solved.

Exercise

1. Consider what skills and knowledge you will need to plan care for a patient?

Check your knowledge and skills against your list and those listed in Box 7.15. Identify any learning needs and/or skills development; discuss these with your mentor and personal tutor.

Box 7.15 Knowledge and skills for care planning

- analytical skills
- problem-solving skills
- knowledge of the illness
- knowledge of anatomy and physiology
- decision-making skills
- negotiating skills
- priority setting.

Identifying problems and needs
Return to Case study 7.1.

> **Case study 7.1** *(continued from p. 218)*
>
> Having undertaken a nursing assessment and taking account of the lifespan, dependency and factors that contribute to health we have now learned that:
>
> Cyril is married to Janet and has three grown-up children. He works for an insurance firm and is looking forward to his retirement in 2 years time. He is a keen gardener and supports his local football team. He lives in a two-storey house, with an upstairs bathroom and toilet. Eighteen months ago he noticed that he was having difficulty in starting to pass urine and stopping. He had also noticed that he was going to the toilet more frequently and he had noticed slight dribbling of urine. This became a problem when he was at work and attending football matches. He believed that the problem was a result of his age and had tried to cope with it. Initially, he was embarrassed and had been reluctant to discuss his problem with anyone. More recently, he had noticed blood in his urine and had been treated by his GP for urine infections with antibiotics. When taking the antibiotics he had also suffered from diarrhoea. On further investigation he had been diagnosed with benign prostatic hyperplasia. He has read some information on the disease and is worried that he may have cancer.

Using the 12 Activities of Living as a framework for assessment the nurse might discover that:

1. *Breathing*
   - Cyril smokes 10 cigarettes a day.

2. *Communicating*
   - Cyril is slightly deaf and wears a hearing aid.
   - He wears spectacles for reading.

3. *Eating and drinking*
   - Cyril has restricted his fluid intake recently for fear of not making it to the toilet on time and becoming incontinent.
   - He normally has a good appetite and eats three meals a day. He has no food allergies or special dietary needs
   - He weighs 90 kg but feels he might have lost a little weight recently.

4. *Eliminating*
   - He has frequency of micturition.
   - He has some incontinence of urine and dribbling.
   - Ward urinalysis shows the presence of blood and protein.
   - He usually has his bowels opened once a day but has experienced diarrhoea when on antibiotics.

5. *Mobilising*
   - He is fully mobile and can manage to climb the stairs to the upstairs bathroom without difficulty.
   - He drives a car.

6. *Expressing sexuality*
   - He is concerned about how his problem would impact on his sexual relations with his wife.
   - He is also concerned about being incontinent during the night whilst sharing a bed with his wife and has moved into a single bed in the spare room.

7. *Personal cleansing and dressing*
   - He is able to shower and bathe independently and usually does so each day.
   - He dresses smartly and is careful about his appearance.

8. *Working and playing*
   - His health problem has impacted on his work, home and social life. He used to like going to the pub to have a drink with his friends.
   - Over the past few months he has purchased some incontinence pads from the local chemist to wear under his underpants.

9. *Maintaining a safe environment*
   - He is pain-free at the moment.
   - He is short-sighted and wears glasses.
   - He is not at risk from pressure ulcer development, his Waterlow score is 10.
   - He has been orientated into the ward environment.
   - A risk assessment reveals he is not at risk from falls but will require a moving and handling risk assessment if he becomes dependent.
   - He understands his medication regime but is concerned that any further antibiotic treatment will result in him suffering from diarrhoea.

10. *Sleeping*
    - He gets up to the toilet two or three times a night. Lately he has experienced some dribbling incontinence at night. He has been tired during the day and in the evening he has been sleeping in his chair in front of the television and is reluctant to go out.

11. *Controlling body temperature*
    - His temperature is normal on admission.

12. *Dying*
    - He has read some information on prostate problems and benign prostatic hyperplasia. He has also read in the newspaper about cancer of the prostate and is worried that he might have cancer.
    - Whilst he does not go to church regularly he regards himself as a Christian and believes in God.

Identifying actual and potential problems

Having undertaken a nursing assessment and reviewed the information it is now possible to consider what actual and potential problems have been identified and how these might be prioritised.

Whilst undertaking the nursing assessment the nurse should be able to detect potential problems which the patient may not be aware of. This is where the nurse's knowledge of the factors relating to ill health, socioeconomic, biological, psychological and environmental is important.

It must be remembered that assessment is an ongoing and interactive process. Having undertaken a thorough assessment you should be able to identify any problems or patient needs and determine the nursing interventions required in order to meet those needs. It is important to stress that such problems and needs must be patient-focused, relate to the nursing assessment and what is needed to aid recovery in the immediate, short and long term. They may be actual or potential problems or needs and should be prioritised to take account of life-threatening situations.

Prioritising problems

Prioritising problems is an important component of care planning. By using the independence/dependence continuum of the model of living we are able to identify and prioritise those problems that patients require nursing care and assistance to regain or maintain their independence, or where the patient is totally dependent on the nurse (Roper et al 1996). You may choose to do this by listing the problems in priority order in the nursing care plan, by dependency or by level of risk. As there may be local systems of prioritising problems it is advisable to check these out with your mentor.

Having now undertaken a thorough nursing assessment you will have already begun to identify a number of potential and actual problems. Taking account of lifespan, and factors which influence the Activities of Living, i.e. psychological, sociocultural, environmental and politicoeconomic, make a list of what you think these might be in relation to the activity of elimination and check your list against those below. This list might not be exhaustive but will give some indication of those you might consider.

Before planning the nursing care, Roper et al (1996, 2000) suggest that the nurse in collaboration with the patient or patient's family determines and agrees the priority of each of the problems. Of course problems that are life-threatening take precedence over those of less importance. The nurse may choose to number these according to the level of priority or simply by listing the problems in order of priority in the nursing care plan. There are a number of ways in which you might do this, for example numbering in order of priority or simply by listing the problems in the nursing care plan in order of importance. However, it is important to take account of the patient's view, as their priority may not be the same as yours (Roper et al 1996).

> **Exercise**
> Review Cyril's nursing assessment, begin to identify any actual and/or potential problems and place them in order of priority.

When determining the priority you must consider the patient's priorities. As a nurse you may have decided that the risk of chest infection, DVT and haemorrhage are potentially life-threatening and therefore given priority. However Cyril's priorities might be very different. He is worried that he has cancer and requires reassurance and information. He may also be concerned and embarrassed about the possibility of being incontinent whilst in hospital and how to gain access to the toilet in time. Box 7.16 provides some possible actual and potential problems which emerged during the assessment of Cyril.

Box 7.16　Actual and potential problems

Activity of Living	Actual problem	Potential problem
Breathing	Cyril smokes and is at risk of developing a chest infection following anaesthetic	Chest infection
Communicating	Cyril has difficulty hearing and needs to have his hearing aid in situ	Misunderstanding of information, advice and instructions aimed at increasing his recovery from surgery
Eating and drinking	Cyril is reluctant to drink fluids due to his dribbling incontinence Difficulty eating in bed due to IVI	Electrolyte imbalance Constipation Nausea due to anaesthetic drugs

Box 7.16 *(continued)*

Activity of Living	Actual problem	Potential problem
Elimination	Cyril is embarrassed about his dribbling incontinence He will have a catheter in situ after surgery Pain from excision site in bladder or catheter	Increased stress levels Blocked catheter due to blood clots Urine bypassing catheter Urinary tract infection Constipation due to period of immobility following surgery
Mobilising	Reluctant to mobilise due to pain	At moderate risk of developing a DVT and PE Constipation
Expressing sexuality	Cyril is worried about the outcome of his surgery on his sexual relations with his wife	
Personal cleansing and dressing	Cyril will be unable to attend to his personal hygiene in the immediate postoperative period	
Working and playing		Anxiety about the impact of his ill health on his ability to earn a living and his future pension
Maintaining a safe environment	Cyril will need to be prepared for theatre and anaesthetic Risk of bleeding from the transurethral site	Haemorrhage Risk of pressure ulcer development due to immobility and surgery
Sleeping	Cyril has difficulty sleeping and gets up two or three times a night	Lack of sleep due to postoperative vital signs, monitoring and pain
Controlling body temperature		Potential drop in body temperature during surgery
Dying	Cyril is worried about his prognosis	Increased stress which might delay recovery

Goal setting

Returning to the main case study and taking into consideration the nursing assessment and actual and potential problems identified, it is necessary to agree long- and short-term goals or outcomes for Cyril's nursing care.

Goals should be realistic, achievable and measurable. It is advisable to include dates and times to indicate when the goal is to be achieved. This enables the nurse to evaluate progress and achievement and demonstrate how nursing has benefited the patient (Roper et al 1996). In some cases it may be necessary to agree long-term goals, i.e. those goals that might take longer to achieve than those that can be achieved within a shorter timescale. Roper et al (1996, 2000) liken goals to signposts on a journey indicating when you have arrived at your destination.

Exercise
1. Revisit Cyril's actual and potential problems.
2. What goals might you identify in relation to the activity of elimination?

Box 7.17 provides examples of how goals might be set.

Statement of intentions/aims

In some clinical areas you might find that nursing staff prefer to identify statements of intentions or aims rather than goals in which case these would be written in a slightly different way. For example, consider problem number 2 in Box 7.17, an aim might be identified as shown in Box 7.18.

Box 7.17 Examples of how goals might be set

Actual problem	Potential problem	Goals
1. Cyril is embarrassed about his dribbling incontinence	Increased stress levels	Cyril states he feels less embarrassed about his dribbling incontinence
2. Cyril is at risk from developing a urinary tract infection due to catheter in situ after surgery	Urinary tract infection	Cyril does not develop a urinary tract infection during his hospital stay
3. Risk of bleeding from the excision site	Blocked catheter due to blood clots Urine bypassing catheter	Cyril's catheter remains patent whilst in situ Urine drains via the catheter and not via the urethra
4. Cyril will be immobile due to surgery	Constipation due to period of immobility following surgery	Cyril states he has his bowels opened and has no pain or discomfort within 2 days following surgery
5. Cyril has undergone surgical excision of his prostate gland	Pain from excision site in bladder or catheter	Cyril states that his pain is controlled postoperatively
6. Cyril is reluctant to drink fluids due to his dribbling incontinence	Dehydration	Cyril is able to explain why he is required to drink 2 litres of fluid a day. Cyril's intake and output are recorded on his daily chart and demonstrate an intake of 2 litres within 24 hours

Box 7.18 Example of how an aim might be identified

Actual problem	Potential problem	Aim/s
2. Catheter in situ	1. Risk of infection	To reduce the risk of infection
	2. Catheter may become blocked due to bleeding from the excision site and blood clot formation in the catheter	To observe for any blockage of the catheter

Whether you decide to use goals or aims you should be able to evaluate the outcomes of the nursing care plan and nursing interventions.

Exercise
1. Now consider Cyril's remaining problems in relation to the other Activities of Living and identify goals or aims that you might set.
2. Discuss these with your mentor or personal tutor.
3. Reflect on how the activity of elimination impacts on the other Activities of Living and vice versa.

Planning care

Having undertaken a nursing assessment and identified actual and potential problems the nurse is now ready to plan the care.

Roper et al (2000) state that the objective of the plan is:

- to prevent identified problems with any of the ALs from becoming actual ones
- to solve identified actual problems
- where possible, to alleviate those that cannot be solved
- to help the person cope positively with those problems that cannot be alleviated or solved
- to prevent recurrence of a treated problem
- to help the person to be as comfortable and pain-free as possible when death is inevitable.

The nursing care plan, in addition to the direct observation of the patient, monitoring of vital signs and verbal report, should guide professional and ethical practice, care delivery, care management and personal and professional development (NMC 2002b).

Availability of resources

When planning the care and determining nursing interventions the nurse must take account of the resources available, including staffing levels, knowledge and skills available, the environment and equipment. It is also necessary to identify and agree, ideally with the patient and other health care professionals, the expected outcomes of these interventions by identifying short- and long-term goals and a date by which an outcome should be achieved. This will enable the nurse to evaluate whether the expected outcome has been achieved.

Care pathways

The introduction of clinical governance into the NHS in the UK (DoH 1998) has placed greater emphasis on ensuring quality care to patients and effective outcomes. A care pathway is a tool that sets out the evidence-based care a patient should receive for an episode of care (Ellis & Johnson 1999). Care pathways are normally developed for high-volume cases. Ellis and Johnson (1999) developed a care pathway for transurethral resection of a prostatectomy (TURP) in Ashford and St Peter's Hospitals NHS Trust. The benefits they identified were that all staff were able to understand how patients undergoing this procedure should be cared for, care was consistent, risks to patients were reduced and auditing by variance reporting informed education and enabled patients to be discharged earlier.

When planning the nursing care of a patient it is necessary to consider where care pathways have been developed and take account of these when determining the nursing interventions and individualising nursing care.

> **Exercise**
> 1. If you are a student nurse undertaking a clinical placement find out if there are any integrated care pathways being used.
> 2. In what way do these take account of the Activities of Living?
> 3. Discuss your findings with your mentor or personal tutor.

Collaboration

Nurses do not work in isolation, they work in teams and in collaboration with others. In hospital nurses are with the patients for 24 hours a day and in many cases they may take the lead role in coordinating the care of the patient, referring if necessary to specialist nurses and health care professionals.

> **Exercise**
> 1. Revisit Cyril's assessment and taking account of the ALs identify other health care professionals who may be involved.
> 2. What would be their role in his care?

You may have considered the following:

- medical staff including Consultant Urologist
- junior medical staff
- Physiotherapist
- Chaplain
- Anaesthetist
- Health Care Assistant.

Other professionals who may input indirectly or at a later date include:

- Pharmacist
- Phlebotomist
- Dietitian
- Social Worker
- Discharge Liaison Coordinator

When preparing a nursing care plan you will need to take account of the input and assessments undertaken by these professionals.

> **Exercise**
> Review Cyril's case.
>
> 1. Reflect on your experience to date. What knowledge and skills do you already possess to enable you to plan his nursing care?
> 2. What knowledge and skills do you need to develop?
> 3. What do you need to see and do to gain the knowledge and skills?
> 4. To what resources do you need access in order to care for this patient?

Nursing interventions

The nursing care plan details the nursing interventions required to achieve the stated goals or aims. The plan should enable other staff including other health care professionals to provide continuity of care for the patient (Roper et al 2000). The nursing care plan may be paper-based or computerised.

When determining the nursing interventions you will need to consider where the patient is on the independency/dependency continuum as identified in the model of living (Roper et al 2000). The nurse provides nursing interventions for a dependent patient whereas nursing interventions in an independent patient aim to encourage and maintain independence. As discussed in part 1 of this chapter dependency may be influenced by the factors associated with living across the lifespan.

Exercise
1. Review Cyril's assessment, actual and potential problems and goals or aims and identify the nursing actions and interventions required.
2. Consider your knowledge and skills to undertake or supervise these nursing activities and interventions. Identify those that you need to develop further with your mentor or personal tutor.

Breathing

Cyril smokes 10 cigarettes a day and is therefore at risk of developing a chest infection following a general anaesthetic. During surgery the patient is unable to cough or sigh and thus expectorate or move any sputum from the lungs. This will pool and become foci for bacterial infection. Patients who smoke should be advised to stop smoking at least 10 days prior to undergoing a general anaesthetic (Rogers 2000). It is important that all patients are referred, prior to undergoing surgery, to a physiotherapist and taught deep breathing exercises and how to clear stagnating fluids from their lungs.

In many cases patients being admitted to hospital for elective surgery attend a nurse-led preassessment clinic where routine investigations are performed and the patient receives information on the procedure and health education advice. If Cyril had attended a preassessment clinic he would have been given advice on giving up smoking and the anaesthetic risks involved (see Chapter 3 for pre- and postoperative care).

Nursing interventions These might include:
- reinforcing information on the risks of smoking prior to surgery
- arranging access to nicotine replacement patches if prescribed
- referring to the physiotherapist for deep breathing exercises
- encouraging deep breathing exercises pre- and postoperatively
- monitoring his temperature, pulse and respirations.

Communicating

Cyril wears a hearing aid. He can hear with difficulty without it and may misunderstand or misinterpret what is being said to him. This may result in increasing stress levels and lack of compliance and cooperation in relation to pre-operative fasting and advice on postoperative recovery (see Chapter 4).

Nursing interventions These might include:
- ensuring that Cyril understands information and does not misinterpret instructions or health advice
- ensuring that Cyril has his hearing aid in place and that it is working when communicating with him
- checking that he has understood any instructions or information

- ensuring that other health professionals are aware that Cyril wears a hearing aid.

Eating and drinking

Whilst Cyril's appetite is fairly good he is reluctant to drink fluids. Cyril will need to have at least 2 litres of fluid a day. An adequate fluid intake is essential to achieve fluid and electrolyte balance prior to surgery. Following surgery Cyril will have an intravenous infusion of fluid in situ. When he has recovered from the anaesthetic he will need to drink at least 2 litres of fluid a day to ensure that the catheter does not become blocked by blood clots and prevent infection, unless medical advice is to the contrary and fluid should be restricted initially due to electrolyte imbalance. The nurse should monitor the patient's intake and output (see Chapter 6).

Nursing interventions These might include:
- encouraging Cyril to drink at least 2 litres of fluid each day when recovered from anaesthetic
- monitoring and recording Cyril's fluid intake and output
- ensuring the safe administration of intravenous fluids
- monitoring the amount and colour of urine drainage from the catheter
- where necessary providing assistance to enable Cyril to eat his meals
- observing any nausea or vomiting.

Eliminating

Initially on admission Cyril will need to be able to find his way round the ward and know the location of the toilets. He will need reassurance regarding his dribbling incontinence and access to any incontinence aids or adaptations. He will also need information on how the activity of elimination will be effected initially postsurgery.

Following surgery he will have a catheter inserted and undergo continuous irrigation until his urine is clear. Preventing infection and maintaining the dignity of the patient are the two key principles in caring for a patient with a urethral catheter (see Selfe 2000, p. 332 for further information on the principles of catheter management). It is essential to maintain a closed system to reduce the likelihood of infection. Cyril's mobility following surgery will be restricted initially and this may result in Cyril becoming constipated.

Nursing interventions These might include:
- ensuring that Cyril is orientated into the ward and knows where the toilets are
- ensuring that Cyril has access to any incontinence aids for his dribbling incontinence prior to surgery
- maintaining Cyril's privacy and dignity when attending to catheter and continuous bladder irrigation
- monitoring and observing urine drainage
- maintaining bladder irrigation as prescribed
- maintaining asepsis when changing urine drainage bags
- attending to catheter toilet

- ensuring that Cyril understands the need for good personal hygiene
- monitoring Cyril's bowel movements and taking action if Cyril complains of constipation
- recording temperature, blood pressure and pulse, and reporting any changes.

Mobilising

Normally Cyril is able to mobilise independently. However, following surgery he will undergo a period of bed rest and his mobility will be restricted by the intravenous infusion and continuous irrigation of fluid. He will also need assistance when mobilising for the first time following surgery. Cyril's privacy and dignity may be compromised due to being catheterised and having to carry around a urine bag.

Surgery and a period of immobility may increase the risk of deep venous thrombosis and pulmonary embolism. Whilst Cyril's risk may be moderate he would benefit from application of compression stockings and advice on leg exercises whilst in bed and early mobilisation (see Rogers 2000). In some cases prophylactic anticoagulants prior to surgery may be prescribed.

Nursing interventions These might include:
- recording Cyril's temperature and pulse and reporting any rise in temperature
- applying compression hosiery prior to surgery
- explaining to Cyril the need for early mobilisation following surgery
- encouraging passive movements whilst in bed
- encouraging gentle exercise following surgery
- referral to the physiotherapist for advice and support pre- and postoperatively
- explaining the hazards associated with mobilising whilst catheter and infusion are in situ.

Expressing sexuality

Cyril is concerned about how his operation will impact on his sexual relations with his wife. Following a TURP most men will suffer from retrograde ejaculation, however, this does not mean that the man will be impotent. It is important that men undergoing this procedure are given adequate information and reassurance and if necessary counselled prior to surgery. Failure to provide this information and support may lead to anxiety and stress. It is important to remember to consider what information his wife will require.

Nursing interventions These might include:
- providing written and verbal information on the side effects of prostatectomy
- listening to Cyril's concerns
- checking that he has understood the information.

Personal cleansing and dressing

Normally fully independent in washing and dressing, Cyril will need help to undertake this Activity of Living in the immediate postoperative period. He may also find it difficult to dress himself as a result of the intravenous infusion and catheter drainage (see Chapter 8).

Nursing interventions These might include:
- assisting Cyril to maintain his personal and oral hygiene
- providing advice on how to manage his catheter care.

Working and playing

Cyril has arranged for sick leave from work. But because of his sickness and absence record any further absences will have financial implications for his family (see Chapter 11).

Nursing interventions These might include:
- referral to social worker for advice on financial support and benefits available during periods of illness.

Maintaining a safe environment

Cyril is scheduled for surgery. He will require preoperative preparation and safe transfer to theatre. Haemorrhage or bleeding from the excision site is a major risk following TURP. Therefore one of the nurse's major roles is to record the patient's blood pressure, pulse and observe the urine for clots and signs of bleeding (see Chapter 3).

Whilst an assessment for the risk of pressure ulcer development showed that Cyril was not at risk, his transfer to theatre, surgery and subsequent recovery period will increase his risk status and it will be necessary to review his score following surgery.

Nursing interventions These might include:
- preparing Cyril for theatre and complete preoperative assessment
- observing for bleeding on return from theatre
- monitoring Cyril's temperature, pulse and blood pressure
- monitoring and observe for bleeding via the catheter
- reassessing risk of pressure ulcer development, providing pressure reduction mattress if required and encouraging Cyril to turn or move regularly
- monitoring and observing pressure points paying particular attention to heel pressure points and ensuring that his skin is clean and dry
- encouraging Cyril to move his position at least 2 hourly, providing assistance where necessary.

Sleeping

Cyril may find it difficult to sleep in hospital at first due to the unfamiliarity of his surroundings, noise and anxiety about his surgery (see Chapter 13). Following surgery postoperative checks carried out by nurses to monitor his vital signs and observe for complications will result in Cyril's sleep being disturbed.

Nursing interventions These might include:
- orientating Cyril into his surroundings and environment
- reducing the amount of noise within the ward wherever possible.

Controlling body temperature

Normally Cyril is able to control his body temperature by thermoregulation. However, during surgery consideration should be given to ensuring a warm environment to prevent unnecessary heat loss and aid recovery. Following surgery his temperature should be monitored. A rise in his temperature may indicate an infection (see Chapter 9).

Nursing interventions These might include:
- monitoring his temperature
- ensuring a warm environment.

Dying

Cyril has indicated that he is very worried about the outcome of his surgery and prognosis. He does not openly talk about dying but when asked he would like to speak to the Chaplain (see Chapter 14).

Nursing intervention These might include:
- referral to the Chaplain
- reassurance and information on the possible outcomes of his surgery.

Implementing nursing care

Successful implementation relies on a thorough initial nursing assessment (Sutcliffe 1990), a comprehensive nursing care plan, well-organised care delivery systems and competent staff.

The nursing care plan provides a written guide and instructions on implementing the care for the patient. It also provides an accurate record of the care given to the patient.

Record keeping is an integral part of nursing care. It is a tool for professional practice and one which should help the care process (NMC 2002b). There is no single model or template for a nursing record but it must follow a logical sequence with clear milestones and goals.

Nursing records are an integral part of the patient's health care record and can be called in evidence before a Court of Law, Health Service Commissioner or in order to investigate a complaint about care at a local level. The NMC Professional Conduct Committee may also use patient records when considering complaints about professional misconduct.

Whilst it is preferable that nursing records are completed contemporaneously, workload pressures, stress and being too busy are reasons given why nurses find it difficult to do so (Mason 1999). Mason also found that the verbal report, direct observation and bedside charts guided practice rather than the nursing care plan. More recently and in response to the concerns expressed, the Department of Health (2001b) has produced a Clinical Practice Benchmark for Record Keeping. You may access these at www.doh.gov.uk.

Exercise

Return to Cyril's nursing care plan.

1. What factors might influence implementation?
2. What knowledge and skills would you need to implement these nursing interventions?

You may have considered the following factors might influence implementation:

- the philosophy of care on the ward or department (beliefs and values, advocacy)
- the nursing model used
- the care delivery system (primary nursing, team nursing, case management or task allocation)
- resources available (skill mix of staff available, equipment, support staff and other health care professionals).

You may have considered that the following knowledge is required when implementing nursing activities:

- anatomy and physiology of urinary and intestinal systems
- psychological effects associated with elimination
- Sociocultural issues relating to elimination
- Environmental issues and concerns
- Political and economic concerns.

You may have considered that the following skills are required when implementing nursing activities:

- caring skills (listening, comforting, reassuring, helping)
- clinical psychomotor skills (catheterisation, intravenous infusions, rectal examination, urine testing, specimen collection, etc.)
- management skills (organisational, supervision, delegation skills)
- counselling skills (listening, problem solving, advising)
- teaching skills
- research skills (literature searching, critical appraisal)
- problem solving skills (problem identification, goal setting, priority setting)
- leadership skills (advocacy, teamwork, transformational leadership skills, networking).

Exercise

1. Reflect on these and assess your current knowledge and skills.
2. Record your reflections in your diary.
3. Identify those areas in which you need further development.
4. Take these to your next tutorial or clinical supervision session. Discuss with your mentor or preceptor how you plan to develop these further.

Evaluation of nursing activities

Evaluation of nursing care is an important part of professional practice and provides feedback on the patient's progress (NMC 2002b). Evaluation is an ongoing process, which should be undertaken by the nurse in conjunction with the patient and his or her relatives or carers and other health care professionals (for further information refer to Chapter 1).

Evaluating care consists of checking the patient's progress against the identified goals and timescales to determine whether these have been fully or partially met or indeed not met at all.

When evaluating the nursing care plan the nurse may seek to establish if the goals or aims have been completely, partially or not met at all. If the goal or aim has not been met or partially met then the nurse must consider if the agreed timescale was realistic. If not then the nurse may decide to extend the timescale. Alternatively the nurse may reassess the problem and modify the plan. Not all goals or aims will be achievable during a hospital stay. Nursing care plans can be a useful tool to provide information on discharge or transfer of care between secondary, tertiary and primary care.

Discharge planning

A comprehensive nursing assessment using the Roper et al (1996, 2000) model of living and model for nursing will also provide the basis of a well-developed discharge plan and facilitate safe and effective discharge back into the community.

Personal and professional development

Having worked through this chapter and the exercises, you need to reflect on what you have learnt and how you might use this to inform your personal and professional development.

You may like to consider your needs under the following headings:

- What do I need to see now?
- What do I need to do now?
- What do I need to know now?
- Who can help me?

Summary points

1. This chapter introduced the fifth Activity of Living – elimination as described by Roper, Logan and Tierney in their model for nursing (Roper et al 1996, 2000). It systematically explored the framework of the model and its application in clinical practice, the use of a case scenario, exercises, and reflection and further reading. It has been impossible within this chapter to cover every aspect in relation to the activity of elimination and health issues associated with elimination. Therefore, it is important that you keep up-to-date with new information and evidence-based practice in order to be able to meet the changing needs of patients and health care delivery.

2. Nurses have a very important role in ensuring the quality of the patient experience, and that patient needs are met in relation to the activity of elimination. Throughout the chapter we have shown how, by applying the Roper, Logan and Tierney model for nursing in practice, the nurse is able to recognise and take account of the patient's individual needs in relation to elimination when assessing, planning, implementing and evaluating holistic patient care.

References

Bandolier Library 2000 Treatments for irritable bowel syndrome. Bandolier Library for Pain Relief Unit, Oxford, pp. 70–75 (www.jr2.ox.ac.uk/bandolier/band79/b79-5.htm)

Beaton S 2001 How foot and mouth disease affected a rural continence service. Nursing Times 97(40): 59, 70

British National Formulary 2002 British Medical Association, Royal Pharmaceutical Society of Great Britain March: 43

Burton G 1996 An assessment of attitudes to incontinence in different migrant groups. Australian Continence Journal March: 4–6

Clarke KW, Gray D, Hampton JR 1994 Evidence of inadequate investigation and treatment of patients with heart failure. British Heart Journal 71: 584–587

Clayton J, Smith K, Qureshi K, Ferguson B 1998 Collecting patients' views and perceptions of continuous services: the development of research instruments. Journal of Advanced Nursing 28(2): 353–361

Continence Foundation 2000 Making the case for investment in an Integrated Continence Service. A source book for continence services. The Continence Foundation, London (http://www.continence-foundation.org.uk)

DoH 1998 A first class service: quality in the new NHS. The Stationery Office, London

DoH 1999 For the record. Health Service circular 1999/053. HMSO, London

DoH 2000 Good practice in continence services. HMSO, London

DoH 2001a Guide to consent for examination or treatment. HMSO, London

DoH 2001b The essence of care: patient-focused benchmarking for health care professionals. The Stationery Office, London

DoH 2001c Reference guide to consent from examination or treatment. The Stationery Office, London

DoH 2001d Modern standards and service models of older people. National Service Framework for Older People. HMSO, London

Effective Health Care Bulletin 2001 Effectiveness of laxatives in adults. NHS Centre for Reviews and Dissemination, The University of York, York. Vol 7(1)

Ellis BW, Johnson S 1999 The care pathway: a tool to enhance clinical governance. British Journal of Clinical Governance 4(2): 61–71

Evans JHC 2001 Evidence based management of nocturnal and enuresis. British Medical Journal 323: 1167–1169

Gastrointestinal Infections in the 1999/2000 Chapter 8 Review of communicable diseases (www.phls.co.uk/publications/annual-review/reviewindex.htm)

Glazener CNA, Evans JHC 2001 Alarm interventions for nocturnal and enuresis in children (Cochrane Review). The Cochrane Library 4, Oxford

Haggar V 1997 Foreign policy. Nursing Times 15: 78

Heaton K 1999 The Bristol stool form scale. In: Understanding your bowels. Family Doctor Series. BMA, London

Henley A, Schott J 1999 Culture, religion & patient care in a multi-ethnic society. A handbook for professionals. Age Concern Books, Glasgow

Herbert J 1999 Faecal incontinence: the last taboo? British Journal of Therapy and Rehabilitation 6(9): 453–458

Hinchliff S, Montague SE, Watson R 1996 Physiology for nursing practice, 2nd edn. Harcourt Publishers Ltd, Edinburgh

Hinds JP, Eidelman BH, Wald A 1990 Prevalence of bowel dysfunction in multiple sclerosis. Gastroenterology 98: 1538–1542

Hunt GM, Oakeshott P, Whitaker RH 1996 Fortnightly review: Intermittent catheterisation: Simple, safe, and effective, but underused. British Medical Journal 312: 103–107

Johanson JJ, Laferty J 1996 Epidemiology of faecal incontinence: the silent affliction. American Journal of Gastroenterology 91(1): 33–36

Kamm MA 1998 Faecal incontinence. British Medical Journal 316: 528–532

Kenworthy N, Snowley G, Gelling C 2002 Common foundation studies in nursing, 3rd edn. Churchill Livingstone, Edinburgh

Mallet J, Dougherty L (eds) 2000 The Royal Marsden Hospital manual of clinical nursing procedures, 5th edn. Blackwell Science Ltd, London

Mason C 1999 Guide to practice or 'load of rubbish'? The influence of care plans on nursing practice in five clinical areas in Northern Ireland. Journal of Advanced Nursing 29(2): 380–387

McDowell BJ, Engberg S, Serika S, Donovan N, Jubeck ME, Weber E, Enberg R 1999 Effectiveness of behavioural therapy to treat incontinence in home bound older people. Journal of the American Geriatrics Society 47: 309–318

McMonnies G 2002 Paediatric continence in children with neuropathic bladders. British Journal of Nursing 11(11): 765–772

Nelson R, Norton N, Cautley E, Furner S 1995 Community based prevalence of anal incontinence. JAMA 274(7): 559–561

Neveus T, Lackgren G, Tuvemo T, Hetta J, Hjalmas K, Stemberg A 2000 Enuresis – background and treatment. Scandinavian Journal of Eurology and Nephrology supplementum (206): 1–44

Norton C 1996 Faecal incontinence in adults 1: Prevalence and causes. British Journal of Nursing 5(22): 1366–1374

Nursing and Midwifery Council 2002a Code of professional conduct. NMC, London

Nursing and Midwifery Council 2002b Guidelines for records and record keeping. NMC, London

Ogden J 1996 Health Psychology: a Textbook. Open University Press, Buckingham

Page A 1999 Twelve years of hell. Nursing Times 95(18): 65–66

PHLS Advisory Committee on Gastrointestinal Infections 2000 (www.phls.co.uk)

PHLS Review of communicable diseases 1999–2000 (www.phls.co.uk)

Powell M, Rigby D 2000 Management of bowel dysfunction: evacuation difficulties. Nursing Standard 14(47): 47–51

Roe B, Doll H 2000 Prevalence of urinary incontinence and its relationship with health status. Journal of Clinical Nursing 9: 178–188

Rogers SE 2000 The patient facing surgery, Chapter 26. In: Alexander MF, Fawcett JN, Runciman PJ (eds) Nursing practice for hospital and home: the adult, 2nd edn., pp. 799–831. Churchill Livingstone, Edinburgh

Rogers J 2001 Fast-track toilet. Training Nursing Times 97(40): 53–54

Rogers J 2002 Managing day-time and night-time enuresis in children. Nursing Standard 16(32): 45–52

Roper N, Logan WW, Tierney AJ 1996 The elements of nursing: A model for nursing based on a model for living, 4th edn. Churchill Livingstone, London

Roper N, Logan WW, Tierney AJ 2000 The Roper Logan Tierney model of nursing based on activities of living. Churchill Livingstone, Edinburgh

Royal College of Nursing 2000 Digital rectal examination and manual removal of faeces. Guidance for Nurses. Royal College of Nursing, London

Royal College of Physicians (RCP) 1995 Incontinence: causes, management and provision of services. Royal College of Physicians, London

Rutishauser S 1994 Physiology and anatomy. A basis for nursing and health care. Churchill Livingstone, London

Selfe L 2000 The urinary system, Ch. 8, pp. 313–348. In: Alexander MF, Fawcett JN, Runciman PJ (eds) Nursing practice for hospital and home (the adult), 2nd edn. Churchill Livingstone, Edinburgh

Shaw C 2001 A review of the psychosocial predictors of help seeking impact on quality of life in people with urinary incontinence. Journal of Clinical Nursing 10: 15–24

Sub-committee of the PHLS Advisory Committee on Gastrointestinal Infections 2000 Guidelines for the control of infection with vero cytotoxin producing *Escherichia coli* (VTEC). The Communicable Disease and Public Health 3: 14–23

Sultan AH, Kamm MA, Hudson CN, Thomas JM, Bartram CI 1993 Anal sphincter disruption during vaginal delivery. New England Journal of Medicine 329: 1905–1911

Sutcliffe E 1990 Reviewing the process progress: a critical review of the literature on the nursing process. Senior Nurse 10(a): 9–13

Swaffield J 2000 Continence, Chapter 24. In: Alexander MF, Fawcett JN, Runciman PJ (eds) Nursing practice for hospital and home: the adult, 2nd edn. pp. 763–782. Churchill Livingstone, Edinburgh

Vickerman J, Whitehead J 2001 Continence management: an occupational therapist and physiotherapist perspective. Nurse May: 34–36

Walsh M (ed) 2002 Watson's clinical nursing and related sciences, 6th edn. Baillière Tindall in association with the RCN, London

Waugh A, Grant G 2001 Ross and Wilson anatomy and philosophy in health and illness, 9th edn. Churchill Livingstone, Edinburgh

Wilkinson J 2002 The psychological basis of nursing. In: Kenworthy N, Snowley G, Gelling C (eds) Common foundation studies in nursing, 3rd edn., pp. 197–224. Churchill Livingstone, Edinburgh

Willis J 1999 The future beckons. Nursing Times 95(18): 61–63

Further reading

Brocklehurst J (ed) 1999 Health outcome indicators: urinary incontinence: report of a working group to the Department of Health. Oxford, National Centre for Health Outcomes Development

Brocklehurst J (ed) 1999 Report to the Department of Health working group on outcome indicators for urinary incontinence. Oxford, National Centre for Health Outcomes Development

DoH 1998b Information for health: an information strategy for the modern NHS 1998–2005. NHSE, London

Royal College of Physicians 1998 Clinical incontinence: A clinical audit scheme for the management of urinary and faecal incontinence compiled by the Research Unit of The Royal College of Physicians. Royal College of Physicians, London

Useful websites

Cochrane Library www.nelh.nhs.uk/cochrane
Commissioning Continence Advisory Services: An RCN Guide www.rcn.org.uk
Continence Foundation www.continence-foundation.org.uk
Department of Health Essence of Care www.doh.gov.uk/essenceofcare/index
Enuresis Resource and Information Centre www.enuresis.org.uk
National Association for Continence www.nafc.org
NHS Direct www.nhsdirect.nhs.uk
Royal College of Physicians www.rcplondon.ac.uk

Personal cleansing and dressing

Karen Holland

Introduction

The way in which people dress and maintain personal cleanliness is inextricably linked to the society and culture in which they live. Clothing is influenced by many factors such as the weather, customs and social expectations of men and women. In Western societies it is also linked to what people can afford. Being 'clean' is also a relative concept, in that it depends on whose standards and beliefs it is being measured against. It is important to take account of this when we are assessing individual needs in both personal cleansing and dressing, in particular as to how it affects the health of the individual.

This chapter will therefore focus on the following:

1. **The model of living**
   - Personal cleansing and dressing in health and illness across the lifespan.
   - Dependence/independence in the AL of personal cleansing and dressing.
   - Factors influencing the AL of personal cleansing and dressing.
2. **The model for nursing**
   - Nursing care of individuals with health problems affecting the Activity of Living: personal cleansing and dressing (i.e. application of Roper et al 1996, 2000 in practice).

THE MODEL OF LIVING

What is meant by personal cleansing and dressing? Roper et al (1996) associate personal cleansing (personal hygiene) with several different activities, i.e. washing and bathing, hand-washing, perineal toilet, care of the hair, care of the nails and care of teeth and mouth. Dressing is used to refer to 'putting on of clothes' which are seen as a medium of nonverbal communication 'and are also essential for living in different environments and social and cultural contexts' (Roper et al 1996, p. 234).

Personal cleansing and dressing in health and illness – across the lifespan

Childhood

When babies are first born they are unable to care for themselves, requiring an adult to both clothe them and take care of their personal hygiene. Clothing is required for both warmth and protection, whilst washing is required to remove urine and faeces from contact with their bodies. This will prevent their skin from becoming sore. As children grow they will come to learn to control their own bladder and bowel activity, learning also to use appropriate toilet facilities depending on the culture in which they live. Children in some cultures will use the more natural environments whilst others will learn to use bathrooms and indoor toilet facilities. The effect of not washing children's skin from urine and faeces can be seen in extreme cases of physical abuse – with severe burns and skin damage through neglect and nonwashing.

Other personal cleansing behaviours learnt by young children include combing or brushing their hair, cleaning their teeth and bathing or showering. Lawler (1991) indicates that our cultural beliefs about the body, its functions and products will be reflected in our practice in managing childhood personal cleansing behaviour.

> **Exercise**
> Reflect on your own childhood.
>
> 1. What were you taught to do with regards to washing and bathing?
> 2. Look at photographs of your childhood and compare with those of parents or other members of your family. How different was their mode of dress?
> 3. Discuss with colleagues their cultural beliefs with regards to how children should be dressed and their personal cleansing needs.

Adolescence

As children grow up their bodies also undergo changes that necessitate additional personal cleansing behaviours. Under-arm perspiration and growth of body hair are two changes that occur at puberty, as are the potential problems of dandruff of the scalp and facial acne. In many societies whole industries have developed, aimed at managing these changes and problems. Products such as shampoo, deodorant and soap have become an essential part of living in the modern world and for many, having to go without these becomes stressful. Roper et al (1996, p. 235) point out that:

> 66 *Adolescence can be the period for experimenting with way out fashions and new hairstyles and provided that they do not cause any harm, tolerance and good humour reap better rewards all round than continual derisory remarks. It can be seen as part of a young person's bid for independence and a means of communication, both with peers and other groups.* 99

Examples of these fashions are nose and lip rings, tattoos and shaved heads. Fashion magazines have a significant influence on how and what we do at all ages but none more so than in young adults. For example one of the major influences is linked to how we express our sexuality (see Chapter 12), in particular the impact on what we do with and to our bodies, both in terms of dressing and personal hygiene.

Exercise

1. Consider your own adolescent years. What kind of clothes did you wear?
2. Discuss with colleagues how your culture expects you to behave in the period before reaching adulthood.
3. Consider the above quote by Roper et al (1996) and consider your views on their opinion of adolescence.
4. Obtain a wide variety of magazines aimed at the 15–19-year-old age bracket. What do they tell you about how we see the body in Western society?

Adulthood

Reaching adulthood will probably require a different lifestyle, as many adults undertake employment, which will give them financial rewards, and the wherewithal to spend money on both clothes and personal cleansing products. The kind of clothes that people wear can tell us much about both their culture and their lifestyle. Henley & Schott (1999, p. 112) state that 'standards of modest behaviour and decency vary enormously' and that 'what is perfectly acceptable to some, shocks others deeply' (see Box 8.1).

Box 8.1 Modesty and health care

Some cultures place a particularly high value on personal modesty. Care must be taken to ensure that people always feel decently covered during examinations, treatments and everyday practical care. It is also important to ensure that the patient's environment takes their requirements for modesty into account.

- Many people, especially women of conservative communities, never undress fully except when they are alone. They may be used to uncovering only the relevant part for a medical examination or for treatment.
- Some people never undress completely even to wash. They shower in their clothes, changing into clean dry clothes afterwards.
- For some people it is important that all intimate treatments, examinations and practical care are carried out by someone of the same sex. When there is no health professional of the same sex, some patients may prefer to be washed or helped with washing and using the lavatory by a family member of the same sex if possible.
- For some people the idea of being seen in bed or in nightclothes by strangers, and particularly by people of the opposite sex, is very shocking. This is especially likely for people who normally have little contact with people outside their own family. Women and some men of many communities may feel immodest and exposed in their nightclothes and in a public area. Some may want to keep their curtains closed all the time so that they are not exposed to public gaze.

From Henley A and Schott J 1999 Culture, religion and patient care in a multi-ethnic society, p. 114.

Exercise

Consider the issues identified by Henley and Schott.

1. How would the issue of modesty be affected in mixed-sex wards or mixed-sex washing and toilet facilities?
2. How would you ensure that cultural practices were taken into account in your health care practice?

It is interesting to note that the current Labour Government in the UK has decreed that mixed-sex wards are no longer appropriate in a modern hospital, and funds were made available to abolish 95% of them by 2002. The National Service Framework for Older People (DoH 2001a) states that: 'mixed sex wards can be embarrassing and for some people culturally insensitive.' (DoH 2001a, p. 57a). This is also outlined in the DoH (2000) Guidance on mixed-sex accommodation for mental health services which will 'ensure that the safety, privacy and dignity of in-patients are protected.'

Old age

As people get older some tasks may become more difficult to undertake. In many cases these difficulties are linked to underlying health problems such as arthritis. Roper et al (1996, p. 235) also state that:

> ❝ *Failing eyesight and shaking hands may make it increasingly difficult for older people to retain their independence with conventional clothing. Back fastenings of garments are difficult to reach and front fastenings are therefore preferable; zips and Velcro tapes are much easier to manipulate than small buttons or hooks and eyes. Many older people more readily feel the cold and may need to wear extra clothing to keep warm. Two layers of thin material (because of the entrapped air which is a bad conductor of heat) are warmer than one thick layer. Adequate warm clothing is a simple but important means of preventing hypothermia, which is a particular threat to old people in severe winter weather.* ❞

Clothes however provide more than physical comfort and protection. They also help provide a positive self-image and clothes that make us 'feel good' about ourselves can boost our sense of wellbeing. This is as important to the older person as it is to other age groups.

Exercise

1. Talk to someone in your family, or a friend, who is over 70 years old and ask them to describe what it is like to be that age in relation to how they dress and how they manage their personal cleansing and dressing activities.
2. Find out what has influenced any changes in their patterns of behaviour or their own personal preferences.
3. Compare their responses with your own experience and discuss with colleagues from different cultural groups to see if there any differences or similarities between age groups.

Dependence/independence in the AL of personal cleansing and dressing

Dependence or independence in this Activity of Living will depend on both age and health and illness status. In infancy there is a total dependence on others, which would also be apparent in later life if the individual was no longer able to physically or mentally cope with their own personal cleansing and dressing needs. Being physically disabled from a traumatic illness e.g. tetraplegia, is one such example, as are the effects of a chronic illness such as multiple sclerosis. Some children may also be affected by such illnesses, thus prolonging their childhood and infancy dependency.

Factors influencing the AL of personal cleansing and dressing

Biological

Roper et al (1996, p. 236) identify the skin 'as the largest physical body structure which relates directly to the Activity of Living of personal cleansing and dressing'. However, as with all Activities of Living, the influence of other physiological systems must be considered. For example we can see that the physiological changes brought about at puberty have a significant affect on adolescent fashion and their body perceptions (see Chapter 12), and that being physically incapacitated by rheumatoid arthritis will prevent the person from being able to dress themselves without help.

The skin

The skin is the largest organ in the body, and has an important role in the defence of the body (Hinchliff et al 2000). It covers a 'surface area of about 1.5 to 2 square metres in adults and contains glands, hair and nails' (Waugh & Grant, 2001, p. 362). Its main structures can be seen in Figure 8.1. Its two main layers are:

- the epidermis
- the dermis.

In addition there is a layer of subcutaneous tissue between the skin and the underlying structures. The skin has many functions:

- protection
- regulation of body temperature
- formation of vitamin D
- sensation
- absorption
- excretion.

An understanding of the structure and function of the skin is important when considering the personal cleansing and dressing needs of individuals both in health and illness. It is also important when considering the needs of patients who experience breakdown in normal skin functions and structure, for example serious burns or the skin disorder psoriasis.

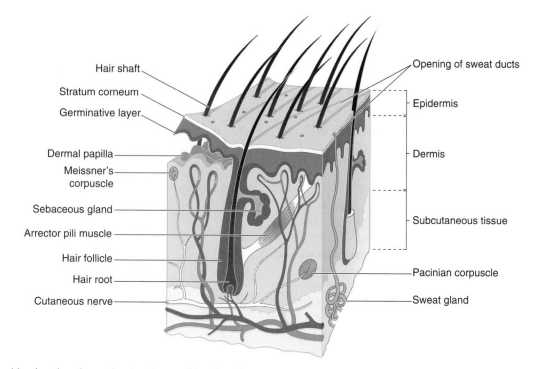

Fig. 8.1 The skin showing the main structures of the dermis (from Waugh & Grant 2001, with permission).

Structure of the skin

As can be seen from Figure 8.1 the skin has many structures in the dermal layers. The epidermis or outer layer:

> *is the most superficial layer of the skin and is composed of stratified keratinised squamous epithelium (see Fig. 8.2) which varies with thickness in different parts of the body. It is thickest on the palms of the hands and soles of the feet. There are no blood vessels or nerve endings in the epidermis but its deepest layers are bathed in interstitial fluid from the dermis, which provides oxygen and nutrients, and is drained away as lymph.*
>
> *There are several layers (strata) of cells in the epidermis that extend from the deepest germinative layer to the surface stratum corneum (a thick horny layer). The cells on the surface are flat, thin, non-nucleated, dead cells, in which the cytoplasm has been replaced by the fibrous protein keratin. These cells are being rubbed off and replaced by cells that originated in the germinative layer and have undergone gradual change as they progressed towards the surface. Complete replacement of the epidermis takes about 40 days.*

(Waugh & Grant 2001, p. 362)

Two health problems where this process is altered are psoriasis and dandruff. Psoriasis is a skin condition 'characterised by rapid and excessive production of keratinised cells

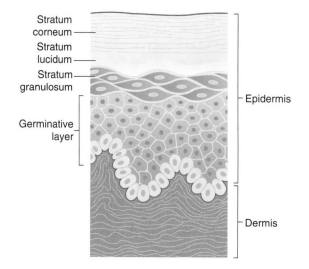

Fig. 8.2 The skin showing the main layers of the epidermis (from Waugh & Grant 2001, with permission).

which form silvery flakes on the skin surface and which result in excessive desquamation' (shedding of skin cells) (Hinchliff et al 1996, p. 625). Dandruff or seborrhoeic dermatitis is 'a minor but unsightly hyperplastic condition of the scalp which results in flakes of keratin being exfoliated' (Hinchliff et al 1996).

Skin colour will vary according to how much melanin (a dark pigment) is in the skin and this varies 'between members of the same race and between races'. Melanin also protects the skin from the harmful effects of the sunlight (Waugh & Grant 2001, p. 362). The observation of skin colour is an important part of a nurse's observation skills and in particular there is a need to understand how certain signs and symptoms of illness need to be particularly observed in both normal and abnormal skin colour. Examples of skin assessment observations can be seen in Box 8.2.

The dermis or inner layer is tough and elastic in structure.

66 *It is formed from connective tissue and the matrix contains collagen fibres interlaced with elastic fibres. Rupture of elastic fibres occurs when the skin is over-stretched, resulting in permanent striate, or stretch marks that may be found in pregnancy and obesity. Collagen fibres bind water and give the skin its tensile strength, but as this ability declines with age, wrinkles develop.* 99
(Waugh & Grant 2001, p. 363)

The main structures found in the dermal layer are:

- blood vessels
- lymph vessels
- sensory nerve endings
- sweat glands and their ducts
- hairs, erector pili muscles and sebaceous glands.

Each of these will be considered in relation to the functions of the skin. It is recommended that you read specialist anatomy and physiology books for more detail in relation to the skin and its structure and function (see Further reading).

Functions of the skin

Protection As well as protecting the deeper and more delicate structures of the body, the skin is an important defence mechanism against: 'invasion by microbes, chemicals, physical agents, e.g. mild trauma, ultraviolet light, dehydration' (Waugh & Grant 2001, p.365).

Regulation of body temperature The normal temperature of the body 'remains fairly constant at about 36.8°C (98.4°F),... although it is slightly raised in the evening, during exercise and in women just after ovulation' (Waugh & Grant 2001, p. 365). In order to ensure this normal measurement the body has to balance heat produced with heat lost from the body. Heat is produced in a number of ways, mainly through muscle activity, liver function and digestion. Heat is lost from the body through the skin, although 'small amounts are lost in expired air, urine and faeces' (Waugh & Grant 2001, p. 365). The mechanisms of heat loss can be seen in Box 8.3 and the control of body temperature can be seen in Chapter 9.

Formation of vitamin D A substance called 7-dehydro-cholesterol found in the skin is converted to Vitamin D by the action of ultraviolet light from the sun. This is then transported in the blood and used in the formation and maintenance of bone (see Chapter 10).

Sensation The dermal layer of the skin consists of nerve endings (sensory receptors) that are 'sensitive to touch, pressure, temperature or pain', and some parts of the body have more of these receptors than others, making them more sensitive, for example the lips and fingertips.

Box 8.2 Physiological assessment (observing skin problems in dark skin)

1. Pallor
There is an absence of underlying red tones; the skin of a brown-skinned person appears yellow–brown and that of a black-skinned person appears ashen, and the lips and nail beds are similar.

2. Erythema
Inflammation must be detected by palpation; the skin is warmer in the area, tight, and oedematous, and the deeper tissues are hard. Fingertips must be used for this assessment, as with rashes, since they are sensitive to the feelings of different textures of skin.

3. Cyanosis
Cyanosis is difficult to observe in dark-coloured skin, but it can be seen by close inspection of the lips, tongue, conjunctiva, palms of the hands and the soles of the feet. Slow blood return is an indication of cyanosis. Another sign is ashen grey lips and tongue.

4. Ecchymosis
History of trauma to a given area can be detected from a swelling of the skin surface.

5. Jaundice
The sclera are usually observed for yellow discolouration to reveal jaundice. This is not always a valid indication, however, since carotene deposits can also cause the sclera to appear yellow. The buccal mucosa and the palms of the hands and soles of the feet may appear yellow.

From Spector R 1996 Cultural Diversity in Health and Illness. Appleton & Lange, Stamford, 4th Edition, p. 206.

Box 8.3 Mechanisms of heat loss

Evaporation
The body is cooled when heat is used to convert the water in sweat to water vapour.

Radiation
Exposed parts of the body radiate heat away from the body.

Conduction
Clothes and other objects in contact with the skin take up heat.

Convection
Air passing over the exposed parts of the body is heated and rises, cool air replaces it and convection currents are set up. Heat is also lost from the clothes by convection.

From Waugh & Grant 2001 Ross & Wilson Anatomy & Physiology, p. 365. Churchill Livingstone, Edinburgh.

Absorption Waugh & Grant (2001, p. 366) state that:

> *This property is limited but substances that can be absorbed include:*
> - *some drugs, in transdermal patches, e.g. hormones used as replacement therapy in postmenopausal women, nicotine as an aid to stopping smoking*
> - *some toxic chemicals, e.g. mercury.*

Excretion The skin is only a minor excretory organ. Substances that it excretes include sodium chloride in sweat, urea and aromatic substances, e.g. garlic.

Other structures associated with the skin are hair, the sebaceous glands and nails. A brief overview is given of these in order to enable them to be considered when assessing patients' needs with regards to personal cleansing and dressing.

Hairs

Hairs are formed of fibrous protein (largely keratin) and are encased in a sheath or hair follicle. Attached to these are the erector pili muscle fibres (see Fig. 8.1). Contraction of these makes the hair 'stand on end' and also raises the skin around the hair, causing a 'goose flesh' appearance (Waugh & Grant 2001, p. 364).

Sebaceous glands

These glands are formed from the same tissue as the hair follicles. They secrete an oily substance called sebum into the hair follicles and can be found all over the body except on the palms of the hand and soles of the feet (Waugh & Grant 2001). It is sebum that keeps hair soft and gives it its shiny appearance. These glands are at their most active at puberty and acne, the scourge of adolescents, is the result of

infection in the hair follicle. There is less sebum produced during infancy and old age, which necessitates extra care and 'oiling' of the skin at these times.

Nails

Nails are also derived from 'the same cells as epidermis and hair and consist of a hard horny keratin plate. They protect the tips of the fingers and toes' (Waugh & Grant 2001, p. 364). The state of the nails can tell us a great deal about an individual's health status, as can the condition of the skin.

Exercise
Consider the structure and function of the skin and discuss the following with colleagues:

1. What happens to the skin when you exercise or sit out in the sun wearing lots of warm clothes?
2. If you cut yourself what does it feel like?
3. What happens when you get sunburn?
4. What happens when you do not wash your hair for a week or more?

Use the above description of the skin and its structure and functions to explore these questions (see also Further Reading). If you can visualise what it feels like for you then it will become easier to empathise with people you may meet with the same problems. For example understanding what it is like to have sunburn which is painful will help you to imagine what the pain must be like with much more serious burns, although one recognises that this can only ever be an imaginary feeling given that every individual experiences pain differently.

Wound healing and skin care

One other important function that the skin performs is that of healing itself when it has been damaged, and knowing the way in which it does this is essential to caring for patients in a variety of situations. The skin can be broken deliberately as in surgery or as a result of other forces for example varicose ulcers due to blood circulation problems. A brief overview will be given in order to facilitate understanding of the process as the basis for assessing the needs of patients with breakdown in skin integrity.

Following injury to the body, 'healing of the wound takes place in order to restore the intact barrier provided by the skin.' (Hinchliff et al 1996, p. 649). It is a process that is closely linked to that of inflammation. Wound healing can be primary or first intention and secondary or second intention. A full explanation of these can be seen in Box 8.4 and the stages of primary and secondary wound healing in Figures 8.3 and 8.4.

Box 8.4 Primary healing (healing by first intention)

This method of healing follows minimal destruction of tissue when the damaged edges of a wound are in close apposition. There are several overlapping stages in the repair process (see Fig. 8.3).

Inflammation

The cut surfaces become inflamed and blood clots and cell debris fill the gap between them in the first few hours. Phagocytes and fibroblasts migrate into the blood clot:

- phagocytes begin to remove the clot and cell debris stimulating fibroblast activity
- fibroblasts secrete collagen fibres which begin to bind the surfaces together.

Proliferation

There is proliferation of epithelial cells across the wound, through the clot. The epidermis meets and grows upwards until the full thickness is restored. The clot above the new tissue becomes the scab and separates after 3 to 10 days. Granulation tissue, consisting of new capillary blood buds, phagocytes and fibroblasts, develops, invading the clot and restoring the blood supply to the wound. Fibroblasts continue to secrete collagen fibres as the clot and phagocytes remove any bacteria.

Maturation

The granulation tissue is replaced by fibrous scar tissue. Rearrangement of collagen fibres occurs and the strength of the wound increases. In time the scar becomes less vascular, appearing after a few months as a fine line. The channels left when wound stitches are removed heal by the same process.

Secondary healing (healing by second intention)

This method of healing follows destruction of a large amount of tissue or when the edges of a wound cannot be brought into apposition, e.g. varicose ulcers and pressure sores (decubitus ulcers). The stages of secondary healing are the same as primary healing and the time taken for healing depends on the effective removal of the cause and on the size of the wound. There are several recognised stages in the repair process (see Fig. 8.4).

Inflammation

This develops on the surface of the healthy tissue and separation of necrotic tissue (slough) begins, due mainly to the action of phagocytes in the inflammatory exudates.

Proliferation

This begins as granulation tissue, consisting of capillary buds, phagocytes and fibroblasts, develops at the base of the cavity. It grows towards the surface, probably stimulated by macrophages. Phagocytes in the plentiful blood supply tend to prevent infection of the wound by ingestion of bacteria after separation of the slough. Some fibroblasts in the wound develop a limited ability to contract, reducing the size of the wound and healing time. When granulation tissue reaches the level of the dermis, epithelial cells at the edges proliferate and grow towards the centre.

Maturation

This occurs as scar tissue replaces granulation tissue, usually over several months until the full thickness of the skin is restored. The fibrous scar tissue is shiny and does not contain sweat glands, hair follicles or sebaceous glands.

From Waugh & Grant 2001 Ross and Wilson Anatomy and physiology in health and illness, pp. 367–368. Churchill Livingstone, Edinburgh.

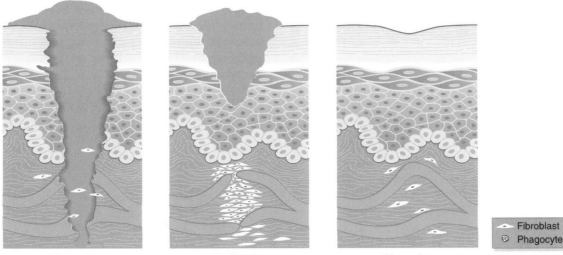

Inflammation   Proliferation   Maturation

Fibroblast
Phagocyte

Fig. 8.3 Stages in primary wound healing (from Waugh & Grant 2001, with permission).

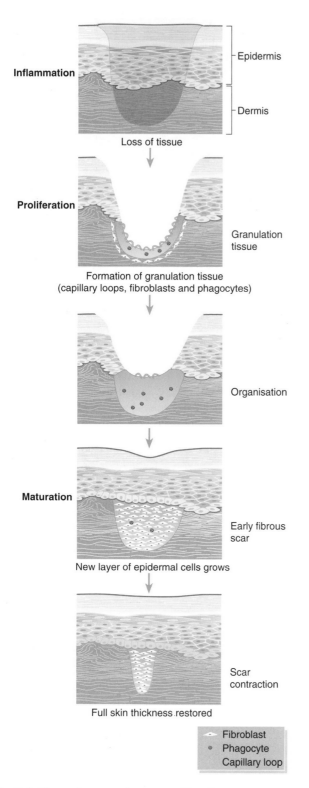

Inflammation

Epidermis

Dermis

Loss of tissue

Proliferation

Granulation tissue

Formation of granulation tissue
(capillary loops, fibroblasts and phagocytes)

Organisation

Maturation

Early fibrous scar

New layer of epidermal cells grows

Scar contraction

Full skin thickness restored

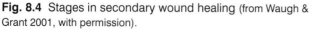

Fibroblast
Phagocyte
Capillary loop

Fig. 8.4 Stages in secondary wound healing (from Waugh & Grant 2001, with permission).

Hinchliff et al (1996, p. 651) identify four factors that delay healing: poor nutritional status, ageing, raised plasma levels of corticosteroids and infection, plus seven criteria for wound healing. These are:

> *1. A moist environment is necessary for epidermal growth.*
> *2. Excess exudates must be removed. This avoids maceration of the wound surface and promotes the remove of debris, toxins and microorganisms.*
> *3. Bacteria must be excluded.*
> *4. The wound must be insulated to provide a constant temperature of 37° C. At every dressing change wound temperature drops with a consequent slowing in the rate of cell division.*
> *5. Vascularisation is promoted in granulation tissue under anaerobic conditions. Occlusive dressing also provides better pain relief.*
> *6. Foreign bodies must not be present since they prolong inflammation. Dressings must not, therefore, shed particles.*
> *7. Dressings should not stick to the wound in any way, nor should new tissue grow into the dressing material, only to be torn away at the next dressing change.*

(Hinchliff et al 1996, p. 651).

Exercise

Consider the facts with regards to wound healing and discuss with colleagues your responses to the following.

1. What could be the concerns of a patient going to the operating theatre in relation to washing and bathing?
2. How would you ensure that infection does not arise as a result of lack of skin care?

Psychological

Personal cleanliness and hygiene are an essential part of a person's wellbeing and health. Different cultures however have different beliefs about this and the nurse needs to be aware of some of these in order to ensure psychological health. Standards of hygiene will also be affected by the mental wellbeing of a person, and it can often be seen that individuals who are depressed may lose interest in their appearance and hygiene. Henley and Schott (1999, p. 117) also note that:

> *People who feel dirty and possibly polluted may become very distressed if they cannot keep clean as they are used to, especially if they are bed-bound and cannot wash themselves. Being dependent on others for washing, bathing and using the lavatory is humiliating for most people. It is important to protect patients' self-esteem and dignity as far as possible by finding out about and trying to cater for their individual habits and preferences.*

For people with compulsive behaviour problems, personal cleanliness norms such as excessive hand washing may become exaggerated.

Sociocultural

Different cultures place different values on personal cleansing and dressing. Consider the questions in Box 8.5 from your own cultural point of view and discuss with colleagues. How will your responses affect your understanding of others' needs?

You may have considered some of the following cultural issues.

Washing and bathing

Many beliefs about washing and bathing are directly linked to religious beliefs. For Hindus:

> *All aspects of bodily functions and emissions are considered impure and therefore polluting. A Hindu's body must be cleansed before worship if they have had contact with impure things. Running water is a purifying agent and Hindus will wish to wash or shower frequently, especially before prayer.*

(Holland & Hogg 2001, p. 197)

Muslims have similar practices:

> *Washing rituals are an important aspect of Islamic prayer. Before prayer the face, ears and forehead, the feet to the ankles and the hands to the elbows are washed. The nose is cleaned by sniffing up water and the mouth is rinsed out. Private parts of the body are also washed after urination and defecation if this takes place before prayer.* (Holland & Hogg 2001, p. 200)

Box 8.5 Cultural values in personal cleansing and dressing

When you were a child, what were you taught about?
- How often you should bath or shower?
- Washing before meals?
- Washing after using the lavatory?
- Washing after touching certain things?

- Do you prefer a bath, a shower or a strip wash?
- Do you oil your skin after washing?
- Do you bath or shower in the morning, at night or both?
- How often do you change your clothes?
- If you go to the doctor's knowing you might be examined, do you wash and put on clean underwear first?
- After using the lavatory do you clean yourself with paper or with water?
- Do you shave some or all your body hair?
- What assumptions do you make about the cleanliness and washing habits of people whose skin colour, culture or religion is different from yours?

Henley & Schott 1999 Culture, religion and patient care in a multi-ethnic society, p. 117. Age Concern, London.

During illness some cultures allow for changes to normal bathing and washing routines. Some Chinese people may choose to 'wash with a sponge and a bowl of very hot water when they are ill to avoid the possibility of getting chilled' (Henley & Schott 1999, p. 118). This practice is linked to their beliefs about health and illness.

Elimination

As seen in the above examples, there is a link between washing and elimination activities in most cultures with the use of running water being very important. Some hospitals ensure that jugs are available in bathrooms and toilets so that patients can pour water when cleaning themselves. Another important custom to note is the use of the right hand. In many 'South Asian and Muslim cultures the left hand is traditionally used for washing after using the lavatory, the right hand is traditionally used for touching clean things and handling food' (Henley & Schott 1999, p. 121). Positioning of lockers and insertion of intravenous infusions therefore become of vital importance to some patients' personal cleansing and dressing requirements.

Skin care

The importance of understanding the structure and function of the skin has already been discussed. In keeping with this is the need to understand how to care for that skin in relation to cultural needs. Older people, for example, are prone to dry skin and they become vulnerable to damage. Those who have black or dark skin are doubly vulnerable as this type of skin can also be dry 'and may be particularly affected by such things as hard water, cold air, air conditioning, certain drugs and by illness and a consequent poor diet.' (Henley and Schott 1999, p. 121). Oil or moisturiser after washing will help to keep it supple and smooth.

Hair care

There are both religious and social considerations to be taken into account when talking about hair care. Hairstyling is as much about fashion as practicality. Visiting the hairdresser becomes a social event for many men and women, and having one's hair 'done' makes a person feel good about themself. Examples of religious considerations can be seen in Henley & Schott (1999, p. 121) statement, in that:

> *Many Muslim and Orthodox Jewish women keep their hair covered. In some cultures long hair is regarded as a symbol of holiness; devout Sikh men and women, particularly those who have taken amrit (confirmation or initiation ceremony), never cut or shave any body hair. Rastafarian women and men keep their hair covered and never cut it. Orthodox Jewish men may wear side locks and beards and keep their heads covered.*

The head itself is sacred in some religions, for example Hinduism, and should not be touched without asking permission. Some Hindu women also wear a streak of red powder (sindur) on the parting in their hair to indicate their married status. It is important to ask men if they want help to shave. Those with beards can be asked if they want it trimmed, washed or brushed, especially if they are unable to do this themselves. Some Sikh men never shave and their beards have to be 'kept rolled and netted' (Henley & Schott 1999, p. 123).

Clothes

Clothes are also seen as both fashion and cultural statements. The clothing industry, for example, thrives on the social need to look good, whether from self perceptions or from the advice given in fashion magazines and the media. The pressure to conform and spend money on clothes which cannot be afforded can lead to both financial and mental health problems, e.g. credit card debt and stress (Sharpe & Bostcock 2002). Modesty is very important to both men and women in many cultures, an important factor to consider when caring for patients at their most vulnerable. Examples of cultural customs are given in Box 8.6.

Exercise

1. Consider how the society you live in and the culture to which you belong affect how you dress and care for your hair and skin.
2. Identify cultural practices that you have also come across in your place of work.
3. Discuss with colleagues their experiences of ensuring that the sociocultural factors are taken account of when considering the personal cleansing and dressing needs of patients and clients in their care.

Environmental

The environment in which one lives will have a significant impact on personal cleansing and dressing behaviour and needs. Where one lives for example will determine what facilities are available to ensure that these needs can be met. In countries where water is scarce there will be none to spare for washing of selves or clothes, in fact there may not be enough for survival. Having access to an adequate supply of water may not even be possible even in those countries with plenty of water, e.g. if one is homeless or lacks finance to pay the water rates. Lack of finance may also stop people from spending money on clothing and other basic personal cleansing items such as deodorant, shampoo or soap. A choice between food and these items may have to be made and these factors need to be considered when giving advice to patients or clients.

The climate will also influence personal cleansing and dressing behaviour. Living in a hot climate for example may require one to wear light cotton clothing which absorbs perspiration more readily, or if in a very cold climate 'garments made from man-made fibres and wool are useful for providing warmth' (Roper et al 1996, p. 239). Continual exposure to sun though can lead to an increased risk of skin

---

Box 8.6 Cultural customs

Hindu beliefs

Women must cover their legs, breasts and upper arms. They usually wear a sari and the midriff is very often left bare. Some Hindu women may wear a shalwar kameez both during the day and night. Women wear jewellery in the form of bracelets and a brooch known as a mangal sutra, which is strung on a necklace. These must not be removed unnecessarily. Men usually wear a kameez and pajamas (trousers with drawstring) or a dhoti. This is a cloth about 5–6 metres in length that is wrapped around the waist and drawn between the legs. Older men may also wear a long coat (Achkan) or a shirt with a high collar and buttons down the front known as a kurta. Some men may wear a bead necklace or other jewellery of religious significance.

Sikh beliefs

As an act of faith Sikhs wear what is known as the 5 Ks.

- Kesh – long hair. Men wear this in a bun (jura) under a turban. Women may wear plaits and cover their hair with a scarf (dupatta or chuni); Sikh boys will usually wear their hair in a bun on top of their head covered with a small white cloth (rumal) or a large square cloth (patka)
- Kanga – small comb worn at all times
- Kara – steel bracelet worn on right wrist
- Kacha – special type of underwear, white shorts
- Kirpa – symbolic dagger/sword.

Women wear the salwar (trousers) and kameez (shirt) with a long scarf (chuni); the salwar and kameez are worn day and night. They will also wear glass or gold wedding bangles that are never removed unless they are widowed. (Their removal symbolises the loss of a husband.) Men wear a kameez and pajama or kurta (a long shirt with a high collar and buttons down the front).

From Holland & Hogg 2001 Cultural awareness in nursing and health care, p. 198, p. 205. Arnold, London.

---

cancer (Jamison 2001, p. 317), whilst in some skin diseases, e.g. psoriasis, exposure to ultraviolet light is one form of treatment. Uniforms and protective clothing are also encouraged in those work areas where people need to be protected from the physical effects of some activities, e.g. men who work with asbestos or coal dust.

Exercise

Examine your own home and work environments.

1. Consider how they affect your personal cleansing and dressing needs.
2. Compare your own living expectations with those of your colleagues and discuss how cultural needs are also influenced by the environment.

Politicoeconomic

The political factors associated with personal cleansing and dressing needs are those associated with both housing and access to employment and therefore financial remuneration. In some countries even providing adequate shelter is all that is possible, for example following a severe flood or other disaster. We have often seen pleas for clothes and blankets as well as money from aid agencies in order to ensure basic protection from the elements. Economic factors are interlinked with the political, for without adequate funds no government can hope to ensure that their policies with regards to meeting basic needs can be implemented. We can also see the economic cost of failing to prevent some avoidable skin problems when we see the cost to the National Health Service of pressure ulcer development. Collier (2002, p. 927) states that the DoH in 1992 and 1993 reported that the cost to the NHS of pressure ulcers was between £60 million and £321 million. The importance of pressure ulcer prevention to the NHS can be seen in the way that it is one of the eight fundamental aspects of care identified in the *'Essence of Care'* report (DoH 2001b). This offers a set of benchmarking standards, underpinned by an evidence base, to help improve the quality of care in relation to pressure ulcer prevention.

Summary points

---

1. Both personal cleanliness and dressing are affected by our culture, gender, age and environment.
2. Personal cleanliness includes caring for our skin, nails, hair, teeth, mouth and hands.
3. Maintaining privacy and dignity for individuals to carry out personal hygiene and dressing activities is an essential part of health care.

THE MODEL FOR NURSING

In order to enhance your understanding of how health and illness affects this Activity of Living the next section will focus on specific case studies, and will utilise the Roper et al (1996, 2000) model of nursing as a framework to assess, plan, implement and evaluate care. (See Chapter 1 for a full explanation of the nursing process.)

Assessing the individual in the ALs of personal cleansing and dressing

It is important to remember that every individual must be considered 'holistically' and that personal cleansing and dressing will be affected by health problems specific to other Activities of Living. The summary of life span, dependence/independence and factors affecting personal cleansing and dressing can be seen in Box 8.7.

Assessing the individual

Assessment involves three phases:

- collection of data when taking a nursing history
- interpretation of the data collected
- identification of the individual's actual and potential health problems.

Collection of data when taking a nursing history

The nursing history will involve all Activities of Living and, as seen in Chapter 1, all must be taken into account in the holistic assessment of individuals. If patients' expectations are to be understood and their problems (whether actual or potential) with this AL are to be addressed then assessment must be undertaken. A résumé of topics addressed in relation to each of the components of the model is provided in Box 8.7 and will serve as a reminder of the many dimensions of the AL of personal cleansing and dressing which underpin nursing assessment.

Assessment of the ALs of personal cleansing and dressing

When assessing the ALs of personal cleansing and dressing the following questions can be considered, which also take account of the whole life of the individual.

Lifespan

- How old is the person?
- Do they have a life history of health problems?
- Is there anything in their life history that may affect the way in which they view their present health problems?

Dependence/independence

- Has the individual experienced any difficulties in relation to independent living?
- Are they able to go out and meet other people or are they dependent on others to transport them?
- Will they experience difficulties in the future as a result of their current health problems?

Factors affecting the AL of personal cleansing and dressing

- What specific health problem are they suffering from?
- What do they understand about their present health status?
- What effect is this having on their other Activities of Living?
- What effect is their health problem having on their emotional wellbeing?
- Are there any cultural needs to be taken into account prior to assessment?
- Are there any specific spiritual or religious needs that the patient may have?
- Does the individual have any environmental needs, which will affect future care?
- What resources could be required to help the individual manage their health problems both in hospital and at home?

Box 8.7 Assessing the individual in the AL of personal cleansing and dressing

Lifespan: effect on personal cleansing and dressing

Infancy
- skin care (incontinent state)
- suitable clothing for mobility/safety
- growth of teeth

Childhood
- developing independence and individuality
- developing concept of modesty
- importance of care of teeth

Adolescence
- increased underarm perspiration
- problems of acne, greasy hair, dandruff
- expression of feelings/individuality/sexuality through clothes, make-up, hairstyle
- puberty (menstruation/ejaculation)

Adulthood
- routines related to working and playing
- reflection of personality in appearance and clothes

Old age
- skin dryness
- difficulties with bathing, care of nails and feet
- difficulties with dressing
- physical disability

Dependence/independence in personal cleansing and dressing
- dependency in infancy/old age/illness
  - on people
  - on aids and equipment

Factors influencing personal cleansing and dressing

Biological
- stage of physical development
- physical changes with ageing
- individual physical differences
- skin state colours bruising/scars/blemishes/dry/moist/ turgid/wrinkled areas of discontinuity cleanliness
- state of hands and nails cleanliness
- hand washing habits

- state of mouth and teeth
- moist dry mouth
- odour of breath
- teeth (number/condition/dentures)
- teeth cleaning routine
- condition/style of hair/type (dry/greasy dandruff/lice/ hair washing routine)
- dress style/appropriateness
- standard of cleanliness/odour/quality
- speciality clothing for work and play
- physical hazards
- physical sex differences
  female – perineal toilet, breast care
      – menstruation, body hair
  male   – cleansing foreskin, shaving

Psychological
- sex differences/sexuality
- standards related to personality/emotional states
- knowledge (e.g. hand washing, dental care)
- intelligence

Sociocultural
- values concerning cleanliness/appearance
- social norms for cleansing/dressing routines
- cultural influences/rules on dress
- religious influences/rules on cleansing, dressing

Environmental
- bath/shower in the home
- piped hot/cold water in home
- exposure at work to substances damaging to the skin
- availability of bathing/hand washing facilities at work
- climate

Politicoeconomic
- adequacy of necessary facilities for low income groups
- personal income for articles for personal cleanliness
- personal income for essential clothing and footwear

From Roper et al 1996 The Elements of Nursing. Churchill Livingstone, Edinburgh

Exercise
1. Reflect on how you have assessed patients' personal cleansing and dressing needs in your practice.
2. Did you use a similar set of questions and a model for nursing?
3. Discuss with your mentor or preceptor how you intend to assess individual patient's personal cleansing and dressing needs by using the Roper et al model for nursing framework and the above questions.

Consider the following case study and using the same approach consider which questions would be appropriate in the assessment of the patient's needs. Given the sensitive nature of her health problem these questions will have to be asked, as with all questioning and all patients, sensitively and with understanding.

Assessment focusing on the ALs of personal cleansing and dressing

A girl, aged 16, attends the Dermatology Clinic in the Outpatient Department for her second appointment. Her GP had diagnosed psoriasis and had referred her to the Consultant at the hospital for further tests and treatment. She is to be seen by both the Consultant and the Specialist Dermatology Nurse. As the Clinic Nurse on the day of her appointment you are required to undertake the initial assessment and history. She is accompanied by her mother.

The following questions might have been asked in relation to the ALs.

Questions as part of the assessment
- When did she first notice the patches of psoriasis?
- Where are the largest ones?
- Do they cause her any irritation?
- Has she been scratching them?
- Has she noticed any scalp irritation or flaky dandruff?
- Has she noticed any flaking of her skin in the bed or on her clothes?
- How does she feel about this?

Box 8.8 Problems reported by patients with skin disorders

Emotional problems
- low self-esteem
- feel body is 'unclean'
- relationships can be problematic
- feel people stare – real and imagined
- regarded as infectious or contagious.

Clothing restrictions
- avoid short sleeves
- avoid dark clothes due to skin shedding
- avoid summer clothes where skin is exposed
- clothes get stained or ruined due to messy creams.

Social restrictions
- skin gets itchy in hot pubs/clubs
- avoid swimming or sports as people stare
- avoid communal changing rooms when shopping.

Financial implications
- routine prescriptions are expensive but essential
- no allowances to replace clothing or bedding
- no allowances available for fuel bills due to extra laundering and bathing, etc.

From: Docherty & Hodgson 2000 Skin Disorders. In: Alexander et al (eds) Nursing Practice – Hospital and Home (The Adult). Churchill Livingstone, Edinburgh, p 475.

- Do any of her clothes make the irritation worse?
- Does swimming make her skin more or less irritable?
- Has she any painful lesions anywhere?
- Has any member of her family the same or similar problem?

Other questions that the nurse or doctor may ask include:

- Has she had a throat infection recently?
- Has she found that being in the sun makes the problem better or worse?
- Has she found that the problem gets worse during menstruation?

The responses to the above questions may also give an indication of how she has been dealing psychologically with the appearance of this skin condition, as well as whether she has been trying to hide lesions which have appeared on her arms and legs (by wearing long sleeve shirts and not going bathing). Assessment may also reveal other problems reported by patients with skin disorders (see Box 8.8).

The following information may be helpful for your assessment of this young girl's needs and also to understand the relevance and importance of some of the questions.

Psoriasis

Psoriasis is a skin disease that causes much psychological distress, mainly because of its appearance and the side effects of some of the treatments. It is a 'chronic, non infectious inflammatory skin disorder, characterised by well demarcated erythematous plaques with adherent silver scales' (Docherty & Hodgson 2000, p. 472). In psoriasis there is an increased production of epidermal cells that do not have time to keratinise completely. This causes 'the build-up of a white waxy silver scale as immature skin cells remain adherent to the skin' (Docherty & Hodgson 2000, p. 472). There is a genetic predisposition to the disease and it occurs in 2% of the UK population. The precipitating factors can be seen in Box 8.9.

Box 8.9 Precipitating factors in psoriasis

- infection – streptococcal throat infection
- drugs – can exacerbate or trigger psoriasis
- sunlight – in some patients, psoriasis improves during the summer and relapses during the winter; however others report that sunlight aggravates the condition
- hormonal – psoriasis can get better or worse during pregnancy
- psychological stress – can exacerbate psoriasis but the condition itself is recognised as a stressful condition
- trauma – creates the 'Koebner effect' where psoriasis is triggered in damaged skin, e.g. surgical scar.

From Docherty & Hodgson 2000 Skin Disorders. In: Alexander et al (eds) Nursing Practice – Hospital and Home (The Adult). Churchill Livingstone, Edinburgh, p. 473.

The link can now begin to be seen between the questions asked at assessment, the underlying physiological changes and precipitating factors. The consultant will then make a diagnosis as to which type of psoriasis she has and the subsequent treatment, which could contribute to further psychological stress. Treatments could include coal tar products, which are messy, smelly and can stain clothes, dithranol (suppresses cell proliferation) which if applied to the skin also stains the skin and clothing and emollients to lubricate and moisturise the skin. Other treatments will depend on the precipitating cause and the type of psoriasis (see Box 8.10). It can be seen from the questions asked at the initial assessment how important it is for the nurse to know not only the nature and cause of the skin condition but also the normal and abnormal physiological responses of the body. Understanding these will enable the nurse to offer support during the subsequent treatment of the patient, in particular when it comes to personal cleansing and dressing activities such as which clothes she might find more comfortable to wear and how she will cope with the possible staining of them by skin preparations. The condition as can be seen is one that has exacerbations and remissions and is unlikely to go away entirely. She will have to live with its presence for the rest of her life and learn how to cope with its visual and systemic appearance.

Undertaking a health history is therefore an essential part of any nursing assessment, and an understanding of the elements of the nursing model that comprise the living aspects will enable you to ensure that the questions directly affecting this young girl will be relevant. However what is not possible within this example is to identify how her other Activities of Living are affected by what is happening due to the fact that we have no further information about her life and health. If it does indicate that she has psoriasis then it can only be surmised at how her life could be affected.

For example, her symptoms may prevent her from going out socially with her friends as she may worry about her skin appearance and wearing the clothes that she would have normally gone out in, e.g. short sleeve shirts (working and playing). Understanding the physiological factors affecting psoriasis will enable you to explain to her why she has the skin problems; understanding about the psychological

---

Box 8.10 Classification of psoriasis

Guttae psoriasis
Presents as drop-like symmetrical lesions on the trunk and the limbs. It is most common in adolescents and young adults and is often triggered by a streptococcal throat infection. It responds well to therapy.

Plaque psoriasis
Presents as well demarcated erythematous plaques covered in dry, white-waxy scale often localised to the knees and elbows. Removal of this build up of keratin leaves small bleeding points. Plaques vary considerably in size and can extend to cover the trunk and scalp. Plaque psoriasis tends to be chronic with exacerbations and remissions.

Flexural psoriasis
Affects the axillae, submammary and anogenital areas and looks different from typical psoriasis. Plaques are sharply defined but the skin has a thin glistening redness, often with painful fissures in the skin folds.

Pustular psoriasis (palmoplantar putulosis)
Localised form of psoriasis affecting the hands and feet. It is characterised by yellow/brown pustules which dry into brown scaly macules. It is a painful and difficult condition to treat.

Generalised pustular psoriasis
Rare and serious form of the disease. Sheets of sterile pustules develop, merging on an erythematous background. These areas of skin shear and the patient will be unwell. It is often triggered when attempts are made to withdraw oral or topical steroids or may just reflect the instability of the condition.

Scalp psoriasis
Can often be the sole manifestation of the disorder. Thick scale adheres to the scalp and can extend to the edges of the scalp margin and behind the ears.

Nail changes
In psoriasis can involve pitting of nails and onycholysis when the distal edge of the nail separates from the nail bed. Treatment is difficult and unsatisfactory.

Erythrodermic psoriasis
Rare but severe form. The skin becomes uniformly red with a high blood volume flushing it. The patient feels unwell and temperature control is difficult. It can be triggered by the irritant effects of therapies (e.g. dithranol, tars) by withdrawal of systemic/oral steroids or by a drug reaction. Erythrodermic psoriasis is an unstable state that is potentially life threatening and warrants urgent hospital admission. The condition can progress to general pustular psoriasis.

Psoriatic arthropathy
Psoriasis can be complicated by psoriatic arthropathy. Psoriatic joint disease occurs in about 5% of psoriasis patients. Joint changes occur in hands, feet, spine and sacroiliac joints. Rheumatoid factor tests are negative. Psoriatic arthropathy is a difficult combination to treat, meriting the combined expertise of a rheumatologist and dermatologist.

From Docherty & Hodgson 2000 Skin disorders. In: Alexander et al (eds) Nursing Practice – Hospital and Home (Adult), p. 473. Churchill Livingstone, Edinburgh.

factors will enable you to give her support to cope with having a skin disease. To be able to explain and offer effective support however will require the nurse to have, and be able to use, good communication skills (see Chapter 4).

Exercise

1. Given the information about the girl's health problem and taking into account the abnormal physiology and types of psoriasis, how would you advise her and her mother about how to manage the condition in the short term and long term?

2. Find current research on the care of patients with psoriasis and other skin conditions you have come across in order to ensure that your practice is evidence based.

Summary points

1. Personal cleansing and dressing is affected by life-span, dependence–independence and biological, psychological, sociocultural, environmental and politicoeconomic factors.

2. Assessment of a patient/client in the daily activity of personal cleansing and dressing needs to be holistic.

3. Sensitive questioning and a knowledge of normal physiology is essential in caring for patients with health problems such as skin disorders which affect personal cleansing and dressing activities.

APPLICATION OF THE ROPER, LOGAN AND TIERNEY MODEL IN PRACTICE

Using all the information in the previous sections of this chapter we will now explore how the model can be used in the care of two patients who have a health problem that affects their personal cleansing and dressing needs (see Case studies 8.2 and 8.3).

Case study 8.2

Focus on health problem in the ALs of personal cleansing and dressing

An evidence-based total care approach

Mrs Joan Wells, an 84-year-old lady, is admitted to hospital with pneumonia.

Case study 8.2 (continued)

Health history

She has a daughter living in Canada and a son living in America, and lives on her own. Her husband Bob had died 5 years previously. She is normally a very physically and socially active healthy person but since she had a fall the previous month she has been unable to look after herself as normal. She had not required hospitalisation but it had made her lose confidence and reduced her mobility. She has been feeling very depressed and has neglected herself. Her present illness has increased this feeling. Her neighbour called the doctor's surgery when she had not seen her for a week and she would not answer the door. Her son and daughter had also contacted her when their mother had not made contact with them as she normally did once a week. When the district nurse and General Practitioner (GP) arrived they were also unable to get a response and the police had to be called to break down the door. They found Mrs Wells in her bed, looking very ill and she was obviously dehydrated. (Her eyes appear sunken and her skin has lost its natural elasticity and is 'wrinkled' in appearance.) Her mouth was encrusted with sores and she had been incontinent of both urine and faeces – due to not having the strength to get out of bed to go to the toilet. She is also slightly confused and it is apparent that she has not been eating either. Her neighbour was also upset to see her in such a mess as she was normally a very fastidious lady and kept herself and her house very clean. The GP decides that she needs admitting to hospital for care and treatment of both the bronchopneumonia and related health problems.

On admission

Mrs Wells is admitted to the ward directly from home following the GP referral and has clearly been unable to maintain her own personal cleansing and dressing needs. Her neighbour has arrived with her and has agreed to contact Mrs Wells' son and daughter regarding their mother, once it has been decided on the course of treatment and care plan. Mrs Wells appears to be confused and cannot remember what has happened to her. She is visibly distressed when she is admitted to the ward.

Exercise

Before assessing her needs on admission identify what issues would need to be considered in relation to:

- lifespan
- dependence/independence
- factors affecting personal cleansing and dressing.

Refer to earlier in this chapter for examples.

You may have considered the following.

Lifespan

Mrs Wells is an older person, and like all patients, requires her personal dignity and modesty to be considered. However, as we can see in the Nursing and Midwifery Advisory Committee Report – *Caring for Older People: a Nursing Priority* (DoH 2001c) – negative attitudes to older people in the acute care sector generally have influenced the way in which nurses ensure this essential care is undertaken. Mrs Wells is very ill with pneumonia and as an older person is more vulnerable to its effects. As a result she has been unable to maintain her normal standards of personal cleansing and dressing. Acknowledgement of her age and her normal capabilities will be vital in restoring her dignity.

Dependence/independence

As seen in the brief profile of Mrs Wells, her neighbour has informed us that she is normally a very active lady who lives on her own. It will be important to determine during the assessment, her normal pattern of independent living and, in preparation for her discharge home from hospital, how she is going to manage during her recuperation from her current illness. She appears to have the support of her neighbour but her immediate family is not available. The way in which she recovers from her present illness will also affect her situation in the future, as it is apparent that her recent depression has contributed to the deterioration in her general health.

Factors affecting personal cleansing and dressing

As we get older there are many physiological changes that occur in our bodies all of which will have an effect on our response to illness. It can be seen that, due to her fall, Mrs Wells has been unable to be as mobile as she is normally. She was fortunate that she had not sustained a fracture, given that osteoporosis is a common occurrence in older women (see Chapter 10).

It can also be seen from the brief health history that the depression that affected Mrs Wells following her fall had contributed to her current state of ill health. Her normal independence was compromised by this. This feeling of isolation can in turn lead to loss of confidence and 'self-worth'. Mrs Wells' son and daughter also live abroad and therefore are unable to offer their immediate support. It is apparent that they are however in regular contact with their mother and have been concerned that she has not been in communication with them. This lack of immediate support from her son and daughter will be crucial when nurses are planning for her discharge home from hospital, as it will mean that Mrs Wells will need to probably rely on the health and social services for her future support. If she owns her own home and has savings it may also mean that she will

have to contribute to her own care. Her home environment will also be a contributing factor in her aftercare – in particular how easy it is for her to use toilet and bathroom facilities, especially as it appears that she has been unable to do so during her prehospital admission. All these factors will influence the assessment of her needs in all areas of her normal living activities.

Exercise
1. Consider Mrs Wells' health history and identify the health and social care services that she may need as support following discharge from hospital.
2. Design a health promotion plan for an older person in a similar situation to Mrs Wells.

Assessment of needs

Using this knowledge of her background and potential influencing factors assess Mrs Wells' individual needs on admission to hospital. Use the questions on p. 243 as a guide.

Collection of data on admission

As well as gathering information from Mrs Wells herself, her neighbour and her GP will also have a contribution to make. It is also pertinent to note that all data obtained concerning Mrs Wells and her care will need to be documented in her medical notes and her nursing care plans. You may work in an environment that has integrated care pathways, in which case the multidisciplinary team will be responsible for documenting care and treatment planned and implemented (see Chapter 1 for further details on care plans).

Assessment of Mrs Wells' actual problems on admission to the ward: using the model for nursing as a framework

Ensuring a safe environment in which to carry out the initial assessment of Mrs Wells' needs will be an important aspect of the nurse's role. It is also important to remember that she is very ill and may be unable to answer questions in the immediate postadmission period. Some details will be essential in order to plan her immediate care but other data can be gathered over the following 48-hour period. Using the questions on p. 243 and her preadmission history we can see that some details have already been obtained from her neighbour, the GP and the district nurse. These are:

- *Lifespan:* she is 84 years old; she is normally a very active healthy person.
- *Independence/dependence:* she has been independent until her minor fall when she appears to have lost her confidence, become depressed and neglected herself to the point that she is now dependent on the health care team.
- *Factors affecting the AL of personal cleansing and dressing:* she has pneumonia which has affected her

ability to care for herself and she has become incontinent of both urine and faeces; it is her previous minor fall that affected her emotional wellbeing initially; we are not aware of her religious nor spiritual beliefs at this stage nor her own health beliefs; as she currently lives on her own, there will be resources, both physical and human that she will require during her stay in hospital and in preparation for her future discharge from hospital.

Based on this initial information an assessment of her needs at various stages of care will now be explored using an evidence-based approach (see Chapter 2). It will be seen that problems in one Activity of Living cannot be easily separated from others, in that each activity is directly linked to another (see Chapter 1 for further information).

Activities of Living: an evidence-based approach
Personal cleansing and dressing

Given that Mrs Wells is seriously ill and has neglected herself as a result of this and her depression, it can be seen that she is unable to care for her own personal cleansing and dressing needs. As she normally did so she will probably be very distressed that she is now dependent on others to manage this for her. An assessment of her tissue breakdown risk also needs to be undertaken as she has been doubly incontinent and her skin integrity is therefore at risk. She has mouth sores and will need mouth care and hygiene. Older people such as Mrs Wells are at a higher risk of developing pressure sores especially if they are also undernourished and incontinent. The nurse may decide to use one of several risk assessment scoring systems available, ensuring that reassessment is undertaken at identified intervals following admission. Bale (2000) argues that 'it is only useful if it is used regularly'. Assessing risk on admission is essential also to ensuring that Mrs Wells has the correct mattress and other pressure-relieving devices as part of her care plan.

Actual problem Mrs Wells is unable to manage her own personal cleansing and dressing activities. She is also at risk from developing pressure sores.

Communication

From the health history it can be seen that Mrs Wells is probably very depressed and may well have withdrawn from communicating with her friends and neighbour. She is normally in contact with her children but has failed to communicate with them recently due to her illness and its consequences. She is also confused on admission, possibly due to the dehydration. This makes it difficult for the nurse admitting her to obtain informed consent to any treatment or care she may require at this stage. The doctor may talk to her next of kin if Mrs Wells continues to be confused and unable to make decisions about her own care. However, the Department of Health (2001d, p. 9), in their publication, *Seeking consent: working with older people*, point out that:

> *If a person is not capable of giving or refusing consent it is still possible for you lawfully to provide treatment and care, unless such care has been validly refused in advance. However this treatment or care must be in the person's 'best interests'.*
>
> *No one (not even a spouse or others close to the person) can give consent on behalf of adults who are not capable of giving consent for themselves. However those close to the incapacitated person should always be involved in decision-making, unless the older person has earlier made it clear that they don't want such involvement. Although legally the health professional responsible for the person's care is responsible for deciding whether or not particular treatment is in that person's best interests, ideally decisions will reflect an agreement between professional carers and those close to the older person.*

Farmer (2000) points out that it is important for confusion to be correctly defined and that causes are many in older people. Treatment will depend on the cause, as in Mrs Wells' situation that has arisen because of her dehydration and her respiratory infection.

Actual problem She is unable to communicate why she has been admitted to hospital. She is unable to articulate her understanding of what is happening to her and to give her informed consent.

Working and playing

According to her neighbour Mrs Wells is normally a very active and healthy lady. However since her fall and her depression she has withdrawn from her normal social activity. This is quite a normal occurrence for someone of her age. The Department of Health Report on caring for older people in acute care areas (DoH 2001c) stresses the importance of assessing the mental health needs of older people and points out that 'older people often (35%) present with co-morbidity of physical and mental problems, most commonly dementia and depression'. They identified a set of standard statements and indicators which could guide nurses in their attempts to ensure that mental health needs were assessed (see Box 8.11).

Actual problem She is unable to undertake her normal social activities.

Expressing sexuality

It is known that Mrs Wells was normally a very fastidious lady, taking pride in herself and her home. She was also very socially and physically active. Her present illness has led to her neglecting her normal personal cleansing and dressing behaviour which would normally enhance her wellbeing and her self-image. She may also be worried about her future and how she is going to cope with caring for herself as she gets older and less able to deal with illness. According to Rutter (2000, p. 204) this is quite often a normal response to coping with the effects of old age.

Box 8.11 Standards in specific clinical aspects of care: mental health needs

Standard statement

The older person's mental health needs form an important part of nursing assessment and care planning, as part of the multidisciplinary approach to care during the acute phase of illness.

Criteria

1. Nursing assessments take account of the older person's mental health status and needs and these are translated into nursing care plans.
2. Nurses work in partnership with other members of the multidisciplinary team to meet the older person's mental health needs.

Indicators

Examples of indicators in each criteria are given below:

1. (i) Local guidance is available on assessment appropriate to the mental health needs of the older person.

This recognises that the person has a biography and that psychological aspects of care are an integral part of assessment in general.

(ii) Nursing staff are aware of local specialist mental health colleagues (e.g. liaison nurse, community psychiatric nurse, dementia care specialist) to whom they refer older people for further assessment and advice.

2. (i) A nurse on each ward or unit is designated to act as a contact point in respect of the mental health needs of the older person and to liaise with other members of the multidisciplinary team and specialists.

(ii) Specialist advice on the mental health needs of the older person is available on the ward/unit.

From Practice Guidance: Principles and Standards and Indicators – a resource tool. Caring for Older People: a nursing priority (Standing Nursing and Midwifery Advisory Committee, DoH 2001c).

In relation to sexual activity (people are sexual beings – see Chapter 12) it is not known if Mrs Wells is still sexually active and this is not immediately relevant to her care. However it cannot be assumed that she has not been sexually active prior to her illness. Roper et al (1996, p. 345) point out that 'although sexual activity generally decreases with age, many older adults continue to be sexually active and human beings do not cease to be sexual beings in old age'. This knowledge would be of value in her post-illness rehabilitation and would possibly be discovered as part of the ongoing care of Mrs Wells. She may, however, decide not to disclose this kind of personal information and that is her right.

Actual problem Mrs Wells has lost interest in her self and her self-image.

Dying

Mrs Wells is seriously ill with pneumonia. She is also suffering from depression and confusion on admission to hospital. She may also have memories of her husband dying in a hospital environment and this may have increased her awareness of her own vulnerability. Roper et al (1996, p. 402) point out that 'for the elderly there is a constant realisation that they are approaching the end of the lifespan and they are made aware of this by an increasing number of deaths in their peer group'. Her religion may also be important to her but because of her confusion and distress this type of information can be obtained at a later time when her condition is improved. She may express her fears of dying to the nurse.

Actual problem Mrs Wells is seriously ill.

Elimination

Mrs Wells has been incontinent of both urine and faeces due to her illness and lack of mobility. This is not normal behaviour for her. On admission the nurse needs to determine the extent of her problem and once the patient is made comfortable offer an opportunity for Mrs Wells to use either a bedpan or commode as soon as possible. The nurse needs to assess her level of confusion at the same time to see whether she is capable of asking for help to go to the toilet. Her skin may already have started to break down. Nurses caring for older people in acute care areas may wish to refer to the published *Practice Guidance: Principles, Standards and Indicators* (Department of Health 2001e) on continence care to support their assessment and subsequent care of patients such as Mrs Wells. These standards are part of a resource tool developed as a result of the findings of the Nursing and Midwifery Advisory Committee report: *Caring for Older People: a Nursing Priority* (Department of Health 2001c, p. iii) which reported that there were 'major deficits in the standards of nursing care given to older patients in acute hospitals, with some of their most fundamental needs remaining unmet' (see Box 8.12 for standards recommended and Chapter 7).

Actual problem Mrs Wells is incontinent of urine and faeces on admission.

Eating and drinking

As Mrs Wells has been unable to care for herself due to her illness and poor mobility she has obviously not been eating and drinking as normal. She has become dehydrated. It will be important for the nurse to determine as soon as possible following admission what her food and drink preferences

Box 8.12 Standards in specific clinical aspects of care: continence

Standard statement

Continence forms an important part of nursing assessment and care planning in relation to the older person. The subject is handled with sensitivity by the nursing staff.

Criteria

1. Nursing assessments take account of the older person's previous, current and desired continence status and health needs and these are translated into nursing care plans.
2. Nurses work in partnership with other members of the multidisciplinary team to meet the older person's continence needs.

Indicators

Examples of indicators for each of the criteria are given below. See also *Good Practice in Continence Services* (DoH April 2000b).

1. (i) A continence assessment is carried out as part of the initial nursing assessment. While the nurse may use a checklist to ensure that the relevant subjects are covered, this is used discreetly with recognition that many older people may find the subject in general a very embarrassing one. Time and as much privacy as possible are allowed for the assessment, to go at the older person's pace and put them at their ease.

   Examples of subjects to be covered include:

   a. current difficulties with continence and nature of difficulty
   b. any accompanying symptoms, e.g. burning, itching or pressure

   c. relevant past medical/surgical history
   d. possibly related areas such as use of medications
   e. activities of daily living: ability to reach and/or find a toilet, finger and wrist dexterity (affecting management of clothing)
   f. usual bowel movement pattern
   g. any recent changes in bowel movement patterns, e.g. constipation or diarrhoea.

   (ii) Where a problem is discovered, a management and treatment plan is started. The named nurse or their substitute acts in an advocacy role for the older person, ensuring that the older person has an explanation of this plan. The nurse introduces the subject sensitively and tactfully, taking time to explain it to the older person and to discuss any psychological issues.

2. (i) A nurse on each ward or unit is designated to act as a contact point in respect of continence care and to liaise with other members of the multidisciplinary team and specialists (e.g. a urologist) about the continence service they provide to older people. The service is reviewed regularly.

   (ii) All nurses are knowledgeable and skilled in the management and promotion of continence and promotion of continence and the continence service provided to older people.

From the Practice Guidance: Principles, Standards and Indicators – a resource tool – Caring for Older People: a nursing priority, DoH 2001e).

---

are, in order to ensure that when she has recovered from the pneumonia her dietary needs are met. What people eat is very often linked to their age and their culture (Department of Health 2001e). Mrs Wells will probably need an intravenous infusion of fluid in order to ensure that her immediate needs are met, which will also improve her confusion if it has been caused by an associated sodium imbalance (Gobbi 2000). An effective assessment of her eating and drinking needs will be key to her recovery. (See Box 8.13 for recommendations and standards of care for older people's nutrition and hydration needs.)

Actual problem Mrs Wells is dehydrated and malnourished.

Maintaining a safe environment

As it is known that Mrs Wells had a minor fall before her present illness and it was a contributing factor in her inability to look after herself, an assessment of how this will put her safety at risk in hospital will be essential. A nursing care plan will need to be devised which will ensure that her need

for independence is taken into account but that this is gradually achieved over time as her illness and her self-esteem improve. She will clearly need to be dependent on the nurses and others until her strength is improved and this will mean ensuring her external and internal environments are safe (see Chapter 1).

Actual problem She is unable to maintain her own safe environment.

Breathing

Mrs Wells has bronchopneumonia (see Box 8.14). She will have difficulty breathing properly and may already have been given oxygen prior to her admission. (See Chapter 3 – Breathing, for details of the normal physiology.) This is also the main cause of her inability to care for herself and her personal cleansing and dressing needs, which are significant considering that she is incontinent of urine and faeces and she will also be sweating due to the pyrexia associated with such an illness.

Box 8.13 Standards in specific clinical aspects of care: nutrition and hydration

Standard statement

The older person's nutritional needs, including hydration, form an important part of nursing assessment and care planning, as part of the multidisciplinary approach to dietary care during the acute phase of illness.

Criteria

1. There is evidence that nursing assessments take account of the older person's physical, cultural and individual preferences when considering nutritional status.
2. Nurses work in partnership with others to meet the nutritional needs of the older person. This includes clinical and nonclinical support staff and involves input from carers, where indicated. It also includes working in direct partnership with the older person.

Indicators

Examples of indicators for each criterion are given below.

1. (i) All older people are screened on admission by nurses to determine their nutritional 'risk' status, using evidence-based protocol. Screening of individual people for past and/or potential difficulties in eating and drinking is also undertaken. This screening needs to include aspects such as:

   a. height and weight
   b. recent weight loss
   c. reduced appetite
   d. eating and digestive difficulties
   e. excessive weakness, apathy, fatigue
   f. other risk factors – infection, recent surgery, radiotherapy, pain
   g. cultural or religious eating habits and taboos.

   (ii) If risk is identified, a dietary care plan is devised with appropriate members of the multidisciplinary team to ensure that older people receive adequate nutrition and hydration. This includes physical assistance with eating and drinking. Nursing staff will ensure that this is provided.

2. (i) A nurse on each ward or unit is designated to act as a contact point in respect of dietary care and to liaise with clinical and nonclinical staff involved in dietary care to review the nutritional service to individual people and to the ward/unit as a whole.

   (ii) All nurses are knowledgeable and skilled in the management and promotion of good dietary care in the context of religious and cultural practices and the dietary care service provided to older people.

From Practice Guidance: Principles, Standards and Indicators – a resource tool, Caring for Older People: a nursing priority (Standing Nursing and Midwifery Advisory Committee, DoH, March 2001e).

Box 8.14 Bronchopneumonia

Pathophysiology

Bronchopneumonia is characterised mainly by patchy areas of consolidated lung tissues. Causative organisms are bacterial and fungal and include staphylococci, pneumococci, streptococci, *Haemophilus influenzae* and Candida. It usually occurs in individuals weakened by other conditions and often in the very old, the very young, and the unconscious and as a result of a pre-existing disease, such as chronic bronchitis, atelectasis or carcinoma in adults or infectious diseases in infants.

Clinical features

These vary in severity depending on the overall condition of the patient but include varying degrees of pyrexia, cough with copious purulent sputum, exhalatory rales, dyspnoea and tachypnoea. Consolidation of the lower lobes is found on auscultation.

Medical management

The causative organism is isolated by sputum culture and sensitivity and appropriate antibiotic therapies are commenced. The patient's general condition is improved by attention to nutrition, hydration and physiotherapy.

Nursing priorities and management

The patient with bronchopneumonia will be very ill and she and her family will need a great deal of comfort and reassurance. Attention to personal hygiene and physical comfort is important. The patient should be turned or encouraged to move regularly. A sitting position, where possible, will make breathing easier and, if oxygen is prescribed, this therapy should be monitored carefully. Aids to prevent pressure sores developing should be selected judiciously.

Bronchopneumonia can be prevented in many hospitalised high-risk patients by thorough nursing assessment and meticulous nursing care.

From Edmond CB (2000) The Respiratory System. In: Alexander et al Nursing Practice – Hospital and Home, 2nd edn, pp 59–86. Churchill Livingstone, Edinburgh.

Actual problem Mrs Wells is having difficulty breathing due to the bronchopneumonia.

Mobilising

Due to the fall she has been unable to be as mobile as she normally is – she is therefore at risk of further falls and immobility. Assessment of her mobility capability will need to be undertaken in order to ensure her safety and also any rehabilitation needs she may have. Her illness will also prevent her from being as mobile and she will probably be dependent on the nurses for many activities, including maintaining her own personal cleansing and dressing needs, until she has recovered. An assessment by the physiotherapist will be essential in order to identify her capability for movement and determine a plan for her physical rehabilitation. At some point an assessment with the occupational therapist will be necessary, in order to determine how she will manage when she is discharged and if she may require aids to help her with her personal cleansing and dressing needs, e.g. bathroom aids such as handles for getting in and out of the bath. As she lives on her own and has been unable to look after herself, it will be essential that an agreement is reached with her and her family prior to her being discharged home as to how her aftercare will be managed. Her immediate family live some distance away.

Actual problem Mrs Wells is unable to mobilise by herself.

Controlling body temperature

The pneumonia will mean she is pyrexial in the early stages of the illness. Observations of her temperature and pulse on admission should reveal the extent of this. As seen in Box 8.14, personal hygiene will be essential to her wellbeing, especially as she will be sweating as a result of the pyrexia (see Chapter 9).

Actual problem Mrs Wells is pyrexial.

Sleeping

Given her health history it is not difficult to imagine that Mrs Wells has been having difficulty sleeping. Older people need less sleep than younger ones (Closs 2000) and anxiety and depression together with physical illness will exacerbate this (see Chapter 13).

Actual problem Mrs Wells may have difficulty in sleeping due to anxiety, depression and breathing difficulties.

Conclusion

Caring for Mrs Wells will require a plan that incorporates every Activity of Living. We can see clearly the difficulties in trying to tease apart the effects of her illness and other predisposing factors. Mrs Wells is a unique individual who has to be seen as a whole person, taking account of the fact that a model for nursing used in the assessment process is there to guide the nurse in ensuring that all her needs are taken into account in the planning, implementing and evaluating stages of her care.

Exercise

Based on the above assessment and an evidence base, plan Mrs Wells' care for the duration of her stay in hospital, with particular reference to her personal cleansing and dressing needs. Refer to Chapter 1 for goal setting and evaluation of care.

Summary points

1. An understanding of the ageing process is essential for assessing the personal cleansing and dressing needs of the older person.
2. Health problems affecting the ALs of personal cleansing and dressing can be seen to be interdependent on other Activities of Living.
3. Effective discharge planning and outcome begin as soon as the patient is admitted to hospital.

Case study 8.3

Health problem in the AL of personal cleansing and dressing

This case study focuses on a health problem not directly connected to ALs of personal cleansing and dressing, but one which has major implications for assessment of need in relation to the individual's specific personal cleansing and dressing functioning.

Mr John Upton a 42-year-old married man is admitted to an orthopaedic ward for amputation of both legs following a car accident in which he sustained a crush injury to both his legs.

Health history

Mr Upton is a self-employed director of his own clothing company. His 38-year-old wife works for him as a fashion buyer and they have two children – boys aged 10 and 15 years. They had just returned from their annual holiday to their villa in the south of France when the accident happened. He plays football for a local team and keeps fit at the sports centre. His work involves meeting different people and he always ensures that his company is promoted by the smart clothes he wears, in particular his sports range and business suits. He is a very social person and enjoys going out with his wife and family for meals and other social events. The family live in a large five bedroomed house with a large garden. He was travelling home from a business appointment when the accident happened. An articulated lorry went out of control on the motorway and hit a number of vehicles. Mr Upton unfortunately became trapped in his vehicle during the 'pile up'.

He has been made aware of the extent of the surgery undertaken to save his life. An above-knee amputation was necessary on both legs.

The following may have been considered:

- knowledge of the anatomy and physiology of the lower limbs, including the blood and nerve supply
- knowledge of what happens during surgery, i.e. the procedure for amputation
- current evidence-based practice for caring for patients who have had amputations
- current medication and treatment for bilateral amputations
- knowledge of care from admission to discharge home and follow-up rehabilitation programmes.

Factors affecting personal cleansing and dressing following bilateral amputation

For any patient removal, or partial removal, of two of their limbs will be a traumatic experience. Mr Upton however has not had the opportunity to be prepared for this eventuality and will therefore require additional support following surgery (Jamieson et al 2000). Consider the issues in relation to postoperative care of a patient, who has been prepared for the eventuality, following amputation of a lower limb (see Box 8.15).

In relation to Point 1 the following have been considered:

- Mr Upton has not been prepared for the surgery.
- He has had two lower limbs amputated at the same time.
- He is severely shocked due to the trauma of the accident and the emergency surgery.
- Mobility will be difficult as he has had two lower limbs amputated.

In relation to Point 2 the following have been considered:

- Mr Upton has been a physically active man who has taken an interest in his own dressing requirements, partly as a result of his own clothing business. He has probably enjoyed swimming as well as playing football and playing with his children. This has now come to an end for the time being, as he is no longer able to stand nor undertake any of the physical activities he was capable of. As we can see in Box 8.15 he will need to adapt his clothing to take account of the fact that until he has his prostheses fitted he will be unable to walk and will be confined to a wheelchair. The clothes that he

---

Box 8.15 Caring for a patient following amputation of a lower limb

Mobilisation

The patient will normally sit out of bed within 12 hours of surgery and may use a wheelchair initially to assist with mobilisation. Practice in standing, and transferring from bed to chair and from wheelchair to toilet will be given. This increases the patient's independence and improves their morale. The physiotherapist will supervise walking. The patient may find that their sense of balance has been temporarily altered, but with advice and support this problem will be overcome.

Clothing

The patients' clothing may need to be adapted temporarily until the prosthesis is supplied. The tucking of an empty arm of a jacket or the leg of a pair of trousers into the body of the garment is an apparent detail but failure to do this can often be the last straw for a patient who until then, has been coping well.

Promoting independence

The patient should be taught how to care for the stump once the sutures are removed by maintaining skin hygiene, moisturising the skin surface if required, and twice daily inspecting the whole stump for any skin discolouration, which may indicate the potential development of a pressure sore. This care will be reinforced during visits to the prosthetic department where information about care of the prosthesis will be given. The patient or a relative should be taught how to apply the stump bandage so that necessary compression is maintained, to help mould and firm the tissue in preparation for fitting the definitive prosthesis at a later date, they must be advised to apply the stump bandage in order to maintain the shape of the stump (Jamieson et al 2000, p. 412). Stump bandaging is an area of changing practice and the elastic bandage soft dressing traditionally used may be replaced by other types of dressing, for example semirigid dressings (Wong & Edelstein 2000).

From Jamieson et al 2000.

previously wore will still be able to be worn, but the trousers will need to be tucked up when he is sitting in a wheelchair. A great deal of his management will depend on how he responds to the postoperative shock of finding he no longer has his lower limbs and that he will be unable to move and exercise as he previously did. The response of his family at this time will also be crucial to how he manages to come to terms with his initial dependence on them and health carers. Caring for his stump, with the help of his wife will also depend on a number of other factors, including how he sees his own sexuality and body image. However, as we can see, making sure the stumps are kept clean and moist will be essential if the prostheses are to be fitted properly.

- Successful rehabilitation in all Activities of Living and caring for Mr Upton and his family will require the involvement of the multidisciplinary team.

Summary points

> 1. Personal cleansing and dressing needs can be affected by indirect health problems in other Activities of Living, e.g. severe trauma causing difficulties with mobility.
> 2. Meeting patient's personal cleansing and dressing needs is the responsibility of the multidisciplinary team and can also involve the patient's family.
> 3. Promoting self-care with personal cleansing and dressing needs is an important part of patient rehabilitation.

References

Bale S 2000 Wound healing. In: Alexander MF, Fawcett JN, Runciman PJ (eds) Nursing practice – hospital and home (the adult), pp. 737–762. Churchill Livingstone, Edinburgh

Closs JS 2000 Sleep. In: Alexander MF, Fawcett JN, Runciman PJ (eds) Nursing practice – hospital and home (the adult), pp. 783–796. Churchill Livingstone, Edinburgh

Collier M 2002 Caring for the patient with a skin or wound care need. In: Walsh M (ed) Watson's clinical nursing and related sciences, pp. 925–959. Baillière Tindall, Edinburgh

Department of Health 2000a Guidance on mixed-sex accommodation for mental health services. DoH, London

Department of Health 2000b Good practice in continence services. DoH, London

Department of Health 2001a National service framework for older people. DoH, London

Department of Health 2001b Essence of care – patient focused benchmarking for health care practitioners. DoH, London

Department of Health 2001c Caring for older people: a nursing priority. Nursing and Midwifery Standing Committee, DoH, London

Department of Health 2001d Seeking consent: working with older people. DoH, London

Department of Health 2001e Practice guidance: principles, standards and indicators – a resource tool – Caring for Older people: a nursing priority. DoH, London

Docherty C, Hodgson R 2000 Skin disorders In: Alexander MF, Fawcett JN, Runciman PJ (eds) Nursing practice – hospital and home (the adult), pp. 467–491. Churchill Livingstone, Edinburgh

Edmond CB 2000 The respiratory system. In: Alexander MF, Fawcett JN, Runciman PJ (eds) Nursing practice – hospital and home (the adult), pp. 58–86. Churchill Livingstone, Edinburgh

Farmer EF 2000 The older person. In: Alexander MF, Fawcett JN, Runciman PJ (eds) Nursing practice – hospital and home (the adult), pp. 999–1013. Churchill Livingstone, Edinburgh

Gobbi M 2000 Fluid and electrolyte balance. In: Alexander MF, Fawcett JN, Runciman PJ (eds) Nursing practice – hospital and home (the adult), pp. 677–696. Churchill Livingstone, Edinburgh

Henley A, Schott J 1999 Culture, religion and patient care in a multi-ethnic society. Age Concern, London

Hinchliff SM, Montague SE, Watson R 1996 Physiology for nursing practice. Baillière Tindall, London

Holland K, Hogg C 2001 Cultural awareness in nursing and health care. Arnold, London

Jamieson L, McFarlane CM, Brown JM 2000 The musculoskeletal system. In: Alexander MF, Fawcett JN, Runciman PJ (eds) Nursing practice – hospital and home (the adult), pp. 393–427. Churchill Livingstone, Edinburgh

Jamison JR 2001 Maintaining health in primary care – guidelines for wellness in the 21st century. Churchill Livingstone, Edinburgh

Lawler J 1991 Behind the screens – nursing, somology and the problem of the body. Churchill Livingstone, Edinburgh

Roper N, Logan W, Tierney A 1996 The elements of nursing. Churchill Livingstone, Edinburgh

Rutter M 2000 Life experiences and transitions in adolescence and childhood. In: Wells D (ed) Caring for sexuality in health and illness, pp. 135–149. Churchill Livingstone, Edinburgh

Sharpe J, Bostock J 2002 Supporting people with debt and mental health problems: research with psychological therapists in Northumberland. Community Psychology 2002 (www.haznet.org.uk)

Spector R 1996 Cultural diversity in health and illness, 4th edn. Appleton Lange, Stamford

Waugh A, Grant A 2001 Ross and Wilson anatomy and physiology in health and illness. Churchill Livingstone, Edinburgh

Wong CK, Edelstein JE 2000 Unna and elastic post-operative dressings: comparison of the effects on function of adults with amputation and vascular disorders. Archives of Physical Medicine and Rehabilitation 81(9): 1191–1198.

Further reading

Jamieson EM, McCall JM, Whyte LA 2002 Clinical nursing practice, 5th edn. Churchill Livingstone, Edinburgh

Walsh M (ed) 2002 Watson's clinical nursing and related sciences. Baillière Tindall, Edinburgh

Hinchliff SM, Montague SE, Watson R 1996 Physiology for nursing practice, 2nd edn. Baillière Tindall, London

Useful websites

www.dohgov.uk/essenceofcare (Essence of Care – Benchmarking Toolkit)

www.alzheimers.org.uk (Alzheimer's Association)

www.icn.ch/matters_ageing (International Council of Nurses)

Controlling body temperature

Susan Walker

Introduction

The body should be considered as being made up of interdependent parts, each part interacting physiologically with others. When one part is impaired in its function, all other body systems are affected. As living individuals, we have homeostatic mechanisms, which assist us to maintain a constant internal environment in the body, so enabling optimum function (see Chapter 3).

Core body temperature is usually maintained within a narrow range of 36.1–37.8°C (Marieb 1999). This is regardless of external environmental temperature or the amount of heat being produced by the body. It is when deviation from this core body temperature occurs that body dysfunction becomes inevitable. With extreme deviations comes the increased likelihood of death.

It is relevant for any interventions to bring the temperature back within normal limits to be based on solid underpinning knowledge. This supports a holistic approach to assessment, planning, implementation and evaluation of care.

This chapter will therefore focus on the following:

1. **The model of living**
   - controlling body temperature in health and illness across the lifespan
   - dependence/independence in the AL controlling body temperature
   - factors influencing the AL controlling body temperature.
2. **The model for nursing**
   - nursing care of individuals with health problems affecting the AL controlling body temperature (i.e. application of the Roper et al (1996, 2000) model for nursing in practice).

THE MODEL OF LIVING

Control of body temperature

Body temperature reflects the balance between heat production and heat loss. Body temperature of 36.1°C–37.8°C

is maintained to enable optimum function by homeostatic mechanisms (Marieb 1999). Extremes of body temperature have an effect on biochemical reaction rates, particularly enzyme activity, which is impaired when temperature changes occur.

An increase in temperature leads to faster chemical reactions. As temperatures rise higher and higher beyond homeostatic range, neurones become depressed and proteins degrade. With a temperature of 41°C convulsions are usually experienced. A temperature of 43°C is likely to precede death (Lloyd 1994).

A decrease in temperature reduces metabolic rate and symptoms associated with the condition of hypothermia may occur. Hypothermia is a condition associated with a body temperature of 35°C or below (Lloyd 1994) (see p. 276).

The vascular system contributes to control of body temperature, with the blood serving as an exchange agent between the core and the shell. When referring to the core body temperature we refer to the organs of the skull, thoracic cavity and abdomen, the skin providing a shell. Whenever the skin is warmer than the external environment, heat is lost from the body through vasodilation. The hypothalamus is the part of the brain most responsible for thermoregulation. Vasodilation is triggered via the parasympathetic (heat loss centre) in the anterior hypothalamus when the temperature of circulating blood rises.

In vasodilation the peripheral blood vessels are dilated to allow more blood to flow to the periphery. This is accompanied by structures called the precapillary sphincters relaxing, allowing blood to flow into peripheral capillaries bringing it close to the surface of the body (Hinchliff et al 1996). Blood flowing through the skin increases, depending upon the need for temperature control.

The skin plays an important role in body temperature control (see Chapter 8). It protects against invading microorganisms and through the processes of radiation, conduction, convection and evaporation, it helps regulate body temperature. These processes are listed on page 258.

Radiation

This is loss of heat in the form of infrared waves. The flow of energy is always from hot to cold. The body can also gain heat by radiation, for example, warming of the skin during exposure to strong sunshine.

Conduction

As in radiation, conduction involves the transfer of heat from the body, but to objects that the body may have contact with, such as a floor or chair. Loss of heat by conduction can be minimised by wearing clothes that are poor conductors of heat. Trapped air provides thermal insulation – so layers of light clothes are better than one heavy garment.

Convection

As heat is generated and transfers from the body surface to the surrounding air it rises and cool air falls. The warm air surrounding the body is constantly replaced by cooler air molecules. Strong winds and electric fans, which move air quickly across the body surface, aid the processes of conduction and convection.

Evaporation

This is the process of converting the water in sweat, to water vapour, by heat production.

Most of the heat lost from the body is through the skin though some heat is lost through excretion in urine and faeces and some through expiration from the lungs. It is the sweat glands in the skin that are the mechanism for heat reduction when the environmental temperature is higher than that of the body, this will be discussed further within this chapter.

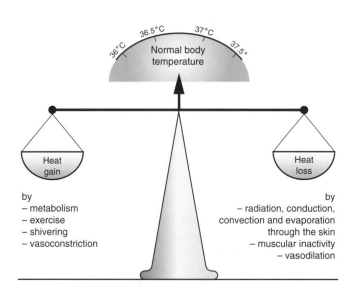

Fig. 9.1 Heat gain/heat loss balance (from Roper et al 1996, with permission).

Vasoconstriction will occur when there is a need to conserve body temperature. This results in peripheral shutdown and is associated with shivering. Shivering is an involuntary spasmodic contraction and relaxation of the skeletal muscles. It contributes to the generation of heat and is associated with the pilomotor reflex, which makes the hairs on the skin surface stand up to trap air producing 'goosebumps'.

Vasoconstriction is triggered via the sympathetic (heat-promoting centre) in the posterior hypothalamus when the temperature of circulating blood falls (see Fig. 9.1 for heat loss/gain balance).

Biological factors related to physiology and temperature control will be discussed throughout the chapter.

Controlling body temperature in health and illness – across the lifespan

Childhood

Body temperature reflects the balance between heat production and heat loss. All body tissues produce heat, those producing the greatest amount being those that are most metabolically active. Infants and young children have higher metabolic rates than adults and smaller body masses. This is relevant as they are generating more body heat, but have a smaller body surface from which to lose it, enhancing the likelihood of temperature deviations. In the newborn infant, heat loss is rapid after birth (Blackburn and Loper 1992, cited in Sganga et al 2000).

Temperature can fall 2–3°C after birth and interventions such as providing warm towels and blankets, skin-to-skin contact, or an incubator are vital (Sganga et al 2000). A young child is dependent on warm clothes, adequate diet and a warm environment to prevent a hypopyrexia.

Fisher (1999) refers to the fact that infants' and children's regulatory reflexes are likely to be underdeveloped, hence an irregular or recurrent rise in temperature may be of little significance. A transient hyperpyrexia may occur following a tantrum, prolonged crying or a physical display of excitement. The resulting discomfort is a hot, sticky and sweaty child, who is dependent on an adult to offer a cold drink, remove an item of clothing and encourage rest, until a child has reached an age where they are able to manipulate their own environment.

Prolonged temperature rise in a child is usually associated with fever as a result of infection from bacteria or viruses.

Fever is recognised as having a positive effect on the immune system. Fullick (1998) refers to the fact that most pathogens reproduce best at 37°C or lower. Therefore a raised temperature will affect reproduction of the pathogen causing less damage. Also, the immune system works better at higher temperatures, and so will be more successful at combating the infection by the raised temperature. By developing knowledge of the immune response and the physiological events that occur during fever we are able to provide appropriate and effective care, recognising when a fever may place a child at risk. Consider the following brief case study.

Case study 9.1

Emma – an 18-month-old baby girl

Emma is an 18-month-old baby girl – normally fit and well. Over the last few days Emma has been unusually sleepy and uninterested in her toys and surroundings. When Emma's mum attempts to encourage food, drink and play Emma becomes distressed, and uncooperative. Sarah, Emma's mum, is 17 and a single parent living in local council accommodation. She is supported by her parents who see her and her baby twice weekly. Recently Sarah and Emma joined a weekly mother and baby group.

Sarah is a sensible and loving parent to Emma. She has checked Emma for a rash and a temperature, neither are noted.

Emma may be reacting to an invading pathogen.

Pathogens and the active immune response
Pathogens are invading organisms that do not belong to the normal body flora. Pathogens transmitted from one person to another result in infectious disease. They may be mild or result in severe illness and death. Human viral disease includes amongst others, polio, influenza and acquired immune deficiency syndrome (AIDS).

Viruses are only able to replicate if inside a host cell. Once inside a cell, the virus will take over the cellular biochemistry and use it to produce new viruses, until the host cell is completely destroyed, leaving the virus free in the circulation to affect other cells (Fullick 1998). Human bacterial diseases include tuberculosis, salmonellosis and cholera. Bacteria can latch on to host cells and live and reproduce independently. Not all bacteria are harmful, and some can help us develop natural resistance (Fullick 1998).

Defence responses to invading pathogens are provided by the immune system. Leucocytes (white blood cells) are manufactured in the bone marrows of the long bones of the body. As they mature they become known as phagocytes. Phagocytes are able to move in and out of capillaries and engulf dead cells and foreign material. Other types of leucocytes are T cells and B cells, these are produced in the lymph glands.

Once a pathogen is inside the body it is recognised by its antigens. These are specific proteins on its outer surface identifying it as foreign material. T cells attach to the antigen and destroy it. Phagocytes will engulf the foreign material. The role of the B cell is to multiply in large numbers and secrete antibodies. Antibodies are proteins specific to a particular antigen, which bind to it and destroy it, the remaining material of destruction being then engulfed by the phagocytes. These immune responses are referred to as the cell-mediated response and the humeral response (see Fig 9.2). As part of the humeral response, B memory cells remain in the body providing a long-term immunology memory. Should the same disease-causing antigen be encountered again, protective antibodies will be released. Fullick (1998) refers to this fact explaining why diseases such as chicken pox or measles are usually only encountered once. (Read Waugh & Grant 2001 Ross & Wilson Anatomy and Physiology in Health and Illness, Chapter 5 – Resistance and Immunity. Churchill Livingstone, Edinburgh.)

You may have considered the following issues.

Flu Influenza is a virus that is highly contagious. It affects the nose, throat and lungs. In the United Kingdom, 3000–4000 deaths are attributed to 'the flu' each year (Gupta 1999). Gupta (1999) goes on to say this figure is increased tenfold during epidemics. There are two strains of the virus, Influenza A, and Influenza B. Type A strain is

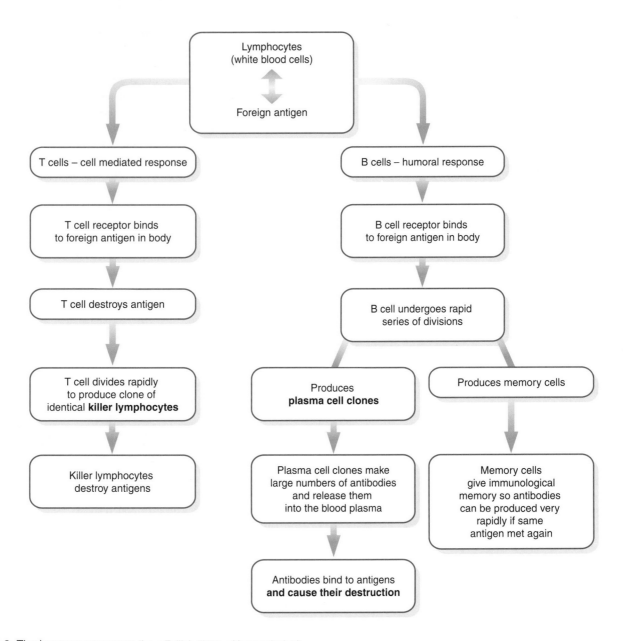

Fig. 9.2 The immune response (from Fullick 1998, with permission).

responsible for more severe illness, often resulting in pneumonia, hospitalisation and death (Miller 2001). The flu viruses are antigenically unstable and mutate constantly (Miller 2001). This is why people contract the flu often, as the immune system will not necessarily recognise the new virus strain.

The Public Health Laboratory Service (1998) states the bigger the change in the viral strain, then the greater the likelihood of a larger outbreak. Management of the flu is largely based on relief of symptoms that have a sudden onset. Symptoms include: headache, coughs, fever, appetite loss, tiredness, aches and pains and chills.

The upper respiratory tract may be affected and you may have experienced the following:

- constant runny nose
- sore throat
- sneezing
- irritated, watery eyes.

Gastrointestinal symptoms may include

- nausea
- vomiting
- often diarrhoea.

When gastrointestinal symptoms occur, it is often referred to as 'stomach flu'.

Miller (2001) states the period of infectiousness from the onset of symptoms is usually 3–5 days in adults and up to 7 days in young children. The World Health Organisation monitors the worldwide influenza situation (WHO 1999). In the United Kingdom, vaccination is available to prevent much of the illness and death attributed to influenza. The vaccine components are dependent on the strains expected to develop in the coming season (Miller 2001).

Symptom management includes rest, increased fluid intake and antipyretic medications to relieve the symptoms of fever. To distinguish flu from other respiratory diseases laboratory tests are necessary. In the United Kingdom, increased surveillance is underway which links laboratory and community data, so that response to any emerging flu epidemic is quick and coordinated. It is the very young and the elderly and those who may be immunosuppressed due to chronic illness that are most at risk.

Immunisation For the newborn infant immunity is provided when antibodies and antitoxins circulating in the mother's blood are passed via the placenta to the fetus. This natural passive immunity usually only lasts a few months following birth. Until the active immunity through immunisation is taken up, the child is vulnerable to infectious disease.

Current controversy exists about the safety of the triple MMR (measles, mumps, rubella) vaccine and its link to the incidence of autism and bowel disease occurring post-vaccination (Patja et al 2000, Taylor et al 1999).

Exercise

1. Talk to parents of young children about decisions they made regarding immunisation of a child.
2. What influenced their decisions regarding immunisation?

MMR protects against measles, mumps and rubella (German measles). Measles is usually a mild disease, however it can cause fever, rash and chest infection. The danger is that if fever is not controlled it may lead to convulsions which if not treated immediately may lead to brain damage. It is a very infectious virus.

In 1987, the year prior to MMR being introduced to England, 86 000 children caught measles and this resulted in 16 deaths. There are now fewer than 100 cases of measles per year reported (NHS 2001).

Mumps is a virus that causes headache, fever and painful swollen neck glands. It can also cause inflammation of the brain and permanent deafness. Due to vaccination, mumps, which is the most common cause of viral meningitis of children under 15 years, has now resulted in hospital admissions for children with mumps meningitis becoming almost irradicated.

Rubella (German measles) is recognised by a rash and can be a mild infectious disease in children, however if contracted by a woman during early pregnancy it can cause serious damage to the unborn baby. Any damage resulting is known as congenital rubella syndrome (CRS) (NHS 2001) (Table 9.1).

Prevention is always better than cure and immunisation of a child against infective diseases that can be prevented is considered vital (see Box 9.1).

Box 9.1 Diseases preventable by vaccination

Anthrax	Poliomyelitis
Cholera	Rubella
Diphtheria	Smallpox
Hepatitis B	Tetanus
Measles	Tuberculosis
Meningitis C	Typhoid
Mumps	Whooping cough

From: Waugh & Grant 2001 Ross & Wilson Anatomy & Physiology in Health and Illness, p. 382. Churchill Livingstone, Edinburgh.

Table 9.1 Childhood vaccination

When to immunise	What is given	How is it given
Two, three and four months old	Polio Diphtheria, tetanus, pertussis and Hib (DTP-hib) MenC	By mouth One injection One injection
Around 13 months old	Measles, mumps and rubella (MMR)	One injection
Three to five years old (pre-school)	Polio Diphtheria, tetanus and acellular pertussis (DtaP) Measles, mumps and rubella (MMR)	By mouth One injection One injection
10 to 14 years old (and sometimes shortly after birth)	BCG (against tuberculosis)	Skin test, then, if needed, one injection
13 to 18 years old	Diphtheria and tetanus (Td) Polio	One injection By mouth

From: NHS (2001).

Tuberculosis Tuberculosis (TB) is an example of a human bacterial disease that can affect anyone at any age. *Mycobacterium tuberculosis* are transmitted from human to human; they cause chronic granulamatous lesions, mainly in the lungs, but often also in bones and the brain.

There has recently been an increase worldwide, and this is reflected in the UK, particularly in respiratory TB, which increased by 13% between 1996 and 1997 (Public Health Laboratory Service 1998 cited in Mallet and Dougherty 2000).

The World Health Organisation predicts that by 2020 nearly one billion people will be infected with TB, of them 70 million will die. TB blackspots include Eastern Europe, South-East Asia and sub-Saharan Africa (BBC News 1999).

Immigrant subgroups have been highlighted as an attributable cause for the increase in the UK (Public Health Laboratory Service 1998 cited in Mallet and Dougherty 2000). This particular group of people prove to be a difficult target for TB prevention programmes due to cultural and language difficulties and ability to access health care professionals. Those who are immunosuppressed due to disease or drugs, along with those suffering with alcoholism or living in poverty are most susceptible to TB, as these conditions tend to predispose its development.

Primarily tuberculosis is spread by inhalation of the bacteria. When an infected person coughs, droplets are produced which can be inhaled by another person. Once infected the host's immune response is activated, it can usually destroy the TB bacilli – preventing development of the disease but producing a calcified granuloma. However, some TB bacteria may survive the host's immune response after primary infection, and lie dormant in any body site, especially the lungs, for many years. They can be reactivated by debilitative disease or by later exposure to TB itself (Medico 2001).

The Department of Health (1998) suggest that TB should be suspected in all people who have a cough lasting for 3 weeks or more, accompanied by weight loss, anorexia, haemoptysis, fever and night sweats. A provisional diagnosis is based on 'smear-positive' findings of acid-fast bacilli in sputum or other bodily fluids. Patients who have a smear-positive result are considered as infectious while those with a smear-negative result are noninfective.

Further investigation is required to identify the specific strain of disease by bacterial growth in culture (Medico 2001).

Prevention and control of spread of TB is necessary. All forms of TB are statutorily notifiable to the consultant in communicable disease control (Medico 2001) or the medical officer for environmental health in the UK. A person with a smear-positive result is a primary source for spread of the disease and contact tracing is an important means of identifying secondary cases (Medico 2001). TB is found in 19% of all contacts; about 10% of notified cases each year are found through contact tracing (Ejidokum et al 1998 cited in Mallet and Dougherty 2000). Besides laboratory testing to diagnose TB, X-rays can be taken. A chest X-ray may show damage in the lungs. A Heaf or Mantoux test to which an individual will react if they are infected or have active disease will be used. This is a common test in children, but is not considered effective in adolescents and adults.

Prevention is through vaccination with Bacillus Calmette–Guerin (BCG). In the UK the vaccine is given to schoolchildren and has been shown to give 70–80% protection lasting at least 15 years. The vaccine is given to new UK entrants from high-risk countries and to infants born to families from these countries (Public Health Laboratory 2001).

Treatment for those found to have infectious (active) TB includes antibacterial drugs. Those who are infectious will also be isolated at the start of the drug therapy. The drugs used to treat TB are: isoniazid, rifampin, pyrazinamide, ethambutol, streptomycin (www.lung.ca.drugs 2001).

A combination of these drugs is usually necessary during treatment, as the TB bacteria can be resistant to one or more of the drugs. Drug therapy can last for 6–8 months. It is essential that the prescribed amount be taken at the prescribed time, for the full length of time prescribed. This is because TB is a slowly developing disease and therefore the desired results may take some time to achieve.

Where severe damage has been caused to an organ of the body, i.e. the lung, surgical intervention may be necessary. This may have a greater long-term effect on an individual and their lifestyle and Activities of Living. For example:

- time spent in hospital
- loss of independence during recovery period
- ability to return to work will all depend on the degree of surgery undertaken and the individual's recovery to the illness and the surgical intervention.

Exercise

1. Find out the incidence of TB in your community.
2. What simple practice can minimise the risk of spread of infection within a community?
3. Discuss with colleagues how you would care for someone with TB.

Adolescence and adulthood

In adolescence and adulthood we experience changes in body temperature as part of the lifecycle or in relation to lifestyle choices we have made.

Around 12 years of age female menstruation occurs, until menopause, which usually occurs when a woman has reached her forties. Gould (1994) refers to the fact that a slight temperature rise may occur at the time of ovulation, but can be as little as 0.3°C. This slight rise in temperature is considered as a method of indicating the time of ovulation and is used by some to aid fertility. There is also a slight temperature rise during the first trimester of pregnancy. These slight variations in temperature are due to the influences of the female sex hormones.

During health diurnal variations can be noted in body temperature. Recordings are lowest in the early hours of the morning, rising steadily throughout the day, reaching a peak in the late evening. This is influenced by the day and night patterns of activity and rest. Roper et al (1996) state that the converse is true for people who regularly work at night and sleep in the day.

It is relevant to note that during adolescence and early adulthood social grouping and social activity are important, as these affect the social activities a young person may choose. Peer pressure should be noted as playing a part in our socialisation.

Some social drugs are known to increase metabolic rate such as nicotine and caffeine, and an increased metabolic rate will lead to a rise in body temperature. Caffeine is legal and socially accepted, but it can be addictive, especially if taken in large amounts. Withdrawal symptoms when coffee drinking stops include lethargy and headache and an inability to concentrate. Nicotine is a mild stimulant, although it is known to cause vasoconstriction of the peripheral blood vessels. This raises the heart rate slightly and leads to an increase in blood pressure. Nicotine is addictive, and when nicotine levels are reduced, there is a physical craving for the drug. Fullick (1998) states withdrawal symptoms include irritability, lack of concentration, restlessness, hunger and sadness or depression, the later 'feeling low' contributing to a reduction in body temperature. (For effects of smoking on the activity of breathing see Chapter 5.)

Alcohol taken in excessive amounts is associated with a lowering of body temperature as cooling is increased due to vasodilatation of blood vessels in the skin (Roper et al 1996).

Freedom of maturity and managing one's own lifestyle may also permit foreign travel. There may be a greater risk of contracting a tropical infectious disease. Chiodini (2001) refers to the fact that the increase in the number of visitors to exotic locations has pushed travel medicine to the forefront of primary care. Access to travel and immunisation advice has become essential. Detailed information can be obtained from the World Health Organisation website at www.who.int.

This chapter has considered the need for immunisation and the body's immune defence system; it now considers general health advice when in a hot climate, at home or abroad. Consider the following scenario.

Case study 9.2

Sarah – 18-year-old

Sarah is 18 years old, a fashion fanatic and a keen sunbather, believing a suntan to be the ultimate fashion accessory. She is planning her first holiday abroad, with friends and is excited about the opportunities for partying and obtaining that ultimate tan.

What advice could you offer Sarah in relation to prevention of sunburn and heatstroke?

You may have considered the following information regarding skin cancer to support your advice.

Skin cancer

If you have revised the function and structure of the skin you will have identified that melanin can provide some protection from the harmful effects of sunlight. Waugh and Grant (2001) state that the amount of melanin in the skin is genetically determined and varies between parts of the body, between members of the same race and between races.

Exposure to sunlight promotes synthesis of increased amounts of melanin and this affects the differences in colour. However, it does not give ultimate protection and exposure to ultraviolet (UV) radiation can damage the skin. UVA ages the skin and UVB burns the skin. Both types of ultraviolet radiation can lead to cancer (jas 2001).

There are three types of skin cancer, basal cell and squamous cell carcinomas are easily treated and rarely fatal, but malignant melanomas grow uncontrollably and these are the most dangerous, and can cause death. About 1500 people die from melanomas in Britain every year (jas 2001). Fortunately melanoma is curable when detected and treated early.

Melanoma cancers contain melanin, which causes them to be mixed shades of brown; they can appear suddenly or may begin in or near a mole or dark skin spot. Melanomas occur on sun-damaged skin and those particularly at risk are those having sudden short bursts of sunlight, on holiday, in places where the sun is very strong (jas 2001).

People most at risk include those with:

- a high number of moles
- red or fair hair
- fair skin or freckles
- blue eyes
- who tan with difficulty and burn in the sun.

It is important for people to recognise that a tan is not healthy, rather that it is indicative of damage to the skin by UV radiation. The melanin moves to the surface of the exposed skin, to provide protection. Remember even dark skin can burn. To reduce risk of melanoma and sunburn requires adaptation of behaviour. This involves:

- avoiding exposure during midday temperatures
- enjoy the sun before 10 am and after 3 pm local time
- wear a wide-brimmed hat to protect eyes, ears, head and neck.
- sit in the shade (remember sand, water and snow all reflect UV radiation) so shade may not give complete protection
- use sunglasses that block UV rays to protect the eyes (UV rays can cause cataracts)
- cover the body with light clothing
- use sun-protective creams/lotions/sprays that guard against both UVA and UVB rays
- protect children – keep them out of direct sunlight as much as possible.

It may be assumed that a person who has little knowledge regarding sunburn, and so places him or herself at risk, is also likely to fail to recognise symptoms of heat-related illness.

Heat stroke

During high environmental temperatures and humidity we are all at risk of heat-related illness and heatstroke without appropriate education and management.

Batscha (1997) refers to three major types of heat-related illness:

- Heat cramps, caused by sodium depletion in the body.
- Heat exhaustion which generally occurs as a result of dehydration and accompanies untreated heat cramps. It is characterised by profuse sweating, fatigue, thirst and headache, which may lead to nausea and vomiting. An elevation in body temperature will be present. It is insidious in onset.
- Heat stroke occurs in two forms. It develops when the body is unable to dispel heat through normal physiological mechanisms. Exertional heat stroke occurs as a result of strenuous physical exercise resulting in excessive internal heat production. Particularly during periods of extremely hot weather. Highest incidence is in the first few days of a heat wave when people have had little chance to acclimatise. Classic heat stroke is often seen in elderly people and the infirm and results from a combination of a hot environment and ineffective heat-loss mechanisms. Heat stroke is considered a medical emergency. It requires an immediate response should it occur; this will be discussed later in this chapter.

Prevention of heat-related illness, again, involves behavioural adaptation such as:

- avoid exercise
- drink plenty of water
- stay cool, by seeking shade and wearing light single-layered clothes
- try to access a heat-conditioned building
- take a tepid shower or bath.

Keeping cool may be more difficult for an overweight person. Reasons for this include the decreased vascularity of adipose tissue which inhibits heat loss by increasing the difficulty of blood moving to the skin surface. Adipose tissue also acts as an insulator (Sidebottom 1992, cited in Batscha 1997). Additional weight also increases the work of the heart when activity is undertaken, which tends to raise body temperature further (Batscha 1997).

Metabolic rate, body temperature and weight control

Fullick (1998) refers to the fact that some lifestyle factors that can cause, or increase the likelihood of suffering, a particular disease or illness are under our control, others are not. Fullick (1998) states babies and young children have little choice about what they eat, yet foundations of diet-related illnesses may well be laid in early childhood.

However adolescents and adults can make lifestyle choices about diet. Food in the diet is required to provide the body with sufficient energy to maintain basic body functioning, and to carry out the Activities of Living. The amount of energy the body requires on a daily basis will depend on the basal metabolic rate (BMR) and the level of activity. The basal metabolic rate can affect body temperature. The BMR is greater in babies and young children, as they use a great deal of energy in growth. In newborn babies brown fat is a form of fat in adipose tissue that is a rich source of energy and can be converted rapidly to heat. It is a useful source of heat production contributing to maintenance of body temperature in babies, where a smaller body surface area can contribute to difficulties with the normal processes of conduction, convection, radiation and evaporation in relation to heat production and heat loss.

This adipose tissue is found around the viscera, the back and the neck. It is controlled by the sympathetic nervous system (Imrie & Hall 1990). The BMR is also related to the total body mass and the lean body mass. People with a higher proportion of muscle tissue require more energy for maintenance than fat. Fullick (1998) states that one reason why men have a higher BMR than women is because they tend to have a higher proportion of muscle to fat.

Marieb (1999) defines the metabolic rate as the sum of heat produced by all the chemical reactions and mechanical work of the body. It can be measured directly or indirectly.

Using the direct method it is necessary for a person to enter an enclosed chamber where heat produced by the body is absorbed by water circulating around the chamber. The rise in the temperature of the circulating water is directly related to the heat produced by the body (Marieb 1999).

The indirect method involves use of a respirator measure of oxygen consumption, which is directly proportional to heat produced. For each line of oxygen used, the body produces about 4.8 kcal of heat (Marieb 1999).

By multiplying the BMR with a factor reflecting an individual physical activity level (PAL) the estimated average requirements (EAR) for energy can be obtained. In the UK a PAL of 1.4 is used for adults (Fullick 1998). If energy intake is not matched to the requirements of the body then weight gain or loss will occur as a result of eating too much or too little.

With a greater body surface area, heat loss to the environment increases and the metabolic rate must be higher to replace the lost heat. With ageing and as the body shrinks in relation to the amount of skeletal muscle, the BMR declines. Decreasing calorie intake can help prevent obesity in later life.

Physical activity and exercise which increase skeletal muscle activity result in the most significant rise in the BMR and body heat production. The combination of increased physical activity and exercise with a reduced calorie intake remains the most acceptable way to reduce weight. This often means a change in lifestyle and/or lifelong habits.

Surface area, age, gender, stress and hormones are all factors influencing BMR. Although bodyweight and size are related, it is body surface area that is the vital factor. A greater body surface area to body volume means a higher BMR, as heat loss to the environment is greater. Body temperature will rise and fall with BMR.

Exercise

Consider the following based on the information presented.

1. Two people weigh the same. One is tall and thin and one is short and fat. Who has the greater BMR? Read up on the hormone thyroxine and its effect on BMR in relation to body temperature, weight gain and weight loss.
2. Assess the amount of physical exercise undertaken by:
   - a school-age child
   - an adult (over 18 years)
   - an older person (over 60 years)

   as part of their normal living activities, e.g. consider exercise involved in work, hobbies, school activities, etc.

Old age

A study conducted on exercise and older people at the University of Indiana's Institute for Aging research (Environmental News Network 1999) reported that older individuals felt less able to engage in exercise, with females being less confident than males. A total of 729 senior citizens spoke with researchers about environmental obstacles that prevented exercise. All respondents were low-income, urban residents.

The elderly people referred to barriers such as bad weather, crime, poor walking paths and facilities, when considering outdoor exercise, whilst those considering indoor exercise were concerned they would experience chest pain or respiratory problems and had fear of injury.

Self-confidence, desire and motivation were also identified as significant factors, even when the person knew that exercise would improve their health and wellbeing.

Researchers at the University's Bechman Institute studied 124 previously sedentary men and women between the ages of 60 and 75 years (Environmental News Network 1999). The group was randomly divided into two, one group gradually worked up to walking an hour a day, three times a week (aerobic exercise), the other group did anaerobic exercises such as stretching and toning. Over the course of 6 months the groups were given a variety of simple tests which measured their ability to plan, establish schedules, make and remember choices and rapidly reconsider them if the circumstances change. The walkers showed an improved ability to complete the tests compared with the nonwalkers.

The researchers were focusing on the areas of the brain responsible for 'executive control processes' these being the frontal and prefrontal lobes of the brain, which are known to be the areas of the brain which decline earliest with ageing.

The better the executive control processes, the better someone can complete day-to-day tasks such as driving, cooking, etc., as these tasks require a person to keep track of more than one thing at once. Hence, the more independent they can be.

The Environment News Network (1999) notes that exercise could help delay the time at which older people become more dependent on others.

In relation to body temperature control ill health and dependency are clearly significant especially when considering an elderly person's ability to respond to variations in temperature. With this in mind, it is important in older age to remain alert and as independent as possible. The thermoregulation system becomes less efficient making it more difficult to detect temperature variations from the norm.

This can be due to a number of factors:

- physiological changes such as a reduction in the ability to constrict peripheral blood vessels, and a possible reduction in the shivering threshold (Collins et al 1977, Macmillan et al 1967, cited in Roper et al 1996)
- increased risk to be medication-dependent
- obesity, increased risk in advanced age due to reduced mobility and exercise
- possible mental impairment affecting judgement and decisions regarding appropriate actions during temperature variations
- possible social isolation, poorer housing.

Old age accompanied by acute or chronic illness/disease will increase the risk of an older person experiencing heat- and cold-related illness.

Exercise

1. Talk to an elderly family member or neighbour about how they adapt to high and low environmental temperatures.

In order to explore the issues of older people and the AL of controlling body temperature consider the following case study.

Case study 9.3

Marjory – a 78-year-old widow

Marjory is a 78-year-old, who has been widowed for 12 months. During the last 12 months she has become increasingly isolated and reliant upon her only daughter for social contact and support. Her daughter makes great effort to visit Marjory every other day.

Case study 9.3 (continued)

Although physically able Marjory has considerably reduced her mobility and spends much time sitting in her armchair, some days not even bothering to get dressed. She has a hot meal on the days her daughter visits and although a meal is left for the next day Marjory chooses to eat something cold. Marjory has seen the doctor at her daughter's request, but has refused any help from social services in the form of a home help or meals on wheels. She insists she is grieving – as confirmed by the doctor, and will come round in her own time. Her only physical complaint is myxoedema for which she takes regular medication (thyroxine).

Christmas is approaching and Marjory has refused to stay with her daughter and family over the Christmas period saying she prefers the peace and quiet of her own home.

Exercise

Consider the following based on the information presented:

1. What physical and psychological factors may increase Marjory's risk of hypothermia?
2. Why are older people considered to be more susceptible to hypothermia?
3. What measures could Marjory and her daughter employ to prevent hypothermia?

Psychological factors

Marjory's psychological state is clearly affecting her behaviour. It is necessary to recognise the effect of an individual's psychological state on body temperature.

When there is an increase or a decrease in the environmental temperature information is sent to the cerebral hemispheres where behavioural and psychological responses are triggered. In response to feeling hot a person may have a cold drink, open a window or remove an item of clothing, alternatively if feeling cold, they may take exercise, walk, or rub hands together in an attempt to create heat and increase blood supply to muscles. They may also add an item of clothing or turn up the heating, however this behavioural response is linked closely to their psychological state. Bringing the environmental temperature back to a comfortable level has the immediate effect of making one feel better.

If an individual's psychological state is impaired through illness such as depression, or affected through medication/drugs such as sedatives, they may neglect to respond appropriately and therefore any increase or decrease in temperature will become exaggerated. The sluggishness, lack of mobility and lethargy associated with 'feeling low' will contribute to a decreased metabolic rate and reduction in temperature, while the increased heart rate and activity associated with the excitement and euphoria of 'feeling good' may contribute to an increased metabolic rate and rise in body temperature.

Other psychological states which may lead to a rise in temperature are anxiety, nervousness, displays of anger and fear. The apocrine sweat glands are those triggered by emotional stimuli. They secrete sweat in the hair follicles of the armpits and groins (Kerry 1999 cited by USA Today (1999)).

Exercise

1. Recall your own psychological state prior to sitting an exam, an important interview, and a visit to the dentist or on your wedding day.
2. What physiological events occurred?
3. Talk to a successful slimmer about the 'feel good' factor related to a weight loss.

Psychological state linked with 'feeling low' leads to consideration of seasonal affective disorder (SAD). This is a type of depression that tends to occur and reoccur during autumn and winter months when there is deprivation of sunshine, daylight hours are reduced, and there is exposure to colder temperatures. Medical recognition of this condition is relatively recent.

Symptoms may include:

- weight gain due to overeating
- feeling low, desperate, anxious
- lethargy
- recurrent infections due to lowered resistance
- behaviour difficulties in children.

The first four of the above-mentioned symptoms might affect body temperature.

It is estimated that 2% of people in Northern Europe suffer with considerable symptoms with more than 10% coping with milder symptoms. Across the world incidence increases with distance from the equator (medicinenet.com 1999). It is thought that bright light makes a difference to brain chemistry. Treatment involves light therapy known as phototherapy and sufferers would obviously benefit from living in brighter, sunnier climates (although this for many is not an alternative).

Environmental factors

Seasonal variations and extremes in environmental temperature can also cause variations in an individual's body temperature, which can cause them to feel hot or cold. These variations may be mild or extreme. The most common conditions related to extremes in environmental temperature are hyperpyrexia (heat stroke) or hypothermia.

Heatstroke is a medical emergency requiring an immediate response. Body temperature may be 40°C or greater, (Hinchliff et al 1996). Hypothermia is defined as a body temperature of 35°C or below (Lloyd 1996).

So why can high and low environmental temperatures have such a profound effect on body temperature?

Worfolk (2000) refers to the fact the body's dominant means of losing heat in a hot environment are radiation and evaporation. But for heat to radiate from the body, the body temperature must be greater than that of the environment. However, when the environmental temperature is higher that that of the body, evaporation of water from the sweat glands forms the only mechanism available for the reduction of body temperature (Green 1989).

Heat is needed to convert water to water vapour. The vaporisation of 1 ml of water needs 0.58 calories (2.4 kcal). The heat is termed the latent heat of vaporisation. This is the amount of heat lost by the evaporation on the skin of 1 ml of sweat. If sweat falls off the skin without evaporating there is no cooling effect (Green 1989). It is the eccrine sweat glands that are triggered by heat and aid cooling (Kerry 1999).

Evaporation is aided by convection. Light winds on an unusually hot day can speed the evaporation of heated moist air next to the body, however on days of extreme humidity, with still air, sweat evaporation becomes impossible. This is because the body's thermoregulatory mechanisms have become overwhelmed. In high heat and humidity it is voluntary acts based on knowledge that will prevent the body temperature rising too high, i.e.

- moving to an air-conditioned building
- turning on a fan
- removing clothing.

Remember these actions are dependent upon a person's ability to respond to the discomfort they are feeling.

In a cold environment, heat production by the body is necessary to maintain core body temperature within normal limits. Heat loss in a cold outdoor environment may be exacerbated by wind chill. This is a term used to describe the rate of heat loss from the body from the combined effect of low temperature and wind. As wind speed increases it carries heat away more quickly. High winds even on cool days can significantly affect body temperature (Noa 2002). Should an individual be exposed to a combination of moderately low temperature, wind and wet, loss of heat from the body is enhanced and the risk of hypothermia is increased. Heat production will depend on internal metabolism, hot food and drink, exercise, and the body's ability to maintain heat through vasoconstriction. Again it is the very young and the very old at risk from extremes in environmental temperature, as this is linked with their perception of temperature change and their independent ability to respond accordingly.

Roper et al (1996) refer to the fact that environmental factors cannot be considered in isolation, they are related to biological, psychological, sociocultural and politicoeconomic factors. They also state that environmental factors influence living throughout the lifespan and have a bearing on the person's independence and dependency status, and influence the individuality in a person's way of living.

Politicoeconomic factors

There is a need to recognise that politicoeconomic factors link clearly to the environment, as living conditions and income clearly play a part. For example, low-quality housing and low income will mean inadequate levels of heating as people worry about being able to 'meet the bills' whilst failure to pay may lead to disconnection, increasing the risk of hypothermia. Low income also dictates diet, and poor nutrition can also affect our ability to keep warm.

According to Help the Aged (www.helptheaged.org.uk) it is difficult to give an exact figure for the number of people affected by hypothermia and cold-related deaths, as other illnesses are more likely to be recorded as the main cause of death should they be present, i.e. heart disease or pneumonia. What is clear is that the risk of hypothermia rises sharply during winter months (see Tables 9.2 and 9.3).

A direct correlation between cold weather and higher death rates is evident from these figures.

Keeping warm costs money. Fuel, food, insulation and upkeep of homes all come at a price, as does social activity such as holidays during winter months to warmer climates, or visiting a luncheon club on regular occasions to ensure a hot meal, good company and a warm environment. Help the Aged (www.helptheaged.org.uk) state that 48% of the households in the poorest tenth of the population are single, retired households.

A recommended room temperature for an older person in the United Kingdom is 21°C compared to that of 18°C

Table 9.2 Deaths related to hypothermia in England and Wales

Year	65+	80+	All ages
1996	365	244	414
1997	215	138	277
1998	212	135	273
1999	225	166	325

Office for National Statistics 1999/2000.

Table 9.3 Excess winter deaths

	1996/7	1997/8	1998/9	1999/2000
65+	38 000	21 000	44 000	45 000
All ages	45 000	23 000	48 000	49 000

Office for National Statistics 1999/2000.

Exercise

Consider the environment in which you work (hospital-based, community staff, those within Schools of Nursing) and

1. if exposed to the outdoors, how do you adapt to environmental temperature variations?
2. if an indoor worker, find out about legislation governing temperatures and ventilation in your work place.

for others. The government offer a winter fuel allowance to all those over the age of 60 years to support older people with fuel bills. A person living alone will qualify for a payment of £200, married couples both eligible for a winter fuel payment should receive £100 each (Department for Work and Pensions 2001).

Outside the United Kingdom for many people politico-economic factors can be considered as the extremes of poverty, isolation and war.

We have seen many images of refugees whose homes have been destroyed, and who exist in refugee camps, living under canvas with little food, water and nonexistent sanitary facilities. (See World Health Organisation for further information on refugee camps and conditions (www.who.int) and the BBC news website for images (http://news.bbc.co.uk)).

Warmth is provided by communal living and sleeping, and by the meagre food, clothing and blanket rations provided. Refugees run the risk of death by hypothermia, as temperatures drop dramatically at night. There is little in the way of sustenance and comfort to prevent it. Poor sanitation, in large overcrowded populations such as those in refugee camps lead to a greater chance of developing an infectious disease and the accompanying symptom of fever.

Politicoeconomic factors clearly have an indirect effect on body temperature control.

Exercise
Think about your own home circumstances and living conditions. Consider:

- the type of accommodation you have
- how much of your (or family) expenditure is spent on food, clothes and keeping warm
- how you keep warm during low environmental temperatures
- how you keep cool during heat waves.

Sociocultural factors

It is easy to make an assumption about sociocultural factors which may influence the AL of controlling body temperature, particularly in relation to customs concerning clothing, religious customs which require full covering of a woman's body despite extreme heat. However, a person may be conditioned regarding behaviour that enables them to cope with the extreme of heat. For example, people may stay indoors in cool stone-built houses in midday temperatures, drink plenty and avoid activity which will increase body temperature further during the greatest heat in the day.

An object's colour and texture as well as its temperature will aid heat loss by radiation (Green 1989). Dark rough surfaces radiate maximally while light smooth surfaces at the same temperature do not lose heat as quickly. The same is said in relation to heat gain by radiation. However, the human skin irrespective of colour is able to radiate heat away from the body. This does not apply to clothes worn.

White clothes are more suitable than black in the tropics where it is very hot (Green 1989).

In a very hot climate there is less heat gained if a person wears white clothing and in a very cold environment there is less heat loss. Remember snow reflects radiation (jas 2001).

Everyone is socialised into acceptance of norms regarding the extent to which clothes can be shed in hot weather. Roper et al (2000) state that this is socioculturally determined rather than by need for comfort and body temperature control.

In the United States where summers are renowned for being hot and humid, great effort is made to prevent heat-related illness. Education regarding application of measures to avoid heat stroke and exhaustion plays a vital part in its prevention. These have been discussed earlier within this chapter. In 1995 Chicago experienced a summer heat wave, which sent 3300 people to the emergency department and killed more than 600 (Dematte et al 1998 cited in Worfolk 2000).

Acclimatisation can produce beneficial physiological changes. Adaptation occurs over 10–14 days of heat exposure. Lloyd (1994) states acclimatisation to heat results in increased work output, endurance, plasma volume and sweat production, with a decrease in heart rate, oxygen consumption, electrolyte concentration and core and skin temperature. This timescale indicates why some of us suffer heat exhaustion whilst on foreign holidays to hot exotic destinations.

But what about countries which have colder winters than the UK? In countries such as Sweden and Canada, there is a much smaller difference between the number of deaths in the summer and in the winter. One reason for this is that houses in these countries are better insulated and heated than homes within the UK.

Sociocultural factors do have an effect on the AL of controlling body temperature, but they are limited. When a person is in good health the homeostatic and physiological mechanisms will assist in the maintenance of a core body temperature which will enable optimum function, but it is important to note that they are connected.

Dependence/independence in the AL of controlling body temperature

In wellness the body is able to regulate its own body temperature. However in infancy and early childhood, the immaturity of the thermoregulatory system and the child's dependency on others to provide suitable clothing and adequate diet, increase opportunities for deviations from normal temperature to occur. In adulthood, in health, changes in body temperature are related to diurnal variations and hormonal influences. Thermoregulation in older age is less efficient and older people are more susceptible to extremes of heat and cold. Nonphysiological contributing factors may be lack of mobility, poor diet and inadequate heating and often underlying pathological disease.

Yet at any age injury or illness can occur, and body temperatures deviating from the norm may be experienced. During this time there is dependence upon others to provide an environment and interventions, which will encourage the body temperature to return within the normal range.

Roper et al (1996) refer to this concept as the dependent/independent continuum component of the model of living.

It is important that the caregiver has an understanding of factors influencing the AL of controlling body temperature to enable them to make an individualised assessment.

Summary points

1. Lifespan
The age of the patient will have great bearing on this Activity of Living. The very young having an immature thermoregulatory system and the elderly possibly an impaired thermoregulatory system. Both groups will have some dependency on others to maintain body temperature. During puberty and menstruation it is important to note there may be some slight rise in body temperature. Also, during female menopause, due to hormonal changes, the person may experience hot flushes and hot sweats that disrupt normal living activities.

2. Dependency
At any time during the lifespan an individual may develop dependency due to ill health.

3. Independence
Linked to health and control of body temperature. It is important to remember that choices are made in health about lifestyle, which may affect body temperature, i.e.

- immunisation
- foreign travel
- diet and weight control
- addictive substances – alcohol, nicotine, caffeine
- amount of exercise taken.

4. Factors affecting control of body temperature
Biological
- age
- underlying pathological illness/disease, i.e. carcinoma, myxoedema, thyrotoxicosis
- trauma
- damage to the hypothalamus or vascular system or skin
- weight and food intake
- physical activity
- medication
- diurnal variations
- puberty, pregnancy, menstrual cycle and menopause
- social drugs.

Psychological
- emotional state – anxiety, depression, fear, euphoria
- seasonal affective disorder.

Sociocultural
- exposure of the skin, traditional clothing linked to religion
- bathing habits (see Chapter 8).

Environmental
- outside temperatures/exposure to heat and cold
- windchill
- exposure to sunlight and UVA/UVB rays
- inside temperatures, air conditioning, draughts, damp.

Politicoeconomic
- standards for living
- housing
- income
- lifestyle choices
- education for health
- political agendas, i.e. war.

THE MODEL FOR NURSING

Using the model for nursing to individualise nursing in the AL of controlling body temperature, this part of the chapter will demonstrate how the components of the model of living are applied in nursing situations in ill health. The case scenarios introduced earlier in this chapter will be developed further. The nursing process (see Chapter 1) will be used to demonstrate application of the Roper et al model for nursing (1996, 2000) in practice.

It has already been demonstrated that in health body temperature is something that is very much taken for granted. Control of body temperature is maintained through a complex feedback system, and behavioural and physiological mechanisms.

So what can cause things to go wrong?

Exercise
1. Review the issues discussed earlier in this chapter in the model of living.
2. List possible causes of disruption to thermoregulation.

Assessment

Assessment of the individual is a dynamic ongoing process. Assessment is the first phase of the nursing process (see Chapter 1) and without this phase it is impossible to proceed with nursing care. Assessment facilitates the collection of information about the individual's past and current health status and life situation. Collier et al (1996) refer to the fact that the extent or depth of assessment may range from being focused to developing a comprehensive database. This will depend upon the situation in which nursing assessment takes place. For example, in an emergency or life-threatening situation rapid, focused, assessment of airway, breathing and circulation may be called for, and identified problems addressed before further comprehensive assessment is possible.

In less acute situations, the nurse will collect data, which will be both subjective and objective in nature. Subjective data are experiences or phenomena experienced by the client and recounted by the nurse. It is an account of how the patient is feeling or a description of symptoms the patient may have experienced.

Collier et al (1996) state that subjective data are not generally observable or measurable by the nurse. The amount of subjective data collated is dependent on the nurse's communication skills (see Chapter 4) and ability to build a therapeutic nurse–patient relationship (Peplau 1952).

The phenomena that can be observed and measured by the nurse are referred to as objective data. The collection of objective data involves the nurse's use of the skills of observation, examination and measurement.

Complete and thorough assessment involves all of these components.

The first part of this chapter (p. 259) introduced Emma, an 18-month-old child. In this section it is disclosed that Emma's health status has deteriorated.

Case study 9.1 (continued)

Emma – 18-month-old baby

18 December 2001   2.00 p.m.

Emma Smith 18-month-old baby girl brought to Accident and Emergency by her mother. No previous medical/surgical history. Normally fit and well. Normal delivery at birth, lives with mother no other siblings. Has social contact with other children.

History of sleeping more than usual over last 3 days, when awake often crying and uninterested in her toys and surroundings. Refusing diet, but taking small amounts of oral fluid. Seen by GP yesterday – no active treatment.

Case study 9.1 (continued)

Today anxious mum, very concerned. This am child vomited ×2, mum noticed shivering. Also number of wet nappies reduced. On examination – she is awake but quiet, skin hot and dry, refusing oral fluids. Her pulse is 108 and tympanic temperature 38.8°C.

Exercise
1. Can you differentiate between the subjective and objective data presented?
2. Can you identify any phases of fever?
3. What nursing interventions may promote patient comfort?
4. At what point would a prescribed antipyretic agent be useful?

The following may be considered.

Fever management in children

Those involved in caring for a child as a parent or a professional will be aware of how quickly a child can become unwell. In children illness is commonly accompanied by a rise in body temperature. When the rise in body temperature is prolonged physical signs and symptoms of fever will be present.

In children under 5 years pyrexia is the most common cause of convulsions. Convulsions are life-threatening, yet early management of symptoms of fever can prevent a convulsion occurring. A temperature above 38°C may place a child at risk. So what is fever?

Porth (1994) cited in Casey (2000) refers to four phases of fever.

The prodromal phase consists of a feeling of being unwell, however body temperature will be normal. A young baby or child may be quiet, wanting to sleep more than usual and refusing food or generally 'cranky' and unsettled.

In this prodromal stage pyrogens (chemicals) are released by inflamed and damaged cells. They travel via the bloodstream to the hypothalamus, which releases prostoglandins which raise the hypothalamic thermostat to a higher temperature.

In the second phase, the chill phase, although the body temperature is now rising the child will complain of cold and shivering will occur. The body is responding to the rise in the hypothalamic thermostat by activating heat-promoting mechanisms, until the higher temperature is reached.

During the flush phase, although the body temperature is elevated, the child may feel better. The skin will feel hot and dry. The child's temperature has reached that of the raised hypothalamic thermostat. To bring the body temperature back within the normal range removal of the causative agent or pharmaceutical intervention is required (Casey 2000).

The body will assist by activating heat-loss mechanisms when the hypothalamus detects an increase in temperature.

The final phase is referred to as diaphoresis. The child will begin to sweat profusely. Sweat needs to evaporate for cooling to occur (Green 1989). Use of fanning and sponging will aid the cooling process. (Further explanation for these interventions is given in the section relating nursing knowledge to best practice for fever management (p. 274).) The skin will be pink and flushed due to vasodilatation.

With the profuse sweating, and evaporation of water from the skin surface, comes the risk of dehydration and electrolyte imbalance. Careful monitoring of the infant/child is paramount.

Exercise

1. Besides shivering which other heat-promoting mechanism will be activated?
2. List the physical signs of dehydration.
3. Consider the effects of a fever on an adult and elderly person as well as Emma.

By applying the information given regarding baby Emma to the model of living it is possible to build a holistic, individualised picture, which supports the nursing approach (see p. 272 for potential Nursing Care Plan for Emma).

Lifespan

Emma at 18 months old is still dependent on an adult to provide a suitable safe environment in relation to body temperature control. Also she is dependent on the provision of suitable clothing for environmental temperature and fluids to promote comfort on hot days and replace fluid lost through sweating.

Dependence

Having developed a fever, Emma is dependent on recognition of her symptoms of illness by an appropriate adult who will provide suitable interventions or seek medical advice.

Independence

For Emma independence in relation to body temperature control is only in relation to biological and physiological feedback systems during health.

Biological

As part of the immune response Emma has developed a fever. Remember fever can play a positive part in the immune response, affecting the ability of the invading pathogen to reproduce and enabling better function of the immune response (Fullick 1998). Emma has recently joined a mother and baby group. She has been exposed to other children through social contact; this may be relevant. Her age will play a part in her ability to respond and should her fever not be well controlled then risk of convulsion is increased. Application of nursing interventions must be appropriate to the stages of fever and the biological and physiological responses of the body.

Psychological

As Emma's temperature increased her thermoregulatory system raised the thermostat to a higher level – this produced a shiver response, as Emma then felt cold, seeing the shiver her mother provided extra clothing, increasing Emma's temperature further. This would result in a hot, sticky and distressed baby. It is imperative that parents are provided with information about fever management to ensure they respond appropriately. Although Emma's mum noted shivering, touch would have told her that Emma was pyrexic.

Sociocultural

Consider the culture that has been created in relation to the use of GPs and emergency services. People must feel comfortable about accessing help and advice. Emma's mum took the correct action in utilising A&E when her child's condition deteriorated.

Environmental

It has already been identified that environmental temperatures can affect control of body temperature. A Health Visitor can be involved to provide further information regarding Emma's home environment. A suitable safe environment is provided in which to nurse Emma. Control of her body temperature to prevent convulsion is paramount. The internal environment of the body in relation to homeostatic mechanisms must be maintained.

Politicoeconomic

This scenario has considered only Emma and her mum. It is relevant to consider the amount of support offered to single parents. Housing, income and lifestyle all need to be considered in the assessment. It is neccessary to ascertain that when Emma is discharged her mum has all the relevant support to continue to care for her daughter to the best of her ability.

Assessment skills

Nurses carry with them unique tools that will aid patient assessment and on-going evaluation in relation to body temperature control. These unique tools are the nurse's ability to utilise interpersonal and communication skills to obtain information. These same skills enable the development of a therapeutic nurse–patient relationship (Peplau 1952). The nurse may also develop an acute use of her special senses to aid assessment.

These special senses involve the use of touch to ascertain if the patient's skin feels hot, cold, dry or clammy. Touch may also enable detection of dehydration should the skin have lost elasticity (usually tested by a skin stretch on the back of the hand). Touch (or movement) of the patient may be associated with pain indicating inflammation.

By using sight to observe the patient, the nurse will notice if the colour of the skin is pink, red, flushed, pale, mottled or cyanosed. The nurse may also notice the presence of a rash, indicating infection, or breaks in the surface of the skin. The nurse will observe and note the level of

Nursing Care Plan for Emma Smith – 18 months

Assessment	Goal/aims	Planning	Implementation	Evaluation
Maintaining a safe environment Emma is dependent on others to keep her safe	Keep safe from harm	Ensure side room is at a constant comfortable temperature and free from draughts Ensure observation is continuous Nurse with cot sides raised Keep mum with child as much as possible Observe intravenous cannula site for signs of infection Maintain IV as prescribed	Mum present with Emma at all times Named nurse identified for continuous observation Document interventions affecting IV site Report and document any evidence of infection	Mum and Emma settled on ward
Breathing Maintaining own airway	To recognise any early disruption with breathing	Record 4 hourly Observe rate, depth Note any audible cough or wheeze	4 hourly observation of temperature, pulse and respiration recorded	Maintaining own airway Breathing rate within normal limits
Communication Emma is quiet and not willing to respond to smiles etc. – possibly due to lethargy Appears content when nursed by mum	To promote positive communication for Emma's stage of development	Observe Emma's communication as temperature returns to normal limits Keep mum in contact with Emma Use gentle tone of voice and smile when talking to Emma Utilise touch to provide comfort Provide information for mum regarding Emma's condition, nursing interventions and treatment	Mum with Emma at all times Side room next to nursing office Tolerating nursing intervention	Good relationship between mum and nursing staff Emma now responding positively with simple words/smile i.e. naming familiar objects and toys.
Eating and drinking Continues to refuse diet, but now taking small amounts of oral clear fluids Not vomiting at time of assessment	For Emma to tolerate fluids and diet	Record input and output Monitor physical signs of dehydration Encourage clear fluids orally Maintain intravenous fluids as prescribed	Tolerating oral clear fluids well Continuing to record input and output Urea and electrolyte balance recorded Intravenous therapy continuing	Now graduated to mixed fluids and light diet. Urea and electrolyte balance within normal limits Intravenous therapy discontinued
Mobilising Able to walk normally unassisted Today prefers to lie still and quiet	To be mobilising as normal	Allow Emma to mobilise as she feels able	Provide a safe environment for mobilisation – keep with adult at all times	Now mobilising
Sleep and rest Awake for short periods of time only Normally sleeps 7 p.m. – 7 a.m. with afternoon nap	Return to normal sleep patterns	Allow to sleep as required Ensure observation Ensure quiet periods Record temperature during rest periods	Nurse in side room	Takes an interest in her surroundings Responding positively to others Still experiencing disrupted nights sleep.
Work and play Uninterested in favourite toys	To be stimulated by play activities	Provide stimulus in the environment, i.e. pictures to look at, mobiles etc. Provide toys which are relevant for Emma's development Keep favourite toy close	Nursed in paediatric side room Environment and toys provided to encourage play when required Favourite toy present	Playing for short periods Still sleeping a little more than normal

Nursing Care Plan *(continued)*				
Assessment	**Goal/aims**	**Planning**	**Implementation**	**Evaluation**
Eliminating One wet nappy today 2.30 p.m. Urine in this nappy observed to be dark in colour and strong in odour	To improve urine output to normal limits	Record output, number of wet nappies Obtain specimen of urine for culture and sensitivity Check bowels moved	Input and output measured Urine specimen obtained for culture and sensitivity	Input and output improved Urine infection isolated Oral antibiotic treatment commenced as prescribed
Expressing sexuality		Allow mum to provide appropriate comfort with love and hugs, etc.	Mum and staff providing comfort with appropriate use of touch	Emma is responding to comfort shown
Maintaining body temperature Raised tympanic Temperature of 38.8°C	To bring temperature back within normal limits 36.5–37.5	Nurse in a suitable environment, free from drafts Give prescribed antipyretic Monitor temperature Promote patient comfort by using tepid sponging at an appropriate time in the fever phase	Paracetemol given as prescribed at 2.10 p.m. Hourly temperature recording implemented skin exposed	Temperature now within normal limits Fever management information provided for mum
Dying Emma due to her stage of development will not be familiar with the concept of death	To promote recovery	Provide information for mum regarding Emma's condition and her treatment. Reassure	Mum informed of all nursing action and involved in care delivery	Responding positively to nursing and medical interventions

activity or lethargy with which the patient presents, and the presence or absence of shivering. The nurse's sense of smell may be used to recognise the presence of infection and excessive sweating. Fetid (stale) breath on the patient may be a symptom of dehydration. The patient may be able to tell the nurse if they feel uncomfortably hot or cold. The nurse must hear the patient and respond accordingly. The nurse may hear moans/cries of discomfort, or the chattering of teeth if shivering is present.

If the patient is conscious the nurse will use her communication and interpersonal skills to ask open and closed questions as appropriate, depending on the patient's ability to respond (see Chapter 4).

The following are examples of useful questions to ask should a patient present with symptoms of fever. They can be adapted for adult or child.

- Are you normally fit and well?
- For how long have you felt unwell?
- How long have you been aware of fever?
- Do symptoms worsen at night and can you describe the symptoms?

- Have you any other symptoms, e.g. cough, cold, headache, sore throat, pain passing urine, stomach pain, vomiting, diarrhoea, joint point, urethral or vaginal discharge?
- Have you recently received a vaccination or travelled abroad?
- Is anyone else you closely associate with unwell?
- How have you managed the fever, e.g. has an antipyretic been taken?
- Is the fever worse at night?
- What is your current fluid intake?
- When did you last pass urine?
- Have you been involved in any new social activity recently?
- Is there any previous history (or family history) of convulsion?

It has been identified that fever can occur whenever the immune system is attacked. It carries greater risk in children as their febrile state may lead to convulsions, but its management in an adult patient is equally important. Consider the following case study.

Exercise

1. List physical symptoms which may lead you to suspect tuberculosis.
2. Identify environmental and politicoeconomic factors which are significant.
3. If Lynn's laboratory test proves 'smear-positive' can you identify those who may require contact surveillance?
4. Using the example of baby Emma – apply the information you have regarding Lynn to the model of living.
5. Devise a nursing care plan for Lynn which addresses her needs on admission to hospital.

Relating nursing knowledge to best practice for fever management

Pyrexia as previously explained is usually the result of an invading pathogen. Watson (1998) states that pyrexia should be considered to be present when body temperature is 38°C or above. If the cause of the pyrexia is bacterial, it can be treated with antibiotics. Should an inflammatory response be present, anti-inflammatory drugs (steroids) will prove useful. Should the invading pathogen be a virus it will need to run its own course. However, the symptoms of pyrexia can be treated regardless of cause, to promote patient comfort. This will require skilled nursing intervention and use of antipyretic medications, with thorough knowledge of the physiological phases of fever (Porth 1994). A mild temperature of less than 38°C in an otherwise healthy person will have a positive effect on the immune system (Fullick 1998) (see p. 260).

A temperature of greater than 38°C carries with it risk of rigors, convulsions in children, electrolyte imbalance and the destruction of body proteins.

In the chill phase of fever, Porth (1994) explained that the body's temperature is increasing to the higher thermostat set point. The patient feels cold and the thermoregulatory system initiates vasoconstriction and shivering (heat-generating mechanisms) until the circulating blood reaches the new temperature set point.

Casey (2000) infers that cooling measures such as tepid sponging are not appropriate at this stage, as cooling the shell of the body will encourage further generation of heat. At this stage pharmacological intervention is recommended to bring the raised thermostat set point back within normal limits. Previous reference has been made to the fact that pyrogens travel via the bloodstream to the hypothalamus, which produces prostaglandins that act on the hypothalamus raising the set point. Casey (2000) states that prostaglandin synthesis can be inhibited by paracetemol and nonsteroidal, anti-inflammatory drugs (NSAIDs).

Paracetamol causes temporary disruption of the enzymes which manufacture the prostaglandins associated with fever and pain responses in the body, and so reduces temperature and helps aid patient comfort. NSAIDs such as aspirin are helpful in reducing fever, but they can cause side effects such as gastric irritation and indigestion. As they act to permanently inhibit the prostaglandins side effects can be widespread throughout the body (Casey 2000).

As body temperature returns to within normal limits during the flush and diaphoresis phases (Porth 1994), nursing interventions may be initiated to quicken the return of normal body temperature. These may be by the use of an electric fan or tepid sponging.

The rationale supporting the use of electric fans is that they encourage convection of heat from the body surface (Watson 1998) so lowering body temperature. This is the same effect as wind-chill, which enhances drops in body temperature during low environmental temperatures. Watson (1998) advises that fans are not directed at the patient as they can cause discomfort, which may lead to shivering and to reflex vasoconstriction that will enhance heat generation. It is only necessary to ensure adequate ventilation, ensuring patients are not in draughts.

Tepid sponging is less aggressive than sponging with cold water, so vasoconstriction is lessened. However latent heat will still evaporate, and cooling will result (Watson 1998). For evaporation to occur the body must be hotter than the temperature of the surrounding environment.

While (2000) states that approaches to treatment for pyrexia lack any robust supporting evidence. Pursell (2000a) reviewed available literature and discovered the nursing intervention of tepid sponging had been studied most extensively, as an addition to paracetamol (Newman 1985, Sharber 1997) but offered little advantage over paracetamol alone. Radiation and evaporation aid immediate heat loss, but this has only a short-term effect (Pursell 2000b). Krikler (1990) states sweating to lose body heat by evaporation tends to occur more at night when the basal temperature is lower. Should tepid sponging promote general comfort for a patient, however, it becomes a relevant nursing intervention. It must be administered at the right time in the phase of the fever.

There are causes of hyperpyrexia that are noninfectious. These include:

- alcohol withdrawal
- drug allergy
- transfusion reaction
- thyrotoxicosis (hyperthyroidism)
- stroke or central nervous system damage
- status epilepticus
- malignant hyperpyrexia
- heat stroke.

Heat stroke was referred to earlier in this chapter. Consider again Sarah who was planning her first holiday abroad. Does she heed the advice regarding the prevention of sunburn and heatstroke?

Case study 9.2 (continued)

Sarah – undertaking exercise (from p.263)

Sarah has spent her morning joining in an exercise class around the pool, at her holiday hotel. She has done this under duress, as she would rather have stayed in bed following a late night of partying and drinking excessive alcohol. It is the third day of the holiday and temperatures have soared in the last week.

During a walk to a restaurant for lunch Sarah complains of headache and nausea. She looks flushed, her skin is dry and her breathing is rapid. On reaching the restaurant Sarah goes straight to the toilet (rest room). Twenty minutes later Sarah has not returned. A friend finds Sarah lying on the rest room floor. She is not responding. Sarah is known to be normally fit and well.

Having made a safe approach and assessment of Sarah's airway, breathing and circulation, all of which are present, consider the following.

Exercise
1. What is the most likely cause of Sarah's collapse?
2. What is the flushed dry skin indicating?
3. How can you initiate cooling until an ambulance arrives?
4. How can blood pressure to vital organs be maintained?
5. Why are antipyretics ineffective in heat stroke (hyperthermia)?

It is necessary to apply some of the information we have gathered regarding Sarah to the model of living as follows.

Lifespan
Sarah is a young adult. She may experience a raise in body temperature due to hormonal changes during menstruation, but other than this, body temperature control is something probably taken for granted. At this time in her life she is probably influenced most by her peers in relation to lifestyle choices.

Dependence
Whilst unconscious Sarah has become totally dependent on others to maintain her life and instigate measures that will bring her body temperature back to within the normal range.

Independence
Quick instigation of nursing and medical care will hopefully return Sarah to a status of independence.

Biological factors
In heatstroke (hyperthermia) the temperature set point in the hypothalamus remains normal, but peripheral mechanisms are affected. This is different from fever, where the set point in the hypothalamus has increased as a result of invading pathogens (Kunihiro & Foster 1998). In hyperthermia the only way to reduce body temperature is by physical cooling. If hyperthermia is not resolved, the thermoregulatory mechanisms are overpowered resulting in a drop in cardiac output. This is what has happened to Sarah. The vessels within the body constrict in an attempt to maintain cardiac output, so leading to further heating of the core and cerebrovascular overload (Batscha 1997). The excessive internal heat depletes energy stores; sweating is nonexistent. The excessive body temperature will break down proteins, resulting in tissue necrosis, organ dysfunction and death (Worfolk 2000). Heat stroke is a medical emergency. Sarah's temperature is likely to be greater than 41°C.

Psychological
The sun and a suntan are often associated with a 'feel good factor'. Holidays are taken to hot, sunny climates to achieve this but it is necessary to know how to keep well in these climates. The psychological state will affect one's ability to respond to environmental temperature changes.

Sociocultural
Sarah is from the UK, so she will not be used to excessively high environmental temperatures. Her youth culture will have contributed to her behaviour and actions whilst away on holiday, i.e. exposure to direct sunlight and alcohol consumption.

Environmental
A combination of high environmental temperature, high humidity, lack of wind, vigorous activity and dehydration will contribute to the development of heat stroke (Lloyd 1994). When humidity reaches 100%, sweat evaporation is inhibited and cooling prevented.

Politicoeconomic
Investment in programmes that educate people about heat-related illness and heat stroke prevention are necessary. Prevention is always better than cure, however education would facilitate early detection and appropriate response,

should heat-related illness be suspected, so preventing the life threat associated with heat stroke.

Whilst waiting for emergency personnel to arrive, it is necessary to begin cooling without delay:

- move the patient to a cool place, lie them down, raise their legs
- remove excessive clothing but maintain dignity
- use cool wet compresses and place them in the groin, axilla and neck
- consider covering the patient with a wet sheet
- observe airway, breathing and circulation
- a fan will be helpful in aiding evaporation and convection.

Worfolk (2000) states that the importance of lowering body temperature cannot be overemphasised. In the acute hospital setting, cooling and careful monitoring of body temperature will be paramount. Cooling will be aggressive with the goal of returning body temperature to less than 37.8°C (Worfolk 2000). Fluid and electrolyte replacement will be necessary and cardiac, pulmonary, neurologic, hepatic and renal functions will be monitored.

The cooling measures used are those of convection and evaporation. In heat stroke, fanning will substantially speed the process of evaporation of moist air next to the body. Sponging will provide the water on the body surface to aid this process (Worfolk 2000).

> **Exercise**
> Devise a nursing care plan for Sarah in her current state of hyperthermia.

Having considered hyperthermia (hyperpyrexia), this section now considers hypothermia. Hypothermia is a condition, which can affect any age group, but carries significant risk for older people.

It has already been ascertained that a core body temperature of between 36.1°C and 37.8°C is required to maintain optimum homeostatic function (Marieb 1999).

Hypothermia is defined as a core body temperature of 35°C or below (Lloyd 1996). Clinical features of hypothermia will vary as the patient's condition worsens, so what are the clinical features and how can sense be made of them physiologically?

Initially clinical features will include pallor, lethargy, feeling cold to the touch, shivering and tachycardia. As the environmental temperature drops peripheral vasoconstriction occurs in response to hypothalamic stimulation, increasing heart rate, blood pressure and cardiac output (Murphy 1998, cited in Kelly et al 2001).

As the person's temperature continues to fall, the shiver response is lost, due to thermoregulatory failure. The patient will develop a bradycardia and a decrease in respiratory effort leading to hypoxia and confusion, often associated with pulmonary and cardiac overload as blood is redirected from the periphery to the major organs.

As body temperature reaches 30°C, the person will be on the verge of unconsciousness. Any responses will be slow, and speech difficult. According to Lloyd (1996) consciousness is usually lost between 32–30°C with occasional exceptions. Pupil reflexes fail and muscle rigidity is increased and cyanosis is evident. They may appear dead. The Advanced Life Support organisation, to this end, advocate that a hypothermic victim should not be considered dead until all reasonable resuscitation efforts have been made and that the hypothermic victim has been rewarmed to 33°C and remained unresponsive at that temperature during resuscitation efforts.

Progressive pulmonary depression can result in respiratory arrest whilst cardiovascular depression and reduction in tissue perfusion increase the incidence of cardiac arrhythmia. Sinus bradycardia is thought to be caused by the direct effects of cold on the pacemaker (sino atrial node) of the heart. Atrial fibrillation and ectopic beats may be present. As cardiac function decreases cardiac output drops (Tinker & Zapol 1992, cited in Keane 2001).

Both respiratory and metabolic acidosis occur. Inadequate respiration causes oxygen retention and decreases tissue perfusion. There is a build up of lactate and this with a fall in secretions leads to a build up of acids in the body.

Cardiac arrhythmias commonly progress to ventricular fibrillation as cardiac output continues to decrease. Cardiac arrest may occur as a direct response, or asystole may result. In the first part of the chapter we were introduced to Marjory who was at risk of developing hypothermia.

> **Case study 9.3** *(continued)*
>
> **Marjory (from p. 265)**
>
> When her daughter next visits she finds Marjory lying on the floor in the hall. Marjory is semi-conscious; she has been incontinent of urine. Her daughter is unable to make sense of Marjory's verbal responses. Marjory has a blue tinge to her lips and hands. She feels very cold to the touch but is not shivering. Marjory's daughter dials for the emergency services to attend. Marjory is transferred to the Accident and Emergency department.

> **Exercise**
> Consider the physiological and objective information you have regarding Marjory.
>
> 1. Without the use of a thermometer, what would you approximate Marjory's temperature to be?

It is possible that a predisposing factor other than a fall has contributed to Marjory's current condition, i.e. stroke, myocardial infarction and infection. Possible causes of collapse must be considered and dismissed accordingly, dependent upon assessment and investigations carried out.

Exercise

Apply the information you have so far in this chapter regarding Marjory to the model of living in the following areas:

- lifespan
- dependency
- independence
- biological
- psychological
- sociocultural
- environmental
- politicoeconomic.

Consideration of all these factors will facilitate a holistic assessment, which will enable the development of a nursing care plan. The plan of care, within implementation and ongoing evaluation should help Marjory reach achievable goals. Goals set for Marjory should promote some independence for her in relation to the Activities of Living. Kelly et al (2001) refer to some key aspects of management for a hypothermic patient and you may wish to consider these as part of Marjory's care.

Exercise

Consider the following then complete the following nursing care plan for Marjory.

Assessment of Marjory's current health status in relation to the Activities of Living has been completed. Now nursing actions such as those in the following lists are required:

- Measurement and monitoring of vital signs. Record rectal temperature regularly to evaluate the effectiveness of interventions.
- Ensure re-warming of the patient is appropriate to the degree of hypothermia.
- A temperature of less than 32°C will require more intense and invasive management.
- Minimise movement of the patient as much as possible to prevent the development or aggravation of cardiac

arrhythmias, electrocardiograph monitoring will aid detection of these.
- Monitor fluid input and output. If the patient is semiconscious always ensure a gag reflex is present. You may consider urethral catheterisation.
- Consider nasogastric intubation and/or antiemetics, if needed.
- Monitor urea and electrolyte levels and blood sugar levels.
- Monitor neurological function.
- Maintain patient safety. Observe for confusion, which may be present if the patient urea and electrolyte or blood sugar levels are low. Confusion may also be present if the patient develops hypoxia.
- Identify and treat any disposing factors.

Complete the following care plan for Marjory.

Assessment	Goal	Plan	Implementation	Evaluation
Maintaining a safe environment Dependent on others to maintain a safe environment and to prevent further reduction in body temperature. Her confused state may lead to injury				
Breathing Maintaining own airway. Respirations are slow and laboured, 8 per min				
Communicating Attempting to communicate verbally but making incomprehensible sounds				
Eating and drinking Maintaining own airway Gag reflex present Taking warm oral fluids with encouragement				
Eliminating Incontinent of urine which is strong in colour and smell No evidence of constipation				

Exercise *(continued)*

Assessment	Goal	Plan	Implementation	Evaluation
Personal cleansing and dressing Unable to maintain own personal hygiene Now in clean, dry, warm night clothes				
Mobilising Moving in the bed/trolley Unable to stand without assistance				
Sleep and rest Drifts occasionally into deep sleep				
Work and play Currently not applicable Reassess when Marjory's condition improves				
Expressing sexuality During episodes of confusion Marjory is attempting to remove bedding and nightclothes. Tolerating rectal temperature measurement				
Maintaining body temperature Rectal temperature 32.5°C Shivering response absent Skin pale slight cyanosis, cold to the touch				
Dying Unable to express fears due to confusion (bereaved 12 months ago)				

Clinical measurement of body temperature

Clinical measurement of body temperature will indicate deviations from normal body temperature, and may be significant in indicating the need for medical and nursing intervention.

Measurement of body temperature can be invasive via the rectum or noninvasive via the mouth, ear, axilla or groin. The method and route chosen should be a direct result of the individualised patient assessment undertaken. The choice of method, route and regularity of body temperature measurement will be part of any nursing care plan.

Peripheral body temperature of the shell varies with changing environmental conditions whilst core body temperature should remain constant, between 36.1°C and 37.8°C (Marieb 1999). Recording body temperature via the mouth, ear, axilla, groin or rectum gives an estimate of the core body temperature, as these sites all have major arteries within close distance (Luckman 1977).

Using a thermometer orally requires placement of the thermometer to be in a pocket on either side of the frenulum, below the tongue (Closs 1987). This facilitates measurement of the temperature of blood in the carotid arteries (Watson 1998). Measurement orally may be by use of glass mercury thermometer, electronic device, or chemical dot disposable thermometer.

Manian and Griesenauer (1998) and Wilshaw et al (1999) cited in Casey (2000) refer to the fact that glass mercury thermometers are still the most accurate standard method of temperature measurement. In the United Kingdom glass mercury thermometers are not the most common method used, due to the risk of breakage and mercury poisoning and the introduction of standards for the Care of Substances Hazardous to Health (COSHH). Woollens (1996) states glass thermometers have been banned in Sweden since 1992 due to the potential harm to both patient and/or nurse.

The placement of glass mercury thermometers sublingually will be determined by the patient's age and ability.

It can be difficult to maintain placement and Casey (2000) states they can take up to 8 minutes for stabilisation, though this is controversial. Edwards (1997) cites studies recommending times for glass mercury thermometer placement from no more than 3 minutes (Pugh-Davis 1986) to 8–9 minutes (Nichols & Kucha 1972). Where there is any indication that the patient may bite, choke or be unable to maintain placement of the thermometer they should not be used. Oral thermometer placement should also be avoided in a nauseous patient for obvious reasons, and also, where closure of the mouth may contribute to any complications with breathing.

Electronic, or chemical dot thermometry has tended to replace the use of glass mercury thermometers in the UK. Electronic thermometers fitted with probes have none of the associated risks with glass mercury thermometers, and the use of plastic probe covers (use once – disposable) reduce risk of crossinfection between patients. Most have a signal, which indicates when maximum temperature is reached (Edwards 1997).

Chemical dot thermometers are now commonly used in the United Kingdom, in clinical areas. They also carry none of the risks associated with the glass mercury method, and they are used once only to prevent crossinfection. The chemical dot thermometer consists of a thin plastic strip with dots of thermosensitive chemicals that change colour to indicate the correct temperature (see Fig. 9.3).

They are placed sublingually for 1 minute. Check individual manufacturer's instructions for use. Common factors which affect the accuracy of oral temperature measurement may include:

- incorrect positioning of the thermometer
- the thermometer being read too soon
- the patient's need to breath through the mouth
- eating and/or drinking hot or cold substances prior to the procedure
- amount of exercise taken prior to the procedure
- smoking.

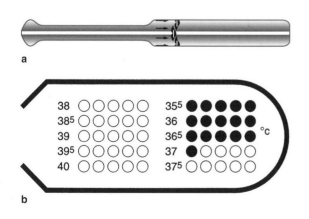

Fig. 9.3 **a** Disposable chemical dot thermometer. **b** Recording area of a disposable thermometer (from Jamieson et al 2002, with permission).

Torrence and Semple (1998) suggest oral temperature should not be recorded within 15 minutes of a patient eating, drinking, smoking or taking physical exercise.

Each of the methods discussed can also be used to record temperature at the axilla or groin. Hinchliff (1996) refers to the fact that axillary temperature is generally 0.5°C lower than an oral temperature reading. This is also relevant when the choice of site is the groin.

> **Exercise**
> 1. Record your own temperature orally, using either a glass mercury thermometer, electronic device or a chemical dot thermometer.
> 2. Then using the same method, record your temperature again via the axilla.
> 3. Is there any marked difference in the measurement recorded?

The axilla may be the site of choice when oral recording temperature cannot be tolerated by the patient for reasons previously highlighted.

Watson (1998) states that whilst the axilla and groin may be less dangerous than the mouth, they may be less efficient in obese and very thin patients. In obese patients this may be due to the excessive fat layer, which prevents the thermometer placement from being close to the underlying artery.

In thin patients, while being held in place, the thermometer may not be in close contact to the skin, but surrounded by air, resulting in an inaccurate measurement of body temperature (Watson 1998). Vasoconstriction will affect accuracy at these sites (Casey 2000).

Tympanic thermometers use infrared radiation to measure the temperature of blood flowing through the tympanic membrane of the ear. This method requires placement of a thermometer probe in the external auditory canal. It is thought to be an accurate method, as the tympanic membrane shares its circulation with the hypothalamus (Casey 2000). The method is quick, convenient and relatively unobtrusive which makes it an acceptable method of measuring temperature in children. Tympanic thermometers use disposable probe covers, which also reduce risk of crossinfection between patients.

Sganga et al (2000) refer to the fact that some evaluations of the tympanic thermometer against other methods cited by Fraden and Lackey (1991) have indicated its reliability as a method of temperature measurement among various ages. However, other studies have questioned its accuracy against other methods (Yetman et al 1993, Wells et al 1995).

Sganga et al (2000) also refer to a study by Pransky (1991) which concluded accuracy of tympanic temperature measurement is increased if an ear tug is used to straighten the ear canal, whilst a 1994 study by Erickson and Woo found an ear tug did not have a significant effect on

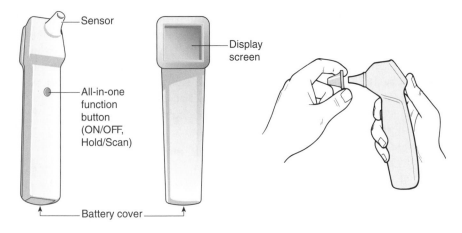

Fig. 9.4 A tympanic thermometer (from Jamieson et al 2002, with permission).

temperature measurement. In their own study comparing four methods of normal newborn temperature measurement Sganga et al (2000) found tympanic temperature measurement correlated poorly with the glass thermometer (see Fig. 9.4).

Rectal temperature measurement is considered to be close to core body temperature, as it measures temperature of blood flowing within the pulmonary artery, due to the rectum being well supplied with blood from the hepatic and portal circulation.

The rectal site was often the site of choice in babies and young children. It carries a risk in relation to injury, bowel perforation and injection. Casey (2000) states there is also cultural distaste for this method. It is also a method that promotes little dignity for the patient no matter what age. Rectal temperature recording is seldom done on paediatric wards in the UK, however Blumenthal's (2000) study found practice nurses still recommend that the rectal route be used in children under 3 years. This raises questions about fever management in children, and how to educate parents regarding the recording of a child's temperature. Noninvasive methods, which cause least distress to the child, are those most likely to be utilised appropriately by parents.

For a patient who is severely ill, or where there is life threat, the rectal route may be used. This involves the placement of a fine electronic probe into the rectum, to facilitate continual body temperature measurement. This is useful in aiding management of cooling or rewarming of a patient, when body temperature deviations need to be returned to within normal limits, in a controlled and measurable way. For example: to rewarm a severely hypothermic patient at 0.5°C per hour.

Exercise
1. Consider the patient scenarios presented within this chapter.
2. Which method and route of temperature measurement is most suitable for each patient?
3. How often should body temperature measurement be undertaken for each patient?

The optimal time to measure temperature is 8 p.m. but this can be affected when patients are hospitalised and pain, trauma and sleep disturbance all affect normal sleeping patterns. Temperatures recorded at other times during the day are equally valuable, but diurnal/circadian rhythms must be considered (Edwards 1997).

Best practice in relation to method, rate and regularity for body temperature measurement will be a direct result of an accurate and individualised patient assessment. Remember assessment is an ongoing process to be performed regularly throughout an episode of patient care.

Summary

1. Caring for a person who has a deviation from normal body temperature involves thorough knowledge of the body's physiological responses. By understanding these physiological responses it is possible to provide safe and effective nursing interventions that promote patient comfort.

Summary (continued)

2. This knowledge also assists in providing advice for others regarding prevention of temperature deviations which can cause great harm. Accurate assessment, followed by the setting of achievable goals, facilitates a plan of care that addresses individualised patient needs. Nursing interventions must be based on best practice, and knowledge of equipment which may be used to measure body temperature is essential. The choice of equipment will be based upon individual patient assessment.

3. Evaluation of nursing interventions must be ongoing, so practice can be altered should the patient's condition change. By using the model for nursing alongside the model of living a holistic view of a person's lifestyle can be developed. Ultimately this should result in an episode of skilled care giving which is beneficial and therapeutic both in the prevention and treatment for illnesses related to deviations in body temperature control.

References

Batscha C 1997 Heat stroke. Keeping your client cool in the summer. Journal of Psychosocial Nursing 35(7): 12–17

BBC News 1999 news.bbc.co.uk/hi/english/health/medical

Blackburn S, Loper D 1992 Maternal, fetal and neonatal physiology. A clinical perspective. WB Saunders Company, Philadelphia

Blumenthal 2000 Fever and the practice nurse: measurement and treatment. Community Practitioner 73(3): 519–521

Casey G 2000 Fever management in children. Paediatric Nursing 12(3): 38–43

Chiodini J 2001 Where do we get our travel health information from? Nursing in Practice 2: 139–140

Closs J 1987 Oral temperature measurement. Nursing Times 83: 136–139

Collier I, McCash E, Bartram J 1996 Writing nursing diagnosis: A clinical thinking approach. Mosby, London

Collins K, Dore C, Exton-Smith AN 1977 Accidental hypothermia and impaired temperature homeostasis in the elderly. British Medical Journal 1: 353–356

Dematte J, O'Mara K, Buescher J, Whitney CG, Forsythe S, MacNamee T, Adiga RB, Ndukwa IM 1998 Near fatal heatstroke during the 1995 heatwave in Chicago. Annals of Internal Medicine 129: 173–181

Department of Health 1998 The prevention and control of tuberculosis in the United Kingdom. HSC 1998/196. Stationery Office, London

Department of Work and Pensions 2001 http://www.dwp.gov.uk/winterfuel

Edwards S 1997 Measuring temperature. Professional Nurse 13(2): 253–258

Ejidokun O, Ramaiah S, Sandhu S 1998 A cluster of tuberculosis cases in a family. Communicable Disease in Public Health 1(4): 245–300

Environmental News Network 1999 (www.enn.com/ennnewsarchive/1999)

Erickson RS, Woo TM 1994 Accuracy of infrared ear thermometry and traditional temperature methods in young children. Heart and Lung 23: 181–193

Fisher B 1999 Walk-in-clinic fever. Practice Nursing 10(15)

Fraden J, Lackey RP 2000 Estimation of body site temperatures from tympanic measurements. Clinical Paediatrics Supplement 30: 65–70

Fullick A 1998 Human health and disease. Heinemann Advanced Science, Oxford

Gould D 1994 Controlling patients' body temperature. Nursing Standard 8(N 35): May 25

Green JH 1989 An introduction to human physiology, 4th edn. Oxford Medical Publications, Oxford

Gupta A 1999 Influenza: Improving uptake of vaccination in older people. Geriatric Medicine 11: 13

Handley AJ, Swain A (eds) 1996 Advanced life support manual, 2nd edn. Resuscitation Council UK, London

Health & Safety Executive 2002 COSHH regulations. http://www.hse.gov.uk/hthdir/noframes/coshh

Hinchliff S 1996 Innate defences. In Hinchliff S, Montague S, Watson R (eds) Physiology for nursing practice, 2nd edn. London, Baillière Tindall

Imrie M, Hall G 1990 Body temperature and anaesthesia. British Journal of Anaesthetics 64: 346–354

jas 2001 (www.jas.tj/skincancer/facts)

Keane C 2000 Physiological responses and management of hypothermia. Emergency Nurse 8(8):26–31

Kelly M, Ewens B, Jevan P 2001 Hypothermia management. Nursing Times 97(9):36–37

Kerry 1999 in USA today at (http://www.usatoday.com/weather)

Krikler S 1990 What to do about temperatures. Nursing Standard 4(25)

Kunihiro A, Foster J 1998 Heat exhaustion and heat stroke. (http://www.emedicine.com/EMERG/tropic236.htm)

Lloyd E 1996 Hypothermia and cold stress. London, Croom Helm

Lloyd E 1994 Temperature and performance II: Heat. British Medical Journal 309(6954):587

Luckman J 1997 Saunders manual of nursing care. Saunders, Philadelphia, PA

Macmillan A, Corbett JL, Johnson RH, Crampton-Smith A, Spalding JMK, Wollner L 1967 Temperature regulation in survivors of accidental hypothermia of the elderly. Lancet 22: 165–169

Mallett J, Dougherty L 2000 The Royal Marsden Hospital manual of clinical nursing procedures, 5th edn. Blackwell Science, Oxford

Manian F, Griesenauer S 1998 Lack of agreement between tympanic and oral temperature measurements in adult hospitalised patients. American Journal of Infection Control 26: 428–430

Marieb E 1999 Human anatomy and physiology, 4th edn. Addison Wesley, California

Medicinenet 1999 (www.medicinenet.com)

Medico 2001 (Medico.uwcm.ac.uk)

Miller D 2001 The flu: current treatments and future strategies. Nursing in Practice 2: 87–90

Murphy P 1998 Handbook of critical care. Science Press, London

Newman J 1985 Evaluation of sponging to reduce body temperature in febrile infants. Canada Medical Association Journal 132: 641–642

NHS 2001 A new guide to childhood immunisation. Health Promotion England, London

Nichols G, Kucha D 1972 Oral measurements. American Journal of Nursing 72(b): 1091–1093

Noa 2002 (www.erh.noa.gov/den/windchill)

Patja A, Davidkin I, Kurki T, Kallio M 2000 Serious adverse events after measles, mumps, rubella vaccination during a 14 year prospective follow up. Pediatric Infectious Disease Journal 19: 1127–1134

Peplau HE 1952 Interpersonal relations in nursing GP Putnam, New York

PHLS Public Health Laboratory Service 2001 (www.phls.co.uk/facts/influenza/flu.html)

Porth M 1994 Pathophysiology – concepts of altered health states, 4th edn. Lippincott, Philadelphia

Pransky SM 1991 The impact of technique and condition of the tympanic membrane upon infrared tympanic thermometry. Clinical Paediatrics Supplement 30: 50–52

Public Health Laboratory Services Communicable Disease Surveillance Centre Supplement 1998 Infectious disease in England and Wales: April 1966–June 1992. Communicable Diseases Report 8(2): 53

Pursell E 2000a The use of antipyretic medications in the prevention of febrile convulsion in children. Journal of Clinical Nursing 9: 473–480

Pursell E 2000b Physical treatment of fever. Archives of Diseases in Childhood 82: 238–239

Pugh Davis S et al 1986 A comparison of mercury and digital clinical thermometers. Journal of Advanced Nursing 11(5): 535–543

Roper N, Logan W, Tierney A 1996 The elements of nursing – a model for nursing based on a model of living, 4th edn. Churchill Livingstone, Edinburgh

Roper N, Logan W, Tierney A 2000 The Roper-Logan-Tierney model of nursing based on activities of living. Churchill Livingstone, Edinburgh

Sganga A, Wallace R, Kiehl E, Irving T, Witter L 2000 A comparison of four methods of normal newborn temperature measurement. The American Journal of Maternal/Child Nursing 25(2):76–79

Sharber J 1997 The efficacy of tepid sponge bathing to reduce fever in young children. American Journal of Emergency Medicine 15: 188–192

Sidebottom J 1992 When it's hot enough to kill. RN 55(8): 31–34

Taylor B, Miller E, Farrington C, Petropoulis M, Favot-Mayaud I, Li J, Waight P 1999 Autism and measles, mumps, rubella vaccine: no epidemiological evidence for a causal association. The Lancet 353: 2026–2029

Tinker J, Zapol W 1992 Care of the critically ill patient, 2nd edn. Springer-Verlag, New York

Torrence C, Semple MC 1998 Recording temperature. Nursing Times 94(3): Practical Procedures for Nursing Supplement

Watson R 1998 Controlling body temperature in adults. Emergency Nurse 6(1): 31–39

Waugh A, Grant A 2001 Ross and Wilson anatomy and physiology in health and illness, 9th edn. Churchill Livingstone, Edinburgh

Wells, King J, Hedstrom C, Youngkins J 1995 Does tympanic temperature measure up? The American Journal of Maternal Child Nursing 14: 88–93

While A 2000 Putting fever in perspective. British Journal of Community Nursing 5(10)

Wilshaw R, Beckstrand R, Ward D, Schaalje GB 1999 A comparison of the use of tympanic, axillary and rectal thermometers in infants. Journal of Paediatric Nursing 4(2): 88–93

World Health Organisation (www.who.int/inf-fs/en/fact.html)

World Health Organisation 2001 International travel and health – vaccination requirements and health advice. Geneva, WHO

Woollens S 1996 Temperature measurement devices. Professional Nurse 11: 541–547

Worfolk J 2000 Heat waves: Their impact on the health of elders. Geriatric Nursing 21(2): 70–77

Yetman R, Coody DK, West MS, Montgomery D, Brown M 1993 Comparison of temperature measurement by an aural infrared thermometer with measurements by traditional rectal and auxiliary techniques. Journal of Paediatrics 122: 769–773

Further reading

Desborough J 1997 Body temperature control and anaesthesia. British Journal of Hospital Medicine 57(9): 440–442

Hinchliff SM, Montague SE, Watson R 1996 Physiology for nursing practice, 2nd edn. Baillière Tindall, London

Jamieson EM, McCall JM, Whyte LA 2002 Clinical nursing practice, 4th edn. Churchill Livingstone, Edinburgh

Jones JG, Needham M, Roberts E, Owen R 1999 A history of Abergele Hospital – confronting the white plague. Gee & Son (Denbigh) Ltd, Denbigh

Mallett J, Bailey C 2000 Manual of clinical nursing procedures, 4th edn. Blackwell Science, Oxford

Useful websites

http://www.helptheaged.org.uk (Help the Aged)
http://www.resus.org.uk (Resuscitation Council)
http://www.age.concern.org.uk (Age Concern)
http://www.statistics.gov.uk (Office for National Statistics)

Mobilising

Julia Ryan

Introduction

A characteristic of living things is the ability to move independently of external forces. Movement is important for many reasons – to find and prepare food, to get away from danger, and to make the environment safe, comfortable and enjoyable. Mobilising is not only about obvious behaviours such as walking, running or swimming – it's also about being able to use a computer keyboard, gardening or painting. Movement provides the means for personal contact with other people and the surroundings.

Many illnesses and injuries can cause mobility problems, diminishing the capacity to move freely around the environment, be that a room, a chair or even a bed. Loss of mobility, even for a short time can have devastating effects on physical wellbeing. Being in control of movement can be a source of autonomy, pride and dignity, so mobility problems can also have significant psychological and emotional effects.

This chapter explores the Activity of Living 'mobilising' described by Nancy Roper, Winifred Logan and Alison Tierney in their model for nursing (Roper et al 1996, 2000). The model of living will be used to look at mobilising in everyday life. Concepts of lifespan, independence/dependence and important factors influencing mobility will be explored. The model for nursing will examine how the Activities of Living can be used in practice.

Using the components of the model, the chapter will focus on the following:

- mobilising in health and illness across the lifespan
- dependence and independence in mobilising
- factors influencing mobilising
- nursing care of individuals with health needs associated with the Activity of Living, mobilising.

This chapter does not intend to be a definitive account of all the knowledge and skills you will need to effectively meet the mobility needs of the patients you will come across in practice – rather the intention is to help you to make sense of your previous experiences, challenge your current ideas, and help you to identify further learning.

THE MODEL OF LIVING

Mobilising in health and illness across the lifespan

Infancy and childhood

Learning how to move independently begins even before birth. Mothers are often all too aware of the movement of their baby in the uterus, and whilst this might mean sleep-disturbed nights, it also indicates that the baby is developing as expected. Fetal movement can be seen on an ultrasound scan in very early pregnancy, and the mother can often feel movement from around 16 weeks gestation onwards.

The newborn human baby is not able to mobilise independently. The development of basic mobility skills is very complex and takes a considerable time, a much longer time, relatively speaking, for humans than other animals. This is principally due to the human infant's immature nervous system which does not allow for purposeful coordinated movement. Throughout infancy and childhood great importance is attached to the development of independent movement. Rolling, crawling, standing, walking and running are greeted with joy by the child's family, and are important milestones noted during the monitoring of a child's development. As children attain greater neuromuscular control, they use their mastery of mobilising to do other Activities of Living such as play, personal cleansing and dressing.

Adolescence and adult

Good mobility habits, as in the early years. Ex element of educatio healthy living skills independence in mobility reflects increasing personal independence. A sign of maturity is the ability to go out into the world; a symbol of this is the young person being given the keys to the car (rather than the keys to the door!). Young adulthood is often seen as a 'risk-taking' time of life. This applies to mobilising as well as other activities and is illustrated by the high levels of road traffic and other accidents and sporting injuries amongst young people.

In adulthood the increasing pressures of work, maybe parenthood or other family commitments, can make regular exercise difficult. This might be especially problematic if one has a sedentary occupation. Mobility as such is taken for granted, and it is only when something happens to reduce one's ability (an accident or illness for example) that the individual might be made aware of how mobility affects many aspects of life.

Late adulthood

Much of the world is experiencing demographic change as both the numbers and proportions of older people increase. In the UK today around a fifth of the population is over 60 years of age. In the future the most significant rise will be in the age group 80 years plus (DoH 2001a). Whilst the majority of older people live fulfilling, independent lives, there are a number of age-related changes that impact on mobility in late life, and increase the likelihood of problems in mobilising. It is for this reason, that much of the material in this chapter will relate to the older adult. As an example, falls are a common occurrence in later life and are associated with significant levels of morbidity (disease and disordered function) and mortality (death) (Stuck & Beck 2001).

Purposeful mobilising depends on a functioning sensory ability, central nervous system coordination and musculoskeletal system. Physiological changes in late life which affect mobilising include: a reduced sense of balance, reduced righting reflex, reduced reaction time and speed of response. Despite these changes, impaired mobility is not inevitable in late life.

There are a number of factors, other than the biological, which impact on an older person's mobility levels. Perceptions and beliefs about levels and types of activity appropriate for older people can be important. Old age can be seen as a time to take it easy and retire to a sedentary life, indeed there is evidence that detraining starts fairly early in the life course. Whilst some physiological changes might be inevitable – the extent to which they impact on mobility and broader function are modifiable. Even a fairly moderate reduction in mobility can have serious implications, for frail older people in particular. Problems with mobilising can mean that the individual can't get out to do the shopping, ~~nd~~ up to cook, or get to the toilet in time. The good ~~that~~ appropriate interventions can increase mobility ~~al~~ independence, and reduce admissions to

> **Exercise**
> Take some time to observe how people move: how they stand, get up from a sitting position, walk or run.
>
> 1. Can you see any similarities and differences in the patterns you observe?
> 2. How are these similarities and differences related to lifespan?
> 3. You might want to think about why people move in the way they do.
> 4. Think about how the way someone stands or sits (posture), or the way they walk (gait) can project an image of who they are (or maybe who they would like to be).

These points may have been noted:

- How a baby learns to stand, balance and walk unsupported. Whilst initially movement is clumsy and the child has to concentrate, movement becomes smooth and automatic.
- Children running, skipping and jumping as they use movement to expend reserves of energy and explore the world around them.
- Young people, as they become more self-conscious are often aware of their bodies and this can affect posture and gait.
- Perhaps you thought about how pregnancy can affect mobility. Try and recall how a pregnant woman stands and walks, especially in the latter stages of pregnancy.
- You might have noticed some differences in gait amongst older people. Older women often develop a narrow base when standing or walking, which leads to a 'waddling' gait. Older men often develop a wider walking base.
- Very old people tend to walk more slowly and deliberately. This might be due to physical changes, but also might be related to a lack of confidence or fear of falling. It's also interesting to think about societal views of mobilising in later life – after all the road sign for 'older people crossing' shows a bent over figure with a stick.
- Some people have a characteristic posture or gait which means you can recognise them even at a distance.

People move in a variety of ways. Some of these differences are due to age, but others are not. They may be due to temporary changes, for example physical factors such as a waddling gait in pregnancy, or psychosocial factors such as the way in which people who are attracted to each other mirror the other's posture. This will be revisited later in the chapter when looking in detail at assessment.

Dependence and independence in mobilising

At a simple level the dependence–independence continuum might be equated with lifespan: dependency existing at both extremes of age, and independence the norm in-between. A wider consideration of mobilising might challenge some notions inherent in this opinion. There is a view that equates physical mobility with independence in its broadest sense – leading to perceptions of people who have impaired mobility as being wholly dependent. Consider a young woman who uses a wheelchair and a modified car to enable her to get to work, go to the pub, or to do her shopping. On one hand she might be considered dependent because she relies on her wheelchair, yet the wheelchair enables her independence in living. Yet again, the young woman might also be an elite athlete with an extremely high level of physical fitness.

It is evident that independence in many of the other Activities of Living is closely related to independence in mobilising.

Exercise

Have you ever had an illness or accident that has affected your mobility? If not, imagine that you are not able to move without help.

1. Make a note of the effects reduced mobility had on your other Activities of Living.
2. What sort of help did you need?
3. How did you feel?

You might have thought about the:

- frustration of not being able to do what you want, when you want
- embarrassment of needing help to go to the toilet, or having to urinate or defecate in bed (have you ever sat on a bed pan? If not then try it!)
- feelings of loneliness with everyone else getting on with their lives whilst you are in bed or in hospital, not able to join in.

Now it might be that you have had or have imagined very different feelings. That is acceptable. It is just worth remembering that even a limited reduction in mobility can have a big impact on one's experience and quality of life (see Case study 8.2).

Dependence in mobility can occur as a result of disease or trauma. For most people this will be temporary and so, with time, mobility will be regained, however for some there will be long-lasting mobility problems. Other people have impaired mobility from birth because of altered body structure and/or function.

There are a number of mobility aids that can be used to support independence in mobilising. Walking aids, such as sticks and crutches can be used to:

- improve balance and stability by widening the person's base
- relieve pain from fractures or arthritis for example by transferring weight through the upper limbs to the ground
- give confidence.

As with any piece of equipment used in patient care, the nurse should understand the principles of use. Walking aids should be of the correct length, so when one is standing and holding the aid the elbows should be slightly flexed (30° angle). The exception to this is a gutter aid, which keeps the elbow at a right angle. Walking aids should be checked regularly to make sure that ferrules (caps) on the end of the aid are tightly fitting and not worn down. Metal aids should be checked for bends in the frame, and wooden ones for splits and cracks.

People might need to use a wheelchair to maintain or restore independence. Each person will have specific requirements, which must be taken into account. Wheelchair use might be temporary, intermittent or regular. There are many types of wheelchair including: self-propelled and electrically controlled, those for indoor use or outdoor use, lightweight or heavyweight, one-arm or two-arm drive, high seat or low seat. From this short list of potential differences it is clearly important to match the person's individual requirements with an appropriate wheelchair.

Exercise

1. What do you think the consequences of inadequate wheelchair provision might be?
2. Have you ever used a wheelchair to transport people? Do you know what to check to make sure that the wheelchair is appropriate and fit for the task?
3. How are mobility aids provided in your locality? Think about walking sticks, crutches, wheelchairs, callipers and prosthetic limbs.

The impact of inadequate provision can be significant as Table 10.1 indicates. In some situations, for example in some nursing homes or rehabilitation wards, there is a pool of wheelchairs that are used for everyone. Not only might these not be suitable for a particular individual, but they might also be poorly maintained and hazardous to both the patient and the nurse.

Factors relating to mobilising

Biological factors

The first question to ask might be 'how do we move?'. To fully answer this question requires a deep understanding of the central and peripheral nervous systems, as well as the musculoskeletal system. It is also important to think about the way that genetics and the external environment can impact upon the anatomy and physiology needed for normal movement.

Table 10.1 Potential consequences of poor wheelchair provision

For the wheelchair user	Impairment or loss of mobility Reduced choice of lifestyle Reduced quality of life Increased dependence Discomfort and pain Pressure sores Poor posture Permanent deformity (especially in children)
For carers	Fatigue Back pain Impact on personal relationship
For service providers	Increased dependency of service user Increased need for care Health problems for wheelchair user and carer

It should also be remembered that we are always moving: your eyes are moving as you read this book, your gut is slowly moving digestive products along its length, the diaphragm and your intercostal muscles are moving your ribcage causing air to move in and out of your lungs. The Activity of Living 'mobilising' is principally concerned with purposeful voluntary movement, and this chapter will provide a basic overview of how bones, muscles and joints work together to produce movement.

The skeleton

The skeleton (see Fig. 10.1) has a number of functions which include:

- providing the body with a supporting framework
- protecting soft vital organs such as the brain, spinal cord, heart and lungs from injury

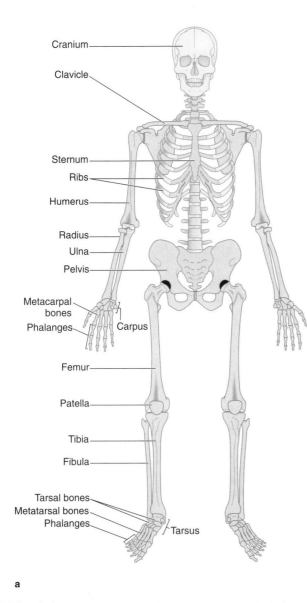
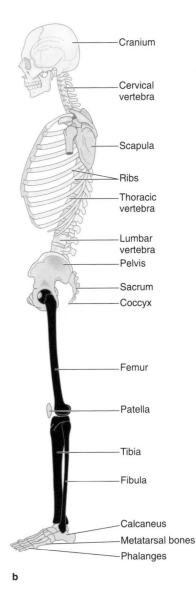

Fig. 10.1 The skeleton (from Waugh & Grant 2001, with permission).

- storing a reserve of minerals such as calcium, phosphorus and magnesium. Around 99% of the calcium content (1 kg) of the body is contained in the skeleton
- developing blood cells in bone marrow
- allowing movement by providing a base for the attachment of muscles and tendons, and the formation of joints.

Exercise

1. Find a model skeleton either in your educational establishment or clinical area.
2. Take your time to look at and handle the bones.
3. Note the shapes of the bones and how they fit together, find out where the main muscles would be attached, and see how and where the joints articulate.

Bone

It is sometimes easy to forget that bone is living tissue. Bone is made up of 20–30% water; so living bones are soft and slightly flexible. Bone has its own blood and nerve supply, which is why fractures are painful and can cause significant blood loss. Bones are not solid, but are made up of small tubes arranged in concentric circles. This means that bone is strong but lightweight, and weight for weight healthy bone is stronger than concrete or steel. If you can, arrange to attend an orthopaedic operation and see for yourself what living bone looks like.

Types and classification of bone   There are two types of bone. Compact bone appears to be solid, but is made up of the tubes referred to earlier, which are closely packed together. These tubular arrangements are called Haversian systems.

Figure 10.2 illustrates the features of a typical Haversian system which consists of:

- a central canal containing blood vessels, lymph vessels and nerves
- concentric plates of bone (called lamellae)
- spaces between the lamellae called lacunae. These are filled with lymphatic fluid and contain osteocytes (bone cells)
- lacunae are linked with the lymphatic system by small channels called canaliculi.

The second type of bone is called cancellous or trabecular bone. The Haversian systems are much larger and there are fewer lamellae than in compact bone. This gives a honeycomb or spongy appearance. Cancellous bone contains red bone marrow.

Bones can be classified, according to shape, as long, short, flat or irregular. Figure 10.3 shows a longitudinal section of a mature long bone. The shaft (diaphysis) is made up of compact bone, and contains yellow bone marrow. The shape of the bone is such that it allows for maximum strength whilst reducing weight. The two ends (epiphyses) have an outer covering of compact bone over cancellous bone. Bone is almost always covered with a fine but tough membrane called the periosteum which gives it some protection. The periosteum also provides for the attachment of ligaments and tendons, and contains cells to help maintain the shape of the bone. At the ends of the bones – where the joint is formed – periosteum is replaced by a tough, smooth substance called hyaline cartilage.

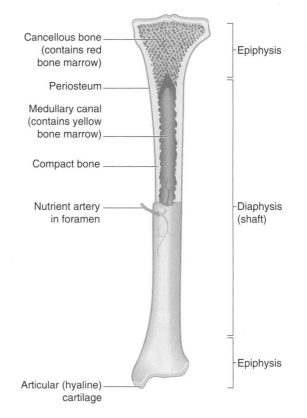

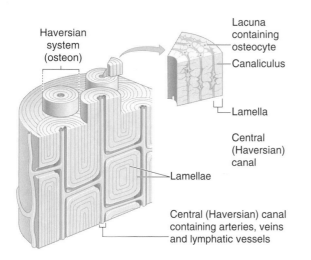

Fig. 10.2 The microscopic structure of bone (from Waugh & Grant 2001, with permission).

Fig. 10.3 A mature long bone in longitudinal section (from Waugh & Grant 2001, with permission).

Short, irregular and flat bones are made up of a thin layer of hard compact bone surrounding an inner mass of cancellous bone. The latter contains red bone marrow.

Bone formation (osteogenesis) and maintenance The development of bone begins before birth and is usually completed by the mid twenties. In the skeleton of a baby many of the bones are made up of cartilage. During childhood the cartilage is replaced by true bone, during which process many bones fuse together, leaving an adult skeleton of around 206 bones. Whilst the number and gross structure of bones normally remains fairly constant in adulthood, bone tissue is constantly being replaced. The rate at which this replacement takes place varies, but can be quite rapid. For example it is estimated that, over a 6-month period, the distal (hip) end of the femur is gradually replaced.

The cells responsible for bone formation are osteocytes (bone cells) and chondrocytes (cartilage cells). There are two types of osteocyte, osteoblasts which build bone up, and osteoclasts which remove bone tissue by reabsorption. As you can imagine, there has to be a fine balance between the activities of these two types of cells so that the structure of the bone is maintained. Imagine the consequences if osteoblasts became more active than osteoclasts (or vice versa).

Balance in the growth, development, and maintenance of bone tissue is governed by hormones. Growth hormone and thyroid hormones are important during infancy and childhood. Excessive or deficient secretion of these hormones can cause skeletal deformities, such as dwarfism, gigantism and acromegaly. During puberty both testosterone and oestrogen play a part in bone development. In adulthood regulation is governed by the action of calcitonin which is released by the thyroid gland increasing bone production, whilst parathyroid hormone which is secreted by the parathyroid glands, causes calcium to be released from bone. It is deficiency in oestrogen in particular which contributes to the development of postmenopausal osteoporosis. Weight-bearing exercise also stimulates local bone growth, and loss of weight bearing results in a loss of calcium from the bone – an important fact to remember when considering the effects of immobility.

Inflamed area

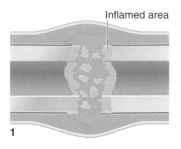

Haematoma and bone fragments

1

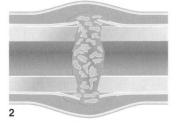

Phagocytosis of clot and debris.
Growth of granulation tissue begins

2

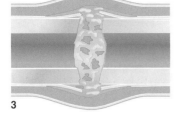

Osteoblasts begin to form new bone (callus)

3

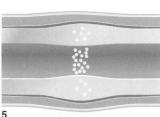

Gradual spread and mineralisation of callus to bridge the gap

4

Bone almost healed. Osteoclasts reshape and canalise new bone

5

Fig. 10.4 Stages of bone healing (from Waugh & Grant 2001, with permission).

Exercise

1. Review what you know about hormones and the way they work.
2. Construct a diagram to illustrate the homeostatic mechanisms involved in bone maintenance in adults. Specifically, identify the role of calcitonin, parathyroid hormones and vitamin D.
3. What effect does weightlessness have on bone formation?
4. Look up the following conditions and find out (a) the cause of the pathology, (b) the effects it has on the individual, and (c) the implications for health and health care:

   - gigantism
   - acromegaly
   - achondroplasia
   - osteoporosis
   - osteomalacia
   - rickets.

Bone healing Following a fracture the broken ends of the bone are joined together by new bone (see Fig. 10.4). This occurs in a number of stages:

1. A haematoma (blood clot) is formed at the site of injury.
2. There is an acute inflammatory response. Large numbers of macrophages (cells which engulf and devour damaged tissue, bacteria and other foreign bodies) enter the injury site and phagocytose (engulf and digest) exudate from the haematoma and small fragments of bone.
3. Granulation tissue develops and new blood vessels infiltrate the site.
4. Large numbers of osteoblasts invade the areas and form new bone or callus.
5. Osteoclasts shape the callus, removing excess bone.

> ### Exercise
> 1. Find out about different types of fracture and their management.
> 2. Identify factors which might hinder bone healing.
> 3. Identify complications which might follow a fracture.

It might have been surprising to learn how much 'broken' bones vary, and how many different factors can influence the rate and effectiveness of bone healing. There are many serious complications associated with fractures, for example fat emboli. The nurse needs to know what to do to promote bone healing, and minimise the risks associated with fractures. Consider Case study 10.1.

> **Case study 10.1**
>
> ### Young man with an injured arm
>
> Pete Marshall, a 19-year-old young man, was on his way home from college when he fell and injured his right arm. Pete is brought to Accident and Emergency by ambulance. It is suspected that he has sustained a fracture. Pete has Down syndrome and lives at home with his parents. He is in pain and distressed.

> ### Exercise
> 1. Review your skills and knowledge in relation to this scenario and the care that Pete may require. Identify any learning needs you might have.
> 2. How would you explain the fracture and the process of bone healing to Pete?
> 3. Pete has a simple fracture of the radius, which is to be treated with a plaster splint. What advice will you need to give him before discharge home?

Joints

A joint occurs where two bones meet. Joints can be classified as:

1. fixed or ossified joints, such as those between the bones of the adult skull
2. slightly movable, cartilaginous joints, such as the symphisis pubis of the pelvis

3. free moving or synovial joints, which are important in movement.

Figure 10.5 illustrates the structure of a typical synovial joint. The bones of the joint are held together by a tough band of fibre (ligament) which is able to give protection to the joint, but is loose enough to allow movement. The articulating surfaces of the bones, which match each other in shape, are covered in smooth durable hyaline cartilage. Synovial membrane lines the internal surface of the joint, and those parts of the bone which are not covered in hyaline cartilage. The synovial membrane secretes a thick viscous fluid (synovial fluid) which provides lubrication. Synovial joints can be further classified according to the range of movements they make (see Box 10.1).

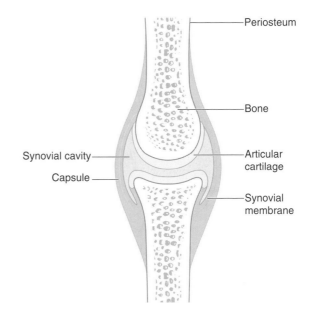

Fig. 10.5 Structure of synovial joint (from Waugh & Grant 2001, with permission).

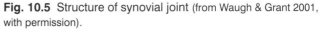

Box 10.1 Terminology used to describe the movement of joints	
Flexion	Movement which decreases the angle between two adjoining bones
Extension	Movement which increases the angle between two adjoining bones
Abduction	Movement away from the mid line of the body
Adduction	Movement towards the mid line of the body
Circumduction	Combination of the four above
Rotation	Movement around the longitudinal axis of a bone
Pronation	Turning down the palm of the hand
Supination	Turning the palm of the hand up
Inversion	Turning the sole of the foot inwards
Eversion	Turning the sole of the foot outwards

Types of joint include:

- ball and socket joints such as the hips and shoulder. They have a wide range of movement – extension, flexion, abduction, adduction, circumduction and rotation

- hinge joints such as the elbows, knees and fingers, which allow both flexion and extension
- pivot joints which allow rotation, such as the joints at the very top of the vertebral column

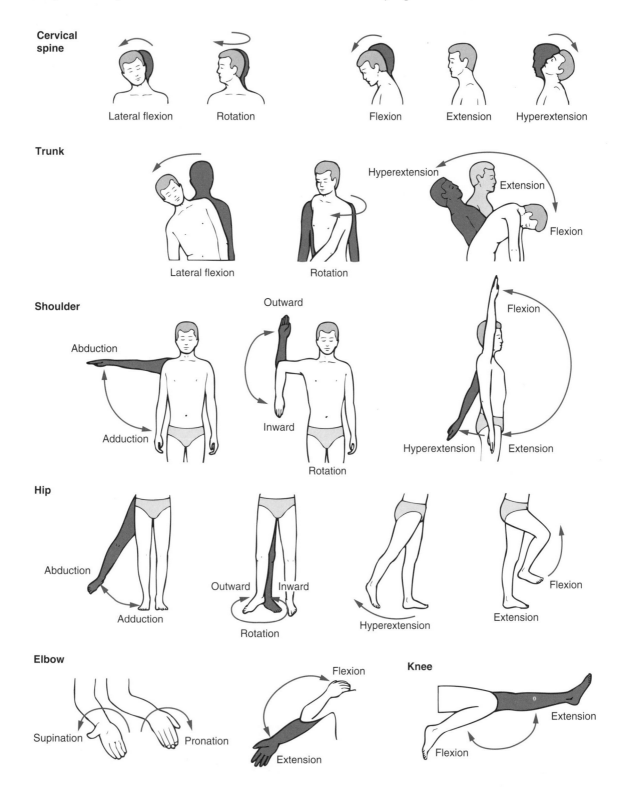

Fig. 10.6 Range of motion exercises (from Boore et al 1987, with permission).

- gliding joints, these are made of two flat surfaces that can slide against each other in any direction. Examples can be found in the hands and feet
- saddle joint, the only example of which in humans is at the base of the thumb. It allows extension, flexion, adduction, abduction and circumduction
- ellipsoid joints are similar to hinge joints but allow movement in two planes, and are found in the wrist and hands (see Fig. 10.6 for range of motion exercises for joints).

> **Exercise**
> 1. Figure 10.6 illustrates normal range of movement of the major joints. Why is it important for nurses to have an understanding of this?

Understanding the underlying anatomy and physiology of joints is a vital component of effective nursing practice.

This knowledge can be applied in many ways, for example knowing how to position someone correctly in bed or in a chair. It is also important to know how to maintain the range of movement when someone is unconscious, or how to support and help someone to exercise a weakened limb.

> **Exercise**
> As with other clinical skills, learning how to do passive or assisted exercise takes practice. You could practice with a colleague! For example, take turns to be the patient. One of you should sit comfortably in a chair with arms. Let one side of the body relax as much as possible. In particular, let your arm relax from your shoulder muscles down to your fingers. Now, whoever is being the nurse should put all the joints in the upper limbs through a full range of movement ten times. Get some (honest) feedback from 'the patient' on how it was for them.

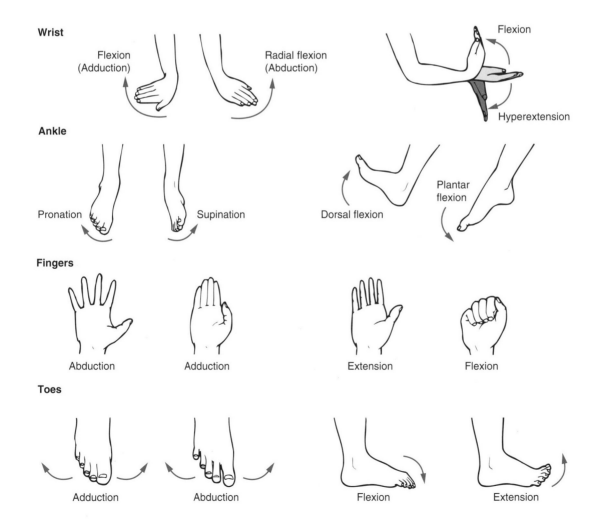

Fig. 10.6 (continued)

Experiencing passive exercise as a recipient should be a useful learning exercise. It might make you think about how you handle and move people in other situations. You might want to think about the amount of time it takes, the speed with which you move people, the pressure and force you use, the importance of supporting joints, and being aware of potential discomforts. Consider the following brief case study.

Case study 10.2

Passive exercise

Brenda Kovic is a 61-year-old woman, who has had an acute stroke (cerebrovascular accident) which has left her with significant brain damage. She has been unconscious for the past 2 days. Regular passive exercises have been planned as part of her nursing care.

Exercise

1. What knowledge and skills do you need in order to implement this care?
2. Imagine you are teaching this skill to a junior colleague.
3. What would you say are the most important principles to keep in mind when performing passive exercise?

If the joints are not moved regularly, or are kept in an abnormal position then there is the risk of permanent damage. You know what it is like to be stuck in one position for any length of time for example sitting at a desk, or at a keyboard writing an essay. If you don't change position regularly and do some stretching exercise, then your neck and shoulders soon start to ache. It is crucially important therefore that you know how to handle, move and position joints correctly. Failure to do so can be devastating for the patient as is illustrated in this exercise.

Exercise

You have just started a placement on a rehabilitation ward. In the report you hear that Mr Collins, who is recovering from a stroke, has 'a subluxation of his right shoulder'.

1. What does this mean?
2. What are the implications of this for Mr Collins?
3. How might this problem have been prevented?

It is important to have an understanding of the common conditions affecting joints which you are likely to come across in practice.

Exercise

1. Review your knowledge about normal joint movements.
2. Use an anatomy and physiology book to familiarise yourself with the names of the major joints.

Exercise (continued)

3. Look up the following conditions and find out (a) the cause of the pathology, (b) the effects it has on the individual and (c) the implications for health and health care:
   - osteoarthritis
   - rheumatoid arthritis
   - gout
   - ankylosing spondylitis.

Muscles

Muscle tissue makes up around 50% of the total body weight of adults. The chief properties of muscle tissue are:

- *irritability* – the ability to respond to a stimulus
- *contractility* – the ability to shorten and thicken
- *extensibility* – the ability to lengthen
- *elasticity* – the ability to return to its original shape.

It is through the contraction and relaxation of muscle that movement is produced. As well as the production of movement, muscle also maintains posture, produces heat, and the contraction of skeletal muscle aids the return of venous blood to the heart.

Type of muscle

Skeletal or voluntary muscles There are about 640 skeletal muscles, which are attached to the skeleton by tendons. It is skeletal muscle that is primarily concerned with mobilising. Movement occurs because as the muscle contracts it pulls on the attached bone (movable point), it then relaxes allowing the bone to return to its former position. In order for this to happen, the moving bone needs to be held steady by being attached to a fixed point. The joint acts as a pivot or fulcrum.

Muscles are often arranged in pairs which enables a push–pull effect. You can feel this in your arm. Place your hand around your upper arm and flex your elbow. You can feel one muscle (the biceps) contract as it pulls in the lower arm. The opposite (antagonistic) muscle (the triceps) relaxes. When the elbow joint is extended, the opposite occurs with the biceps relaxing whilst the triceps contracts. This is illustrated in Figure 10.7.

Under a microscope skeletal muscle has a striped appearance and so is sometimes called striped or striated muscle. It is innervated by the voluntary part of the nervous system. Skeletal muscle movement is rapid and fatigues easily.

Visceral or involuntary muscle This is found throughout the body and makes up internal organs such as the stomach, intestines, bronchi, bladder and blood vessels. It is innervated by the autonomic (involuntary) nervous system. Under a microscope visceral muscle does not have stripes and so is sometimes called unstriated or smooth muscle. It contracts slowly, using less energy than skeletal muscle and is slow to fatigue.

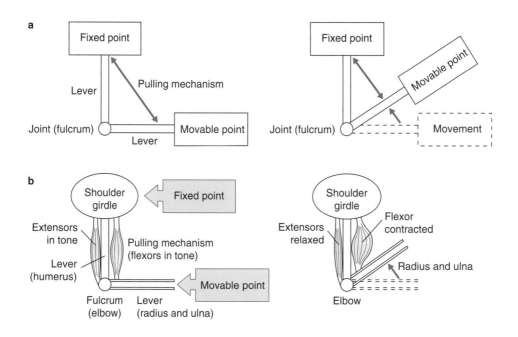

Fig. 10.7 Principles of movement: theoretical components in relation to movement of the forearm (from Chilman & Thomas 1987, with permission).

Cardiac muscle This highly specialised muscle is found only in the heart and at the cardiac ends of the great vessels. It has some features of both skeletal and visceral muscle. It is innervated by the involuntary nervous system. Cardiac muscle has innate rhythmical activity and is able to contract without fatigue.

Fatigue in skeletal muscle can be demonstrated through a simple exercise. Clench your fingers into fist, and then open them out again. Keep repeating the action. How long is it before your muscles start to ache and become tired? The contraction of muscle requires lots of energy. This energy is obtained from glucose, or its storage product, glycogen. As part of the energy-releasing process, these products are converted to pyruvic acid. If there is plenty of oxygen available, pyruvic acid is converted into carbon dioxide and water, which can be easily excreted. However, if there is insufficient oxygen available, the pyruvic acid is converted into lactic acid, which is less easily excreted. If lactic acid builds up in the muscles, the individual experiences the muscle pain and fatigue we call cramp. The removal of accumulated lactic acid can be aided by gentle exercise; this is why athletes always do warm-down exercises.

Muscle structure Skeletal muscle is made up of numerous fibres (muscle fibres). These fibres are of varying length and lie parallel to each other. Each muscle fibre is filled with a special cytoplasm (sarcoplasm) which contains many nuclei. The outer membrane of the muscle fibre is called the sarcolemma. Each muscle fibre contains many fine threads (myofibrils) which run along its length (see Fig. 10.8).

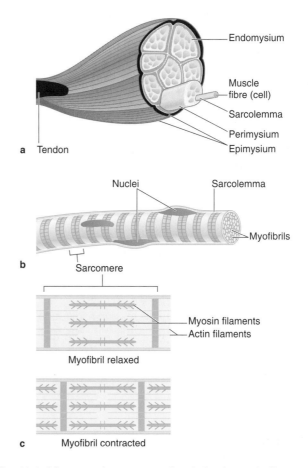

Fig. 10.8 Microscopic structure of a skeletal muscle fibre (from Waugh & Grant 2001, with permission).

When viewed through an electron microscope, the structure of the myofibril is revealed as consisting of sets of thick and thin filaments. The thick filaments are made up of a protein called myosin, and the thin filaments of a protein called actin. Muscle contraction is caused by the interaction of these proteins. Contraction is also affected by the concentration of calcium in the fluid in the cell.

Actin and myosin have a natural attraction for one another. Where filaments of actin and myosin overlap, they bond to form crossbridges. The sliding filament theory of muscle movement proposes that when a bond forms the myosin crossbridge bends, pulling the myosin filament along the actin filament. The conversion of the chemical ATP to ADP releases the energy needed to straighten the myosin crossbridge to its former position. This means the myosin can reattach to the actin filament further along its length. This repeated action pulls the two ends of the muscle fibre together, causing it to contract (see Fig. 10.9).

Muscles have a very rich nerve supply. Motor neurones (nerve cells) travel from the central nervous system and carry an electrical impulse to muscle fibre. The impulse is transferred from the motor neurone to the muscle at the neuromuscular junction or motor end plate through the release of a chemical (acetylcholine) which stimulates the contraction of the muscle fibre.

Under normal circumstances, at any one time, some muscle fibres will be contracted, whilst others will be relaxed. This state is called muscle tone. Muscle tone is particularly important for maintaining posture. Disorders of muscle tone are often the result of muscular or neurological disorders. Loss of muscle tone means the muscles are floppy or flaccid. Flaccid muscle tone can be the result of prolonged reduced mobility (such as bed rest for example). Excessive muscle tone results in spasticity which can cause the formation of contractures.

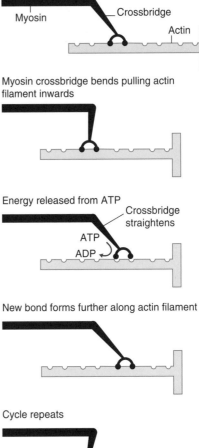

Bond forms between actin and myosin

Myosin   Crossbridge

Actin

Myosin crossbridge bends pulling actin filament inwards

Energy released from ATP

Crossbridge straightens

ATP

ADP

New bond forms further along actin filament

Cycle repeats

Fig. 10.9 How the making and breaking of actin and myosin bonds causes muscle contraction (ATP = adenosine triphosphate, ADP = adenosine diphosphate) (from Rutishauser 1994, with permission).

Exercise

1. What are the effects of exercise and endurance training on muscle?
2. What effects do steroids have on muscle?
3. What are the short- and long-term effects of lack of muscle use?
4. What happens in rigor mortis?
5. Look up the following conditions and find out: (a) the cause of the pathology, (b) the effects it has on the individual (c) the implications for health and health care:

   - motor neurone disease
   - Parkinson's disease
   - myasthenia gravis
   - myopathy
   - myositis.

Mobilising therefore is a complex process which depends on the coordinated functioning of nerves, bones, joints and muscles. Further reading may be necessary to gain sufficient knowledge of biological factors influencing mobilising and a range of recommended texts are given at the end of the chapter.

Psychological factors

There are many psychological factors that can influence how an individual mobilises. Further, impaired mobility can have serious psychological and emotional effects.

The ability to mobilise allows infants and young children to discover who they are and where they fit into their environment. Lack of ability or opportunity to explore can affect psychological wellbeing. Even for adults movement can act as an outlet for emotional expression. Indeed the link between our emotional state and mobility is complex. Think of the behaviours you might see in someone who is anxious – an archetypal picture might be someone who is not able to keep still, who is pacing up and down, 'like a cat on hot bricks'. People who are depressed often feel a desperate lack of energy, overwhelming fatigue and lack of motivation, which prevents them from mobilising.

People may hold beliefs and attitudes which influence mobilising patterns. In the past, beliefs about people with physical disabilities underpinned exclusion from mainstream society. It was commented on earlier that there are beliefs regarding mobility in late life, which can impact on the lives and wellbeing of older people. It might be that the relationship between beliefs and mobilising is best illustrated by considering attitudes to exercise. Roper et al (1996) draw attention to the increasing mechanisation evident in contemporary industrialised societies. The effect of an increasingly sedentary life on health has been well recognised. The 1998 Health Survey for England (DoH 1999a) identified that seven out of ten women, and six out of ten men were not taking sufficient exercise to maintain general health and wellbeing. The positive benefits of physical activity are increasingly well established (DoH 1995, USDHHS 1996, Biddle et al 2000) The positive benefits of exercise are summarised in Box 10.2.

In order to gain a health benefit physical activity needs to be regular and sustained. In some cases people might not be aware of the benefits simple, moderate regular exercise (such as 30 minutes brisk walking per day) can bring. The Department of Health in the UK has developed a framework for exercise referral systems, which identifies the role of the nurse in initiating, facilitating and supporting exercise programmes (DoH 2001b). It also suggests that nurses should act as role models, and that practitioners who are themselves physically active are more effective health promoters (McKenna et al 1998).

Exercise

1. Reflect on your own levels of physical activity. Do you achieve the recommended level of 30 minutes of moderate intensity activity at least five times per week?
2. What factors increase or decrease the amount of physical activity you undertake?

It might be that you already reach the recommended levels of physical activity. Well done! Keep it up! Thinking of factors in your own life that might make you more or less likely to exercise can help you to recognise how you can help others. There are many reasons why people do not take sufficient physical activity: lack of opportunity, lack of resource, lack of time, interest or motivation. The idea of 'fitness' can be off-putting if linked to the achievements of elite athletes, or the membership of an expensive gymnasium or health club.

Sociocultural factors

It is important when considering sociocultural factors affecting mobilising to examine societal attitudes to dependency and disability. Physical dependency in mobilising is often equated with both emotional and cognitive impairment. The classic manifestation of this is the person in the wheelchair being ignored, whilst their companion is asked 'Does he take sugar?'. This stems from a paternalistic perception that 'the disabled' need to be looked after as dependent children, rather than treated as autonomous adults.

Exercise

Have you ever had to use a wheelchair yourself, or taken someone out and about in one? What are your recollections?

1. You are in the queue at a shop; the person in front of you is in a wheelchair. How do you respond to them? How do you feel?
2. You notice someone with a visual impairment waiting at the side of a road. What do you do? How do you feel?
3. Ask your friends what they would do, and how they might feel in the same situations.

People often behave differently when faced with people with obvious mobility or sensory problems. Some will distance themselves and will ignore the disabled person, whilst others will be over-protective.

In 1980 the World Health Organisation published the International Classification of Impairments, Disabilities and Handicaps (ICIDH). It is useful to review these terms as

---

Box 10.2 The preventative effects of exercise

Regular physical activity can:

- decrease the risk of death from cardiovascular disease generally
- decrease the risk of death from coronary heart disease in particular
- prevent or delay the development of high blood pressure
- reduce blood pressure in people with existing high blood pressure
- help people control body weight
- help control diabetes
- reduce the risk of colon cancer and maybe other forms of cancer
- enhance the immune system
- have positive effects on mental health, reducing the risk of depression and anxiety, and enhancing mood and self-esteem
- help in the prevention and treatment of low back pain.

Specific forms of physical activity can:

- reduce the risk of falls and other accidents by improving the health of bones, maintaining body strength, balance and co-ordination and cognitive function.

From: DoH 2001b.

they are still commonly used. *Impairment* is defined as a psychological or physical abnormality which may or may not lead to a disability. *Disability* is defined as a loss of function experienced by the person which might (or might not) lead to a handicap. *Handicap* occurs when someone is disadvantaged in some way because of the disability. So it is possible to be disabled without being handicapped. For example an individual may have an impairment of the shape of their eyeballs causing a disability of severe short-sightedness. However, by wearing spectacles they are not handicapped by this. Or consider someone who has had a stroke (impairment) which has left them unable to walk (disability). They will be handicapped by the inaccessibility of many buildings. From this you can see that the individual's experience of handicap in mobilising is related to sociocultural, environmental and politicoeconomic factors. Challenging handicap means challenging the attitudes and beliefs of individuals, institutions and governments.

The ICIHD has been revised (ICIDH-2 1999) with a greater emphasis on the context of the person in a social context. The language has been altered to reflect this, for example handicap has become 'participation' and is concerned with the social roles, whilst 'disability' has become 'activity' and is concerned with function or behaviour (Wade & de Jong 2000) (see Chapter 11 for further information on issues of disability).

Exercise

1. Reflect on your own cultural background and experiences.
2. What beliefs, attitudes and practices have you experienced relating to
   - mobilising?
   - people with impaired mobility?
3. Find out about the beliefs, attitudes and practices of people from other cultural backgrounds.
4. What implication might there be for nursing practice?

All Activities of Living are influenced by cultural and ethnic identities. Many desired activities such as personal prayer, ritual washing and attendance at communal worship can be affected by impaired mobility.

Mobility can also be important in enabling people to fulfil social responsibilities and roles. These may be within the family group or the wider community. An inability to maintain cherished roles can have a negative impact on the individual's sense of self-esteem and self-worth.

Environmental factors

The environmental factors influencing mobilising are many, and include the home, work and community space. Transport issues are obviously relevant. Income plays a large part in determining transport choices. Access to good, accessible public transport is essential for some groups of people. Older people in particular rely on public transport,

and need transport services that are accessible, available, safe and inexpensive (Atkins 2001).

Local communities may have resources aimed at those people who have difficulty in accessing public transport. These might be supported by local government, but are often provided by the voluntary sector. If you don't know already, find out what transport services are available in your community.

With current levels of traffic all pedestrians need both agility and speed to safely negotiate the roads. For people with impaired vision, or those who use mobility aids, dealing with street furniture can provide enough hazards, before contemplating finding an appropriate road crossing. The built environment can also help or hinder mobility. High-rise housing might mean that youngsters cannot get out to play. Even living on the second floor might confine a frail older person to their home. On the other hand, a positive planned environment can encourage mobility. Access to safe parks and open areas not only support individual mobility but can also foster a sense of community and belonging, thus combating the social isolation felt by many people who have mobility problems.

Fear of crime can prevent people from mobilising freely. Although statistically younger people are the most common victims of street crime, older people are the most fearful. There are reports that indicate that some women from minority ethnic groups living in the UK rarely leave their homes because of the fear of racial abuse.

It is useful to also think of the care environment and the extent to which it affects mobilising. For example, people with mobility problems who are able to live independently in their everyday lives, can be disabled in a hospital environment which prevents them from managing their Activities of Living in their usual manner.

Politicoeconomic factors

In the United Kingdom, local government has responsibility for some elements of the local environment. For example the provision of low-level kerbs, user-friendly road crossings and good street lighting, which all promote safe mobilising. The Local Authority also has responsibility for the provision of parks, swimming pools and leisure and fitness centres, all of which can provide opportunity for physical activity. A key issue here is the extent to which these services are accessible and appropriate to all sectors of the community.

Increasing urbanisation is leading to a reliance on the private car as a principal means of transport. This is exacerbated by the proliferation in many industrialised countries of 'out of town' shopping. The closure of small, local facilities such as banks, post offices, chemists and other shops disadvantages those people without private transport. This can contribute to the sense of social exclusion in many disadvantaged communities.

Back pain and back injury have a significant personal and economic cost. It has been estimated that in 1998 the economic cost of back pain in the UK was over £1632 million.

In a national survey in Great Britain, 40% of adults said they suffered from back pain lasting more than 1 day in the previous 12 months (DoH Statistics Division 1999). Nurses are an occupational group at significant risk of back injury. In some fields of practice the nurse undertakes numerous handling and moving activities, increasing the likelihood of developing back problems (Pheasant 1998).

Moving and handling activity can be defined as 'any transporting or supporting of a load (including the lifting, putting down, pushing, pulling, carrying or moving thereof) by hand or bodily force' (HSE 1998). Throughout the European Community there are a range of legal requirements in relation to moving and handling. These international requirements are supported by national legislation and guidelines, and local policies.

> **Exercise**
> 1. Find out what the legal requirements for safe moving and handling are in your country.
> 2. Find any national policies or guidelines which support the implementation of the above. These guidelines might be developed by government, trades unions, professional associations, for example.
> 3. Now look at local policy and procedure, to see how the legal framework and national initiatives can affect everyday practice.

When this exercise has been completed you might want to spend some time reflecting on your own moving and handling practice.

In the UK, moving and handling is regulated through The Manual Handling Operations Regulations 1992 (HSE 1998), under the terms of the Health and Safety at Work Act (1974). These comply with EU directives aiming to standardise the various and varying national safety directives/legislation. The directive makes clear what can be reasonably expected of employers and employees. Employers should, as far is reasonably practicable:

- avoid the need for employees to undertake manual handling which involves the risk of injury
- take appropriate steps to reduce risk of injury to the lowest level possible
- make sure that a 'suitable and sufficient' written assessment is undertaken by a designated person of all manual handling operations that involve the risk of injury. The assessment must take into account: the task, the load, the working environment and the capabilities of individuals involved
- provide suitable equipment and training in its use.

Employees must:

- use the process and implement policy as designed
- use equipment in accordance with their training
- report any hazards and changes in circumstances which may impact upon the assessment. This includes

individual or personal changes (for example back injury or pregnancy).

For a moving and handling activity to be successful, it needs to address two objectives, minimal effort on the part of the handler and the experience of minimal discomfort for the patient (Mallet & Dougherty 2000). This is dependent on a comprehensive and accurate assessment. The RCN Code of Practice for Patient Handling (RCN 1996a) makes clear the importance of a detailed assessment and clear recording and communication of the subsequent plan of action (RCN 1996b).

There are some key principles to remember whilst moving and handling. When you stand at rest, most of the force of gravity is applied through your head, trunk, and spinal column. You need exert little effort to maintain stability, and there is little damaging pressure on the spine. When the trunk moves away from this midline, the spinal column experiences harmful shearing forces. So any twisting motion can exert harmful pressure on the spine and seriously damage the vertebral discs. So when moving and handling any load (not only people) you need to think about:

- moving with the natural curves of the spine maintained as much as possible
- holding the object as close to the body as possible
- making use of large, strong hip and thigh muscles, rather than the muscles of your back and arms
- keeping a wide stable base to help maintain your balance and reduce the risk of twisting your spine.

> **Exercise**
> 1. What factors must you think of when planning to move/handle a patient?

The following might have been considered:

- assessing the patient need
- assessing risk
- recognising your own level of skill and expertise
- working as a team
- using appropriate equipment
- communicating and gaining cooperation
- using touch and recognising any taboos on touch
- conveying respect, developing trust and promoting the patient's dignity.

Individuality in living

Individuality in mobilising is a result of the ways in which influencing factors come together. The capacity for mobilising depends on the possession of physical ability, the motivation to move and the provision of a nonrestrictive, enabling environment. Alterations in any of these elements can affect an individual's mobilising behaviour.

The model of living framework gives us an idea of how and why people mobilise in the way they do. It also highlights the complexity of the model and the extent to which the individual Activities of Living are interrelated. Consider the following case study and undertake the exercise.

Exercise

1. Read through the case scenario given below.
2. Use the components of the model to consider individuality in the Activity of Living mobilising.

Case study 10.3

Individuality in mobilising

Three generations of the Abram family live together. Cilla, aged 70, is the grandmother. She worked as a nurse before she had to retire at the age of 56. Cilla has osteoarthritis, which particularly affects her spine and hips making it difficult for her to walk. Whilst she manages to mobilise in the house and garden, she often uses an electrically powered wheelchair outside. Jeanie is her daughter, she works full time as a nursing sister on a rehabilitation ward. Craig who is 13 and Paula aged 10 make up the family.

You might have considered the following points:

Lifespan

The Abram family represent a range of ages across the lifespan. The expectation is that all members of the family would be independent in mobilising. Although joint stiffness and some discomfort might be perceived as 'normal' ageing, Cilla's degree of mobility impairment is greater than the majority of people her age expect. Jeanie has a busy job which although active, does not guarantee sufficient physical exercise. Her work and family commitments might make it difficult for her to maintain healthy levels of physical activity. The young people will be expected to take part in physical activity at school.

Dependence/independence

Cilla is dependent upon members of her family for help with mobilising, and some other Activities of Living. However, Jeanie depends on her mum to provide childcare and emotional support. The interdependence of the family unit is an important factor to consider. Cilla uses a wheelchair to aid her independence.

Factors influencing the Activity of Living

Biological The changes associated with 'normal' ageing. Osteoarthritis is a painful, long-term, degenerative condition that restricts mobility. Cilla's mobility is likely to become more impaired in the future.

Psychological Higher risk of depression in older people with long-term health problems. Attitudes of family members to physical activity.

Sociocultural Maintenance of social roles in the family. Beliefs about disability and handicap.

Environmental The impact of domestic and community space on Cilla's mobility, and the ability of the family to undertake joint activities. Accessibility of safe transport for all members of the family.

Politicoeconomic Financial concerns for the future. Ability to access appropriate services and facilities. Jeanie at risk of back injury.

Summary points

The information and the exercises in this chapter so far should have demonstrated a number of important aspects to this Activity of Living. These are summarised below. It is important that you understand the model of living, as this is the basis for individuality of care using the model for nursing.

1. Mobilising is a complex activity.
2. Individuality in mobilising can be illustrated through the components of the model of living.
3. Mobilising is affected by all the other Activities of Living.
4. Mobilising affects all the other Activities of Living.
5. Problems in mobilising can have a detrimental effect of health, wellbeing and quality of life.

THE MODEL FOR NURSING

Introduction

The aim of the model of living is to identify individuality in Activities of Living leading to individuality in nursing care. In the model for nursing, the role of the nurse is to provide person-centred nursing care which can prevent, alleviate, solve or help people come to terms with problems (actual or potential) related to Activities of Living. Chapter 1 of this book gives more detail on the overall model. This chapter will now focus on how you can use the model for nursing to care for people with actual or potential mobility problems.

This section also uses the nursing process as a vehicle to discuss the organisation and delivery of nursing care. It is intended to use the nursing process as a way of illustrating how you might 'think' about assessing, planning, implementing and evaluating the nursing care for an individual, rather than completing specific documents or care plans. Chapter 1 provides a more detailed description of the nursing process.

In this part of the chapter Miss Roberts and her experiences will be used as a case study to explore how to use the Activities of Living model in practice (see p. 302). Miss Roberts is based on the story of an older woman who was a participant in a research study on the nurse's role in rehabilitation (Long et al 2001). Permission has been given to share her story in this context. Miss Roberts' path, from admission to hospital after fall, through treatment and care for a fractured hip to her discharge home will be explored. The case study will look at the process as it relates to mobilising, it is not intended to give a comprehensive account of Miss Roberts' care. The interrelatedness of both the Activities of Living and the stages of the nursing process will be illustrated – demonstrating the complexity and skill of nursing practice.

Before starting to think about using the model in more detail, it might be useful to think broadly about some of the health problems related to mobilising.

Exercise

Using the components of the Activities of Living model, your life experiences and clinical experience to date, note down a list of health problems people might have in relation to the activity of mobilising.

1. Reflect on these and identify your learning needs.
2. You may wish to discuss these with your teachers to identify a learning plan to meet these needs.

Table 10.2 gives a list of some of the health problems you might have identified. You can probably add to this list from your own. What this exercise illustrates is the wide range of health problems that can cause (or be caused by) reduced or impaired mobility. It also gives an indication of the depth and breadth of knowledge and skill needed by the nurse in order to deliver effective nursing care to people with a range of mobility problems.

Assessing the individual

Whilst this chapter is looking specifically at mobilising, it must be borne in mind the extent to which mobility problems affect other Activities of Living and vice versa. A comprehensive nursing assessment must also address all the other Activities of Living. It is through understanding a person's individuality in living that the nurse is able to provide individualisation in nursing (person-centred care).

Box 10.3 provides a summary of factors related to individuality in mobilising and their relationship to assessment.

The core processes in assessment are:

- collecting data
- reviewing and interpreting the data
- identifying problems related to Activities of Living
- identifying priorities amongst identified problems.

The primary source of information in any assessment is the patient. Secondary sources include the patient's family and friends, other professionals and the patient's records and notes. There are two types of information collected as

Table 10.2 Components of the Activities of Living model and health problems related to mobility

Lifespan	Congenital problems, e.g. congenital dislocation of the hip, congenital dystrophy Hormonal effects on development Trauma Sports injury Osteoporosis
Dependence–independence	Use of mobility aids Effects of the environment
Biological factors	Arthritis Infections Trauma Tumours Neurological disease (e.g. stroke, Parkinson disease)
Psychological factors	Fear of falling Learning disabilities Cognitive impairment Depression
Sociocultural	Lifestyle choices Lack of exercise Social isolation
Environmental	Road traffic accidents Falls Limited local amenities for exercise
Politicoeconomic	Work-related injury Finance Limited access to resources and services

part of the assessment process, biographical data and data related to the Activities of Living. The main methods of data collection are interview, observation and measurement.

It is important to remember that assessment is a continuous process and an initial assessment often needs to be built upon. For example, if somebody is suffering an acute exacerbation (worsening) of rheumatoid arthritis, they are likely to be in pain and extremely tired, and it may be neither possible nor desirable to undertake a comprehensive assessment in one sitting. Patients must also be reassessed in relation to change in condition or as a result of the evaluation of care.

The nurse also works in collaborative ways with other members of the multidisciplinary team to deliver comprehensive care based on comprehensive assessment. There is a danger that the patient can become overburdened with duplicate assessments (DoH 2001a). In Miss Roberts' case, for example, she was assessed a number of times by people who asked some identical questions. Failure to share information gained through assessment can also lead to the patient failing to receive the most effective and appropriate package of care (Nolan & Caldock 1996).

Box 10.3 Assessing the individual in the AL of mobilising

Lifespan: relationship to the AL of mobilising
- infancy and childhood – increasing skills
- adolescence and young adulthood – peak performance
- later years – decreasing agility and stamina.

Dependence–independence in mobilising
- increasing independence in childhood, to adulthood
- dependence on another person
- body-worn aids/external aids (for aided independence)
- transport mode – to school, work, shops, for leisure.

Factors influencing mobilising
Biological
- adequacy of musculoskeletal and nervous systems
- body posture/gait
- muscle strength/mass/tone
- congential/hereditary interference with function
- effects of trauma, disease.

Psychological
- intelligence, temperment, values, beliefs, motivation
- knowledge about benefits of exercise and prevention of injury

- general attitudes
- attitudes to dependence and disability.

Sociocultural
- social class, tradition, religion
- work activities/transport
- effects of mechanical advances on lifestyle
- dependence affecting role in relation to family, work, leisure.

Environmental
- housing conditions and environs
- local climate and terrain: influence on work/hobbies
- effect of man-made energy on transport of people and goods.

Politicoeconomic
- community amenities
- safety of streets/crossings and prevention of injury
- legal requirements for access to and mobility in buildings
- availability of exercise facilities for leisure.

From Roper et al (1996), p. 293.

Collecting and interpreting data

The aim of the assessment process is to answer the following questions in relation to the Activity of Living:

- What was the person's previous routine?
- What can the person do independently?
- What can't the person do independently?
- What were the person's previous coping behaviours?
- What actual and potential problems does the person have?

Exercise

1. Using the components of the model, identify the sort of data you need to conduct a comprehensive assessment of an individual with an actual or potential mobility problem.
2. What sorts of skills and knowledge do you need?
3. Reflect on your current knowledge and skills base and identify your learning needs. Write these in your learning plan.

A range of ideas will have been generated on the sorts of data you might need. Obviously, assessment in practice has to be relevant and appropriate to the individual person and the context of care, but initially think very broadly about the most complete and comprehensive data collection you might ever make in relation to mobilising! To begin with, think about the questions to ask.

Lifespan
- How old is the person?
- How might age influence their mobility?
- Does the person have a history of mobility problems?
- How have they managed mobility problems in the past?
- Is there anything in their life history that might influence their current experience?

Dependence–independence continuum
- How dependent/independent is the person in mobilising?
- What form does any dependency take?
- What effect does this have on the other Activities of Living?

Biological factors
- Are there deficits or deficiencies in the bones, muscles or joints?
- Are there any deficits or deficiencies in any other body system that might affect the person's mobility, or experience, or possible treatment?
- When/how does the individual undertake physical activity?

Psychological factors
- What is the person's level of knowledge and understanding about their current problem?
- How is the mobility problem affecting their psychological wellbeing?

- How is the mobility problem affecting their personal relationships?
- What is the person's level of knowledge and understanding of the relationship between health and mobility?

Sociocultural factors

- How is the mobility problem affecting the person's usual roles and behaviours?
- How might the person's cultural background influence their experience of a mobility problem or any possible treatment or intervention?

Environmental factors

- What effect is the mobility problem having on the person's ability to mobilise in their own social environment, at home and in their community?
- What access does the individual have to forms of transport?

Politicoeconomic factors

- Does the mobility problem affect the person's ability to work or play?

You might want to reflect on how and when you might ask these questions and the skills you need (see Chapter 4).

Some elements of data collection will now be considered in a little more detail. A large amount of data can be collected about an individual's mobility through observation. Other sorts of physical data also need to be identified, for example from examination and measurement. However, in order to undertake an effective and comprehensive assessment, the nurse not only needs to know what to look for, but also what a particular piece of data might mean.

> **Exercise**
> Look at Table 10.3.
>
> 1. Fill in the third column. You need to find out what the observational data might mean.
> 2. You might want to add other observational data of your own.

It is evident that there is a wide range of data available when assessing an individual's mobility. For some observational data (these may be referred to as cues), there might be a number of possible explanations. A core skill of nursing practice is the ability to integrate and interpret a number of cues and so come to an understanding of exactly what the patient's problem is and what has caused it.

Table 10.3 Observations made during the assessment of the AL of mobilising

When you observe	You might see	Which might mean
Posture	A lateral S curve (scoliosis) A rounding of the thoracic spine (kyphosis) An increase in the curve at the lumbar spine causing the shoulders to be thrown back (lordosis)	
Gait	Poor balance Unsteadiness Irregular movements Weakness and fatigue	
Joints	A restricted range of movement Instability or stiffness Swelling Tenderness Nodules Crepitus	
Muscles	Differences in muscle strength Changes in muscle tone	
Limbs	Differences in size and shape of hands, feet, arms, legs, digits Alteration in reflexes	
Skin	Pallor Cyanosis	
Pulses	Faint or absent pulse	

Standard assessment scales which assess aspects of mobility and/or function may also be used. Examples of such assessment tools are given in Table 10.4 which can be used to grade the degree of spasticity in an affected part, and Table 10.5 which can be used to assess the degree of contracture.

A more detailed view of assessment can now be examined using a case study.

Table 10.4 The modified Ashworth scale for spasticity

0	no increase in muscle tone
1	slight increase in tone (catch and release)
2	slight increase in tone (catch and resistance through less than half of the range of movement)
3	marked increase in tone through most of range of movement
4	considerable increase in tone (passive range of movement difficult)
5	rigidity (flexion or extension) of affected part

From Davies and O'Connor (1999).

Case study 10.4

Assessment following a fall

Elizabeth Roberts is 84 years old. She is single and until recently lived with her brother. He died about 6 months ago and now she lives alone. Miss Roberts has been admitted to a medical ward from Accident and Emergency following a fall which left her lying on the floor for several hours. You have been told there is no bony injury, but that Miss Roberts is bruised, distressed and remains very unstable when she tries to walk.

Exercise

You have been asked to assess her.

1. What sort of data will you want to collect? Why do you want that data? How will you collect it?
2. What sort of knowledge base will you need to undertake the assessment?
3. What sorts of skills will you need to use?
4. Identify any learning needs in relation to the case study and develop a learning plan to meet these needs.

Table 10.5 Contracture assessment scale

Area	Severe (3)	Moderate (2)	Mild (1)	None (0)
Pain	Pain most of the time, with or without movement. Overt facial signs of pain Guarding while performing passive ROM exercises. Analgesia may not relieve.	Pain with passive ROM exercises. Sometimes pain at rest, relieved by analgesic.	Pain at end of range of passive ROM exercises, resolved by rest. Activity may be slowed. Analgesia not usually required.	Occasional or no pain.
Function	No function possibly due to lack of innervation or fixed nature of the contracture. No active of purposeful movement.	Limited function. Poor coordination due to limited movement. Random joint movements may be present. Limited grasp and release but no strength.	Independent function possible. Gross movements are easy, finer movements may be difficult. Some incoordination may be present. Movements may be uncoordinated. Adaptive devices my be used.	Independent function without assistive devices. Fine movement unimpaired.
Ease of movement	Fixed joints or limbs. Passive range of movement absent or very limited (less than 25%).	Some passive joint movement (up to 50%). May or may not be able to initiate movement. Joint returns to contracted position.	Nearly full range of passive movement. Some resistance at the end of the range.	Full range of active movement.
Nursing	Very difficult to clean skin and to prevent breakdown. Nail cutting impossible. Skin may be macerated.	Difficult to complete skin care and reposition after care. Odour may be present.	Skin care is easy. Limited ability to reposition.	Easy to clean skin and to reposition after care.

From Davies and O'Connor (1999).

A wide range of data needed for a comprehensive assessment of Miss Roberts should have been identified. In addition, recognition of the knowledge and skills base needed to support your assessment. Part of that knowledge base is an understanding of falls, particularly as experienced by older people.

Knowledge for practice: falls in later life

Falls are a major public health issue in all industrialised societies. They are associated with high levels of morbidity and mortality. In 1997 in the UK around 67% of accidental deaths in females over 65 years of age were due to falls. A fall is often a sign that there is something wrong, and should always be taken seriously and followed up.

There is evidence that falls can be prevented. The National Service Framework for Older People (DoH 2001a, www.doh.hov.uk/nsf/olderpeople.htm) identifies the prevention and effective management of falls as a key target. The primary prevention of falls focuses on a number of population-based initiatives. These include raising awareness of safety amongst the general public, encouraging life-long healthy eating habits, and healthier levels of physical activity and exercise.

Central to the prevention of falls and related injury is the identification of those individuals who are at high risk of falling. Whilst the NSF for Older People (DoH 2001a) states that there will be prospective screening as part of the over 75s' health check, good clinical practice should also incorporate opportunistic screening. This means that all nurses coming into contact with older people should be able to undertake a rigorous, evidence-based falls risk assessment. Alongside this there is the identification of people who have, or who are at risk of developing, osteoporosis.

Osteoporosis is a common disease. It is associated with pain, disability and death. Osteoporosis is the consequence of a reduction in bone mass, due to osteoclast activity (so there is more bone reabsorption than there is bone building). Compact bone becomes thinner, the Haversian canals enlarge and the bone becomes fragile and more porous. The disease develops over many years, it is often symptomless, and many older people are not aware that they are at risk. More women than men develop osteoporosis. High alcohol intake and tobacco consumption are both associated with the development of osteoporosis.

Osteoporosis carries a high risk of fracture. Nursing interventions for people with osteoporosis include the prevention of further bone loss and fractures, encouraging a diet rich in calcium and vitamin D, and supporting cessation of smoking. Exercise has been found to have a preventative effect on fracture rate (Law et al 1991).

There are multiple risk factors for falls and osteoporotic fracture which are illustrated in Table 10.6. Look at the risk factors in relation to the previous exercise. Is there anything you want to add to your data collection?

It is already known that some older people are more at risk of falling. They are those who are admitted to acute hospital care, or who are in nursing or residential care. Falls in hospital are a worldwide problem, and a falls risk assessment is increasingly part of routine practice. A systematic review of studies of hospital falls (Evans et al 2001) identified the at-risk patient to be one with impaired cognition, with special elimination needs, impaired mobility and a history of previous falls. This report stated that whilst older people are more likely to fall than younger people, this was a function of factors such as poor mobility or confusion rather than simply age itself.

The consequences of a fall are numerous. Physical injury is common, including fracture of the neck of the femur. Psychologically, the older person's confidence can be undermined and the fear of falling severely curtails mobilising. This can lead to functional deterioration and even institutionalisation.

Exercise

Find out what resources are available in your locality for the prevention and treatment of falls.

1. On your next practice placement ask about the process used for falls risk assessment.
2. If there is a specialist falls service find out how it works. Identify what the referral mechanisms are to and from the falls service.
3. Identify the nurse's role in the prevention and treatment of falls in the primary, secondary and tertiary care settings.

Table 10.6 Falls and osteoporotic fracture: risk factors

Risk factors associated with falls	Risk factors associated with osteoporotic fracture
• Impaired gait, balance or mobility	• Evidence of bone thinning (osteopoenia)
• Polypharmacy (particularly drugs acting on the central nervous system or those causing hypotension	• Loss of height associated with vertebral deformity
• Visual impairment	• Previous fragility fracture
• Impaired cognition	• Prolonged corticosteroid treatment
• Depression	• History of early menopause
• Stroke, Parkinson's, lower limb disease	• History of maternal hip fracture
• Postural hypotension	• Smoking
• Home environment	• Low body mass index

Now, return to the assessment of Miss Roberts. Review and add to the notes from the last exercise and include the process of falls risk assessment.

As part of the data collection process the following questions might have been asked:

- Have you fallen before if so, when? how often? what happened?
- Tell me about this latest fall?
- Do you normally have any trouble walking or getting around?
- Do you ever feel like you are losing your balance?
- Do you use anything to help you walk? inside the house? outside the house?
- Are you afraid of falling?
- Are there any activities you would like to do but don't because you can't get around?
- Do you ever have pain or discomfort in your joints and/or muscles?
- Are you seeing the doctor for anything at the moment?
- What medications are you taking?
- How much exercise do you get? (in particular weight-bearing exercise such as walking)
- How much do you smoke and drink?

In order to identify the risk of osteoporosis the following might have been considered:

- Do you have any blood relatives who have, or have had, osteoporosis, or who have had fractures late in life?
- Have you had any fractures in adult life?
- Do you take any vitamin D or calcium supplements?
- Have you ever had your bone density measured?
- Do you take any medication for osteoporosis?

These observations might have been undertaken:

- height measurement and compare to peak height
- lying and standing blood pressure
- observe walking, posture and gait pattern
- observe moving from lying to sitting, and from sitting to standing
- cognitive ability
- sensory impairment.

The following may have been noted:

- any medical condition which is associated with falls or osteoporosis
- any medication that might increase the risk of falls (including over-the-counter medicines)
- hazards in the environment (e.g. lighting, flooring, furniture)
- when and where to refer to other colleagues for expert assessment, advice and treatment.

From the assessment therefore, identification should have been made of:

- Miss Roberts' history in relation to mobilising, in particular:

  – usual routines and habits
  – usual level of independence
  – established coping mechanisms
- Miss Roberts experience of and feelings about her current mobility problem
- factors which may have contributed to her current fall
- risk factors related to future falls
- risk factors related to osteoporotic fracture.

As part of any comprehensive, holistic assessment it will also be necessary to look at how the actual/potential mobility problem might affect the other Activities of Living.

Exercise

What data related to the other Activities of Living would you need to collect in order to produce a holistic assessment of Miss Roberts?

This exercise illustrates how the Activities of Living are interrelated. A number of ideas may have been generated here – some of these are related to the mental picture of 'Miss Roberts' that may have been formed in your mind. For example, the following may have been considered:

1. *Maintaining a safe environment*
   - How well does Miss Roberts understand her medication and possible side effects?
   - What is her normal home environment? Does she leave the house/how does she manage in the external environment?
   - Does Miss Roberts have any pain?
   - Does Miss Roberts have any problems with seeing and hearing?
   - Are there any risks of pressure ulcer development?
   - Will there be a need for moving and handling?

2. *Communicating*
   - What language does Miss Roberts speak?
   - Has she any impairment in speech and/or hearing?
   - What is Miss Roberts' usual ability to communicate?
   - Has/how has admission to hospital affected this?

3. *Breathing*
   - Does Miss Roberts smoke?
   - Does she get out of breath or feel uncomfortable when undertaking physical activity?

4. *Eating and drinking*
   - How does Miss Roberts do her shopping and cooking?
   - What are her usual eating and drinking habits?
   - What is her appetite like since her brother died?
   - Has there been any weight loss or gain?
   - What is Miss Roberts usual fluid intake?

5. *Eliminating*
   - How does Miss Roberts usually manage her elimination needs?

- Has she experienced any problems with eliminating?
- Can/is she able to get to toilet on her own in the current environment?
- What sort of help might she need whilst in hospital?

6. *Personal cleansing and dressing*
   - How does Miss Roberts usually bathe, wash and dress?
   - What effect has her mobility problem had on her usual routine?
   - What sort of help might she need whilst in hospital?

7. *Controlling body temperature*
   - Does Miss Roberts have a low temperature due to being left on the floor all night?

8. *Working and playing*
   - What are Miss Roberts usual work and play activities?
   - Does she usually require any assistance with household tasks? Is so, what?

9. *Expressing sexuality*
   - Has her current mobility problems affected her ability to maintain personal and/or intimate relationships?
   - Has it affected her body image/self-image?

10. *Sleeping*
    - Can Miss Roberts get in and out of and move around the bed on her own?
    - What is her usual sleep routine?
    - Has she any difficulty in falling asleep?
    - Does she feel fully rested?

11. *Dying*
    - How has Miss Roberts coped with the changes in her life since the death of her brother?
    - Has she any fears for her own future?

The above list is just an indication of some of the questions you might want to answer as part of your assessment of Miss Roberts. The overall outcome should be that you have sufficient data to identify Miss Roberts' actual and potential problems with her Activities of Living.

Identifying and prioritising problems related to mobilising

The end point of the assessment process should be the identification of the patient's actual and potential problems with the intention of establishing goals for care and determining nursing interventions. The Activities of Living model identifies four categories of mobility problems:

- a change of independence/dependence status
- a change in mobilising habit
- a change in environment or routine
- pain associated with mobilising.

Obviously these are only broad categories and it is important to be clear and specific in writing problem statements.

Problems can be described as actual, that is existing at the present time, or potential, that is there is a clear risk that in the present circumstances a problem is likely to develop (see Chapter 1).

A return to Case study 10.3 is necessary. Through the assessment the following has been learnt about Miss Roberts.

1. *Lifespan* Miss Roberts celebrated her 84th birthday last month. She had a 'small' party attended by a number of her friends from the local church and neighbourhood, and by her nieces, nephews and their children and grandchildren. Miss Roberts says 'I'm lucky to have so many good friends and a lovely family'. She considers her general health 'quite good for my age … I've always looked after myself'. She has never been in hospital before ('except as a visitor, and that was enough').

2. *Dependence–independence* Miss Roberts considers herself to be very independent, although she has found it more difficult since her brother died. For all her adult life she lived with either her parents, or with two of her brothers. She appears to have well-established social networks, and access to local resources. Miss Roberts makes no use of either health or social care services.

3. *Maintaining a safe environment*
   - wears bifocal spectacles. Says that her eyesight has become worse in the past 6 months
   - no apparent hearing problem
   - Waterlow score of 18 which puts her at risk of developing pressure ulcers
   - no history or current evidence of cognitive impairment
   - has some pain as she banged her head, knee and arm when falling
   - has dizziness when rising from sitting to standing and intermittent dizziness when walking
   - pulse rate 92 and regular, blood pressure is 180/100 sitting, drops to 130/80 when standing
   - other vital signs/neurological observations are normal
   - feet cold and her skin is dry and tissue-paper-like, foot pulses are present she says her feet 'always feel cold'
   - takes regular medication for high blood pressure ('blood pressure tablets and a water tablet'). Takes regular anti-inflammatory pain-relieving medication. No other prescribed medication. Understands her medication.

4. *Communicating*
   - speaks English
   - is able to communicate verbally and nonverbally
   - appears to understand instructions and information.

5. *Breathing*
   - has never smoked

- gets a little out of breath when walking rapidly, or doing 'heavy' housework such as cleaning windows
- for the past 3 months has become increasingly dizzy.

6. *Eating and drinking*
   - appetite normally fine, but not so good since brother died. Does her own cooking, enjoys cooking for members of the family
   - has been cutting down on fluids to reduce risk of urinary incontinence
   - can get to the local shop unaided. Goes to the supermarket with a family member once a fortnight. Local grocer and butcher will deliver
   - wears dentures which fit well. No signs of oral infection
   - appears of average build, says she has lost weight, 'about a dress size' since her brother died.

7. *Eliminating*
   - experiences feelings of urgency and occasionally has urinary incontinence
   - feels very embarrassed about this 'I haven't told anyone. It's all I can expect at my age'
   - has to get up to go to toilet at least twice in the night
   - takes regular over-the-counter medication to prevent constipation
   - urinalysis normal.

8. *Personal cleansing and dressing*
   - usually has a shower independently – uses a shower stool
   - doesn't have bath – worried about not being able to get out
   - independent in dressing and personal grooming
   - likes to look 'smart', always wears make up.

9. *Controlling body temperature*
   - body temperature 36.4°C
   - usually independent

10. *Mobilising*
    - is usually independent in her home and the local environment. Does not use a walking aid. Tries to go out for a walk for at least half an hour every day
    - has fallen twice in the past few weeks, didn't tell anyone. Has been using the furniture to steady herself in her home. Was getting worried about going out in case she fell and broke a bone
    - got up in the night to go to the toilet, felt dizzy, tripped over a tear in the carpet, fell and couldn't get up
    - usually has some joint discomfort and stiffness, especially when getting out of bed
    - some rounding of the thoracic spine, says she has lost height as she has got older
    - poor balance and very unsteady when walking
    - is fearful of falling, grips tight onto the nurse's hand
    - does not know of a family history of osteoporosis. Two maternal aunts died in hospital after fracturing a hip.

11. *Working and playing*
    - worked as a book-keeper for a local firm, whilst she retired from full-time employment at the age of 70, she continued some part time work until the age of 78
    - plays important role in the local church. Helps with the children in Sunday School, and twice-weekly drop-in groups
    - works two afternoons a week at a local charity shop
    - family and friends help with household tasks
    - no support from outside agencies.

12. *Expressing sexuality*
    - never wanted to get married, work and family have always come first
    - no current close, intimate relationships
    - self-image, has always felt independent, now feels lost and powerless.

13. *Sleeping*
    - usually goes to bed about 10.30 – does not take a sleeping pill. Reads for an hour or so and listens to the radio. Gets up about 8 o'clock.
    - feels tired sometimes can't get back to sleep
    - gets up in the night to go to the toilet.

14. *Dying*
    - is still upset about the death of her brother
    - worried that she might not be able to go home and about dying in hospital
    - has a strong faith in Christianity.

> **Exercise**
>
> From the information given above, identify and list Miss Roberts actual and potential problems in relation to mobilising.

To identify problems, you need to go through a process of analysing and interpreting the data you have collected. This involves reviewing the data, identifying important cues and looking for patterns and groupings of the cues. It might be that some problems are simple to identify. This should be because you have sufficient data to confirm the problem. However you must be wary of making assumptions, that is jumping to conclusions that you know what an individual's problems are. Assumptions are often based on stereotypes. For example, ageist stereotypes of older people include assumptions of dependence, disability, confusion and asexuality – which means that older people may be assumed to have some kinds of problems (for example being disabled or being lonely), but not to have others (such as sexual problems).

It might be that you feel you need more data than already given in order to identify Miss Roberts' problems. This underlines the on-going nature of assessment, and the way in which data collection and analysis feed into each other. However, you should at least be able to make some preliminary identification of Miss Roberts' problems related to mobilising. The problems you have identified in relation to mobilising might include:

- Miss Roberts is unable to mobilise safely and independently due to unsteady gait, dizziness and change in environment.
- Miss Roberts is at high risk of future fall and injury.
- Miss Roberts is very afraid of falling again.
- Miss Roberts experiences discomfort and joint stiffness, especially on first moving.

Exercise

From the information given above, identify and list Miss Roberts' actual and potential problems in relation to other Activities of Living. Remember that you should consider all the components of the model – lifespan, dependency, and all the factors influencing the Activities of Living.

A number of actual and potential problems will have been identified related to the other Activities of Living. These might have included:

- pain and discomfort
- anxiety regarding the future
- recent loss of appetite
- occasional urinary incontinence
- potential problem of constipation.

You might also identify where you need to collect more data to confirm or disregard a possible problem. For example, Miss Roberts has had a loss of appetite, developed sleeping problems, feels tired on waking and feels that she will never recover from the loss of her brother. Together these cues might suggest a possible problem related to low mood or depression. Depression is commonly experienced by older people who are admitted to hospital, and is often not recognised.

Roper et al (1996, 2000) suggest that the next step of the process is to prioritise the problems. This should be done in collaboration with the individual and/or their family. It is clear that problems that are actually or potentially life threatening take precedence. Thereafter one is often dealing with competing priorities. The dependency/independence component of the model can be used to prioritise problems, with the most urgent problems being those in which the patient is completely dependent.

Exercise

1. Review the list of actual and potential problems generated in the previous two exercises and put them in order of priority.
2. What criteria are you using to decide the relative priority of problems?

When you review the problems identified in relation to Miss Roberts' mobility you need to consider the impact of the problems on Miss Roberts' dependency, and the degree of harm likely to result from (currently) potential problems. The highest priority problems therefore are those related to her inability to mobilise safely and independently, and her high risk of falling and sustaining a serious injury. Of medium priority is Miss Roberts' fear of falling, which has the potential to affect a range of Activities of Living other than mobilising. Lowest priority at this time is Miss Roberts' joint discomfort and stiffness, long-standing problems which do not usually significantly impair her independence.

So far the case study and exercises have looked at how Miss Roberts might be assessed and identify and prioritise her needs. Her case might appear at the outset to be fairly simple and uncomplicated, however you should by now be aware that she has some complex needs for nursing. Older people often present with complex multiple pathologies, where there is coexisting chronic and acute health breakdown (physical and mental) and social needs, on top of the 'normal' changes associated with ageing. This underlines the importance of a comprehensive and accurate assessment.

Planning nursing care to meet needs/problems in mobilising

Planning nursing care involves a number of processes including:

- setting short-term and long-term goals
- deciding what nursing actions to take
- documenting the plan.

Setting goals

Goal setting can only be based on an accurate assessment and identification of problems and needs. Goals should refer to the expected outcomes of nursing interventions. They should be measurable, realistic and achievable within the individual person's circumstances. They might be immediate, short term (hours or days) or long term. As far as is possible, goals should be understood by and agreed with the patient (see Chapter 1 for more detail on goal setting).

Exercise

1. Set a goal for each actual and potential problem identified for Miss Roberts in the exercises on pp. 306 and 307.
2. Are the goals observable? measurable? realistic? achievable?

Goals need to be observable and measurable if possible. This is important as goals are used to monitor and evaluate both the patient's progress and the effectiveness of nursing interventions. Goals that are not realistic and achievable will be discouraging for the patient and you. In some circumstances it might be relevant to identify long-term and short-term goals. Long-term goals may refer to desired outcome in weeks, months or years to come. In Miss Roberts' case, long-term goals can be set in relation to her care after discharge from hospital. For example: 'Miss Roberts will be able to mobilise safely and independently in her home environment.'

However, a number of short-term goals might be needed in relation to her care in hospital, such as: 'Miss Roberts will identify the need for and request assistance in moving and transferring' and/or 'Miss Roberts will demonstrate the use of an appropriate walking aid'.

Thinking about goal setting can help to identify challenges in planning effective individualised care. For example, Miss Roberts' ability to mobilise safely and independently is impaired, yet she wishes to mobilise independently as quickly as possible so that she can go home. You need to think about a plan of nursing care that will reduce the risk of her falling, yet not compromise her feelings of autonomy.

Deciding on nursing interventions

The Activities of Living model for nursing identifies four levels of helping:

- solving or alleviating the problem
- preventing a potential problem from becoming an actual one
- preventing a solved problem from reoccurring
- developing positive coping strategies for any problem that cannot be solved.

Exercise

1. List the factors you need to take into account when planning nursing care.
2. Reflect on your current knowledge and skills in relation to planning nursing care.
3. Identify any learning needs and develop a learning plan to meet those needs.

A long list of potential factors should have been identified, which might influence your plan of care. The list probably included:

- your own knowledge of normal movement
- your own knowledge of normal living and dependency across cultures
- your own knowledge and experience of mobility disorders
- your understanding of the evidence base for nursing practice
- your knowledge of alternative interventions
- the accuracy of the assessment
- your skill of observing, interpreting and prioritising data
- your understanding of the work with others in the multiprofessional team
- the physical environment of care and access to physical and human resources

- the patient's ability to participate
- the patient's personal knowledge and beliefs.

Planning all the proposed nursing interventions needed to achieve the stated goals is necessary. The written plan needs to be in sufficient detail so that it can be used by others to deliver the care. Also remember that this is the patient's plan and so should be written so that they can understand it.

Exercise

Miss Roberts falls whilst walking to the toilet unaided. She complains of severe pain in her right hip and leg. She looks extremely pale and frightened, her pulse rate is raised. Miss Roberts cannot move her right leg voluntarily. On observation her right leg appears shortened and is externally rotated. You now need to:

- re-assess
- identify Miss Roberts' immediate problems (actual and potential)
- prioritise the problems you have identified
- set relevant, measurable and achievable goals
- identify what nursing interventions will be needed to:
  – solve or alleviate actual problems
  – prevent potential problems from becoming actual ones
- compare and contrast your assessment and problem identification for Miss Roberts before and after this injury.

Note the differences between assessment in an emergency and nonemergency situation. For example, the differing sources of data might have been considered in the assessment process. After this latest fall Miss Roberts is in considerable pain and distress, so the amount of verbal information you can expect will be reduced. Add to this the disorientation that can occur to anyone who is injured and frightened. A number of actual and potential problems including pain, shock, immobility and anxiety will also have identified .

Exercise

Following an X-ray it is seen that Miss Roberts has sustained a fracture to the neck of the femur on her right leg. Miss Roberts is transferred to an orthopaedic ward. It is over 16 hours later that she is transferred to the operating theatre. During this time, her mobility is severely restricted.

1. Review your knowledge on the potential hazards of prolonged immobility using Table 10.7.
2. What is the nurses' role in preventing problems associated with immobility?
3. What nursing interventions need to be planned for Miss Roberts during this preoperative period?
4. What skills and knowledge do you need in order to plan nursing care for Miss Roberts in this preoperative period?
5. Identify your learning needs and develop a plan to meet these needs.

Table 10.7 Preventing the potential complications of prolonged impaired mobility

Potential problem	Nursing intervention (see Exercise p.308)	Rationale
Loss of independence		
Disorientation		
Depression		
Isolation		
Lack of venous return		
Venous stasis		
Reduced lung expansion		
Bronchial pneumonia		
Deep vein thrombosis		
Pulmonary embolism		
Contracture		
Flexion deformity		
Loss of muscle strength		
Orthostatic hypotension (drop in blood pressure on standing)		
Hypothermia		
Loss of appetite		
Dehydration		
Constipation		
Urinary stasis		
Pressure ulcers		

From Table 10.7 it can be seen that there are a number of serious potential problems associated with enforced reduced mobility, many of which the nurse can prevent or alleviate. It is important that the risk of any of these complications occurring is recognised and does not only relate to the extent and duration of reduced mobility. For example, there are a number of factors that increase Miss Roberts' risk of developing a deep vein thrombosis:

- her mobility has been restricted for some time previously
- her age
- major surgery on the hip joint.

In planning Miss Roberts' nursing care needs before she goes to the operating theatre, the following should have been recognised:

- identifying and providing appropriate intervention for actual problems
- preventing any potential problems preoperatively and minimising the risk of postoperative complications
- effective preoperative preparation
- ensuring Miss Roberts knows what to expect postoperatively·
- maintaining privacy, dignity and promoting choice and participation.

Exercise

Miss Roberts is transferred to theatre where she has an internal fixation of the fracture using a dynamic hip screw. After the operation, Miss Roberts is transferred to an orthopaedic ward for the first 5 days of recovery.

1. Write a plan of care for Miss Roberts
   - in the immediately postoperative period
   - during early mobilisation (first 5 days postoperative).
2. What knowledge, skills and resource will you need to plan and deliver the care Miss Roberts needs?
3. Identify your learning needs and write a learning plan to meet those needs.

In the exercises on pp. 308 and 309 a wide range of skills and knowledge needed in order to plan Miss Roberts' nursing care should have been identified. These should have been included:

- general perioperative care
- the specific perioperative needs of older people
- the management and care of fractures – in particular fractured neck of femur
- pain management for older people
- wound care and wound healing
- mobilisation techniques
- roles of multiprofessional team
- psychosocial support.

It is important that you are confident in the general principles of perioperative care (see Mallet & Dougherty 2000). You should also be able to recognise any specific considerations that need to be given to older patients. For example, the effects of normal physiological ageing, such as a reduction in physiological reserve capacity, mean that older people are particularly vulnerable to a range of stressors. There is a higher incidence of chronic conditions such as diabetes, anaemia and cardiac failure in later life, and multiple pathologies need to be taken into account when assessing and planning care. Acute confusion is not uncommon perioperatively and is usually due to low oxygen levels in the blood (hypoxaemia) (see Chapter 3 for further information on pre- and postoperative care).

Fractures

A fracture is a loss in the continuity of bone tissue, usually due to traumatic injury. There are many ways of classifying fractures and you should familiarise yourself with these. Box 10.4 highlights the signs and symptoms of fractures, although these will vary according to the site and severity of the fracture.

The immediate management of the fracture includes: immobilising the affected part by use of splints, reducing pain and oedema, assessing and observing the affected part (see Box 10.5) and observing for signs of systemic shock. Subsequent management aims to fix the fractured bone in the correct anatomical position.

Box 10.4 Common signs and symptoms associated with a fracture

- Pain
- Loss of normal movement
- Loss of sensation
- Obvious deformity
- Change in the curvature or length of the bone
- Crepitus or a grating sound on movement of the limb
- Soft tissue oedema
- Warmth over the affected areas
- Bruising (which might not be apparent for a number of days)
- Further signs and symptoms of shock related to severe pain, blood loss and tissue injury.

Box 10.5 Neurovascular assessment

A circulation check or neurovascular monitoring is an essential component of care following neuromuscular trauma, after the application of bandages, casts or splints, or postoperatively. The frequency with which the assessment takes place will depend on the situation. In the case of trauma or postoperatively it may be carried out every 15 minutes. The key elements of the assessment can be remembered as the 5 Ps:

Pulselessness, **P**araesthesia, **P**allor, **P**uffiness, **P**ain.

Data collection
Subjective: complaints of pain, numbness or tingling (paraesthesia).

Objective: cool, pale or cyanotic skin above or below the damaged site.
- Absent or faint pulses
- Oedema
- Capillary bed refill time over 2 seconds

Fracture of the hip

Fractures of the distal/head end of the femur are commonly referred to as hip fractures. Hip fractures are extremely common in all industrialised countries, especially amongst women. Women are more at risk of hip fracture, which is linked to a higher incidence of osteoporosis. The lifetime risk of a woman having a hip fracture is 1:6 (Ethan & Powell 1996). Such fractures are often the result of an impact trauma such as a twist or a fall. In the UK, it is the most common fracture which is treated as an inpatient.

Hip fractures can be classified into three main types: femoral neck, intertrochanteric and subtrochanteric. The first two are the most common amongst older people. Surgical management will depend not only on the type of fracture but on the amount of displacement and whether the fracture is complete or incomplete. It is important that surgery occurs soon after fracture, preferably within 24 hours. The aim of surgical intervention for both femoral neck and intertrochanteric fractures is to achieve a stable reduction of the fracture whilst allowing weight bearing as soon as possible. Undisplaced femoral neck fractures are fairly straightforward and are likely to be treated by internal fixation with pins or cannulated screws. Displaced fractures have a much higher rate of necrosis and nonunion and are so more likely to be treated with primary prosthetic replacement femoral head whether alone (hemiarthoplasty) or more rarely a total hip replacement. Intertrochanteric fractures are usually stabilised using a sliding or dynamic hip screw.

The Audit Commission report *United they stand* (1995) looked at the treatment and care of people with a hip fracture in a range of settings from Accident and Emergency, through orthopaedic and rehabilitation wards to home and community services. The report made the following points.

- The majority of staff had little specific education and training regarding the care of older people, despite the numbers and proportion of older people in the care settings examined.
- Assessments were often incomplete. Problems associated with this include the cancellation of operations, inappropriate rehabilitation plans and delayed discharge.
- Misdiagnosis occurred, for example temporary confusion (due to pain, injury, the effects of the operation or medication) being seen and treated as dementia.
- Deficiency in hydration and nutrition.
- The mismanagement of incontinence, in particular the overuse of catheters.
- Failure to assess and manage pain.
- Development of pressure sores.

Hip fracture also carries a high risk of infection (chest, wound and urinary tract), deep vein thrombosis and hypoxia. The prevention of such complications and early mobilisation are vitally important components in the care of someone with a fractured hip.

Miss Roberts undergoes early postoperative rehabilitation and early mobilisation. This requires a whole-team approach. Care pathways are often used to indicate who does what, and which interventions have a shared responsibility (for example identifying who will be deciding if the patient can weight bear). Weight-bearing restrictions are not standardised, they can be affected by the type of fixation used, the location and type of fracture, the integrity of the bone, the patient's cognitive and functional ability.

The following is indicative of a fairly standard protocol for early mobilisation after surgery for a fractured hip.

1st postoperative day
- hip movement precautions (after replacement of the femoral head some movements are prohibited, e.g. flexion beyond 90°, adduction past the midline and internal rotation)
- active range of movement for other limbs
- isometric exercises of the affected limb to strengthen quadriceps and gluteal muscles.

2nd postoperative day
- observe hip precautions
- practice transfers and mobility in bed
- assisted standing whilst observing weight-bearing restrictions.

3rd postoperative day onwards
- walk short distances using walking aid
- observe weight-bearing restrictions.

Whenever assisting someone to move, there are certain simple interventions which you need to establish as routine. Firstly, before anything else, check the environment and make sure that you, the patient, and anyone else involved knows what they are doing. Check that any chair you might be using is of the right height and has arms. It's really difficult to get up from a sitting position without chair-arms to push down onto. Make sure that the person's footwear, shoes or slippers are of a good fit and offer some support to the foot. It is better if shoes have a low heel, with the heels as wide as the heel of the foot.

The movement from sitting to standing can be problematic, especially for frail older people. Without the ability to make this movement it is difficult to transfer or to walk. Being able to successfully achieve what appears to be a simple task can have a significant effect on levels of independence – and achievement might be the key to enabling someone to live in their own home. Firstly make sure that the patient's feet are pulled back and in a stable position. Whilst pushing up from the thighs, the patient should also push down on their hands to provide extra impetus. Make sure the patient bends forward from the hips, with the head well forward, and then push to rise to a standing position. When the person is standing, you must make quite sure that they have got their balance before they start to walk.

When assisting someone to walk, try to use as little direct intervention as possible. If it is helpful, ask the patient to talk through what they are going to do before they start to move. When the patient is mobilising observe them carefully then you can give feedback to the patient and to colleagues. Give direct instructions only when they are needed, and then only one instruction at a time. If you need to demonstrate a skill do not make it too complex or complicated. Identify a specific task and break it down into steps.

When the patient starts to walk you shouldn't hover around or hold onto them unnecessarily. You should position yourself close against the patient's shoulder and remember to walk at their pace and encouraging the patient to take steps of an equal length. If you are worried about someone's balance you can place one hand on their lower back to support their centre of gravity. Alternatively, have someone behind you pushing a wheelchair which the patient can sit in if needed.

Remember also that people need to learn how to take a few steps backward, a skill sometimes needed to sit down and to open doors safely. It is important that people learn how to open and close doors without reaching forward and possibly overbalancing. It's also important that people learn to walk on different surfaces, coping with gravel, slopes and getting up and down pavements. It is important therefore to have knowledge of the person's home, social environment and lifestyle to equip them with the necessary mobilising skills.

A standard walking frame enables the distribution of weight through the arms so reducing weight on the affected leg. It also slows and steadies the gait. Some patients may move from a standard to a wheeled walking frame which allows more rapid movement and helps establish a normal gait pattern. Further progression might be made to a single point cane, which should always be used in the hand opposite the fractured leg.

Exercise

1. In order to achieve her long-term goal of going home, Miss Roberts' short-term goals relate to knowing how to safely:
   - move about in the bed
   - get on and off the bed
   - get on and off chairs
   - get on and off the toilet
   - walk using a frame including negotiating doors and stairs.
2. Review your knowledge and skills in relation to the above?
3. Find out what interventions can be used to support the development of mobilising activities.
4. What role would you play in helping Miss Roberts achieve these long- and short-term goals?

Documenting the nursing care plan

The nursing care plan might be written using a range of differing documentation, or a computerised record system. It should include a record of the assessment and the plan of care which directs nursing activities to achieve the desired goals.

Interprofessional case management and care pathways may be used to support the delivery of a coordinated service. An effective care pathway should inform everyone (including the patient) what is going to happen, which should enable contribution and cooperation. It is increasingly common for hip fracture to be managed using a clinical pathway (www.nelh.nhs.uk/carepathways).

Exercise

Look at the interventions you have identified in the exercises on pp. 308, 311.

1. Reflect on
   - your original assessment and problem identification of Miss Roberts
   - your updated assessment and problem identification after her fracture
   - any new knowledge you have gained.
2. Review the plan of intervention you have devised and make any changes you think are needed.
3. Identify the rationale (what is the evidence) for the interventions you have chosen.

Implementing care

It is important that you remember that gathering and analysing data, identifying problems, and setting goals is always going on. This is particularly obvious during the implementing phase of the nursing process, when you are constantly observing the effects of nursing actions. Implementing care provides the opportunity to gather data and note changes, responses and so on. Benner (1984) discusses the intuitive aspect of practice, which is born of expertise and experience. This intuitive ability enables the expert practitioner to identify nursing problems as they develop and be able to formulate and deliver a response.

Exercise

List the sorts of skills and knowledge you might need to implement the nursing care planned for Miss Roberts.

The following might have been considered:

- direct care-giving – doing and thinking
- delegating and supervising care
- managing of care
- professional responsibility and accountability
- interpersonal skills – listening, talking, observing, helping
- analytical skills
- problem-solving skills
- decision-making skills
- evidence-based practice
- research knowledge and skills
- knowledge of the factors affecting the Activities of Living
- understanding of pharmacology and other treatments
- beliefs, values and attitudes
- creativity
- critical thinking
- decision making
- resources – skill mix, equipment, support services.

Implementing care in practice often means having to work closely with others. The importance of this can be demonstrated by considering the role of the nurse in rehabilitation.

Exercise

Miss Roberts is transferred to an orthopaedic rehabilitation ward where she makes a good recovery and is discharged home to the care of a community rehabilitation service, 18 days after her operation.

1. Identify the role of the nurse, and other members of the multiprofessional team:
   - during Miss Roberts stay on the rehabilitation ward
   - in planning her discharge from hospital
   - following her discharge.

Rehabilitation is currently seeing an increase in attention from providers of healthcare. This can be traced to the increasing incidence of chronic disease and disability and rising population of older people worldwide. Effective rehabilitation is proposed as being a way of reducing demand on hospital beds, preventing admission to hospital and reducing long-term care costs, as well as improving survival rates.

There is little consensus in the numerous definitions of rehabilitation (Young et al 1999). Some definitions support a 'restricted model' of rehabilitation, with focused periods of goal-centred therapy aimed primarily at restoring function. Others propose a 'social model' which centres on user choice and control, the enablement of independent living or optimal functioning within our own environment (Robinson & Batstone 1996).

Wade and de Jong (2000) suggest a definition of specialised rehabilitation service related to structure, process and function.

Structure A rehabilitation service is made up of a multidisciplinary team who:

- have appropriate knowledge and skills
- work together towards shared goals for each patient
- can address the most common problems likely to be experienced by the patient
- involve and educate the patient and family.

Process Rehabilitation is an active, educational, patient-focused process involving:

- assessment – to identify the patient's problems and those factors relevant to the patient's experience
- goal setting – involving the patient and family
- intervention – to either influence the process of change or maintain the patient's quality of life, safety or both
- evaluation – to check on the effects of the intervention.

Outcome The aim of rehabilitation is to:

- maximise the ability of the patient to participate in their social environment
- minimise the stress/distress experienced by the patient and family.

Using the definitions given above, you should be able to see how the Activities of Living model, with its focus on enabling and facilitating individuality in living, can be used in rehabilitation nursing.

Davies and O'Connor (1999) review the applicability of the Activities of Living model to rehabilitation practice. They conclude that some aspects of the model fit well, namely:

- the focus on Activities of Living, and the role of the nurse in enabling people to achieve a balance between needs and abilities
- the 'relativist' definition of health (that is a definition that focuses on the individual optimum)
- the importance of the environment as being something which can be manipulated by the nurse to help the person.

However they also recognise limitations in the model, in particular the extent to which focus in practice has been on the physical to the neglect of the other components of the model (Davies and O'Connor 1999).

Defining the role of the nurse in rehabilitation is not straightforward. Rehabilitation nursing can be described as 'hands off' rather than 'hands on'. Whilst this might be an oversimplification this is something that some nurses experience as tension between what they see as between 'doing for' (caring) and 'standing back' (rehabilitation) (Long et al 2002). The research project in which Miss Roberts was involved identified six key interlinked aspects to the role of the nurse in rehabilitation:

- assessment
- coordination and communication
- technical and physical care
- emotional support
- involving the family
- therapy integration and therapy carry on.

Figure 10.10 illustrates the dimensions of therapy carry on and therapy integration. Therapy carry on has a limited focus with the nurse carrying out prescribed interventions such as using hot and cold packs, or applying splints. Therapy integration is much broader and has two aspects:

- creating a therapeutic environment which facilitates rehabilitation
- integrating therapy into the Activities of Living.

Discharge home

Effective, timely and appropriate discharge relies on good assessment and team working, and the nurse's role can be vital. This is particularly so when complex packages of care are required. In the NHS in the UK it is a requirement that all hospitals must have a clear discharge policy. Parker et al (2002) report a lack of evidence regarding the impact of specific discharge processes. They comment on the extent to which older people and carers complain about discharge arrangements – despite there being a range of legislation and guidance on the issue.

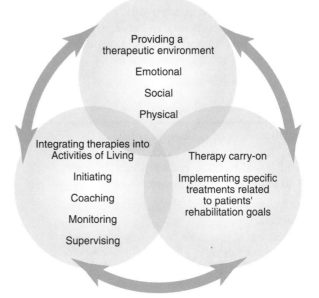

Fig. 10.10 Therapy integration and therapy carry on.

Whilst discharge planning should be multidisciplinary and multiagency, it is good practice that an identified individual coordinates the discharge process. Discharge should not occur unless the postdischarge arrangements are in place, and written information and advice should be given to the patient and carer. Liaison between community and hospital services is essential.

It might be the case that some patients are left with a long-term or permanent impairment in the activity of mobilising. The nurse has an important role to play in enabling the individual to adapt to this change in their lives.

It is important to recognise the varied potential reactions of the person, including a sense of loss or low self-esteem. Box 10.6 gives some potential effects of long-term

---

Box 10.6 Potential effects of impairment and disability in mobilising

Physical
Loss of power, energy, impaired function

Psychological
Mood swings (patient and family), boredom, depression, aggression, frustration

Sociocultural
Impact on family and personal relationships, changed ability to fulfil roles, cultural interpretation of suffering as good, bad or punishing

Environmental
Creation of dependence and handicap

Politicoeconomic
Change in/loss of employment, reduced income

impairment. It is important that you, as the nurse, can develop a trusting relationship with the patient; your attitude towards and acceptance of her/him is very important. You should always support participation and choice, enabling people to make decisions about their own care and their own lives.

Evaluating

Systematic, rigorous evaluation enhances the overall quality of care. It enables us to understand what works and what does not work. Evaluation emphasises the responsibility and accountability of nursing practice.

> **Exercise**
> 1. How would you evaluate Miss Roberts care?
> 2. What sorts of skills, knowledge and resource might you need?
> 3. Identify any learning needs and develop a learning plan to meet your needs.

When evaluating, you should review the extent to which the nursing interventions you have planned and implemented have met the goals set. The skills needed to evaluate include:

- observing
- questioning
- examining
- testing
- measuring.

Miss Roberts achieved her overall goals – she went home to carry on her life much as before. She used a walking frame for about 6 weeks, then used a stick only when she went outside. Within 3 months she was fulfilling the same social roles she had previously. Her family replaced old and worn out carpets throughout her house. Her blood pressure medication was changed and she no longer felt dizzy and 6 months after discharge had suffered no falls or trips.

Conclusion

Mobilising is a complex Activity of Living, the understanding of which requires a depth and breadth of knowledge. This complexity is reflected in the knowledge and skills needed to assess, plan, implement and evaluate effective, individualised nursing care. It is hoped that in working through part or all of this chapter, you have been able to recognise and value the knowledge and skills you already have and in addition that you have learned something new, and identified where you need to learn more.

References

Atkins WS 2001 Older people: their transport needs and requirements. Department of Environment, Transport and the Regions, London

Audit Commission 1995 United they stand: co-ordinating care for elderly patients with hip fracture. Audit Commission, London

Benner P 1984 From novice to expert. Addison-Wesley, California

Biddle SJ, Fox K, Boutcher S 2000 Physical activity and mental health: A national consensus. Routledge, London

Boore JRP, Champion R, Ferguson MC 1987 Nursing the physically ill adult. Churchill Livingstone, Edinburgh

Chilman AM, Thomas M 1987 Understanding nursing care, 3rd edn. Churchill Livingstone, Edinburgh

Davies S, O'Connor S 1999 Rehabilitation nursing foundations for practice. Baillière Tindall, Edinburgh

Department of Health 1995 More people, more active, more often. Physical activity in England: a consultation paper. HMSO, London

Department of Health 1999 Health survey of England 1998. HMSO, London

Department of Health Statistics Division 1999 The prevalence of back pain in Great Britain in 1998. Government Statistical Service, London

Department of Health 2001a National service framework for older people. HMSO, London

Department of Health 2001b Exercise referral systems: A national quality assurance framework. HMSO, London

Ethan K, Powell C 1996 Rehabilitation of the patient with hip fracture. Reviews in Clinical Gerontology 6: 371–388

Evans D, Hodgkinson B, Lambert L, Wood J 2001 Falls, risk factors in the hospital setting: a systematic review. International Journal of Nursing Practice 7: 38–45

Health and Safety at Work Act 1974 Stationery Office, London

Health and Safety Executive 1998 Manual handling operation regulations: guidelines on the regulations, 2nd edn. HSE, Sudbury

ICIDH-2 1999 International classification of functioning and disability. WHO, Geneva (www.who.int/icidh; accessed August 2002)

Law MR, Wald NJ, Meade TW 1991 Strategies for the prevention of osteoporosis and hip fracture. British Medical Journal 303: 453–459

Long A, Kneafsey R, Ryan J, Berry J, Howard R 2001 Teamworking in rehabilitation: exploring the role of the nurse. Researching professional education, research reports series number 19. English National Board for Nursing Midwifery and Health Visiting, London

Long AF, Kneafsey R, Ryan J, Berry J 2002 The role of the nurse within the multi-professional rehabilitation team. Journal of Advanced Nursing 37(1): 70–78

Mallet J, Dougherty L 2000 The Royal Marsden manual of clinical nursing procedures, 5th edn. Baillière Tindall, London

McKenna J, Naylor PJ, MacDowell N 1998 Barriers to physical activity promotion by general practitioners and practice nurses. British Journal of Sports Medicine 32: 242–247

Nolan M, Caldock K 1996 Assessment: identifying the barriers to good practice. Health and Social Care in the Community 4(2): 77–85

Parker SG, Peet SM, McPherson A 2002 A systematic review of discharge arrangements for older people. Health Technology Assessment 6: 4

Pheasant S 1998 Back injury in nurses – ergonomics and epidemiology. In: Lloyd P (ed) Guide to the handling of patients, 4th edn. National Back Pain Association/RCN, London

RCN 1996a Code of practice for patient handling. Royal College of Nursing, London

RCN 1996b Manual handling assessments in hospitals and community. Royal College of Nursing, London

Robinson J, Batstone G 1996 Rehabilitation: a developmental challenge. Kings Fund working paper. Kings Fund, London

Roper N, Logan W, Tierney A 1996 The elements of nursing: a model for nursing based on a model for living, 4th edn. Churchill Livingstone, Edinburgh

Roper N, Logan W, Tierney A 2000 The Roper–Logan–Tierney model of nursing based on activities of living. Churchill Livingstone, Edinburgh

Rutishauser S 1994 Physiology and anatomy: a basis for nursing and health care. Churchill Livingstone, Edinburgh

Stuck A, Beck JC 2001 Preventing disability and death in old age. International Journal of Epidemiology 30(4): 900–901

US Department of Health and Human Services 1996 Physical activity and health: a report of the Surgeon General. Centre for Disease Control, Alabama

Wade DT, de Jong BA 2000 Recent advances in rehabilitation. British Medical Journal 320: 1385–1388

Waugh A, Grant A 1996 Ross and Wilson anatomy and physiology in health and illness, 8th edn. Churchill Livingstone, Edinburgh

World Health Organisation 1980 International classification of impairments, disabilities and handicaps: a manual of classification relating to the consequences of disease. WHO, Geneva

Young J, Brown A, Forster A, Clare J 1999 An overview of rehabilitation for older people. Reviews in Clinical Gerontology 9: 181–196

Further reading

Effective Healthcare 2000 Acute and chronic low back pain. NHS Centre for Reviews and Dissemination, The University of York, York (available at http://www.york.ac.uk/inst/crd last accessed August 5 2002)

Hinchliff SM, Montague SE, Watson R 1996 Physiology for nurses, 2nd edn. Baillière Tindall, Edinburgh

Hoeman SP (ed) 2002 Rehabilitation nursing: process, application, and outcomes, 3rd edn. Mosby, St Louis

Lloyd P (ed) 1998 Guide to the handling of patients, 4th edn. National Back Pain Association/RCN, London

Rutishauser S 1994 Physiology and anatomy: a basis for nursing and health care. Churchill Livingstone, Edinburgh

Smith M (ed) 1999 Rehabilitation in adult nursing practice. Churchill Livingstone, Edinburgh

Useful websites

The Association of Rehabilitation Nurses website http://www.rehabnurse.org (accessed August 5, 2002)

Cochrane Rehabilitation and Related Therapies Field http://www-epid.unimaas.nl/cochrane/field.htm (accessed August 5, 2002)

Essence of Care Benchmarking Standards – DoH http://www.doh.gov.uk/essenceofcare

National Electronic Library for Health http://www.nelh.nhs.uk/carepathways

RCN website for policy on patient handling http://www.rcn.org.uk

Reports for the Health Technology Assessment Programme, including Cameron et al 2000 available at http://www.hta.nhsweb.nhs.uk (accessed August 5, 2002)

Working and playing

Susan Whittam

Introduction

The activities of work and play are central to human development and motivation, influenced by individual opportunity, ability, necessity and desire and as such there are enormous variations in the degree to which the activities are carried out. Through the lifespan people experience significant changes in their lives that are marked by events such as starting school, starting work, changing jobs and reaching retirement. Although there are many differences throughout the world, there is a sense that work takes priority over play, play being more commonly associated with childhood. As societies have developed and work has become an important feature of life, in the interests of health and wellbeing, there has been a growing recognition of the need to ensure that work and play are suitably balanced. In the UK this is referred to as the work–life balance, and in March 2000, the Prime Minister himself launched a national campaign to help employers make changes to traditional working practices (Department of Trade and Industry 2000). In the context of nursing, the use of the model helps related health and wellbeing issues to be explored and understood.

The importance of considering this activity is central to the notion that on average most people spend about two-thirds of their day engaging in activities that are associated with working or playing. The activity is complex and has many dimensions that are influenced by many factors such as age, gender, physical and intellectual ability, social organisation, culture, opportunities and experience. By using the Roper, Logan and Tierney model(1996, 2000), it becomes possible to broadly but systematically explore the activities that are associated with working and playing in order to develop an understanding of normal everyday living, the changes that occur during ill health and the impact this has on other Activities of Living (ALs). This chapter will therefore focus on the following.

1. **The model of living**
   - working and playing in health and illness across the lifespan
   - dependence and independence in the activity
   - factors influencing the activity of working and playing

2. **The model for nursing**
   - nursing care of individuals with health problems that are affecting their ability to undertake the activity of working and playing.

THE MODEL OF LIVING

Working

It is important to appreciate that the word 'work' does not necessarily relate to a paid job. For example housework, schoolwork and voluntary work, whilst making a valuable contribution to the lives of individuals and society, do not result in financial gain. Given this understanding, work is best described as a meaningful, regular activity for which a person has responsibility, indicating their status, purpose and/or a sense of achievement. Whether the work is paid or unpaid, the activity provides a degree of daily structure, personal organisation and in most cases, contact with other people. Paid work is generally associated with economic sufficiency and a means of providing for essential living needs. The type of work that is chosen is based upon individual abilities, circumstances and the availability and supply of jobs; hence there are many different attitudes towards the value of work. For many people work is a necessity rather than a desire and is often viewed and experienced negatively. For some people however, financial gain is not the only key driver for work and some people are able to combine paid work with their particular skills, interests and ambitions, for example musicians or artists. As a paid activity, generally speaking, work features throughout the lifespan, beginning in adolescence through to adult life and gradually reducing in old age. Terms such as unemployment and retirement are used to describe cessation of paid employment and may be indicative of some loss of financial independence.

Throughout the world, there are many factors which influence the activity of working, based upon individual motivation, personal needs and circumstances, economic and social influences, and these will be discussed throughout this chapter.

Playing

Within the context of the model the activity of 'playing' is considered to be important at every stage of the lifespan, focusing upon activities that are pursued in the spare time that is not taken up by work. The importance of play in childhood development remains undisputed, but the model goes further to explore the importance that play has in adult life. Changing patterns of employment and wealth have increased the pursuit of leisure activities that have led to a significant growth in the leisure industry, providing facilities for sport, relaxation, hobbies, holidays and other personal interests.

The discussion so far has demonstrated that the degree to which individuals choose to, or are expected to, engage in work and play activities, are influenced by many factors. The differences that occur will now be explored through the framework of the model, in order to help you develop your understanding of the following:

- why the AL is important to health and wellbeing
- what factors influence individual behaviour and choices within the AL
- how individuals might be affected by a temporary or permanent inability to carry out the activity
- why this knowledge and understanding is important to the quality of nursing care.

The topic is very broad and has close links to the AL of maintaining a safe environment. It will be necessary for you to refer back to Chapter 3 from time to time and further extend your knowledge by consulting the recommended reading list at the end of this chapter.

Working and playing in health and illness across the lifespan

Childhood/adolescence

The capacity for and importance of play in childhood is closely associated with learning and development. Through play a child learns to develop physically, intellectually, interpersonally and socially (McArdle 2001). Opportunities for play are provided through contact with other people and the provision of appropriate play equipment, toys, games, imaginative play and other stimulating environments both within and outside the home (Slater & Lewis 2002). The activity of play remains predominant into adolescence and early adulthood, but the notion of work takes on gradual emphasis as a child progresses through their school life, whereupon activities are referred to as 'schoolwork'. By the time a child completes their school career they will have been encouraged to achieve a basic level of knowledge and skill to prepare them for working life. Throughout childhood there will have been opportunities to engage in a vast number of play, sport and leisure activities, influenced by either school or the family. By the time an individual reaches adolescence, they are likely to have developed a preference for the type of play they enjoy, which they may then continue to pursue into adulthood. The presence of illness and disability will place some restrictions upon the ability to fully engage in some work and play activities.

However, there is a growing appreciation and requirement by law in some countries for schools, employers and leisure facility providers to ensure that individuals have equal opportunity and access to work and play activities.

Adulthood/old age

In adult life there is generally a clear distinction between working life and leisure time, with the exception of those people who have the opportunity to combine their leisure activities or interests with paid work such as sportsmen and women, actors, musicians, authors and scientists. The ability to secure and sustain employment is a central feature of adult life, the nature of which will influence how much spare time, income and motivation there is to pursue leisure activities. It is estimated that most adults will spend more than half of their lives in work, the experience of which will vary enormously, dependent upon individual capability and actual availability of work. Some people will spend all of their working life pursuing one career path, whilst others may frequently change directions acquiring new knowledge and skills accordingly. By contrast unemployment and redundancy are common events that can have devastating effects upon individuals and their families. Whilst unemployment and retirement creates a greater opportunity to pursue leisure activities, a lack of income or physical health can restrict the ability to make the most of the available time. In the UK retirement from paid work usually takes place at the time when the state pension becomes available which is the age of 65 years. Retirement prior to this is commonly associated with ill health or disability, however other issues such as financial security and the desire to improve the quality of life in retirement have become of equal importance (University College London 2001). In the UK the average life expectancy is 74.3 years for men and 79.5 years for women (Department of Health (DOH) 1999), indicating that on average only 11.9 years will be spent in retirement.

Preparation for life in retirement means that individuals will need to prepare and cope with changes in health, work, social and leisure pursuits and financial security (Hartnell 2000). The conventional view of retirement is that people are no longer required or able to undertake paid work, which contributes to the negative views of ageism. The World Health Organisation (WHO) point out that the reality is that in their millions throughout the world, older people are making a valuable but often invisible contribution to national economies carrying out community voluntary work and more importantly health and social care support within the family (WHO 1999).

Dependency and independency in relation to the activity of working and playing

Children and adolescents spend most of their lives being dependent upon either the family or society to help them develop the skills that enable them to engage in work and play activities for the remainder of their lives. For individuals with learning difficulties, physical or mental health disabilities, a degree of dependency upon the family or public services will to a certain extent remain, although the focus should always be to optimise independent living.

In adult life, there is an interdependency between employers and employees to provide work opportunities and reasonable working conditions, while in return employees can offer their knowledge, skills and experience. In old age particularly, where there are risks to health or safety, there can be a gradual return of dependence upon the family, friends and/or public services. It must be pointed out however that many older people do live quite independently through their older life. Although there are a number of reasons why independence at any given time across the lifespan might be affected, health and financial self-sufficiency is the common link.

Individual attitudes towards independence may also vary, for example some may view retirement as a loss of independence in terms of income, whilst others may see it as a welcome opportunity to pursue hobbies and leisure activities.

Exercise

How does society value people who are retired?

1. Consider your own personal views about retirement – what has influenced your views?
2. Think of someone who you know has been retired for some time. Ask them for their views about retirement as follows:

   - How well were they prepared for their retirement?
   - What different activities have they pursued since retirement?
   - How easy has it been to cope with retirement?

Factors influencing the AL of working and playing

Given that the nature of the AL of working and playing has been identified through the common events that might occur across the lifespan, the next section will help you to understand the differences that exist between individuals. This should help you to acknowledge the range of different circumstances that patients may face within the AL when they become ill and enable you to provide effective care that supports maximum individuality and independence.

Biological factors

All work and play activities will have some degree of biological link in relation to the following:

- physical ability to carry out work and play activities
- the extent to which activities are interrupted due to ill health.

It is important to understand that work and play activities will probably be associated with a number of body systems and that no one specific biological system can be aligned to this AL. However, work and play activities will essentially rely upon normal growth and development of all body systems, particularly the senses, movement, balance and coordination. Different activities will require varied degrees of physical health and fitness. Some activities are extremely physically demanding and the individual must have the required strength, energy and fitness to be able to sustain the activity over time. For a variety of reasons the ability to undertake the activity can be limited by disability, disease, injury or the ageing process. People who develop limitations within the AL may need help and support to engage in alternative activities that are compatible with their needs and abilities. Employers and leisure facility providers can make a range of adjustments to improve access to work and play activities by improving access to buildings, providing a range of specialised equipment and ensuring that staff have access to disability awareness training. Staff training plays an important part in changing attitudes towards disability and ensuring that individual needs and appropriate resources are provided. For some work and play activities, regular health checks may be required, in order to ensure that the individual can safely carry out the activity; for example, pilots, train drivers and individuals who join health and sports clubs. In sport, athletes undergo rigorous health checks, to detect if they have been taking drugs to enhance their sporting performance.

Exercise

Consider the following health problems:

- A hay fever sufferer?
- A person who requires regular renal dialysis?
- A person with a hearing difficulty?
- A person with irritable bowel problems?

1. How might their symptoms affect the AL?
2. What could be done in the work and play environment to accommodate their needs?
3. What advice could you give to each individual?

It will have been seen that even the most minor ill health problems can influence the AL and that in all cases some adjustments within either the work or play environments would be required. It is important to recognise that disabilities are not only associated with mobility issues and by increasing your awareness and understanding about the effects that ill health can have upon the AL of working and playing, you will begin to appreciate the importance of a holistic approach to nursing care.

Psychological factors

There are many different factors that influence an individual's choice of work and play activities, which are essentially related to levels of intelligence and personality. From birth emotional and intellectual development is continued through play, to gradually help the development of communication and interpersonal skills that are essential to the AL (Sheridan et al 1999).

In the world of work some jobs will require a certain level of knowledge and specific qualifications, whilst for others there may be a greater emphasis upon practical skills and experience. Many organisations are recognising the importance of recruiting the right staff and use a variety of psychological selection techniques ranging from simple interviews to sophisticated assessment exercises (Torrington & Hall 1998). Some employers go to great lengths to appoint employees with the right knowledge, skills and experience to undertake the work, but also with the attributes to ensure organisational success. In the UK and across Europe, the concept of lifelong learning in the workplace is gaining momentum, as employees need to be able to develop new knowledge and skills in order to respond and adapt to constant changes (Longworth 1999). To this extent many organisations now recognise the

importance of providing education and training to support employee development. In 2001, the NHS launched a specific strategy for lifelong learning to support its modernisation plans (Department of Health 2000, 2001a). To support work choices, careers advisers and job centres are available to help both schoolchildren and adults identify careers that best suit their knowledge, skills, experience and personal attributes.

The ability to take part and be safe in play and leisure activities will similarly rely upon individual skills, abilities, interests and personality. Essentially there is a greater freedom of choice over play and leisure activities, although physical strength and in some instances financial cost may restrict participation. It is important that, in the pursuit of leisure, individuals remain safe and do not take risks that may endanger themselves or others; although, for some individuals it will be the risks that are the motivating factor for pursuing the activity, for example motor car racing, mountaineering and extreme sports.

Stress related to work and play

The subject of stress and its effects upon the body were introduced in Chapter 3. In relation to work, every individual has their own range of coping mechanisms, which helps us to understand why one person's stress can be another person's energiser. The subject of stress has been studied from many perspectives, and whilst it remains complex, the causes, effects and costs of work-related stress nationally, organisationally and individually are very well documented (Holmes 2001). Stress in the workplace occurs when an individual feels overwhelmed and overburdened, resulting in a variety of physical and psychological illnesses. Certain types of jobs can cause workplace stress, related workload, working conditions, working relationships, career opportunities, organisational culture, gender differences and the ability to sustain a work–life balance (Lundberg & Frankenhaeuser 1999). The effects of stress in the workplace can result in decreased job satisfaction, low morale, boredom, low performance and productivity, increased absenteeism and high staff turnover rates (Mullins 1999). However it is important to recognise that stress is not exclusive to adults in the workplace. People who work at home, often in isolation such as housewives, are also known to suffer from stress, resulting in many associated physical and mental health problems (Lombardi & Ulbrich 1997). Equally there is growing concern about stress experienced by young people resulting in a reported increase of self-harm and suicides (Anderson 1999).

By contrast unemployment caused by the inability to secure work, redundancy or retirement can be equally as stressful leading to poor health and altered psychosocial behaviour (Ferrie 2001).

Coping with stress

There are a number of measures that both individuals and organisations can engage in to combat the causes and effects of stress, many of which are linked to the 'playing' element of the AL (Iwasaki et al 2001). In recognition of the problem employers and governments have been prompted to tackle the problem, by developing long-term strategies to prevent and reduce the effects of stress. In the UK the Health and Safety Executive (HSE) has produced guidelines for employers to change their attitudes towards stress, adopt new management styles and provide training and resources to combat the effects. In recognition of stress in the NHS all health care organisations will be expected to achieve targets outlined by the *Improving Working Lives National Audit Instrument,* which sets out a framework of good employment practices (DoH 2001b). At an individual level people can manage their own stress by learning to recognise the signs and adopt healthier lifestyles by acknowledging the importance of balancing work and leisure more effectively.

Effects of the absence of work and play

Absence from work can be caused by a multitude of factors such as illness, injury, retirement, redundancy and unemployment. In all cases there will be an immediate impact upon psychological wellbeing, which may a loss of self-esteem, confidence and social status. Research has shown that this leads to increased prevalence of physical and mental illness and premature death through suicide (Kposowa 2001, Richardson 1999). Not all absence from work however is viewed negatively. For some people redundancy and retirement provides them with the opportunity to make lifestyle and career changes that they would not have otherwise made. Given support and advice people can be assisted to make the necessary psychological adjustments to enable them to enjoy this aspect of living (Bass 2000, Rosenkoetter & Garris 2001).

Exercise

1. Consider what lifestyle changes you would have to make if you were to lose your job tomorrow?

   - How do you think it would affect your health?
   - What impact would your situation have upon those around you?

2. What plans have you made towards your own retirement?

   - Try to imagine what it might feel like.
   - What would be your main concern?

Sociocultural factors

The structure and culture of a society has considerable influence upon the type of work that is both available and undertaken, and many differences can be seen throughout the world. For some societies, work remains central to ensuring the self-sufficiency of a whole community of people, such as in remote tribes where there will be long-established traditions governing the nature of work which will have

---

Box 11.1 Registrar General's Social Class classification

I	Professional occupations
II	Managerial and technical occupations
III(N)	Skilled occupations: Nonmanual
III(M)	Skilled occupations: Manual
IV	Partly skilled occupations
V	Unskilled occupations

From: Roper et al 1996.

---

changed little over time. By contrast in the industrialised world, it has become necessary for individuals to constantly learn new skills in order to maintain the supply of goods and services to sustain an established national economy. In the UK the type of work undertaken determines a person's social status as described in Box 11.1. This classification system equates social class with occupational skill and employment status. In the UK The Office of Population Censuses and Surveys (OPCS) use the classification to collect information about health and demography.

Influence of beliefs upon working and playing

Prevailing beliefs, values and traditions held by individuals or societies can have a strong influence upon the AL of working and playing. For example, in some societies culture will influence the type of work that men and women traditionally undertake and which can also influence play, sport and leisure activities. As countries have become more industrialised many traditional values and beliefs, relating particularly to work, have also changed. Today there are many examples in the Western world of a reversal of traditional roles, where women have become the main earner of the family income and men have taken primary responsibility for caring for the family at home. Because cultural beliefs can be so strong, many of the changes that have occurred have required support from equal opportunity legislation, to ensure that, for example, women and people with disabilities have access to equal pay and opportunities in the workplace. Despite these changes it is often possible to observe cultural values in the play of children. The different games that boys and girls play are often gender-specific and have the potential to influence work choices in adult life. In adult life the pursuit of leisure activities is generally influenced by the amount of spare time or finance that is available.

Social change and the effects upon work and play

In relation to the activity of working and playing there is a need to understand the significant impact that change can have upon the AL, especially in relation to health and wellbeing. Over the last century, life for many people has changed rapidly, both in terms of pace and technology and today the effects that this has had upon health are widely recognised. Throughout the world many physical and psychological ill health problems are directly attributed to the type of work that people undertake. Over time this has forced employers not only to ensure the safety of their staff, but also change their attitudes towards improving their working lives, such as providing protective equipment/clothing and better working conditions. So rapid are the changes in the workplace that globally organisations are experiencing many skills shortages. As a result many people are working longer hours and engaging in education and training activities, but ultimately this reduces their leisure and relaxation time. However, it is worth pointing out that in some countries, many children and adults are exploited in the workplace and have little to no access to any kind of leisure or play activities, neither are there any laws to help relieve their plight (Parker & Bachman 2001).

By contrast there is growing concern that where changes in a society's play and leisure activities have occurred, there is also an increase in sedentary lifestyles, which may cause health problems for the future (Seefeldt et al 2002). In recognition of the growing need to balance work, play and health, there has been substantial growth in the leisure industry, providing activities for people at every stage of the lifespan. The ability to pursue many of the activities available is influenced by many factors such as affordability, availability and physical health and capability. If safety is to be maintained it is important that individuals are aware of the dangers that some pursuits may have for them and carefully choose activities that meet their individual needs and circumstances (Mullineaux et al 2001). For example Schnohr et al (2000) highlight the dangers that exist for men who take up jogging in an effort to keep fit, only to find that this may be actually detrimental to their health.

Changes in society are also linked to changes in the behaviour of people and one of the growing concerns in the UK, is the increasing reports of antisocial behaviour affecting people of all ages across the lifespan. Within the workplace there appears to be an increase in the incidence of violence, unfair treatment, sexual harassment and bullying, although the increase is associated with greater awareness and reporting of incidents (Cortina et al 2001). In the UK and Europe this has prompted the introduction of a number of laws governing the responsibility that employers have to protect their staff. Schools are similarly reporting an increase in antisocial behaviour, exposing teachers as well as students to attack. This has prompted many education authorities and schools to take positive action to combat the rising problems (Karstadt 1999). In communities there are increasing reports of attacks upon individuals of all ages and racially motivated attacks and rioting. There is recognition that a lack of recreational facilities for young people, combined with boredom and a lack of parental control, is leading to an increase in juvenile crime (Rutter et al 1998). Unfortunately many of these crimes are also associated with an escalating rise in drug, alcohol and substance abuse, causing misery to thousands of people across the lifespan. Over time a combination of government intervention and public pressure often prompt the introduction of new laws, policies and regulations in an attempt to reduce and solve the problems.

Exercise

1. Discover how the values and traditions about work and play have changed over time within your own family.
2. Try to determine what factors might have influenced these changes.
3. How might these values differ from someone of another culture?
4. How might values change in the future?

Environmental factors

In the work environment as discussed in Chapter 3, there is an equal responsibility for individuals and organisations to ensure health and safety. To support this many countries have legal requirements for organisations to have procedures in place that enable risks to be identified and as far as possible prevented. In the UK the Health and Safety at Work Act 1974 serves to ensure that organisations take steps to assess and identify risks and provide essential information, policies, guidelines, equipment, training, skills, environments and facilities in an attempt to reduce accident rates. To reinforce compliance with the law the Health and Safety Executive (HSE) exists to provide a comprehensive information, audit, research and investigation service that constantly informs good practice in ensuring health and safety. The HSE provide information about the health risks associated with a whole range of industries and occupations that range from physical injury to genetic disorders, infertility, stress, tumours, skin, cardiac and respiratory disorders, through exposure to harmful substances and unsafe environments. The development of new technologies within the workplace means that new risks and hazards are emerging all the time for example the problems that are now known to be associated with computer work such as the injury to the wrist known as repetitive strain injury (RSI) and headaches and visual problems associated with the use of visual display screens.

It is important to recognise that not all work and play activities are governed by legislation and the individual takes sole responsibility for their own health and safety. People who are self employed would be expected to take individual responsibility to identify risks and provide themselves with personal insurance to protect themselves financially in the event of an accident. Housewives, home workers and retired people are often at risk from accidents and stress, yet do not benefit from employer protection. For children and young adults, the responsibility for health and safety lies with the parents or guardians. Recently there have been a number of incidents where children have been injured and killed in coach crashes, fairgrounds and outdoor pursuits whilst on organised activities, bringing into question the need to provide adequate supervision and assessment of risks. For adults pursuing leisure activities it would be expected that there would be equal responsibility upon the individual and activity provider, to consider the risks that might be involved.

To support the needs of disabled people, The Disability Discrimination Act 1995 and The Disability Rights Commission (DRC) Act 1999 guide the requirements for employers and service providers to make environmental adaptations to reflect the changing nature of work, daily living and leisure activities. Retail and leisure industries such as hotels, leisure clubs, banks, supermarkets and shopping centres are adapting services such as lowering counters, cash machines and providing electronic shopping vehicles to improve access and independence for disabled people.

Exercise

Think about the places you visit regularly in your day-to-day life and identify where adaptations have been made or could be made to meet the needs of the following disabilities?

1. mobility difficulties
2. visual difficulties
3. hearing difficulties
4. decision-making and problem-solving difficulties.

A variety of access adaptations, facilities and special services are available, particularly for people with mobility and other commonly known disabilities. You may have recognised that further improvements could be made to reflect the diversity of disabilities.

Politicoeconomic factors

The purpose of work in society

The ability to earn an income has two purposes; firstly, to sustain an individual lifestyle and secondly to contribute collectively towards the national economy. At a national level work enables the production of goods and services that can be widely traded (industrialisation) and forms the basis of national wealth. The way in which the national economy is sustained is the business of governments and concerns ensuring that a country has a sufficiently skilled workforce. This involves recognising the impact that changing working trends may be having upon society such as 24-hour services or new technologies and putting in place a range of systems and services to support labour market requirements. The following are examples of systems and services, which over time have been provided in the UK to support the AL of working and playing:

- minimum age of employment
- minimum wage
- working time directives
- sickness and maternity pay
- paid holiday leave

- child, family and incapacity benefits
- unemployment benefits
- retirement age and pensions
- health services
- education services.

In an industrialised country those who are in work contribute to the provision of the services through income tax and national insurance payments. These payments contribute to national services such as health and social care, education, unemployment and sickness payments and retirement pensions. When balancing the national economy it is vital that there are enough people in work in order to continue to provide such services.

At an individual level, paid work provides an income to provide for personal and family needs. In the UK a person's wage or salary is generally associated with their occupation and social class (Box 11.1 on p. 321), and pay increases are generally negotiated through trade unions or linked to individual work performance. None-the-less the link between poverty and ill health is well documented and developed countries seek to support low pay through a variety of health and social care services.

The changing nature of work

Over the last 50 years there have been significant changes in the nature of work influenced by some of the following:

- introduction of new electronic technologies
- introduction of information communication technologies
- increased number of women in the workforce
- increase in part-time working
- increase in early retirement.

With such rapid changes, it can be difficult to predict how the future workforce should look. Trade markets can be unstable and the effects of new technologies may not be fully understood, the impact of which results in unemployment or skills shortages. In the UK the NHS is just one example of how organisations worldwide are having to modernise themselves in response to the changes created by the impact of new technologies, service delivery, staff and skills shortages (Department of Health 2000). What is happening in the NHS is of course not unique and many organisations are facing similar issues, highlighting the need for employers and employees to work together to create flexible attitudes to work. In order to continuously sustain national social and economic health, governments introduce policies and initiatives to influence education and employment, in an attempt to ensure that workforce skills are available. In the UK this has led to the introduction of the following:

- Reform of the Education Act (1998)
- Improving Working Lives (DoH 2001b)
- The learning age, a renaissance for a new Britain (1998)
- Investors in People (1991).

Support for the activity of working

As discussed earlier in this chapter, health and safety legislation exists to protect individuals at work, but in addition, there is also a range of other employment laws that have been introduced to reflect changing needs, such as:

- The Employment Rights Act 1996
- The Industrial Tribunal Act 1996.

These acts outline the responsibilities of employers to provide good employment environments and working relationships covering issues related to disability, equality and diversity, race, sexual orientation, religion and beliefs and age. By way of additional support the following services and organisations exist.

Trade unions Trade unions have a responsibility to act in the best interests of their members to negotiate nationally and locally not only on issues of pay but also to ensure fair employment rights and conditions as follows (Boeri et al 2001):

- worker health and safety education and surveillance
- development of national and local policies
- worker education and training
- support for workers in dispute with employers.

Exercise

1. Find out which trade unions are associated with health care in the UK.
2. What services do they provide for health care staff?
3. What support could a health care worker expect to receive from the trade union regarding a personal health problem due to working conditions?
4. If you are living and working in another country find out what the laws are with regards to trade unions and their activities.

Occupational health services Occupational health services consist of specifically trained occupational health doctors and nurses and other health specialists and therapists such as stress counsellors who are employed by organisations to provide comprehensive employee health screening and health promotion services to staff. The range of services available include pre-employment screening, prevention and management of occupational/workplace disorders, surveillance and research (Edling & Waldron 1997, Oakley 2002).

Employment services In the UK there are a wide range of statutory and voluntary services that help people to secure suitable work. This begins in schools with careers advice and includes job centres, employment and recruitment agencies for those seeking to change jobs or find alternative employment following a period of unemployment.

Employment legislation also supports the provision of services to help people seek and secure work. The legislation works to ensure that organisations provide fair and equal opportunities for people who might otherwise have been unequally paid, dismissed, or excluded from employment on the grounds of their gender, race or disability (Department of Trade and Industry 2002).

Exercise

Locate the Department for Education and Skills website www.dfes-uk.co.uk to find out what employment services, schemes and benefits are available for young people and adults.

Support for play in society

The importance of play in society is central to enjoyment and viewed as complementing working life. It is influenced by the standard of living and may be dependent upon the provision of appropriate facilities. Across the lifespan there are a variety of reasons why one individual may have more time for play or leisure than another and this is largely influenced by social class, income, culture and social provision.

During childhood and adolescence, encouraging human growth and development through play has many benefits to society that have been highlighted throughout this chapter. Schools may provide the foundation for introducing sport and leisure activities, but the extent to which these are pursued in later life is influenced by a number of individual, social and economic factors. Just as legislation has improved attitudes and access to work opportunities, so too has it influenced changes in attitudes and improvements for access to play, sport and leisure. This has led to improvements in facilities for disabled people to access local sports facilities to participation in international events such as the Paralympic Games, which are now held in conjunction with the Olympic games every 4 years. As a result of increased disability awareness there has been a growing recognition of the need to widen the access to recreational activities such as holidays, theatres, cinemas, adventure centres, theme parks, museums, restaurants and hotels, through the provision of ramps, lifts and provision of specialised equipment.

For families, changing work patterns have led to a growing demand for child care and leisure services such as nurseries, play schemes and out-of-school clubs which in turn have increased the demand for accredited child care and play specialists (Office for National Statistics 2002). In addition there has also been a rapid increase in the provision of family-orientated recreational services such as holidays abroad, holiday centres, theme parks, various sporting activities, cinemas and eating out, which only a few years ago would not have been available. Similarly for adults there is a vast array of sport, leisure and recreational activities available, but a lack of finance, time and physical ability remain the main obstacles for not engaging in these activities. As services and opportunities have increased so too has the requirement to ensure public service standards and safety as discussed in Chapter 3. To this extent governments become obligated or pressurised to introduce or amend legislation and services.

A lack of opportunity to engage fully in recreational activities has an impact throughout the lifespan ranging from boredom in children and young adults, the adoption of adverse recreational habits (poor diet, smoking, increased use of alcohol and recreational drugs) to the social deprivation of elderly people (Office of the Deputy Prime Minister 2000). Ultimately changes begin to impact upon individual and community health, safety and wellbeing to such an extent that action to remedy situations is required either through political will, pressure groups or high-profile media coverage such as the sale of drugs and the problem of children as young as 8 years old vandalising housing estates late at night in some of Britain's towns and cities.

Conclusion

The framework of the model of living has been used to demonstrate how the model can be used to guide your understanding of how the AL of working and playing in everyday life is influenced and why the AL is important to health and individualised patient care. It is hoped that by engaging in the exercises provided throughout this chapter that you began to appreciate the interrelatedness of the other ALs. The final two exercises provide you with two mini case studies that will help you begin to apply the model in practice. These exercises will enable you to identify what is influencing a change upon the AL of working and playing and how this is impacting upon the other Activities of Living.

Effects upon the activity of working and playing

Exercise
Read through Case study 11.1 and consider how the activity of working and playing is being influenced from a lifespan, dependence/independency and factors affecting health perspective.

Case study 11.1

Individuality in the AL of working and playing

Gill, a former company secretary, is 39 years old and has suffered from a back problem for many years, the result of which is that she is now registered disabled and constantly needs to use a wheelchair. Gill is a single mum bringing up her son aged 17 and daughter aged 19.

The following points may have been considered:

Lifespan
Gill would normally be expecting to live a full and active life, enjoying her family and freedom to pursue leisure time. She would have developed expertise in her job and possibly be looking to increase her income or career aspirations.

Change in dependency
There is potential for loss of financial and personal independence. Gill will need to consider alterations to her environment to promote independent living.

Factors affecting health
Biological
- loss of mobility with the potential to affect other physiological functions such as eliminating, personal cleansing and dressing, expressing sexuality.

Psychological
- risk of depression and stress
- loss of self-esteem and confidence.

Sociocultural
- risk of social isolation and exclusion
- increased dependence upon children, family and friends and support agencies
- may need to give up leisure activities and identify new activities.

Environmental
- may need adjustments to home and work environment
- may have difficulties driving or using public transport.

Politicoeconomic
- may have difficulties continuing in employment
- may have concerns regarding family income
- may have anxieties about securing social benefits
- may have little knowledge about support mechanisms available.

Exercise
Consider for a moment if Gill had been a patient in your care in a general hospital ward.

1. Without the use of the model, how thorough would your assessment of her individual needs have been?
2. How is Gill's problem impacting upon the other ALs?

Exercise
Read through Case study 11.2 and identify the impact of a change in health status upon the Activities of Living.

Case study 11.2

How altered working and playing activities may impact upon other ALs

Mike is a 23-year-old man who works as a car mechanic for a small local company. He is due to be married in 6 months. He has sustained a crush injury to his right foot, whilst at work. He is the top striker for his local football team.

Effect on other Activities of Living

1. *MSE*
   - safety issues at work may prevent him returning until he is fully recovered
   - risk of delayed healing through further injury or infection if returns to normal work and play activities.

2. *Communicating*
   - may be angry and upset
   - may feel isolated by altered contact at work or friends
   - may need to discuss financial worries with appropriate people/agencies.

3. *Eating and drinking*
   - may need to ensure diet is conducive to healing and medication
   - may increase weight during period of reduced activity.

4. *Eliminating*
   - may have difficulty due to reduced mobility.

5. *Mobilising*
   - normal activities reduced due to injury
   - may require extensive physiotherapy intervention
   - unable to go to work or take part in football.

6. *Expressing sexuality*
   - may affect relationship with fiancée
   - may feel body image is altered.

7. *Maintaining body temperature*
   - risk of infection may increase body temperature.

8. *Sleep and rest*
   - may be interrupted due to pain and discomfort.

9. *Dying*
   - dependent upon seriousness of injury or recovery complication.

Summary points

The two exercises demonstrate the following: •

1. Working and playing can be affected by all the factors affecting health.
2. Working and playing can be affected by all the other ALs.
3. The lack of ability to engage fully in this activity can have detrimental effects upon health and the quality of life.
4. Engaging in this activity presents many risks to health and wellbeing.

THE MODEL FOR NURSING

Individualising nursing for the activity of working and playing

The application of the model for nursing is based upon integrating the components of the model of living with each of the four phases of the nursing process (assessing, planning, implementing and evaluating) as shown in Figure 11.1.

This part of the chapter will now concentrate upon helping you to understand how the information from the model of living can be applied to nursing practice. In the first part of this chapter, the model of living helped you to understand how the activity of working and playing is usually carried out, a summary of which can be found in Box 11.2.

By systematically integrating the model of living as shown in Box 11.2 to each stage of the nursing process you will be able to increase the individuality of the nursing care plan. It is important to remember that when considering the holistic needs of patients, some or all of the other ALs may also be affected, particularly the AL of maintaining a safe environment. You will need to refer to other AL chapters as appropriate. By working through the exercises and case scenarios that follow you will gain an appreciation of the interrelatedness of all of the ALs. Whilst working through this section and when encountering individual patients in practice, you may find it useful to refer back to the information contained within the first part of this chapter, remembering the importance of keeping up to date with related information in order to ensure that patients always receive a high standard of care. The use of the model also helps to identify nursing interventions that are associated with the activity of working and playing, which in general will be related to the following:

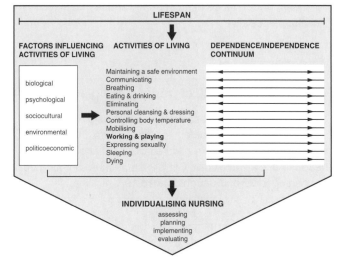

Fig. 11.1 Diagram of the AL of working and playing (from Roper et al 1996, with permission).

Box 11.2 Summary of the model of living in health – working and playing

Lifespan
- normal activity expected for age group

Dependence/independence
- expected level of dependence/independence related to lifespan
- identified level of dependence related to other Activities of Living.

Factors affecting working and playing
Biological
- general physical health
- age and general physique/fitness or energy levels.

Psychological
- level of intelligence
- personality, temperament and self-discipline
- emotional stability and ability to cope with stress and changes within the AL
- motivation
- attitudes to work and play.

Sociocultural
- recognition of individual personal attitudes, beliefs and values, religious beliefs
- social class
- gender differences
- attitudes to work and play.

Environmental
- identification of risks and hazards
- provision of adequate protection.

Politicoeconomic
- availability of work/job security
- personal economic status
- access to relevant social systems and legislation
- support from employment legislation preventing discrimination and promoting equality
- affordability of leisure activities.

- teaching patients about health and safety at work and at play
- preventing accidents and ill health associated with working and playing
- supporting patients to cope with altered health states
- providing care to support individual needs
- helping patients to adapt to change and adopt healthier lifestyles

Assessment of needs and problems

Assessing the individual using the model for nursing

The application of the model begins by using the components of the model of living to collect the following information:

1. the patient's normal habits and routines within the AL of working and playing
2. the factors that may be causing the activity to be altered
3. identification of actual and potential problems related to the AL.

The initial assessment of individual needs is important, as it provides essential information upon which all other aspects of the nursing care are to be planned. It is important to recognise that whilst the process of nursing begins with an assessment, it is a continuous activity that should be undertaken regularly in order to support the changing needs of patients through their entire care episode.

Collection of specific information related to the AL of working and playing

Prior to the assessment

Assessment begins by using the components of the model of living to act as a framework for assessing the patient's normal habits and routines, in order to identify the extent to which ill health is influencing the ability to carry out the activity of working and playing. When conducting an assessment the following points must be considered:

1. The actual or potential problem identified may be more specifically aligned to another AL (demonstrating the interrelatedness with other ALs).
2. Collaboration with other professional groups or agencies may be required in order to fully solve or alleviate the problem.

Identification of ill health problems associated with working and playing

In order to identify the individual needs of patients, it is important to be able to determine the extent to which the AL has changed. Box 11.3 summarises some common issues that bring about a disruption in the AL.

Exercise
1. What employment and social services are available in your area to support the issues identified in Box 11.3?
2. What recreational activities are available in your area for young people?
3. Identify your learning needs and produce an action plan that you can discuss with your mentor/preceptor.

Box 11.3 Factors which may alter or disrupt the AL of working and playing

Lifespan
- presence of illness, injury or disability preventing normal expected activity at lifespan stage.

Dependency/independency
- inability to fully undertake activities at any stage of the lifespan caused by a change in personal health, social and financial circumstances.

Factors affecting health
Biological
- presence of physical ill health or injury
- presence of disability (physical or sensory).

Psychological
- stress, inability to cope with changes
- changes in personality, mood and behaviour
- lack of motivation
- lack of knowledge to promote independency
- inability to acquire new knowledge and skills.

Sociocultural
- changes in domestic and employment circumstances
- culture, harassment and violence at work
- antisocial behaviour/disruption
- cultural restrictions.

Environmental
- exposure to risks and hazards
- lack of adequate protection
- change in work environments
- lack of recreational facilities

Politicoeconomic
- redundancy/retirement
- high unemployment
- restricted access to social support systems
- lack of education and training opportunities.

The patient assessment

The ability to provide individualised nursing care is based upon the knowledge of a person's individuality. As demonstrated in the model of living, the activity of working and playing is extremely complex and highly individualised, requiring careful assessment and support. When assessing the activity it is important to determine the following:

- the extent to which ill health is affecting the activity
- the extent to which a change in the activity is influencing ill health.

For example patients are not usually admitted to hospital as a result of not being able to undertake the AL of working and playing, but the activity may be seriously disrupted and require adaptation due to a problem associated with another AL. Hence a thorough assessment is vital in order to ensure that the subsequent care plan is relevant to what the patient can realistically achieve and should aim to address the following:

- how actual problems may be solved
- how to prevent potential problems becoming actual ones
- how to prevent solved problems from recurring
- how to alleviate problems which cannot be solved
- how to help the person cope with temporary or permanent altered states.

Data collection

In relation to working and playing you will need to base your assessment on the following:

- What are the individual's experiences or attitudes to work and play?

- In which kind of working and playing activities does the person normally engage?
- How much time does the individual spend working and playing?
- What factors are influencing the individual's approach towards work and play (ability, knowledge, experience, resources)?
- Has the individual had to make any previous adjustments to work or play in the past?
- What identifiable problems or difficulties is the individual currently experiencing?
- How are current problems or restrictions impacting upon normal activity?

When undertaking an assessment you will need to utilise the following skills:

- interviewing skills
- observation skills
- listening skills.

Exercise

Consider what assessment skills you have and the ones you need to develop when undertaking an assessment of working and playing.

Interviewing
- asking open and closed questions about work and play experiences
- determining the priority of questions to be asked
- giving information and checking understanding
- involving relatives.

Exercise *(continued)*

Observation
- verbal and nonverbal responses
- mood and personality
- body language
- physical ability and health for activity
- stress, pain and anxiety.

Listening
- act on verbal and nonverbal cues
- use of own body language to reassure and encourage the patient.

By using the components of the model of living with the identified assessment skills, a systematic assessment of the patient can take place. Regular use of the model in this way will help you to develop an effective assessment style and ensure that patients receive a thorough and professional assessment. The components of the model in relation to conducting an assessment of working and playing will now be considered as shown in Box 11.4.

Patient assessment exercise

Using the assessment guide outlined in Box 11.4 consider the information that you might gather from Case study 11.3.

You can record the information on the Patient Assessment Sheets provided in Appendix 2. This case study will be used as the main scenario for the chapter. Other short case studies will be used to help you transfer your understanding of working and playing to other individual situations and other ALs.

Case study 11.3

Working and playing–main case scenario

John is a 45-year-old sports teacher at a local comprehensive school and was admitted to hospital 4 days ago following an acute myocardial infarction (AMI). He is married with three teenage children. John is highly committed to his work and has been under pressure lately with teaching and team management responsibilities, as well as arranging league games with other schools. He is presently making a good recovery from the MI but is having difficulty identifying how to adopt a healthier lifestyle in order to prevent further health problems. John believes that his interest in sport would enable him to stay healthy particularly as his own father died of a heart attack in his early 60s. John eats a healthy diet, has never smoked cigarettes and only drinks alcohol occasionally.

Box 11.4 Working and playing assessment guide

Lifespan
- At what stage of the lifespan is the patient?
- Does the patient have an understanding of the importance of work and play and associated risks/hazards?
- What are the individual's normal occupational/leisure activities?
- How physically demanding are the individual's normal activities?

Dependency/independency
- What constraints are influencing dependency (e.g. age, ill health)?
- How is the individual coping with changes within the AL?
- How might the individual manage the AL in the future?

Factors affecting health
Biological
- Is the patient in good physical health?
- Is there presence of a disability?
- How is the individual's current health status affecting the AL?

Psychological
- Does the individual have sufficient understanding/ information to manage the AL safely, i.e. avoid stress and hazards?

- Does the individual have sufficient knowledge to receive and be motivated by appropriate information?
- What is the individual's reaction to current health status, e.g. boredom, agitated, anxiety?
- What are the individual's reactions to other life events, e.g. retirement, redundancy?

Socioeconomic
- Is the individual's social role altered/compromised by current health status?
- To what extent are the individual's family, social or work obligations altered?
- What support does the individual require to maintain the AL?

Environmental
- Does the individual have sufficient knowledge and understanding of safety issues?
- Is the individual aware or able to assess risks/hazards in the environment?
- Does the person need help or advice?

Politicoeconomic
- Does the individual have any economic concerns?
- Does the individual require help or advice from other agencies?
- Is a lack of resources compromising health or recovery?

Using your knowledge and experience identify what John's individual working and playing needs are, as follows:

1. Identification of normal lifespan stage/lifestyle expectations, level of dependence and the factors which have led to the health breakdown.
2. Identify the actual and potential needs/problems associated with the AL of working and playing.
3. Identify which other ALs are affected.

Assessment of lifespan, dependency and factors contributing to health breakdown

Using these components of the model will enable you to determine the individual's normal habits and routines and identify where the patient is vulnerable within the AL. This aspect of assessing working and playing focuses upon the following:

- health expectation against stage on the lifespan
- usual routines and habits
- normal dependency capability
- previous coping mechanisms.

By using the components of the model again it becomes possible to also identify the factors that have contributed to John's health breakdown as shown in Box 11.5.

From a working and playing perspective it is possible to determine that as an individual John has the following problems, which have resulted in a health breakdown:

- an acute cardiac problem which will require him to readjust his lifestyle
- a potential predisposition to heart disease
- a health education need in relation to physical activity and stress management
- a health promotion need to adopt a healthier lifestyle.

Identification of actual and potential problems associated with working and playing

Having identified the problems or needs that are individual to John, the next stage is to determine which of the problems are actual and require solving or those which are potential and require prevention. By continuing to use the factors affecting health as a framework, it becomes possible for you to apply your knowledge of health to the patient's individual situation and identify where the patient may need support to carry out the activity in the immediate and long term. Upon identification of the problem(s) it is important to recognise that nursing activities may need to be complemented with a range of other health and social care agencies.

Physical problems

Physical problems associated with the AL of working and playing are generally linked to physical health, strength, mobility and sensory function, resulting in either a temporary or permanent effect upon independence. Broadly

---

> **Box 11.5 Assessment of lifespan, dependency and factors contributing to health breakdown**
>
> **Lifespan**
> - AMI is a common medical problem in adult life, exacerbated by a stressful lifestyle.
> - Under pressure at work and home. Need to identify why John has not been able to identify or make changes to his current lifestyle.
>
> **Dependency**
> - High degree of dependence currently being experienced. Dependent upon medical, nursing and pharmacological care. Normally very independent coping with work, home and social responsibilities
>
> **Factors leading to health breakdown**
> *Physical*
> - Family history of heart disease
> - Lifestyle has exceeded physical health.
>
> *Psychological*
> - Stress from work overload
> - Unhealthy work behaviours and inability to reduce or recognise the dangers.
>
> *Sociocultural*
> - Personal health beliefs
> - Strong work ethic and family values
> - High drive to achieve success.
>
> *Environmental*
> - Able to combine work with leisure interests, but to the detriment of not balancing work and relaxation.
>
> *Politicoeconomic*
> - Pressure to achieve success for school (work) and meet targets
> - Pressure to work to provide income for family.

speaking physical dependence in the activity is associated with being young, old or unable to carry out aspects of the AL without assistance from other people, equipment or services. An understanding of the issues that alter independence are essential, in order to support the needs of patients in the nursing context. In modern societies there is an increasing emphasis upon helping people to optimise their abilities to engage in work and play activities (Rimmer 1999).

Physical disability A wide range of impairments and chronic health conditions cause physical disabilities, but it is important to recognise that they extend far beyond mobility and sensory impairment difficulties such as blindness or deafness. In the UK it is estimated that at least 8.5 million people are classified as being disabled by a range of problems such as asthma, diabetes, epilepsy, heart problems and mental illness (Department for Work and Pensions 2002b). As a result disabled people often face many barriers and discrimination that can have an impact upon their ability to engage fully within the activity of working and playing. In the UK in 1997 the government set up a Disability Rights Taskforce in order to identify the issues and advise upon what action should be taken to promote the rights of disabled people (see www.disability.gov.uk).

The degree to which disabled people may be restricted within the AL will be dependent upon the particular disability and the provision of appropriate access, equipment and services. Unfortunately in many cases it will be society's attitudes towards disability that create the greatest barrier.

Exercise

1. Identify one work and one play/leisure activity that require physical fitness.
2. Could the activities you have identified continue if a person had either of the following:
   • breathing difficulties
   • mobility difficulties.
3. What adjustments would be required in order to help the person continue with the activities?
4. How could you, as a nurse, help the patient to achieve the adjustments?

Initially you may have considered it difficult for the activities to continue, but with some adjustment, very often activities can continue but in different ways. As a nurse it is important to have an understanding of how other agencies can help patients achieve the required adjustments.

Sensory loss or impairment The loss of hearing, sight, smell and sensation can be either temporary or permanent, capable of causing a range of minor to serious effects upon the individual's ability to carry out the AL of working and playing. Actual and potential problems with loss of sensation may also impact upon other ALs such as MSE, communication and mobility and these will be further discussed in the appropriate chapters. For most people who encounter problems, a period of adjustment is required, which sometimes involves the use of new equipment and skills. The huge development in electronic equipment, such as computers and sensory devices, has enabled many people with sensory difficulties to increase their independence and enjoy new aspects of life and work. Problems with hearing and sight can occur suddenly or gradually resulting in partial or complete loss of ability, caused from birth through a genetic disorder or throughout life by injury or disease. Problems with speech can range from mild to severe and may be related to development and learning difficulties from childhood to changes caused by injury or disease.

Exercise

Identify what common diseases, accidents or injuries are associated with the following:

• loss of sight
• loss of hearing
• loss of speech.

Psychological problems

Psychological problems relating to the AL of working and playing have two dimensions. One is that the mental health of patients may become disrupted as a result of changes or demands within the AL and the other is that an underlying health problem may be affecting the ability to carry out the AL effectively. As a result it is likely that any psychological problems identified will be closely related to other ALs. Ultimately psychological problems within the AL will relate to personal safety, self-motivation issues and may also impact on other ALs.

It is important to recognise that special consideration must be given to those individuals who have intellectual limitations or difficulties, in order to ensure that their needs are accurately identified.

Exercise

Identify possible psychological differences between the following:

• a person who has been made redundant
• a person who has been out of work for 2 years
• a person who cannot pursue a career choice through disability
• a person who recently retired on the ground of ill health
• a person who has to cease a lifetime leisure activity through ill health/injury.

You may have identified that whilst the situations are different they may trigger similar kinds of ill health problems such as stress, depression and loss of confidence and self-esteem. The extent to which patients react to any of the situations will depend upon their individual personalities, experience and motivation as well as having access to available support mechanisms and services.

Sociocultural problems

The purpose of identifying problems related to sociocultural aspects of living is twofold. Firstly to establish an understanding of how the individual normally carries out the AL and secondly to determine how the AL has become affected by ill health or injury. For individuals who may need to adapt their lifestyle either temporarily or permanently there may be considerable anxiety surrounding personal beliefs, values and social status.

Environmental problems

Assessment of environmental problems associated with working and playing involves consideration of the following:

1. That the environment within which the individual carries out their normal activities may have resulted in a problem occurring.
2. That the problem identified may relate to activities being restricted because the environment cannot be adapted to meet their immediate or future needs.

It is also important to recognise that some of the aspects of care related to this AL may extend beyond the scope of nursing. For example, patients may need specialist advice regarding employment, state benefits or environmental adaptations. It is therefore vital that nurses have a good understanding of the roles and functions of other multidisciplinary agencies in order to ensure that appropriate and timely referrals are made.

Politicoeconomic problems

There is a need to determine if there are any politico-economic factors that are contributing towards an inability to fully engage in the AL. Problems experienced may limit recovery and a return to normal activities. For example working overtime to provide sufficiently for the family may have resulted in health breaking down in the first instance. Consequently a return to this way of working may compromise a full recovery and future health for which social support may be required to alleviate the problem.

Defining actual and potential problems

Returning to Case study 11.3 it is possible to identify what John's actual and potential problems might be as shown in Box 11.6.

Identification of impact on other ALs

In reality, rarely would one AL be affected in isolation. Whilst this chapter concentrates upon working and playing it is important to consider the impact that a change in activity might have upon the other ALs. Box 11.7 demonstrates how the problems identified from Case study 11.3 may impact upon the remaining ALs.

Box 11.6 Actual and potential problems identified for the main case scenario

Maintaining a safe environment	Actual problems	Potential problems
Physical	Is unable to work or continue leisure pursuits due to having suffered an acute myocardial infarction	May be unable to resume previous work and leisure activities
Psychological	Is anxious about his health and ability to carry out a full and active life	May be agitated and bored by being in hospital
Sociocultural	Concerned about being dependent upon others	May be concerned about career prospects
Environmental	Anxious/frustrated about his health state and the impact upon work and home	Concerned about his ability to change/reduce activities
Politicoeconomic	Concerned about his responsibilities	May be concerned about longer-term financial issues

---

Box 11.7 Impact of actual and potential working and playing problems upon other ALs

Activity of Living	Actual problems	Potential problems
Maintaining a safe environment	Stress at work and family history of heart disease may have contributed towards suffering the AMI	At risk from subsequent cardiac problems if lifestyle not adjusted
Communicating	Will be anxious about current health state and implications for the future work and play activities and require information and reassurance	May be unable to come to terms with future adjustments
Breathing	Pain, altered respirations and oxygen therapy will limit activity in hospital	Concern that work and play activities may cause breathing problems and pain
Eating & drinking	Loss of appetite due to anxiety or reduced activity	May need to alter diet and take regular medication to prevent further problems

Box 11.7 *(continued)*

Activity of Living	Actual problems	Potential problems
Eliminating	May experience problems due to reduced activity and medication	May experience some problems if lifestyle becomes too sedentary
Personal cleansing & dressing	Will require assistance until fully recovered and mobile	May neglect self if becomes depressed about personal situation
Mobilising	Reduced mobility will prevent normal activity	Physical strength may become affected due to change in activities
Sleep & rest	Difficulties in sleeping due to change in environment, pain and/or anxiety	Difficulties in sleeping due to altered activity and worry
Expressing sexuality		May be anxious about body image and self esteem
Maintaining body temperature	May notice changes in body temperature due to reduced activity	
Dying	Is concerned about dying	Worried about future activity and life expectancy

Exercise

Using the information presented so far in this chapter consider how different your assessment and identification of working and playing might be with the following brief case studies. Check your answers against the information in Boxes 11.8, 11.9 and 11.10.

1. A 46-year-old engineer whose job requires a considerable amount of physical strength, lifting, crouching and climbing, has over the last 4 years begun to develop chronic arthritis (see Box 11.8).

2. A 21-year-old man with a promising career ahead of him is severely brain injured in a motorcycle accident. He has made a good recovery but his speech and left-sided coordination have been permanently affected (see Box 11.9).

3. A patient who is in despair from being unable to secure a job and support his family has attempted to take his own life with an overdose (see Box 11.10).

Box 11.8 Engineer with chronic arthritis

Physical
- How limiting are his mobility problems in relation to work and play and other ALs?
- How has he been managing his symptoms?

Psychological
- How has he been coping?
- What is his mood and outlook on life?

Sociological
- How important is work and leisure to him?
- What support is he getting from home, family and work?
- What restrictions are being experienced?

Environmental
- Can any adaptations be made to improve/support activities?
- Is safety compromised?
- Are there any environmental factors that have contributed to the health breakdown?

Politicoeconomic
- What financial pressures exist forcing the need for activities to continue?
- Is the individual aware of resources or agencies which could help?

Box 11.9 Motorcyclist with a head injury

Physical
- What activities will he be able to take part in?
- Are there any other identifiable physical risks?
- How are other ALs being affected?
- How physically fit are his carers?

Psychological
- To what extent can he express his needs?
- How is he able to communicate?
- How is his family coping with the situation?

Sociological
- Is it possible to identify his own current views and expectations?
- What are the views of his family?
- What personal support is there available?
- What social support is available?

Environmental
- What facilities exist for him to engage in work and play activities?
- Do any adjustments need to be made at home, work or for recreation?
- What risks and hazards are there?

Politicoeconomic
- What activities and facilities are there to maximise independence?
- What agencies are available to support employment and independent living?

NB Additional information would need to be obtained, from the family and other health, social and employment care agencies.

Box 11.10 Patient who has taken an overdose

Physical
- What are the risks to physical wellbeing?
- Are there any side effects from the overdose?
- What has been the effect of unemployment on his physical health?

Psychological
- What is his current mood?
- What are the risks of a further suicide attempt?
- How long has he been feeling suicidal?
- How are other ALs being affected?
- What have been his coping mechanisms to date?
- Does he have sufficient knowledge of how to get help?

Sociological
- What support has he been getting from family, friends and other agencies?
- How has his social life changed through unemployment?
- What other social risks are there?

Environmental
- What are the risks of being isolated at home?
- What activities are available to improve his situation?

Politicoeconomic
- What is the extent of the financial problems?
- How has he managed financially so far?
- Is he aware of agencies that can help?

Planning nursing activities

Planning nursing activities involves the following

- identifying the priorities
- establishing short- and/or long-term goals
- determining the nursing actions/interventions required
- documenting the nursing care plan.

Planning nursing care accurately and effectively begins with exploring the actual and potential problems that have been identified and determining the nursing interventions that are required to achieve the following:

- to solve actual problems
- to prevent potential problems occurring
- to prevent solved problems from reoccurring
- to develop positive coping strategies for any problem which cannot be solved.

Throughout the planning phase it is important that the nurse remains focused upon the patient's problems and what is appropriate to the patient's recovery in the immediate, short and long term.

Factors influencing the planning stage

It is important to recognise the factors which can influence the planning stage which in relation to working and playing may be as shown in Box 11.11.

Identification of priorities

Having undertaken a comprehensive individualised assessment, the next stage is to plan the nursing care. The initial assessment will have helped to identify a range of actual and potential problems within the AL and give an indication of the impact this is having on the other ALs. In order to plan effective care focused upon solving actual problems and

Box 11.11 Factors influencing planning care for the AL of working and playing

Nurses	Patients/clients
• Knowledge of normal living and dependency across the lifespan in various cultures • Knowledge of normal physiology required for a range of work and play activities • Knowledge of how the activity of work and play might disrupt normal physiology • Knowledge and skill in required evidence base for nursing interventions • Skill in observation and assessment • Skill in determining priorities • Knowledge of a range of multiagencies to support health and social care including employment services and legislation • Staffing levels, skill mix, supervision and ongoing professional development	• An understanding of the importance of health in relation to work and play • Personal beliefs, values and experiences • Ability to communicate needs and describe expectations and feelings • Anxiety concern about coping mechanisms • Ability to discuss very private and personal aspects of life

preventing potential ones from occurring, you will need to determine the priorities for nursing care. Initially life-threatening problems associated with other ALs may take priority over working and playing problems, but as the patient begins to make good progress towards a physical recovery it is important that any problems associated with working and playing are given priority. By using the dependency/independency element of the model it is possible to develop priority criteria to help determine the degree of altered dependency that the patient is experiencing. Box 11.12 shows an example of dependency/independency criteria.

It is important to recognise that dependence/independence can change and this requires continuous assessment. In relation to Case study 11.3 review the actual and potential problems identified and determine the priority against them (see Box 11.13).

The priorities identified amongst the other ALs are described in Box 11.14.

Box 11.12 Dependency/independency priority criteria

Priority 1	Completely independent in the AL/independency maintained
Priority 2	Potential problem in the AL/remains mostly independent
Priority 3	Actual problems identified within more than one AL/some dependency noted but remains mostly independent
Priority 4	Existence of actual and potential problems in a number of other ALs with associated increasing dependency
Priority 5	Life-threatening actual and potential problems/total dependency

Box 11.13 Priority of actual and potential working and playing problems related to main case scenario

Working and playing	Actual problems	Priority	Potential problems	Priority
Physical	Has an excessive workload and social commitments which limit relaxation time	3	At risk from subsequent cardiac problems if lifestyle not adjusted	5
Psychological	Is anxious about his health and ability to carry out a full and active life	3	May be agitated and bored by being in hospital	3
Sociocultural	Concerned about being dependent upon others	3	May be concerned about career prospects	3
Environmental	Anxious/frustrated about his health state and the impact upon work and home	3	Concerned about his ability to change/reduce activities	3
Politicoeconomic	Concerned about financial circumstances and career prospects	3/4	May be concerned about longer-term financial issues	3

Box 11.14 Identification of main case scenario priorities in all other ALs

Activity of Living	Actual problems	Priority	Potential problems	Priority
Maintaining a safe environment	Overwork has contributed towards suffering an AMI	4	At risk from subsequent cardiac problems if lifestyle not adjusted	4
Communicating	Will be anxious about current health state and implications for the future work and play activities and require information and reassurance	3	May be unable to come to terms with future adjustments	4
Breathing	Pain, altered respirations and oxygen therapy may limit activity in hospital	4	Concern that work and play activities may cause breathing problems and pain	4
Eating & drinking	Loss of appetite due to anxiety or reduced activity	3	May need to alter diet and take regular medication to prevent further problems	3
Eliminating	May experience problems due to reduced activity and medication	3	May experience some problems if lifestyle becomes too sedentary	2
Personal cleansing & dressing	Will require assistance until fully recovered and mobile	2/3	May neglect self if becomes depressed about personal situation	2/3
Mobilising	Reduced mobility will prevent normal activity	3/4	Physical strength may become affected due to change in activities	2/3
Sleep & rest	Difficulties in sleeping due to change in environment, pain and/or anxiety	3/4	Difficulties in sleeping due to altered activity and worry	3/4
Expressing sexuality			May be anxious about body image and self-esteem	2/3
Maintaining body temperature	May notice changes in body temperature due to reduced activity	3		
Dying	Is concerned about dying	3	Worried about future activity and life expectancy	3/4

It will have been seen from this exercise that John's problems in relation to work and play would not, in the immediate phase of his care, take priority over other physical life-threatening problems such as the potential for cardiac arrest and associated psychological needs. As John begins to make a physical recovery and prepare for discharge concerns about his return to normal living will take on an increasing priority. The information in Boxes 11.13 and 11.14 also illustrate the interrelatedness between the ALs which is important to recognise in order to ensure that holistic care is provided.

Exercise
You may wish to return to the brief case studies and identify the actual and potential problems associated with each (Case studies on p. 333).

Goal setting
Goal setting in relation to the AL of working and playing is dependent upon the extent to which normal activity is altered and the anticipated timescale for returning to an agreed level of independence. For example, a relatively minor problem may result in a patient being able to resume normal activities within hours, whilst for some patients they may never return to the previous level of activity and require complete readjustments to the AL, which may take many years. The goal statement is important as it describes what the patient is expected to, or has agreed to, achieve. In relation to working and playing the overall goal(s) may need to be broken down into immediate, short and long term, recognising that optimum dependence within the AL may take place over a period of time. When setting goals, it is important to ensure that information about individual normal habits and routines, identified during the assessment

Box 11.15 Identification of short- and long-term goals for working and playing problems for Case study 11.3		
Problem	**Short term**	**Long term**
John is currently unable to work or continue leisure pursuits due to having suffered an acute myocardial infarction	To identify the lifestyle changes that are required to enable recovery and consideration for a safe return to work and play activities	To return to work having recognised own physical safety limits and adopt healthy work and recreational behaviours that limit physical exertion to limit further cardiac problems

phase, are acknowledged and integrated into the goal statement. This will help to ensure that goals are both realistic and achievable and wherever possible goals should be agreed with the patient (see Chapter 1). The more realistic, measurable and observable the goal(s), the easier it becomes to monitor and evaluate the progress the patient is making. Box 11.15 outlines the short- and long-term goals identified for John that are central to:

- helping him to understand why his AMI occurred
- helping him to recognise what activities may cause further symptoms
- helping him to adopt an altered lifestyle.

Box 11.15 gives an example of the short- and long-term working and playing goals set for John.

Once the short- and long-term goals have been set the appropriate nursing actions can be planned to enable the goals to be achieved.

> **Exercise**
> You may wish to return to the brief case studies and identify the short- and long-term goals associated with each patient.

Implementing care to meet working and playing needs and problems

Having identified the actual and potential problems and agreeing where possible with the patient and/or significant carer the desired goals, the next step is to produce and implement a care plan. By using the factors affecting health as framework, a range of nursing interventions, specifically associated with the activity of working and playing can be identified. The aim of the nursing interventions being to help individual patients resume a lifestyle that is as healthy and normal as possible.

This next section will outline the most common interventions under the headings of the five factors affecting health, broadly describing the dependency, comforting and preventative aspects of nursing as outlined by the Roper et al model (1996). It is essential that as a nurse you constantly up-date your knowledge and skills in the areas outlined as follows in order to ensure that patients receive quality care.

Nursing interventions related to physical factors influencing ill health

The object of nursing actions related to the patient's physical problems within the AL of working and playing are central to:

- helping restore optimum physical health and lifestyle
- helping to prevent further complications
- helping the patient to cope with any physical and lifestyle changes.

For every different type of work and play activity, some kind of physical ability is required. Many chronically disabling diseases and common accidents which impact upon the ability to carry out the AL will basically require the cardiopulmonary, nervous and musculoskeletal systems. The many activities that have been identified so far highlight, as with the AL of maintaining a safe environment, that no one single biological system can be aligned to the AL of working and playing. When planning care for individual patients, it is essential that the systems affected are fully identified and that you have sufficient understanding of any associated biological function. To this extent all the other AL chapters will contain information that may be appropriate to the AL of working and playing, demonstrating once again the interrelatedness of the model.

Physical disability

Every day nurses encounter patients with disabilities and altered activity, be this either temporary or permanent, but for the patient this can be a very frightening experience. A physical disability is often defined by the medical diagnosis, which creates an emphasis upon physical and medical needs. In doing so, the potential exists for patients to adopt what is referred to as the *sick role*. This is characterised by an increased dependence upon carers, social withdrawal and a reduction in the ability to adapt to new lifestyles (Harris 2000). Whilst it is vital to ensure that the patient's physical and medical needs are met, it is equally important to ensure that working and playing needs are not neglected at the expense of other priorities. The nurse must remember that for patients there may be considerable concern related to this AL and that failure to identify or provide adequate support for needs may ultimately effect recovery. Regaining independence in the AL may, of course, take weeks, months or even years to achieve, requiring support from a variety of different health and social care professionals. To this extent it is important that all professionals work effectively as a team, but it may be the nurse who is pivotal in ensuring that accurate and appropriate referrals are made as soon as possible. To be effective in supporting patients with disabilities the nurse should concentrate upon the following actions:

- supporting the patient's physical recovery from injury or disease
- making appropriate and timely referrals to other professionals and agencies
- helping the patient/family come to terms with their disability
- helping patients determine what limitations the disability places upon them
- helping patients/families to make decisions, priorities and identify needs
- providing sufficient information.

For some patients with severe physical problems it may not be possible for them to live independently without the support of family, friends, specialised equipment and/or facilities. Box 11.16 gives an example nursing care plan to meet John's physical needs.

Nursing actions associated with psychological factors influencing ill health

Illness and injury within AL of working and playing can have a radical impact upon the lives of patients and their families, causing extreme stress and anxiety, especially when newly faced with permanent disabilities. Many patients experience feelings of disbelief, anger, grief and a sense of hopelessness, which they may find difficult to express. The scope of nursing care is to anticipate the patient's feelings and handle situations that arise as sensitively and honestly as possible (Brillhart & Johnson 1997). At the same time it is also important to encourage as much patient independence as possible in order to prevent adoption of the sick role. Early detection of any signs of depression and immediate referral to the appropriate specialist is essential if the patient's recovery is to be optimised. Patients should be encouraged to balance activity and rest during their recovery period. Some patients however may feel agitated and bored

during their recovery and will need access to appropriate activities. Introduction to activities such as relaxation techniques can help patients to plan how they might manage necessary lifestyle changes. There should always be a broad range of activities available to meet the patient's physical and individual needs. These are commonly books, board games, television, music and access to the telephone. Providing that health and safety is not compromised the patient can be supported to maintain a limited amount of work and domestic responsibilities, as often the anxiety of being isolated can cause additional strain. This has the advantage of making some observations about how the patient might cope beyond discharge.

For some people with learning difficulties or mental health problems it may not be possible for them to gain or maintain full independence in the AL. Community living and rehabilitation services exist to help individuals learn how to cope and be valued within society. Many voluntary organisations, training centres and employers provide support and opportunities for even the most profoundly disabled people to gain work, leisure and life skills. (See useful disability websites at the end of this chapter.) The psychological care identified for the main case scenario is illustrated in Box 11.17.

Nursing actions associated with sociocultural factors affecting ill health

Nursing care related to sociocultural factors involves supporting patients to maintain as normal a lifestyle as possible, from the onset of illness through to discharge and beyond. For many patients a return to normal activity will take place within a matter of weeks, as soon as healing has taken place and physical strength is regained. Some patients however will need to make significant changes to their work and lifestyle. If patients are expected to achieve their recovery goals, it is vital that their individuality within the AL is fully appreciated and that social care as well as health care needs are provided for, by involving a range of professionals such as therapists, social workers and other specialist advisors. The aim of nursing care from the outset is to encourage optimum independence associated with the effects of being isolated and a loss of personal influence and control due to

---

Box 11.16 Nursing care plan to support identified physical needs in relation to the working and playing main case scenario

Problem	Goal	Nursing intervention
Has an excessive workload and social commitments which limit relaxation time At risk from subsequent cardiac problems if lifestyle not adjusted	To help the patient identify the lifestyle changes he needs to make in order to promote a full recovery and prevent further complications	Identify short- and medium-term physical limitations Assess lifestyle, make decisions and priorities Identify changes to work and recreational activities to limit physical exertion Plan individualised mobilisation programme Plan recovery programme and identify changes/support at work

Box 11.17 Nursing care plan to support identified psychological needs in relation to the working and playing main case scenario		
Problem	**Goal/aim**	**Nursing intervention**
John is anxious about his health and ability to carry out a full and active life John may be agitated and bored by being in hospital	To minimise anxiety and promote independence	Encourage John to express concerns to staff and family Listen carefully and observe nonverbal communications Deal with issues sensitively and honestly Record progress accurately and report/refer concerns immediately Identify activities to relieve boredom/agitation

illness or injury. As previously mentioned the nurse must acknowledge the risk that patients can become overly dependent upon their carers, be that nurses or family members. To limit this it is important to set independence goals that the patient can work towards, that are realistic and achievable. Alternatively some patients may have difficulty in coming to terms with being cared for by someone else and a flexible and creative approach to meeting the patient's needs will be required. By recognising the disruption that illness or disability can cause within the AL, it is possible for the nurse to recognise how situations might be adapted. The aim being to help patients maintain a reasonable and safe amount of social, work and recreational activity, even though they may be restricted by their physical state or environment. Providing creative solutions for patients not only promotes independence but also provides the nurse with the opportunity to make some observations about how the patient may cope during recovery and after discharge.

When the AL of working and playing is disturbed through illness or disability, normal day-to-day contact with family, friends and other work and social groups alters. In the family this can create difficulties particularly if the family members are themselves normally dependent upon the patient, for example a young mother with children or an elderly husband who looks after an infirm wife. By recognising the needs of patients to maintain some control over their responsibilities, a flexible approach to care can be maximised through flexible visiting arrangements. Access to telephones is another important way of helping patients keeping in touch with family, friends and work colleagues. Increasingly the use of text messaging and email is used. In some hospitals patients may be able to access email through computers that are sited in public places such as main reception areas and cafés.

In the home patients are able to control visitors, but in hospital the activity can be restricted by organisational rules and regulations. The nurse must recognise the importance that visiting plays in supporting the sociocultural needs of the patient, in order to minimise some of the problems that are associated with the experience of isolation and separation. However it is also important that patients have sufficient periods of rest and there will be some occasions when the nurse will need to advise the patient and family, particularly if this is having an adverse effect upon the patient's

recovery. Over the years many visiting regimes have been relaxed and replaced with more flexible arrangements, for example some patients are able to go home at weekends or even go to work whilst remaining in hospital in the evening (Wilkinson 2000).

Essentially nursing care associated with the patient's sociocultural needs concentrates upon preparation for discharge and needs to involve the family and significant carers. It is important to bear in mind that standard discharge information needs to be tailored to specific needs, for example men and women often have different needs and support mechanisms which must be taken into consideration.

Exercise

What individual recovery differences might there be for the following patients who have undergone abdominal surgery:

1. A 40-year-old married man with a physical job.
2. A 36-year-old single parent with two children under 12 years and a part-time job.
3. A 70-year-old lady who lives alone.

It may have been noted that each of the patients in the exercise will have different levels of support available to them. Differences in age, domestic, social and financial circumstances will all influence the extent to which standard discharge guidance will be followed. Discharge information therefore should not only be clear but also relevant to each individual taking into consideration the following:

- individual ability
- age
- gender
- interests/habits and routines
- personality
- previous lifestyle
- work environment
- home environment
- leisure environment.

For some patients, however, a return to a previous lifestyle is not possible and whilst this is daunting there is often the opportunity to gain new skills and interests. The

Box 11.18 Nursing care plan to support identified sociocultural needs in relation to the working and playing main case scenatio

Problem	Goal/aim	Nursing intervention
John may have concerns about work and home life	To minimise anxiety and encourage contact with family and work colleagues to promote a safe recovery	• Encourage John to express concerns with family and to staff • Encourage family to discuss concerns with staff • Listen carefully and observe nonverbal communications • Support contact with work in conjunction with John and his family in order to reduce anxiety • Ensure financial concerns are properly referred • Agree with John a recovery plan central to his work and recreational activities

impact of chronic illness or disability can severely restrict social roles and functions causing patients to withdraw from domestic, social and recreational activities. Patients may also be fearful of social attitudes towards them, causing them to withdraw even further. Often patients can benefit from counselling and psychotherapy to help them develop personal confidence and self-worth, assertive skills and stress management techniques (White & Johnstone 2000). In order to help patients and their families achieve as normal a life as possible, nursing care must be based upon preserving patient individuality and dignity. In addition it is vital that the nursing care plan reflects the interventions that specialists from other agencies can make towards enhancing patient care helping both patients and their families live as normal a life as possible. Box 11.18 identifies the nursing interventions associated with John's sociocultural needs.

Nursing actions associated with environmental factors affecting ill health

Ill health and disability often limit mobility and subsequently restrict activities, particularly outdoor activities. In hospital it can be difficult to provide patients with a range of activities sufficient to their needs of promoting independence and preventing boredom. The role of the nurse is to help the patient identify a range of activities that can be carried out whilst either confined to bed or the immediate ward area, such as the dayroom. Some patients may be well enough to use other facilities available within the hospital such as a shop, café, gardens, play areas, library, churches or mosques. There may also be other activities that are arranged as part of the patient's recovery or rehabilitation programme such as physiotherapy and occupational therapy sessions. The nurse has a responsibility to identify any risks that might be associated with any activities and ensure that reasonable action has been taken to prevent any accidents or incidents occurring. In hospital a certain amount of equipment and staff will be available to promote activities, but in the home patients may require adaptations to be made, before independent living can be optimised (see Chapter 3, p. 57). In the workplace employers are encouraged to provide appropriate facilities and flexible approaches to helping people back to work. In order to engage fully in work and play activities, patients may require a range of appliances and adaptations to be available either in the home, at work or in places for play, education or leisure. Without proper support and resources patients are at risk from being increasingly isolated in their own homes.

For children, admission to hospital can be strange, frightening and even dangerous. The natural curiosity of children in play has the potential for accidents to happen and again the nurse must be able to identify and prevent risks. If necessary an education service can be provided within the hospital and play coordinators and therapists provide specialist support for play in accordance with the individual needs of the child. Paediatric units recognise the importance of supporting family-centred care in order to enhance normality for the child but also support the coping needs of parents.

Box 11.19 describes the nursing interventions associated with environmental needs for the main case scenario.

Nursing actions associated with politicoeconomic factors affecting ill health

When patients become ill or disabled it is important to acknowledge that not all their anxieties will be related to their physical health and that they may have greater concerns about their financial circumstances and ability to return to work. For some people an absence from work may affect promotion or training prospects and a chronic illness or disability may even lead to the patient having to change jobs and possibly retrain. It is important that nurses are aware of the information and agencies that are available to support the patient's individual needs in order to reduce anxiety and promote independence. At the most basic level patients should be provided with information regarding their recovery and supported to identify how their health status may affect normal working and playing activities. If patients need financial support they should be given accurate information about how to claim for sickness benefits.

Patients who are likely to be away from work for long periods or unable to return to their original type of work will need specialist advice from a range of agencies. However

> **Box 11.19 Nursing care plan to support identified environmental needs in relation to the working and playing main case scenario**
>
> | Problem | Goal/aim | Nursing intervention |
> |---|---|---|
> | John may feel agitated and constrained by the reduced activity due to confinement to the ward | Ensure safety and promote independence in preparation for discharge | • Familiarise John with the ward and any routines and equipment
• Point out safety measures and risks
• Show John how to call for assistance if required
• Agree types of activities that can be undertaken safely during the recovery period
• Discuss with John how he might assess risks within the home or work in preparation for discharge |

navigating the way through the variety of employment agencies that are available can be very daunting and confusing. By having an understanding of the types of statutory and voluntary agencies that are available both in the hospital and the community, nurses can ensure that appropriate and timely referrals are made.

> **Exercise**
>
> Think about some of the legislation and agencies that you have been introduced to within this chapter and consider the following:
>
> 1. What other professionals or organisations could you contact to help?
> 2. How can you keep up to date with legislation and service developments?
> 3. How might you best provide patients with information?
> 4. If you live outside the UK consider these questions in relation to your own country.

By understanding the politicoeconomic needs associated with ill health and injury nursing care can focus upon ensuring that the patient has access to accurate information and advice regarding employment and health promotion.

Promoting health

It is important to recognise that when promoting health there may be a cost implication that may prevent the patient from achieving set goals. For example patients who need to purchase special foods or medications may appear to be noncompliant with their treatment when in fact there is an underlying financial implication. In addition nurses need to recognise that ill health may be directly linked to working life. For example it may be difficult for patients to avoid factors which are contributing towards their ill health because they cannot afford to change jobs or learn new skills. Alternatively patients may become ill as a result of being unable to work and an exploration of this with the patient may reveal that health problems such as increased alcohol intake, increased smoking, drug dependency, poor diet, stress and insomnia may be linked directly to unemployment (Mathers & Schofield 1998). It is therefore important

that nurses recognise early how the patient's health and lifestyle might have been affected over time by work activities and the need to secure an income.

Access to work and play

Following an episode of ill health or an injury, most patients will return to normal individual activities fairly quickly, without any complications. Patients with long-term health problems or disabilities however will need support to find alternative activities and possibly learn new skills. One of the greatest problems facing individuals with disabilities is discrimination and a lack of understanding and opportunity on behalf of employers. In recognition of the rights of disabled people to secure and retain employment and enjoy recreational activities many pieces of legislation have been introduced.

- Disability Discrimination Act (1995)
- Chronically Sick and Disabled Persons Act (1970)
- Community Care Act (1989)
- Human Rights Act.

The legislation is geared not only to assist disabled people to gain access to work and leisure but also change public and employer attitudes towards recognising the value and contribution that disabled people can make. In the UK employers have been actively encouraged through the 'Positive about Disabled People' initiative to review recruitment and employment policies, so as to increase awareness and provide opportunities to employ people with disabilities (see Department for Work and Pensions website listed at the back of this chapter). In addition there are a variety of government services and agencies that exist to help people find suitable employment, redeployment and access to financial support. In addition a range of specialist living, employment and training centres exist nationally to provide information, education, equipment and support within communities and nurses need to be aware of what services are available within their areas.

Within the nursing care plan it is important not to ignore the play and recreational needs, remembering that these activities provide a balance to the whole AL. For children in the UK most hospitals and other health and social care environments recognise the importance of providing resources either in terms of personnel or equipment to prevent boredom or support continuing developmental and social needs. The range of activities therefore needs to cater for babies right through to adolescents. Providing such a range of resources can be expensive and often this depends upon donations and fundraising activities. All equipment requires careful consideration, particularly if they are potentially a safety hazard in relation to falls, ingestion or cross-infection. Other equipment may be expensive and pose security risks, such as playstations, mobile phones, etc. The nurse will need to assess carefully each particular child's needs in relation to the following:

- age
- physical, psychological and social developmental stage
- length of stay
- safety knowledge and needs.

Upon discharge from hospital parents and families often require detailed advice about play and return to school. Advice needs to be practical and realistic and related to what is known about family circumstances. For example it may be difficult for a parent to take extended leave from work to look after a child and this may have a financial impact upon the family. The nurse has an important role in ensuring that parents have access to accurate information and other services in order to prevent financial difficulties.

Provision of recreation resources for adults equally requires careful attention and the nurse should not presume that all patients can have their needs met through watching television, reading or doing jigsaws. Supporting patient's recreational needs begins with the nurse identifying what the patient's usual recreational activities are and find some way to support individual needs whilst in hospital and if necessary beyond discharge. Often the onset of illness and disability reduces independent access to some of the most basic personal resources such as money to buy newspapers or snacks or make telephone calls. The nurse needs to recognise that this can have detrimental effects upon a patient's recovery as shown in the following exercise.

Exercise

Eve is an 83-year-old retired school teacher who has no immediate relatives. She has suffered with rheumatoid arthritis for many years and has been admitted to hospital with a fractured femur. Her usual daily recreation is to read the *Times* newspaper. The staff on the ward are concerned that she is becoming increasingly withdrawn.

1. Why do you think Eve is becoming withdrawn?
2. What might be the economic factor influencing her recovery?

You may have discovered one of many things about Eve as follows:

- Eve's preferred daily activity of reading the newspaper enables her to keep in touch with world affairs.
- Her individual need to read a newspaper had not been assessed or met.
- Due to being an emergency admission she does not have any money with her.
- It may be some time before she has a visitor.
- She may not have reading glasses with her.
- She may have been too embarrassed to ask for help or money.
- Observations of withdrawal are in relation to social deprivation.

This exercise demonstrates the importance of acknowledging and assessing the economic factors that can influence health and its recovery. In the home the patient would make more independent choices about the types of activities they could engage in, but in hospital the provision of more individualised resources can be difficult.

Many hospitals now have cash machines available at a central site and are installing individual bedside telephones and pay per view televisions. However not all patients use cash cards and some may not have enough money to spend on such amenities and the issue of security for personal belongings becomes a cause for concern.

The issues raised in this section have highlighted the importance of assessing the politicoeconomic factors affecting health in order to ensure that nursing care is appropriate to individual needs at a variety of stages in the patient's recovery. Box 11.20 describes the issues that John from Case study 11.3 might have in relation to politicoeconomic factors and his current ill health state.

Implementing working and playing nursing activities

The delivery of quality care is dependent upon the quality of the information detailed within the nursing care plan. In the care setting a variety of health professionals will need to refer to the nursing care plan and it is essential that the plan is conducive to the delivery of consistency in care standards. Prior to the implementation of nursing activities the following must be in place:

1. A detailed written care plan and verbal handover to ensure that all staff are aware of patient progress, goals to be achieved and skills required to deliver the care.
2. Competent practitioners are identified to safely deliver the planned care.
3. Nursing actions and patient progress are recorded and goals are evaluated.

Box 11.20 Nursing care plan to support identified politicoeconomic needs in relation to the working and playing main case scenario

Problem	Goal/aim	Nursing intervention
John may have concerns about financial issues	To reduce any anxieties	• Discuss any concerns with John and his family • Provide accurate and timely information • Make appropriate and timely referrals to specialist agencies and advisors

The nursing plan is a document, which guides the required nursing activities to help the patient achieve the identified goals. The plan should be constantly reviewed and updated to record the following:

• when a goal/desired outcome has been achieved
• when nursing intervention has been changed to support goal achievement
• when the goal needs to be modified
• when the evaluation date needs to be changed
• when problems change or develop.

Factors influencing implementation of working and playing nursing actions

To ensure the effectiveness of implementing the working and playing plan it is important to identify the factors, which might influence this.

Knowledge
• normal health and the impact of illness on the AL
• psychological health and requirements for engaging in the AL
• social and cultural implications for poor health or recovery
• environmental influences and concerns
• political and economic influences and concerns

• knowledge of care and services outside of the sphere of health (social and employment services).

Skill and competency
• philosophy of care and attitudes to patient care
• communication/interpersonal skills
• observation skills
• problem-solving skills
• technical/caring skills
• management/leadership skills (directing, coaching, delegating, supervising skills)
• teaching skills
• research skills.

Resources
• appropriate skill mix
• sufficient equipment
• sufficient support services
• knowledge of and access to specialist agencies.

Working and playing and medically derived care
In addition to the identified nursing care plan it is also important to consider the impact that medical or other health care intervention can have which requires the nurses to integrate into the plan as described in Box 11.21.

Box 11.21 Identification of medical and social care associated with working and playing

Medical and social derived care	Nursing intervention/support
Specific medicotechnical intervention	• Knowledge skill and competency to manage equipment, observe results and report changes. • Knowledge and skill to describe to patients the effects upon the AL of working and playing
Specific pharmacological intervention	• Knowledge and skill regarding action and side effects • Knowledge and skill to describe to patients the effects upon the AL of working and playing
Specific nutritional intervention	• Knowledge and skill to support patient information • Knowledge and skill to describe to patients the effects upon the AL of working and playing
Specific physiotherapy intervention	• Knowledge and skill to provide 24 hour continuing physiotherapy care • Knowledge and skill to describe to patients the effects upon the AL of working and playing
Specific social, occupational and employment service intervention	• Knowledge of available services and professional specialists. Skill in assessment and referral • Knowledge and skill to describe to patients the effects upon the AL of working and playing

Evaluation of nursing activities

The evaluation stage provides the basis by which to determine if the patient is making the desired progress and provides the mechanism for judging the effectiveness of the nursing actions. Evaluation activities should be ongoing and take place on a continuous, hourly, daily or shift basis in accordance with the level of disturbance associated within the AL.

To evaluate effectively the following skills are required:

- observing
- interviewing
- listening
- analysing
- measuring.

The steps in evaluating are as follows. It is recommended that where possible the patient is involved in describing the progress/achievement made.

1. Check the identified goals against patient progress:
   - Have the goals been partially or completely met?
2. Is the timescale realistic?
3. Record the progress as follows:
   - goal completely met, state the evidence to support this and discontinue the problem
   - goal partially met, then decide if there is a need to extend the timescale or modify the plan
   - goal not met, then decide if there is a need to extend the timescale, change the plan or reassess the whole problem.

Box 11.22 provides you with an evaluation of John's care and identifies the evidence and nursing skills that would be required to make an accurate evaluation.

Plan review

If the goals are achieved, nursing actions effectively become redundant. Where goals are not achieved the following questions need to be asked:

1. Is more information required to determine goal achievement?
2. Should the nursing plan be adapted to enable the goal to be achieved?
3. Has the problem changed?
4. Can the planned nursing care be stopped?
5. Has the problem worsened?
6. Should the goal and intervention be reviewed?
7. Was the goal inappropriate?
8. Does the plan require intervention from other health care professionals?

John's plan recognised that long-term goals could not be realistically met during his hospital stay. Therefore upon discharge information regarding his progress and continuing care needs would need to be accurately forwarded to the appropriate professional who will be involved in John's care as shown in Box 11.23.

Summary points

> 1. The model is intrinsically linked to the model of living.
> 2. The AL of working and playing can be affected by ill health and also be the cause of health-related problems.
> 3. Individualised nursing care can be accomplished by using the four stages of the nursing process in conjunction with the components of the model.
> 4. Accurate, continuous assessment is vital as all other stages are dependent upon it.
> 5. All stages can be influenced by various situational factors relating to the nurse, the patient, relatives and the environment.
> 6. A variety of skills and other professionals are required to deliver optimum care to patients.

Box 11.22 Evaluation skills and evidence related to the main case scenario

Goals/aims	Evaluation skills	Evaluation evidence
To help John identify the necessary lifestyle changes that he will need to make in order to continue work, family and recreation activities, that meet his needs and prevents further cardiac problems	Communication skills Interviewing skills Observation skills Information finding skills Assessment skills Negotiation skills Problem-solving skills Creative skills	• John will be able to express some confidence about his recovery and return to independent living • John asks questions freely and demonstrates control over his recovery and return to work and home • John will be able to discuss the information and help he has been given • John will have been able to maintain contact with work and home without this having a detrimental affect upon his health • John's family will express confidence about his discharge from hospital • John is able to identify activities and situations which may create health problems

Box 11.23 Plan review for the main case scenario

Goal	Evaluation	Plan review
To help John identify the necessary lifestyle changes that he will need to make, in order to continue work, family and recreation activities that meets his needs and prevents further cardiac problems	John has made a good recovery from his AMI He is confident about his discharge from hospital and is able to describe how he will adapt his lifestyle accordingly John will need to continue medical treatment and cardiac rehabilitation	Care and observation will continue as an out-patient May need referral to appropriate health, social and employment specialists for example: • Stress Counsellor • Practice Nurse/GP • Social Worker • Cardiac Support Group • Employment services • Physiotherapist • Occupational Health • Dietitian

References

Alexander MF, Fawcett JN, Runciman PJ 2000 Nursing practice – hospital and home, 2nd edn. Churchill Livingstone, Edinburgh

Anderson M 1999 Waiting for harm: deliberate self-harm and suicide in young people – a review of the literature. Journal of Psychiatric and Mental Health Nursing 6(2): 91–100

Bass SA 2000 Emergence of the Third Age: toward a productive aging society. Journal of Aging and Social Policy 11(2–3): 7–17

Boeri T, Brugiavni A, Calmfors L 2001 The role of unions in the twenty-first century. Oxford University Press, London

Brillhart B, Johnson K 1997 Motivation and the coping process of adults with disabilities: a qualitative study. Rehabilitation Nursing 22(5): 249–256

Cortina LM, Magley VJ, Williams JH, Langhout RD 2001 Incivility in the workplace: incidence and impact. Journal of Occupational Psychology 6(1): 64–80

Department for Education and Employment 1998 The learning age a renaissance for a new Britain. The Stationery Office, London

Department of Health 1999 Saving lives: our healthier nation. HMSO, London

Department of Health 2000 The NHS plan: a plan for investment, A Plan for Reform. HMSO, London

Department of Health 2001a Working together – learning together a framework for lifelong learning in the NHS. HMSO, London

Department of Health 2001b Improving working lives standard. HMSO, London

Department for Work and Pensions 2002a Becoming a disability symbol user. (http://www.jobcentreplus.gov.uk/cms.asp?Page=/Home/Employers; last accessed July 2002)

Department for Work and Pensions 2002b Disability rights taskforce. (http://194.202.202.185/drtf/index.html; last accessed July 2002)

Department of Trade and Industry 2000 Work–life balance campaign. (http://164.36.164.20/work-lifebalance; last accessed July 2002)

Department of Trade and Industry 2002 Employee relations. (http://www.dti.gov.uk/er/index.htm; last accessed July 2002)

Disability Discrimination Act 1995 (http://www.hmso.gov.uk/acts/acts95)

Disability Rights Commission (DRC) Act 1999 (http://www.legislation.hmso.gov.uk/acts/acts1999)

Edling C, Waldron HA 1997 Occupational health practice, 4th edn. Butterworth Heinemann, London

Employment Rights Act 1996 (http://www.hmso.gov.uk/acts/acts1996)

Ferrie J 2001 Is job insecurity harmful to health? Journal of the Royal Society of Medicine 94(2): 71

Harris M 2000 The patient in need of rehabilitation. In: Alexander MF, Fawcett JN, Runciman PJ (eds) Nursing practice – hospital and home, 2nd edn., pp. 983–998. Churchill Livingstone, Edinburgh

Hartnell C 2000 The retirement handbook. Age Concern, London

Holmes S 2001 Work-related stress: a brief overview. Journal of the Royal Society of Health 121(4): 230–235

Industrial Tribunal Act 1996 (http://www.hmso.gov.uk/acts/acts1996)

Investors in People 1993 (http://www.IIPuk.co.uk)

Iwasaki Y, Zuzanek J, Mannell RC 2001 The effects of physically active leisure on stress-health relationships. Canadian Journal of Public Health 92(3): 214–218

Karstadt L 1999 The school bullying problem (research into school bullying, holistic management and the role of the school nurse). Nursing Standard 14(11): 32–35

Kposowa AJ 2001 Unemployment and suicide: a cohort analysis of social factors predicting suicide in the US National Longitudinal Mortality Study. Psychological Medicine 31(1): 127–138

Lombardi EL, Ulbrich PM 1997 Work conditions, mastery and psychological distress: are housework and paid contexts conceptually similar? Women and Health 26(2): 17–39

Longworth N 1999 Making Lifelong Learning Work: learning cities for a learning century. Kogan Page, London

Lundberg U, Frankenhaeuser M 1999 Stress and workload of men and women in high-ranking positions. Journal of Occupational Health Psychology 4(2): 142–151

Mathers CD, Schofield DJ 1998 The health consequences of employment: the evidence. The Medical Journal of Australia 1684: 178–182

McArdle P 2001 Children's play (significance of play and its relevance to development). Child Care Health and Development 27(6): 509–514

Mullineaux DR, Barnes CA, Barnes EF 2001 Factors affecting the likelihood to engage in adequate physical activity to promote health. Journal of Sports Sciences 19(4): 279–288

Mullins LJ 1999 Management and organisational behaviour, 5th edn. Financial Times Management, London

Oakley K 2002 Occupational health nursing. Whurr Publishers, London

Office for National Statistics 2002 Social trends 32. The Stationery Office, London

Office of Population Census and Survey (OPCS) (http://www.statistics.gov.uk)

Office of the Deputy Prime Minister 2000 Our towns and cities: the future – delivering an Urban Renaissance. The Stationery Office, London

Parker DL, Bachman S 2001 Economic exploration and the health of children: towards a right-orientated public health approach. Health and Human Rights 5(2): 92–118

Reform of the Education Act 1998 (http://www.hmso.gov.uk/acts/acts1998)

Richardson VE 1999 Women and retirement. Journal of Women and Aging 11(2–3): 49–66

Rimmer JH 1999 Health promotion for people with disabilities: the emerging paradigm shift from disability prevention to prevention of secondary conditions. Physical Therapy 79(5): 495–502

Roper N, Logan W, Tierney AJ 1996 The elements of nursing. A Model for Nursing Based on a Model for Living, 4th edn. Churchill Livingstone, Edinburgh

Roper N, Logan W, Tierney AJ 2000 The elements of nursing. A Model for Nursing Based on Activities of Living. Churchill Livingstone, Edinburgh

Rosenkoetter MM, Garris JM 2001 Retirement planning, use of time and psychological adjustment. Issues in Mental Health Nursing 22(7): 703–722

Rutter M, Hagell A, Giller H,1998 Antisocial behaviour by young people. Cambridge University Press, Cambridge

Schnohr P, Parner J, Lange P 2000 Mortality in joggers: population based study of 4,658 men. British Medical Journal 321(7261): 602–603

Seefeldt V, Malina R, Clark M 2002 Factors affecting levels of physical activity in adults. Sport Medicine 32(3): 143–168

Sheridan MD, Harding J, Meldon-Smith L 1999 Play in Early Childhood from Birth to Six Years. Routledge, London

Slater A, Lewis M 2002 Introduction to Infant Development. Oxford University Press, London

Torrington D, Hall L 1998 Human resource management, 4th edn. Prentice Hall, London

University College London 2001 Predictors and consequences of early exit from the workforce: findings from the Whitehall II cohort Health and Social Research group. (www.ucl.auk/hssrg/nuffield.html; accessed August 2002)

White MA, Johnstone AS 2000 Recovery from stroke: does rehabilitation counselling have a role to play? Disability Rehabilitation 22(3): 140–143

World Health Organisation 1999 Myth No 5: Older people Have Nothing to Contribute. WHO, Geneva

Wilkinson S 2000 Relative values. Nursing Times 96(2): 20–22

Further reading

Alexander MF, Fawcett JN, Runciman PJ 2000 Nursing practice – hospital and home, 2nd edn. Churchill Livingstone, Edinburgh

Trade Union Council 2000 The Employment Relations Act: a TUC guide. Trade Union Council, London

Useful websites

Disabled Living Centre Council www.dlcc.org.uk
Disability Living Foundation www.dlf.org.uk
Department for Education and Skills www.dfes.gov.uk
Disability Alliance www.disabilityalliance.org
Department for Work and Pensions www.dwp.gov.uk
Health and Safety Executive www.hse.gov.uk
Investors in People UK www.IIP.co.uk
Royal College of Nursing www.rcn.org.uk
UNISON www.unison.org.uk
World Health Organisation www.who.int/peh/

Expressing sexuality

Karen Holland

Introduction

Human beings are sexual beings and how an individual manages their sexuality in health is determined by many factors. Biological differences in sex and sexual development and the influence of society and culture, including sexual behaviour across the lifespan, are fundamental to this management. It is essential if a holistic approach to care is to be adopted that there is also an understanding of how these factors can affect the care given to patients who are ill (see Chapter 1 for further information on the factors).

This chapter will therefore focus on the following:

1. **The model of living**
   - expressing sexuality in health and illness (see model of living – Chapter 1)
   - dependence/independence in the AL of expressing sexuality
   - factors influencing the AL of expressing sexuality.
2. **The model for nursing**
   - nursing care of individuals with health problems affecting the Activity of Living: expressing sexuality (i.e. application of Roper, Logan, Tierney (1996, 2000) in practice).

THE MODEL OF LIVING

Before examining the different aspects of expressing sexuality as an activity it is important to define both sexuality and sexual health. Roper et al (1996) view sexuality as more than sex and sexual intercourse, which they see as 'an important component of adult relationships'. Human sexuality they believe is also expressed in personality and behaviour. They state that:

66 *Femininity and masculinity are reflected not only in physical appearance and strength but also in style of dress; in many forms of verbal and non-verbal communication; in family and social roles and relationships and in choices relating to work and play.* 99

(Roper et al 1996, p. 22)

How do others view sexuality?

McCann (2000, p. 134) states that 'people are sexual beings all of the time, whether they are healthy, ill or disabled' and offers two quotations from the literature that he believes help us to understand the 'human aspects of a person's sexuality'.

Adams (1976, p. 166) for example states that:

66 *The definition of sexuality can be as narrow as the act of intercourse or as broad as seeing the entire universe. Each individual determines the answer to defining his or her sexuality. Sexuality is a celebration of oneself, a voyage into body, mind and spirit. It is based on one's cognition, emotions and physical functioning.* 99

Stuart and Sundeen (1979, p. 356) argue that:

66 *Sexuality is an integral part of the whole person. Human beings are sexual in every way, all the time. To a large extent human sexuality determines who we are. It is an integral factor in the uniqueness of every person.* 99

It can be seen from all these possible explanations of sexuality that it is a complex, yet important, part of who we are. An awareness of this is essential when considering patients' or clients' needs in a holistic way. Ensuring sexual health is part of meeting these needs. The World Health Organisation defines sexual health in the following broad terms:

66 *Sexual Health is a personal sense of sexual well-being as well as the absence of disease, infections or illness associated with sexual behaviour. As such it includes issues of self-esteem, self-expression, caring for others and cultural values. Sexual health can be described as the positive integration of physical, emotional, intellectual and social aspects of sexuality. Sexuality influences thoughts, feelings, interactions and actions among human beings and motivates people to find love, contact, warmth and intimacy. It can be expressed in many different ways and is closely linked to the environment one finds oneself in, the environment can hinder or enhance sexual expressions.* 99 (WHO 2000)

Box 12.1 Reproductive health: WHO goals

People should be able to exercise their sexual and reproductive rights in order to:

- Experience healthy sexual development and maturation and have the capacity for equitable and responsible relationships and sexual fulfilment
- Achieve their desired number of children safely and healthily when and if they decide to have them
- Avoid illness, disease and disability related to sexuality and reproduction and receive appropriate care when needed
- Be free from violence and other harmful practices related to sexuality and reproduction

From: World Health Organisation (1998) Reproductive health: meeting people's needs (WHO/RHT/98.17).

In keeping with World Health Organisation guidelines Jamison (2002) states that sexual health can be 'largely regarded as:

- a capacity to enjoy and control sexual and reproductive behaviour in accordance with a social and personal ethic
- freedom from psychological factors such as fear, shame, guilt and false beliefs inhibiting the sexual response and impairing sexual relationships
- freedom from organic disease, disorders and deficiencies that impair sexual and reproductive functioning' (Jamison 2002, p. 163)

The World Health Organisation have also adopted the term 'reproductive health' to encompass a whole range of goals which include those related to sexuality and sexual behaviour (see Box 12.1). Expressing sexuality as an Activity of Living is therefore an essential part of existence as human beings.

Expressing sexuality in health and illness – across the lifespan

Childhood

Sexual identity begins at birth, i.e. boy or girl, and many societies attach great importance to this. Boys for example may be more welcome in societies where men are considered to be more important than women. Understanding the differences between cultures and their views and behaviour regarding sexuality is essential for ensuring that the needs of patients are considered holistically.

How sexuality is expressed will depend in a large part on experiences at different ages. Babies will have enjoyed being cuddled and young children may have enjoyed playing games such as mothers and fathers, where gender roles are imitated and acted out. However, given that in many countries children are now being brought up in a single-parent household the image of two parents living together is no longer always the norm.

There are also other problems with children coming to realise the complexities of human sexuality and the different ways in which men and women behave, these will often have major repercussions later on in life and during illness. Sexual abuse of children is an example and the trauma of such an experience may seriously affect their personality and their sexual development.

Exercise

1. Reflect on your own childhood. How did you learn about the gender and sex differences between men and women?
2. Find out what children in different cultures learn about how men and women are supposed to act.

In some South Asian communities for example there are very strict codes of behaviour for men and women (Henley & Schott 1999, p. 454). They may not mix with each other in public, and often visit ill relatives or go shopping separately. Children may therefore very rarely see their parents touching each other in public. Children brought up in an Orthodox Jewish home will come to know that men and women do not touch each other whilst the woman is menstruating as it is considered unclean or 'polluting'. This belief is also to be found in Muslim, Hindu, Sikh and Traveller–Gypsy cultures (Holland & Hogg 2001).

An area where it is also possible to see the effect of adult sexual behaviour on the child is in the area of HIV/AIDS where it is estimated that '13 million children currently under the age of 15 have lost one or both parents to AIDS, most of them in sub-Saharan Africa' (UNAIDS 2002). It is also estimated by UNAIDS that by the end of 2000 '1.3 million children were living with HIV/AIDS and that 4.3 million had already died of the disease' (UNAIDS 2002). Many of these children will have become infected through their mothers as the HIV virus may be transferred from an infected mother to her infant before, during or after birth through breast milk (Alexander et al 2000). The other modes of transmission for HIV can be seen in Box 12.2.

Exercise

1. Using the worldwide web as a resource, find out how caring for children with AIDS is taking place in different countries.
2. Share and discuss your findings with colleagues.

This will enable you to see how very often the politico-economic and environmental factors have a major influence on how AIDS is managed and how sexuality is perceived in the country in which you live.

Box 12.2 Mother to child transmission

This form of transmission is known as 'vertical transmission, i.e. down 'from' an infected mother to her child in the womb or during delivery, when the mother's blood and the child's blood become mixed. There is a possibility that transmission through amniotic fluid and ('horizontally') through breast milk can also take place (Mok 1993, Carlisle 1998).

From birth until 11–18 months, the baby will carry the mother's HIV and other antibodies. Therefore, all babies born to HIV-infected mothers are found to be HIV antibody-positive. At about 11–18 months, the baby will lose the mother's antibodies and go on either to being HIV antibody-negative (not carrying the virus) or to developing his own antibodies (being infected in his own right). A few go on to become HIV antibody-negative but positive to another test which isolates antigen (particles of the actual virus) so that they are carrying the virus but not the antibodies.

At the beginning of the HIV epidemic it appeared that about 50% of children born to HIV antibody-positive mothers became infected in their own right.

In countries where there are good antenatal facilities and the mother remains well throughout pregnancy, the rate of transmission from mother to child is dramatically lower. The babies still carry the mothers' antibodies, but only about 20% appear to go on to being infected in their own right.

Atkinson J 2000 The Person with HIV/AIDS, p. 1036.

Adolescence

Most societies have a way of defining age groups as part of the social organisation of people. This is often linked to groupings based on gender. In Western society one such group is adolescents. Adolescence is heralded by the onset of puberty (in young men) and the menarche (in young women) resulting in the capability for fertilisation/conception.

Exercise

1. Consider your own adolescent years. How did you learn about what was happening to your body at this time. Who explained what was happening to you?
2. Discuss with colleagues what it was like to be 12 or 14 years of age?

Sex education for young people is of paramount importance given the increase in sexually transmitted disease and a rise in teenage pregnancy (www.doh.gov.uk/nshs). For example in the UK:

> *In 1997 the conception rate for girls under the age of 16 was 8.9% per 1000. For girls aged 15–19 the rate was 62.3 per thousand. These are the highest rates of teenage pregnancy in Western Europe.*

> *Half of under-16 conceptions and more than a third of conception to 16–19 year olds end in abortion.*

> *Virtually all the sexually transmitted diseases are increasing. The commonest conditions are genital warts (some types of which can be associated with the subsequent development of carcinoma of the cervix), chlamydia and gonorrhoea, which if untreated can result in ectopic pregnancy and infertility. Chlamydial infection seen in clinics has risen by 21% between 1996 and 1997 and a further 135% from 1997 to 1998 (latest figures). Population surveys have reported rates of chlamydia as high as 20%, particularly in young women.*

> *There has been no reduction in the annual number of new diagnoses of HIV made and the latest annual figures (1999) saw the highest number of new HIV diagnoses ever recorded.* (DoH 2000)

In response to this the Government is committed to developing a National Sexual Health and HIV Strategy (DoH 2000) and the strategy group has been set up to address HIV, teenage pregnancy and sexual health issues. This is an example of how political and social factors influence daily living and tries to ensure that combating health problems in the early years will prevent further breakdown in adulthood and old age.

Adulthood

Adulthood in Western society can be described as having three stages following the end of the adolescent period (see Table 12.1).

In other societies it is achieved at puberty and the menarche, and is celebrated through rituals and initiation ceremonies to mark the occasion as a life transition. This is very often linked to complex belief systems that are essential for that cultural group to live together. La Fontaine (1985, p. 130) describes one such initiation.

> *The initiation of Wogeo boys takes place in a number of stages. All children, girls and boys, have their ears pierced at the age of about three "to assist their growth". This is an informal event for a girl, but for a boy it is the first ritually assisted step on the road to manhood. At about nine or ten he will be formally taken from his mother and introduced into the men's clubhouse; at about the age of puberty he undergoes a further ceremony designed to enable him to play the flutes (a symbolic act); and then a final stage which permits him to wear the head-dress which is the sign of an adult man. The purpose of all the rites, which can be seen as an extended initiation, is to ensure that the boys will grow into men: that is, natural growth is seen as weak and likely to fail unless strengthened by the rites.*

(La Fontaine 1985, p. 130)

Table 12.1 Summary of aspects of the development of sexuality throughout the lifespan

	Prenatal	Infancy (0–5 years)	Childhood (6–12 years)	Adolescence (13–18 years)	Young Adulthood (19–30 years)	Middle Years (31–44 years)	Late Adulthood (45–64 years)	Old Age (65+)
PHYSICAL SEXUAL DEVELOPMENT	DETERMINATION OF SEX	Growth of sex organs		♂ PUBERTY ♀ MENARCHE	Continuing sex differences in body build and strength Completion of development of secondary sex characteristics	**Changes of pregnancy ♀**	MENOPAUSE ♀	Physical and hormonal changes may cause decline in libido and potency
PSYCHOSEXUAL DEVELOPMENT		Establishment of sexual orientation (masculine/feminine)		Consolidation of sexual self-image	Development and modification of sexual self-image and attitudes towards sex, sexual relationships, sexual behaviour and sex-related roles and functions			
SEXUALITY AND SOCIAL ROLES		Sex differences in roles and functions within family, school and community, settings		Problem of unwanted teenage pregnancy	Sex differences in family roles ♂ as FATHER ♀ as MOTHER Sex differences in social roles Sex differences in occupational roles			Decreasing differentiation of role and function according to sex
INTERPERSONAL/ SEXUAL RELATIONSHIPS		Mainly confined to FAMILY relationships	Friendships with same and opposite sex	Homosexual liaisons Heterosexual friendship and partnerships	ESTABLISHMENT AND DEVELOPMENT OF ADULT SEXUAL PARTNERSHIPS: Temporary liaisons or long-term mateship/marriage (heterosexual or homosexual)			Possible loss of sexual partner through death
SEXUAL BEHAVIOUR		EARLY SELF-STIMULATORY SEX PLAY		MASTURBATION Various forms of noncoital behaviour with same and opposite sex	ADULT SEXUAL BEHAVIOUR PATTERNS Attracting/courting behaviours Self-stimulatory activities Sexual intercourse			Possible decline in sexual behaviour and in libido
SEXUAL REPRODUCTION				CAPABILITY FOR EJACULATION AND FERTILI-SATION CAPABILITY TO CONCEIVE ♀	♂ EJACULATION AND FERTILISATION OF FEMALE ♀ CAPABILITY FOR CONCEPTION AND REPRODUCTION (i.e. FERTILE)		♀ Incapable of conception after menopause	

From Roper et al 1996

An example that may be considered is the bar mitzvah – practised by the Jewish culture. Transitions can also occur in later adult life. The onset of the menopause (or cessation of menstruation), for example, can occur at any time from the late thirties to the early sixties, the effects of which can vary in terms of its physical and emotional effects on both women and men. Consider the following description by Rutter (2000a).

> *Women's responses to the menopause are, to a large extent, shaped by their previous psychosexual relationships; their attitudes towards themselves and their sexuality; and their current situation and career/work commitment. For those with high self-esteem, in a happy partnership, enjoying a satisfying sexual relationship, the menopause usually constitutes a relatively easy transition. For others, who have never enjoyed sexual intercourse and have viewed it as a 'chore' or 'duty' there may be a sense of relief since they can use the menopause as an excuse not to have sex. However, even when women have previously enjoyed their sexual lives, there may be a feeling that after the menopause it is no longer 'proper' to enjoy sex. For some sexual satisfaction is bound up with procreation, and it may be difficult to feel a sexual person when fertility ceases.*
>
> (Rutter 2000a, p. 166)

Old age

The age when one is considered old varies from culture to culture and unlike those societies where age is considered to be of value, in Western society old age is considered by many as a time to be prevented at any cost. This has the potential to affect the way in which people act in relation to their health and wellbeing (see Box 12.3).

Given the changing balance of older people in UK society, i.e. are living longer and healthier, many may well be entering into marriage for the first or second time. This can bring with it uncertainties and anxiety. Consider the following case study.

Box 12.3 Transition to older age

There are cultures in which old age is regarded as ideal, and is equated with wisdom and dignity so that older people are treated with respect. However, in our society there is a great deal of emphasis on youth, so that older people either feel or are seen by others as having reduced power, with consequent negative effects on self-esteem. Views on our changing biology have led to an expectation of declining health and competence in old age. Of course there is an element of reality in these expectations. Extreme old age tends to be accompanied by failing memory, reduced vision and hearing and restricted energy and mobility. But the stereotype is seriously misleading for four different reasons:

1. In most cases, the decline does not take place (at least in marked form) until a person is in their 80s and 90s rather than in their 60s and 70s.
2. There are huge individual variations in the effects of age.
3. Decline is much influenced by the extent to which individuals remain active physically and mentally.
4. Old age may bring new experiences with opportunities for growth and achievement. Personal development is as much a feature of later life as it is of other years. (Baltes et al 1999, Wells, 1999.) Cited in Rutter (2000b, p. 204).

Case study 12.1

Age and sexual health

Mrs Jones, aged 67, attended the well-woman clinic asking for a check up. When I asked her what sort of check up she was hoping for she appeared uncertain and anxious. 'I'm too old for a smear test, aren't I, but I just wondered if you could see if I'm alright there?' I asked her if she felt something was wrong. 'Well, I'm not sure. I'm a bit worried – I haven't had sex for over 10 years since I lost my first husband and I'm just going to get married again. I feel a bit scared about starting sex again. I've no idea what my vagina's like now. I've never taken HRT and I wonder if it's all dried up?' She was relieved when I said we could do a vaginal examination together. She agreed I would examine her first and then she said she would like to feel herself. She was relaxed and easy to examine and her vagina and pelvic floor felt normal with reasonable muscle tone. She was relieved to hear this and agreed that she would examine herself with me close at hand. This she did and to her surprise said: 'I never thought it would be so easy and normal – I think I'm alright, aren't I?' We continued to talk about her plans for her new life and she showed her excitement and happiness. It appeared that she was in touch again with her vagina and the prospect of her renewed sexuality. (Rutter 2000a, p. 168)

You may have considered the way in which body image is viewed, for example the fashion journals focusing on the young rather than older age group. Despite a growing awareness of sexual behaviour and needs of older people, it is not well represented in either men's or women's journals and is often linked to health problems such as male impotence or effects of the menopause.

A summary of the aspects of the development of sexuality throughout the lifespan can be seen in Table 12.1.

Dependence/independence in the AL of expressing sexuality

Children and adolescents will be dependent on adults and older people for guidance in relation to sexual activity and sexuality. They are dependent on being protected from sexual, emotional and physical abuse and will need to be taught, in a sensitive way, about the dangers of going with strangers and in the case of adolescents placing themselves in potentially dangerous situations when going out socially or otherwise.

Independence can only be achieved through knowledge and understanding, and then behaving appropriately and safely. Effective sex education is essential to this learning and not only applies to the young but also to older people who require information about safe and enjoyable sexual practices in health and illness. Those with specific needs in this area are people with learning and physical disabilities. By definition having learning difficulties means that their capacity for learning is slower than others. For example, adolescent girls may not be able to cope with menstruation and most importantly neither young boys nor girls with learning difficulties may be able to cope with contraception or contraceptive advice. Those with physical difficulties may be dependent on using different mechanical devices in order to enjoy as independent a life as possible, e.g. a false penis or a vibrator.

Factors influencing the AL expressing sexuality

In order to demonstrate the interconnectedness of the factors this section will focus on two themes.

1. Anatomy and physiology related to expressing sexuality (biological factors).
2. Expressing sexuality in society (sociocultural, environmental, psychological, politicoeconomic factors).

Anatomy and physiology relating to expressing sexuality

In order to be able to promote health and nursing care for individuals who are ill it is essential to be able to understand the structure and function of the body in both health and illness. In relation to expressing sexuality this initially refers to the reproductive system and the breast. It is important however to note that in illness which directly stems from these, that other Activities of Living will also be affected (see Case study 12.3, p. 364).

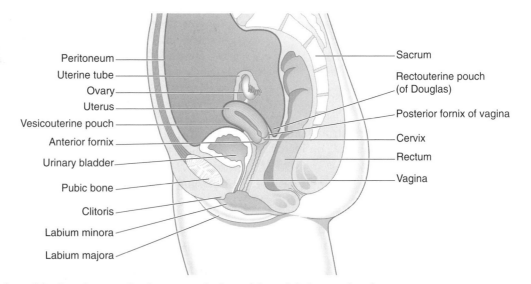

Fig. 12.1 Lateral view of the female reproductive organs in the pelvis and their associated structures (from Waugh & Grant 2001, with permission).

Male and female reproductive systems and the breast
The male and female reproductive systems differ, both in terms of structure and function. Their prime function 'is the propagation or continuation of the human species' (McQueen 2000).

The female reproductive system The female reproductive system comprises of the following structures. The internal organs, namely the ovaries, uterus, the uterine tubes (fallopian), the vagina and the external organs, namely the vulva and the mammary glands or breasts (see Figs 12.1, 12.2, 12.3).

Women have two ovaries, one on each side of the uterus. These have two functions – to produce ova (eggs) and hormones. The age at which the ovarian cycle begins is normally around 12–13 years of age, however this can be earlier or later in some girls, e.g. 9 or 16 years. The hormones secreted are progestogens and oestrogens and it is the delicate balance of these hormones that establishes the pattern found in the woman's menstrual cycle (ovarian and endometrium cycles) (see Fig. 12.4).

The menstrual cycle (menarche) prepares the body for fertilisation of the ovum, if this does not occur the body responds by getting rid of the prepared endometrial lining and results in a menstrual blood loss. This is normally around 50 ml, although it can vary between 10 and 80 ml

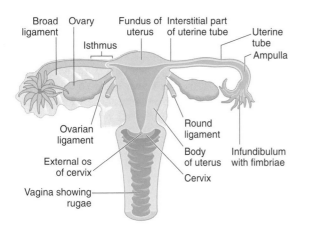

Fig. 12.2 Anterior view of the female reproductive organs (from Waugh & Grant 2001, with permission).

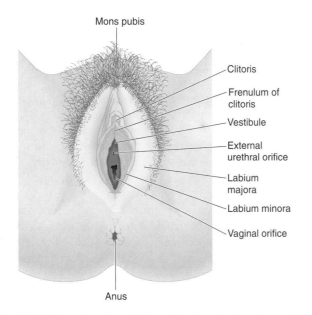

Fig. 12.3 The external genitalia of the female (from Waugh & Grant 2001, with permission).

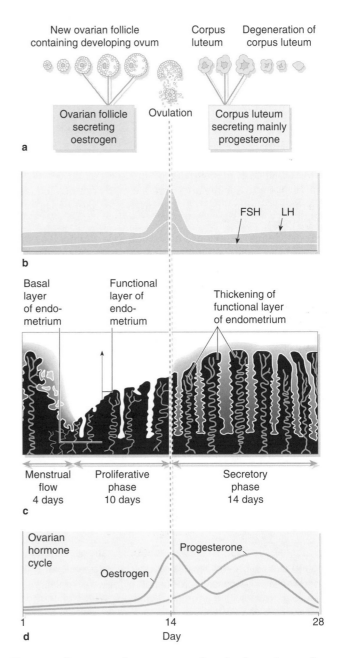

Fig. 12.4 Summary of one menstrual cycle: A ovarian cycle, B anterior pituitary cycle, C uterine cycle, D ovarian hormone cycle (from Waugh & Grant 2001, with permission).

(Hinchliff et al 1996). Clotting of menstrual blood is not normal, due to the fact it contains no fibrinogen and is 'therefore incapable of clotting', although 'sometimes small darkly coloured "clots" of blood are observed in the menstrual blood, but these are usually aggregations of red blood cells in a mass of mucoid material or even glycogen' (Hinchliff et al 1996, p. 705). Normally, menstruation causes no problems other than a monthly blood flow – which for some women is 'artificially' created when taking the contraceptive pill (see Box 12.4 for examples in normal variation). Cessation of menstruation is defined as the menopause and is only one of many changes taking place in the woman's body in the phase of life known as 'the climacteric' (see Box 12.5).

Box 12.4 Menstruation and associated problems

Excessive menstrual flow, menorrhagia, can lead to iron deficiency anaemia due to depletion of iron stores. The iron status of women seems to be very delicately balanced. A woman taking a normal diet with a haemoglobin concentration of 12 g/dl and a roughly regular cycle, will remain in iron balance only if her blood loss does not exceed 65 ml (Wilson & Rennie 1976). Thus, women that experience heavy menstrual bleeding may need to be advised to take intermittent courses of iron therapy. Women with an intrauterine contraceptive device in situ often experience an increased menstrual loss and thus may become iron deficient.

The absence of menstruation or amenorrhoea is usually a sign of failure to ovulate and there are many possible causes. The most common cause of secondary amenorrhoea is pregnancy.

Some women experience mood changes and unpleasant physical symptoms during the 10 days prior to the onset of menstruation. This has been given the name premenstrual tension (PMT) or, more commonly, the premenstrual syndrome (PMS). The clinical features can include a varying and complex range of symptoms, including lower abdominal discomfort and distension, nausea, giddiness or vertigo, breast discomfort, general 'bloated' feeling, weight gain of up to 3 kg, frequency of micturition, increase in acne, headaches, joint pains, depression, fatigue and decreased libido.

The other common problem is dysmenorrhoea or painful menstruation. Some pain at the time of menstruation is almost universal, but a few women have severe and disabling pain. About 45% of menstruating women report moderate or severe dysmenorrhoea. The pain is lower abdominal, either suprapubic or literalised. Dysmenorrhoea is described as being cramp-like or as a dull ache. It is most severe on the first day of bleeding and in some young women may be associated with fainting, nausea and vomiting. The incidence decreases with age and after childbearing.

From Hinchliff et al 1996, pp. 705–707.

Box 12.5 The climacteric and menopause

The word climacteric comes from the Greek word *klimacter,* meaning a step or rung of a ladder. This signifies a step or phase in life from the child-bearing years to a period of infertility associated with age-related changes. The process of the climacteric is usually gradual and may extend over several years. Most women experience the climacteric or perimenopause over a period of 2–3 years, but it may extend over 10 years. During this time the body adjusts to lower levels of oestrogen.

The ageing process of the ovaries results in ripening of fewer follicles and a decreased stimulation by the pituitary hormones. The ovaries atrophy and less oestrogen is released into the circulation. Initially this reduced oestrogen level in the blood results in excessive production of follicle-stimulating hormone (FSH) from the anterior pituitary gland and this feedback mechanism can continue for several years. The withdrawal of oestrogen and the increase in pituitary hormone contribute to the changes associated with the climacteric.

The menopause is sometimes confused with the climacteric. However, the menopause is defined as the cessation of menstruation and is marked specifically by the date of the last menstrual period. It follows then, that the time of the menopause or last menstrual period can only be identified in retrospect some months after the event. The menopause is only one effect of the climacteric. 'Postmenopausal' is a term applied to events occurring after menstruation has stopped for at least a year.

The menopause (last menstrual period) signifies the end of a woman's reproductive capacity. This normally occurs between 45 and 55 years of age, with the mean age for cessation of periods being 51 years. This has remained constant for many years (Abernathy 1997).

A premature menopause is one that occurs before the age of 40 years. This can occur naturally or may be induced iatrogenically. The age of menarche, socioeconomic factors, race, use of oral contraceptives and number of pregnancies appear to have no effect on whether a woman has an early or late menopause (Abernathy 1997).

From: McQueen (2000, p. 224).

(see Box 12.6 – Asian women and the menopause)

Exercise

Imagine you are working in a women's health unit and you have to explain to:

1. a young woman of 18 how the contraceptive pill is going to affect her normal menstruation cycle
2. a woman of 50, the onset of the menopause.

- What would you need to inform each of them?
- How different would your explanation have to be to women of different cultures?

In relation to 1 you may have considered the following:

1. Explained the purpose of contraceptives and the different types.
2. Side effects of the contraceptive pill and what it does to the normal menstrual cycle.
3. The importance of regular health checks whilst taking the contraceptive pill and to report any side effect which affected their daily living activities.

In relation to 2 you may have considered the following:

1. Explained what the menopause is and how it will affect the body.

2. Discussed with them their understanding of what happens at the menopause (see Box 12.6 – Asian women and the menopause).
3. The importance of regular health checks and reporting any change in pattern following cessation of menstruation periods.

The needs of women from different cultures will vary considerably, depending on a whole range of values and beliefs. Schott and Henley (1996, p. 182) for example state that: 'Contraception is a delicate and highly sensitive topic which can touch on people's deepest feelings about their sexuality and self-esteem, their relationships and their perceptions of themselves and of their families.' They also point out that the reasons why contraception is used will also vary in different countries. In Western cultures 'children are expensive and are the focus of strong consumer pressure. They can often be more of a worry and a drain than a pleasure, especially to parents on low incomes with restricted options and poor housing and other facilities' (Schott & Henley 1996, p. 182). In Third World countries, the opposite is seen – 'children are an important economic asset, i.e. they can help on the farm, in the home or wherever help is needed' (Schott & Henley 1996, p. 182), but in some countries contraception becomes a political issue and

---

Box 12.6 Asian women and the menopause

Findings from interviews with six British Asian (Punjabi–Sikh) women.

The women have come to the UK in their childbearing years. In the ensuing two to three decades they had acquired a wealth of experience, knowledge and information about pregnancy and fertility issues. As will be seen from the excerpts, each woman had certain knowledge of the Punjabi myths associated with menopause.

Menstruation folk speech (Golub 1992, Davis 1986) exists universally. Punjabi euphemistic expressions illuminating menstruation are: visitor/monthlies/bleeding/unwell/cloths are here, time of the month, my turn has come, rest days. Similarly the menopause is referred to in Punjabi folk speech as 'all those woman's troubles are now finished', 'monthlies have gone', and 'now I have started my old woman phase'. Meanings of menopause were articulated by the women in terms of others' experiences, symptoms, changes of lifestyle and other concepts.

'When you change, your face becomes spotty, your hair turns white.' (Manjit)

'The old ones always have headaches; you know women who are a bit soft can go mad. I don't want to go mad.' (Satto)

'They say once your monthlies stop, you body is less energetic and softer … the skin is soft like cotton wool and marks easily (meaning bruising).' (Satto)

'Menopause is the time for leisure … daughters are married … daughters-in-law are in charge of housework.' (Sukh)

'I was so pleased to finish with this dreadful business of periods. I thanked God a million times. It gives me freedom.' (Sukh)

'When I lived in India, I never knew anybody who had the menopause. When I got married I was nearly 18, my youngest brother was three (referring to her parents sexuality). I don't know how old my mother or aunts were at their menopause.' (Gurdip)

There was certain vagueness about the meanings and myths of menopause for these women. One reason for this may be that, having migrated to the UK in their childbearing years, as a group these women did not observe their older relatives' experience during menopause. Lack of reference to loss of reproductive ability was unexpected. These women were from a culture that encouraged them to consider their reproductive ability as the most important contribution of their lives (Greer 1991), yet they were very accepting of the functional change of their body from fertility to nonfertility. Further discussion indicated that loss of biological fertility was compensated by grandparenthood.

From: Mayor 1996, pp. 120–139.

means of social control, e.g. China, where a 'one child' policy has been enforced.

Culture and beliefs therefore are a major deciding factor in both choice of contraception and the decision to use any. In the same way, what women know and understand about their bodies and how it functions will affect how they manage the menopause. Mayor's (1996) study of British Punjabi–Sikh women's experiences of the menopause offers an excellent insight into how understanding cultural beliefs would be of value in explaining how the menopause affects daily living (see Box 12.6)

The male reproductive system The male reproductive system comprises the following. Those structures responsible for the production, maturation and delivery into the female reproductive tract of spermatozoa necessary for the fertilisation of ova. The essential organs of this system are the two testes, in which spermatogenesis occurs. The accessory organs, which support the reproductive process, include:

- the genital ducts – the epididymis (2) vas deferens (2), ejaculatory ducts (2) and urethra, which convey the sperm to the exterior
- the glands – the seminal vesicles (2), the prostate gland and the bulbourethral (Cowper's glands) (2) which produce fluid as a vehicle for sperm
- the supporting structures – the scrotum, penis and spermatic cords. (Selfe, 2000: 317) (see Figs 12.5, 12.6).

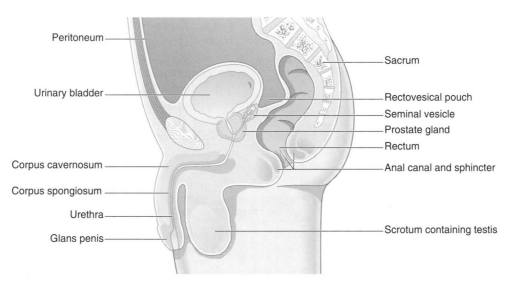

Fig. 12.5 The male reproductive organs and their associated structures (from Waugh & Grant 2001, with permission).

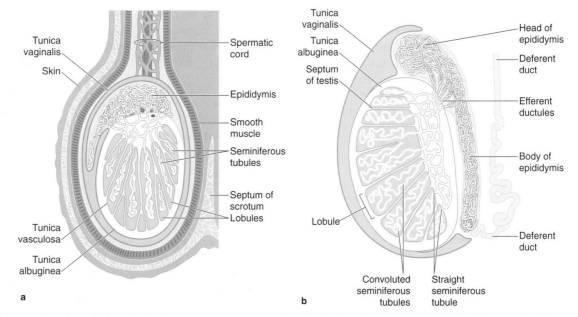

Fig. 12.6 The testis: A section of the testis and its coverings, B longitudinal section of a testis and a deferent duct (from Waugh & Grant 2001, with permission).

The testes

> *The testes are oval organs 4–5 cm in length and weighing 10–15 g each. They are suspended in the scrotum by the spermatic cords. Each contains 200–300 lobes, within which are tightly coiled seminiferous tubules. It is here that the primitive sex cells (spermatagonia) present in male babies at birth become transformed into spermatozoa. This process starts at puberty and continues throughout life.*
> (Selfe 2000, p. 317)

The testes also produce hormones, the most important being testosterone. This promotes, among other things, 'maleness and male sexual behaviour and the development and maintenance of male secondary characteristics and the functions of the accessory organs' (Selfe 2000, p. 318). These organs are the seminal vesicles (secrete seminal fluid – 30% volume), prostate gland (secrete alkaline fluid – 60% seminal fluid volume) and bulbourethral glands (secrete lubricating mucus – less than 5% seminal fluid volume). 'The temperature of the testes is 2–3 degrees centigrade below body temperature which helps to preserve sperm viability' (Selfe 2000, p. 319). Sperm are transported in the seminal fluid into the woman's vagina via the penis, during sexual intercourse. The alkaline nature of the fluid reduces acidity of seminal fluid and vaginal secretions, and 'is an important reproductive function, as the motility and viability of sperm are greatly reduced in an acid solution' (Walsh 2002, p. 768), this has implications for men who have removal of their prostate gland (prostatectomy).

Exercise

1. Imagine you are working in a men's ward specialising in genitourinary health problems. A man of 50 years asks you to explain what will happen to his ability to have sex with his wife following removal of the prostate gland.
2. Discuss your patient education plan with a colleague and justify your decisions with an evidence base.

The breast The breast plays a major role in how both men and women express sexuality and sexual behaviour. It is the 'human organ of lactation which develops in puberty to enable a mother to feed her offspring. In Western society the breasts are strongly associated with femininity and sexuality as well as with motherhood' (Burnet 2000, p. 279). Because of this breasts play an important part of women's body image and any illness that may cause disfigurement or alteration could have profound effects on the woman's wellbeing, for example breast cancer.

In order to understand how breast cancer and treatment affect the physical appearance of women, it is important to understand the anatomy and physiology of the breast (see Fig 12.7 for lateral cross-section of the breast).

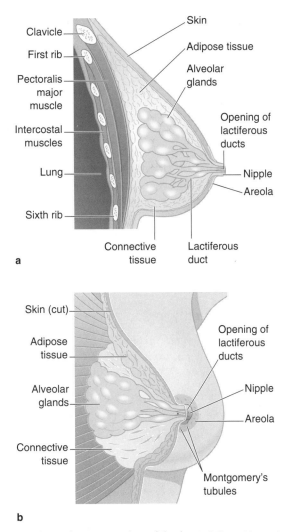

Fig. 12.7 Lateral cross-section of the breast (from Alexander et al 2000, with permission).

Structure of the breast

> *The breast is made up of glandular, fatty and fibrous tissue and is covered by skin. Men and women both have breast tissue, but in the male it remains rudimentary and does not develop in puberty. The glandular tissue of each breast is divided into 12–20 lobes or segments. Each is made up of hundreds of lobules, which are activated during pregnancy to produce milk. They are connected by terminal ducts that join to form lactiferous ducts before ending in around 10 openings in the nipple. Breast tissue is supported by Cooper's ligaments, which may contract when affected by a tumour causing dimpling of the skin (peau d'orange). With increasing age and weight these ligaments stretch, causing the breast to droop, which is otherwise known as ptosis. The nipple contains smooth muscle and becomes erect when stimulated, allowing a baby to suck more easily. It is surrounded by the areola, on the surface of which are Montgomery's tubercles. These lubricate the nipple during breast feeding.* (Burnet 2000, p. 279)

The breasts are very vascular structures and contain many lymph nodes. They are also positioned close to muscles such as the pectoralis major and minor, which are essential to ensuring the shoulder girdle is stabilised (see Fig. 12.8).

Exercise

Consider the role and structure of the breast and the implications for:

1. A young woman of 30 years, with two children who has been diagnosed as having breast cancer. She would like to have more children and breast-feed them.
2. How would your knowledge of structure and function of the breast help you to care for this young woman?

Expressing sexuality in society

66 *Sexuality is broadly defined as the becoming and being a man or woman and as such, adult sexuality has four major divisions.* 99 (Walsh 2002, p. 782).

These being, biological sex, core gender identity, sex role imagery and sexual behaviour (see Box 12.7).

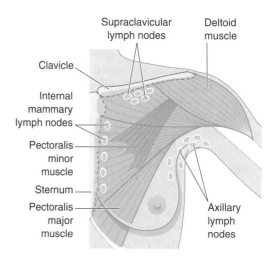

Fig. 12.8 The breast and associated structures (from Alexander et al 2000, with permission).

Exercise

Consider the issues outlined in Box 12.7 and discuss with colleagues how:

1. nurses are viewed in relation to sex role imagery (sociocultural factors)
2. beliefs about sexual behaviour influences their role as nurses.

Box 12.7 Sexuality

Biological sex
Biological sex refers to the individual's physical attributes. This is based on the genotype (XX, XY or other combinations) and includes internal and external genitalia with the corresponding underlying hormonal, neural, vascular and physical components.

Core gender identity
This refers to one's inner sense of being a man or a woman, and is established early in life, usually by 3 years of age. At this age, the child knows he or she is a boy or a girl. In most cases the core gender identity corresponds to the physical attributes of the individual.

Sex role imagery
This refers to the learned behaviour that the particular society subscribes to their men and women. Sex or gender role imagery is complex because it includes the myriad beliefs about what is often labelled feminine or masculine by a society. It also conveys the image of appropriate sexual conduct for particular social groups. Some examples of those beliefs are: trousers are worn by men, skirts by women; women are passive; men are active. Sex role imagery is of great interest because it represents much of the learned behaviour which influences human choice and lifestyle.

Much stereotyping of human behaviour has resulted from the need for society to set up expectations by which to guide and judge sex role behaviour. These roles can be used to set the parameters of a culture's moral agenda. The learning of sex role imagery begins in infancy and continues throughout most of life. This learned behaviour, combined with personal experience, is internalised and becomes the individual's personal belief about sexuality.

Sexual behaviour
This refers to sexual expression and is the acting out of sexual feelings and beliefs. It includes a broad spectrum of human behaviour and varies from how one walks, to how and with whom one performs the sex act. For example, a person may choose to have sex with a member of the opposite sex or stay within his or her own sexual groups, whilst a range of various sexual aids may be incorporated into sexual behaviour.

These four aspects of sexuality are interrelated and reinforcing. Biological make-up and learning promote a core gender identity which influences acceptance of specific sex roles. Sexual expression reflects biology, gender identity, sex role and behaviour.

From: Walsh M 2002, p. 783.

In relation to (1) you may have discussed the way that female nurses in the past were not allowed to wear trousers in their working environment or the way in which female nurses have been seen as subservient to male doctors. The way in which nursing has always been seen as a traditionally female occupation has also had an effect on recruitment of men.

In relation to (2) you may have discussed how you find it difficult to imagine having sex with someone from your own sexual group, i.e. a man or woman, but that you know that it cannot be allowed to interfere with how you care for or treat patients. Stewart (1999) found that there were still some negative attitudes towards the diagnosis of AIDS 'but no longer with homosexuality' (see Box 12.8).

Clifford (2000) cites the following case study that demonstrates the importance of sensitivity to gay and lesbian people:

> *Alice, who was caring for her dying partner, spoke of the relief she felt when together they told one member of the hospice staff of their lesbian relationship. They wanted other staff to know and so gave their permission for the practitioner to inform her colleagues. Then, like other couples they could be supported by the staff, privacy was ensured and Alice shared in the intimate care of her loved one.* (Clifford 2000, p. 39)

Box 12.8 Research study

The threat of an AIDS epidemic in the early 1980s saw the emergence of strong negative attitudes from both the public and health care professionals alike. Certain 'high-risk' groups in society who were considered as susceptible to the disease, homosexuals and intravenous drug users in particular, became the victims of prejudice and discrimination. More recent research has indicated a possible shift to a more positive orientation, although the findings are far from conclusive. In this current study the Prejudicial Evaluation and Social Interaction Scale (PESIS) was administered to four separate cohorts of student nurses approximately a year apart in training (N = 192). Each cohort was divided into four groups, each one completing the PESIS after reading a version of a vignette that described either a person with AIDS or leukaemia and who was either homosexual or heterosexual. Overall the results showed that the student nurses held positive attitudes although they reported a significantly greater prejudice towards AIDS. No significant differences were found for sexual orientation. Additionally significantly greater levels of blame and responsibility were associated with the person with AIDS but again there was no effect for sexual orientation.

From: Stewart (1999) Journal of Advanced Nursing, 30(3): 740–748.

What is acceptable in one culture however may not be in another, and the sanctity of marriage between heterosexual partners makes it very difficult for gay and lesbian women and men to express themselves sexually. Henley and Schott (1999, p. 349) discuss the 'conflicting and irreconcilable pressures they face – which may become intolerable' and cite the following example of an extreme outcome.

> *A young Bengali man came under great pressure from his mother to marry and have children. She could think and talk of nothing else and said that if her son loved her he would agree to get married. People in the community were beginning to talk and she was ashamed among her friends, all of whom had married sons. The young man's partner, who was white, wanted him to leave home so that they could live openly together. He could not understand why the young man didn't just make up his mind and do what he wanted. If his mother didn't understand, that was her problem. Both the mother and the partner became more and more insistent. Eventually the young Bengali man committed suicide.* (Henley & Schott 1999, p. 349)

Being aware of sociocultural factors, such as beliefs and values, is essential if one is to ensure culturally appropriate care. Nowhere is this more clearly visible than in the attitudes and behaviour surrounding HIV/AIDS and Henley & Schott (1999, p. 349) state that 'negative attitudes, especially when combined with racism, place an unendurable burden on people who are coping with a fatal disease and who may already have watched loved ones die of infection.' They use the term 'double jeopardy' to describe the way in which people with HIV/AIDS who are also from a black or minority ethnic group are disadvantaged. They also point out that a new language (for previously taboo and secret aspects of our lives), has had to become socially acceptable and this will have implications for the assessment of patients and their needs (see Box 12.9).

How sexuality is expressed in both public and private spheres of our lives is also an influencing factor. For example, the sexual act between two consenting adults is one that is normally kept in the private sphere, except where it is portrayed in the media on film or in photographs. However even here there are standards and rules about what is acceptable and unacceptable behaviour, with pornography (obscene writings or publications intended to provide sexual excitement, usually produced commercially – Penguin Concise English Dictionary definition) being at the unacceptable end in most societies. This is especially the case of child pornography. Sex can also be work for many women and men – and 'those living in the "sex industry" are vulnerable to HIV/AIDS and other sexually transmitted diseases, as well as violence' (Roper et al 1996, p. 355).

There are laws however about sexual relations. It is still a criminal offence in some countries 'to have sexual relationship with a consenting adult of the same sex' but in some European countries prostitution has been decriminalised.

Box 12.9 Language and sexuality

Difficult terms

'Terms such as penetrative sex, anal sex, safer sex and condoms are now in common usage. Bisexuality and alternative sexual practices are talked about in ways that would have been unthinkable two decades ago. Nevertheless, many people, including many health professionals, find them embarrassing or distasteful and have difficulty in raising them or discussing them in a calm and objective way.

Language can even be more of an obstacle in more conservative communities. In most South Asian languages, for example, there are no socially acceptable words for parts of the body between the waist and the knees and no appropriate words other than offensive slang for different sexual identities and sexual activities. Where such words have not become at least partially accepted, it can be very difficult to discuss intimate personal and sexual matters.

In communities where homosexuality is strongly disapproved of, lack of vocabulary may not be the only problem. Men who have sexual relationships with men may simply not identify with words such as gay, homosexual or bisexual. It is important to think in terms of behaviour rather than categories, and to talk, for example, about 'men who have sex with men'.

From: Henley and Schott 1999.

Box 12.10 Methods of contraception

Spermicidal agents
- Foam, gels, jelly, pessaries suitable for use with barrier methods. Not adequate when used alone.

Barrier methods
- Condom
- Femidom (female condom)
- Cervical cap
- Diaphragm.

Hormonal contraception
- Oral contraceptive pills
- Depo-Provera injections
- Norplant system – recently discontinued but some women may have the system in place until 2004.

Intrauterine devices (IUDs)
- Mirena intrauterine system (progestogen-only intrauterine contraceptive device)
- Gyne T Slimline.

Surgical methods
- Tubal ligation
- Vasectomy.

Emergency contraception (EC)
- Yuzpe regime EC
- Progestogen-only EC
- IUD insertion.

From Walsh 2002 p. 811.

Incest on the other hand is a criminal offence, which may well be a reason for the underreporting of its occurrence. Rape is also deemed a criminal offence but, like incest, the number of victims who report the occurrence to the police is thought to be many less than the number of offences (Roper et al 1996, p. 356).

Government health policy on free contraceptives, morning-after pills and sexually transmitted diseases are examples of the way in which politicoeconomic factors influence our sexuality. They are issues however that are dealt with differently according to the country in which people live.

Exercise
1. Using the examples in Box 12.10 find out what contraceptives are freely available in your own country and consider the factors that influence their use.
2. What laws are there in your country regarding pornography, rape and homosexuality?
3. If you have met individuals involved in pornography or rape (both as victims and perpetrators) how did you manage to deal with your own feelings and undertake your role as either a student or qualified practitioner?
4. Discuss with your colleagues.

The World Health Organisation website (www.who.int) offers a valuable information resource that you can access to read research and opinion papers on a range of topics such as the following:

- violence against women – rape and sexual assault (July 1997).
- Module 4 – understanding sexual and reproductive health including HIV/AIDS and STDs among streetchildren – a training package in substance use, sexual and reproductive health including HIV/AIDS and STDs (www.who.int/substance_abuse/PDFfiles).

Summary points

1. Sexuality encompasses sexual knowledge, attitudes and behaviour and is shaped by our culture and family, education and personal experiences.
2. Adult sexuality encompasses biological sex, core gender identity, sex role imagery and sexual behaviour.
3. Education about sex and acceptable sexual behaviour is strongly influenced by the society in which people live.

THE MODEL FOR NURSING

Using the model to individualise nursing for the Activity of Living – expressing sexuality

In order to enhance your understanding of how health and illness affects this Activity of Living the next section will focus on specific case studies, and will utilise the Roper et al (1996, 2000) model for nursing as a framework to assess, plan, implement and evaluate nursing care (see Chapter 1 for full explanation of the nursing process).

Assessing the individual in the AL of expressing sexuality

It is important to remember that every individual must be considered 'holistically' and that expressing sexuality will be affected by health problems specific to other Activities of

---

Living. For example, if a patient is unable to move due to an accident causing paralysis then they may be unable to be dependent in expressing their sexuality. The summary of how lifespan, dependence/independence and factors affecting expressing sexuality can be seen in Box 12.11.

Assessing the individual

Assessment involves three phases:

- collection of data when taking a nursing history
- interpretation of the data collected
- identification of the individual's actual and potential health problems.

Collection of data when taking a nursing history

The nursing history will involve all Activities of Living and, as seen in Chapter 1, all must be taken into account in the holistic assessment of individuals.

If patient's expectations are to be understood and their problems (whether actual or potential) with this AL are to be addressed then assessment must be undertaken. A resume of topics addressed in relation to each of the components of the model is provided in Box 12.11 and will serve as a reminder of the many dimensions of the AL of expressing sexuality, which underpin nursing assessment. Examples of health problems which could affect the AL of expressing sexuality, can be seen in Box 12.12.

Assessment of the AL of expressing sexuality

When assessing the AL of expressing sexuality the following questions can be considered, which also take account of the whole life of the individual.

Lifespan

- How old is the person?
- Do they have a life history of health problems?
- Is there anything in their life history that may affect the way in which they view their present health problems?

Box 12.11 Assessing the individual for the AL of expressing sexuality

Lifespan
- Consider the effect of age on sexuality and sexual behaviour.

Dependence/independence
- Dependence is linked to lifespan and age, e.g. childhood
- Dependence is linked to specific needs, e.g. learning difficulties
- Ill health affects the dependence–independence balance, e.g. trauma, paralysis.

Factors affecting expressing sexuality
Biological
- Stage of physical sexual development
- Gender differences in body structure and function.

Psychological
- Attitudes to sexuality
- Emotional state
- Sexual orientation, e.g. homosexuality

Sociocultural
- Sociocultural similarities/differences
- Society views
- Media portrayal
- Sexual practices.

Environmental
- Home circumstances.

Politicoeconomic
- Legal factors, e.g. age of consent for sex
- Effects of work on sexual behaviour.

Adapted from Roper et al (1996).

Box 12.12 Health problems affecting the AL of expressing sexuality

Lifespan
Childhood congenital abnormalities, e.g. spina bifida.

Dependence–independence
For example rheumatoid arthritis, multiple sclerosis, paraplegia and tetraplegia, trauma.

Factors affecting health
For example breast cancer, surgery – leading to colostomy/ileostomy formation, HIV/AIDS, sexually transmitted infections, e.g. chlamydia, surgery – leading to hysterectomy, cervical cancer, testicular cancer, abortion/miscarriage, prostate problems.

Independence/dependence

- Has the individual experienced any difficulties in relation to independent living?
- Are they able to go out and meet other people or are they dependent on others to transport them?
- Will they experience difficulties in the future as a result of their current health problems?

Factors affecting the AL of expressing sexuality

- What specific health problem are they suffering from?
- What do they understand about their present health status?
- What effect is this having on their other Activities of Living?
- What effect is their health problem having on their emotional wellbeing?
- Are there any cultural needs to be taken into account prior to assessment?
- Are there any specific spiritual or religious needs that the patient may have?
- Does the individual have any environmental needs, which will affect future care?
- What resources could be required to help the individual manage their health problems both in hospital and at home?

Exercise

1. Reflect on how you have undertaken to assess individual needs in relation to the above questions in your practice to date.
2. Identify specific situations where you could include these in your assessment of the AL of expressing sexuality for individuals in your care.

Consider the following case study and using the same approach decide which questions would be appropriate in the assessment of his needs. Given the sensitive nature of his health problem these questions will have to be asked sensitively and with understanding.

Case study 12.2

Assessment focusing on the AL expressing sexuality

A young man, aged 24, arrives at the Accident and Emergency Department with painful micturition and a urethral discharge.

You may have decided to ask the following questions in relation to the ALs.

Questions as part of the assessment

- How long had he had the problem?
- Had he experienced anything like it before?
- What kind of pain is he experiencing?
- What helps the pain?
- What makes it worse?
- When did the problem start?
- Did the pain start at the same time as the discharge?
- Does the discharge smell?
- What does he think the problem is?

The above questions should highlight issues that may be an indication of whether he has experienced anything like this before and due to other health problems. From this a decision can then be made about this history, whether to continue with more sensitive questions around the young man's sexual behaviour that will be essential if the care he is to receive is appropriate.

Additional sensitive questions

- Has he had any sexual relations recently?
- If yes, when?
- Was this with a regular partner or not?
- Did they take precautions? E.g. condoms.
- Would he be willing for you take a swab for identification of any infection?

The following information may be helpful in caring for this young man and will indicate why these questions have been identified as relevant to his care.

Sexually transmitted diseases

Despite the increased availability of health education and protection during sexual activity the number of people with sexually transmitted diseases is not decreasing. Examples of sexually transmitted diseases, their signs and symptoms can be seen in Box 12.13.

Undertaking a health history is an essential part of any nursing assessment, and an understanding of the elements of the nursing model that comprise the living aspects will enable you to ensure that the questions directly affecting the young man's sexuality and sexual behaviour will be relevant. However what is not possible within this example is to identify how his other Activities of Living are affected by what is happening, due to the fact that we have no further information about his life and health. If it does indicate that he has a sexually transmitted disease then we can only surmise at how his life could be affected.

For example – his symptoms may prevent him from going to work or going out socially (working and playing), he has painful micturition (eliminating), he has a urethral discharge and will need to bathe more frequently than usual (personal cleansing and dressing). Understanding the physiological factors affecting sexual health will enable you to explain to him why he has painful micturition and a urethral discharge; understanding about the psychological factors will enable you to give him support to cope with having a sexually transmitted disease.

Box 12.13 Sexually transmitted diseases

Gonorrhoea

Cause of infection: *Neisseria gonorrhoea*. Transmitted almost exclusively by sexual intercourse.

Effects on the patient:

- Symptoms appear 3–7 days after initial content.
- Men may experience inflammation of the urethra (urethritis) and a purulent discharge. Some itching and burning around meatus is present, and urethral meatus is red and oedematous. Can be asymptomatic in 2% of men.
- If untreated an ascending infection of prostate, seminal vesicles, bladder and epididymis may occur.
- Diagnosis confirmed from smear taken from site of infection, e.g. endocervical, pharyngeal, rectal and urethra
- The female vagina is resistant to gonococcus, therefore vulnerable areas are vestibular glands, the urethra and endocervix. The glands become red, swollen and sore. A purulent discharge may drain from the urethra and ducts of the glands. Dysuria and frequency can occur. Fifty per cent of women may have vague and mild symptoms.
- Treatment: Penicillin or for drug-resistant strain – spectinomycin or a cephalosporin, e.g. ceftriaxone.
- Partner notification and treatment are required.

Chlamydia trachomatis

Cause of infection is a parasitic sexually transmitted infection of the reproductive tract.

- The woman may present with symptoms of increased vaginal discharge, intermenstrual spotting and vague pelvic pain. Unfortunately the woman is often asymptomatic and the infection may go unnoticed and untreated for several years.
- Chlamydia is a common cause of pelvic inflammatory disease as well as an increasing cause of infertility.
- Diagnosis is confirmed via an endocervical swab for cells using a Chlamydia-specific antigen swab.
- Doxycycline 100 mg twice daily for 7 days is an effective treatment. Azithromycin, one 1 mg tablet by mouth provides an equally effective cure and significantly reduces patient error regarding compliance.
- Sexual partners of the woman require treatment as well.

Human papillomavirus infection (HPV)

Cause of infection is condylomata acuminata or genital warts. Previously thought to be benign but recently associated with several genital cancers in both men and women.

- Risk factors for acquiring the virus are early age at first intercourse (less than 17 years old), multiple sex partners, a history of sexually transmitted diseases, poor personal and sexual hygiene, a sexual partner with similar history, a history of anal intercourse, and immunosuppressive drugs or immunodeficiency for any reason. Sexual intercourse is the method of transmission.
- The infection may be silent.

- Those presenting with external warts will be screened for other sexually transmitted diseases and if present they will be treated.
- A colposcopy examination and smear tests will be done and the partners of infected patients should also be examined and treated if necessary.
- Treatment: external warts are treated with podophyllin 10–25% in tincture of bezoin. This caustic agent is applied with a cotton applicator and washed off in 4 hours. The surrounding skin is coated with petroleum jelly before application of the podophyllin. It is not used on internal warts. Cervical and vaginal warts may be bathed in an 85% solution of trichloracetic acid. This produces a stinging sensation; a vaginal discharge follows for about 1 week as the tissue sloughs away.

Syphilis

Cause of infection is the spirochaete *Trepenoma pallidium*. It is a serious disease – less common than gonorrhoea.

- Incubation varies between 10 and 90 days. In most cases the disease is spread by sexual intercourse. It does not survive outside the host.
- In the untreated condition three stages are distinguished.
- Primary lesion – small painless chancre or ulcer. It is deep and has indurated edges. Usually this heals spontaneously giving the false impression that the disease is cured. It appears most commonly on the penis of the male and the labia, vagina or cervix in the female.
- Secondary stage – usually characterised by a rash appearing all over the body. This may be accompanied by condylomata lata on the female vulva. This is a cauliflower-appearing collection of flat grey vulval warts. As are all lesions of syphilis they are teeming with spriochaetes and are highly infectious. The rash is usually accompanied by fever and malaise. This soon regresses and patient enters latent stage (absence of symptoms). Three outcomes now possible: patient enters third stage immediately or after delay of 10–30 years; the disease remains latent for the rest of person's life; or a spontaneous cure occurs.
- In the tertiary stage – bones, heart and central nervous system, including the brain can be affected. Personality disorders arise and typical ataxic gait of the tertiary syphilitic appears. A large ulcerating necrotic lesion known as a gamma now occurs.
- Treatment: penicillin is drug of choice (usually by injection as oral medication is not effective).

Human immunosuppressive virus infection (HIV)

Cause of infection (can occur through non-sexual contact) is human immunodeficiency virus, which causes damage to the immune system. It is associated with a spectrum of disease ultimately presenting as acquired immune deficiency syndrome (AIDS).

Box 12.13 *(continued)*

- The virus infects the cells – primary target is T4 or T helper cells of the immune system–and destroys them. The body's immune system is weakened making the individual prone to a variety of opportunistic infections, malignant diseases and neuropsychiatric complications.
- HIV transmitted by sexual intercourse, inoculation of infected body fluids through skin or onto mucous membranes, transplantation of tissues and transfusion of contaminated blood. HIV may also be transmitted from mother to baby either through the placenta or during delivery. Transmission of HIV has occurred through blood, semen, vaginal fluids and occasionally breast milk.
- Symptoms: some people may develop an acute illness 2–6 weeks after infection. Symptoms include fever, myalgia, arthralgia, headache, diarrhoea, sore throat, lymphadenopathy and a maculopapular rash.
- It is estimated that 40% of HIV-infected individuals will have developed AIDS 8 years after antibodies to the virus in the blood are found (seroconversion), 95% after 15 years.
- The most common opportunistic infection in individuals with AIDS is *Pneumocystis carinii.* The most common neoplasm is Kaposi's sarcoma, which is most likely to develop in homosexual or bisexual men.
- Treatment: antiviral drugs can work at several points in the life cycle of the virus. Azidothynidine (AZT) is the most widely used. The development of a vaccine to prevent HIV infection remains to be achieved.

Adapted from Walsh 2002, pp. 790–791.

Exercise

1. Given the information about the young man's health problem and taking into consideration the above issues, identify a plan of action for his care, both during and after being seen by the doctor in the Accident and Emergency department.
2. What confidentiality issues will you need to consider when planning any care or treatment for this man?

Summary points

1. Expressing sexuality is affected by lifespan, dependence–independence and biological, psychological, sociocultural, environmental and politicoeconomic factors.
2. Assessment of patient/client in the daily activity of expressing sexuality needs a holistic approach.
3. Sensitive questioning is essential in caring for patients with health problems related to expressing sexuality.

APPLICATION OF THE ROPER, LOGAN AND TIERNEY MODEL IN PRACTICE

Using the information in the previous section of this chapter we will now explore how the model can be used in the care of two patients who have a health problem, which affects the AL of expressing sexuality.

Case study 12.3

Focus on health problem in the AL of expressing sexuality (an evidence-based total care approach)

Razia Bibi, a 40-year-old woman is admitted to the gynaecology ward for a hysterectomy.

Health history

Following attendance at an Asian Well Women's Clinic a cervical smear revealed that she had cervical cancer, which had invaded the upper vaginal wall (Stage 2 carcinoma). She had been complaining of irregular vaginal bleeding, associated with sexual intercourse and a vaginal examination by a woman doctor had also revealed an ulcerated area on the cervix. A vaginal discharge was also present and this was now offensive. She was very upset by her symptoms and she had found it very difficult to tell her husband about her problems, especially as it affected her ability to help out in the family shop. This was her first cervical smear.

Her oldest daughter Nafisa, aged 22, had noticed her mother was not well and had advised her to go to the clinic for help. She had attended with her. Razia had five other children aged 20, 16, 14, 9 and 4. All were boys except the oldest and the youngest. She had tried to use the intrauterine contraceptive device (IUCD) after her fifth child but had to have it removed due to it causing increased bleeding at menstruation. Since her last child she has also begun to experience some urinary incontinence – when coughing or sneezing. This has added to her stress about the cancer and need for surgery.

On admission

Razia Bibi was visibly distressed on arrival on the ward with her eldest daughter. Although her mother did not speak much English Nafisa offered to translate.

Case study 12.3 (continued)

She was a trainee interpreter at another hospital, but also worked in her father's clothes shop. She was interested in health care. She explained that her mother was worried about her children and who would take care of them whilst she was in hospital, and also if anything should happen to her.

Exercise

Before assessing her needs on admission identify what issues would need to be considered in relation to:

- lifespan
- dependence–independence
- factors affecting sexuality.

Refer to section 1 of this chapter for examples.

The following may have considered .

Lifespan

Razia Bibi is a Muslim woman and as such will have been subject to the beliefs and expectations of her culture. In certain Muslim communities men and women are segregated (purdah) but the degree of segregation varies. Henley and Schott (1999) state that:

> *In some Muslim families and communities in Britain, though not all, strict purdah is regarded by both men and women as the right way to live, and is a matter of pride and family honour. A good husband is expected to try to enable his wife to live in purdah. Many women in these families rarely leave their homes, going out only to visit other family members, either on foot or by car (rarely by public transport). Family visits are often a very important part of their role, and at certain times – illness, a death, a birth, a wedding – visiting is an absolute obligation.*

(Henley & Schott 1999, p. 513).

This need for male–female segregation will affect her communication with the wider social community, in particular the health service. We have seen that she has attended an Asian Well Woman's clinic rather than a general one but not all Asian women will be able to do this. This service may not be available in other local communities. We have also seen that her eldest daughter does not stay home all the time, preferring instead to work in the interpreting service, which will bring her into contact with men and women from other cultures.

Beliefs about menstruation will have a major impact in relation to her care needs and nurses need to be aware of these in order to be able to explain the outcomes of having a hysterectomy on her daily life. For example, Dahmi and Sheikh (2000, p. 51) point out that:

> *Whilst menstruating, women are exempt from some of the important religious rites, such as ritual prayer, fasting and Hajj. Sexual intercourse is prohibited at such times. All other forms of physical contact between husband and wife for example, hugging and kissing are allowed. A period therefore may have a number of social and psychological ramifications. There are also a number of possible implications for clinical care. Women may be reluctant to attend for gynaecological symptoms, cervical smear tests or coil checks for fear of bleeding following pelvic examination. Many Muslim women are unaware that traumatic bleeding of this kind is quite distinct from menstrual bleeding and hence the same religious constraints do not apply.*

The impact of no longer having menstrual periods will therefore be very significant to Razia Bibi's daily life as a Muslim woman.

Dependence–independence

Razia Bibi is obviously very dependent on her daughter in relation to health problems and communication with health professionals. She needs to have a good relationship with her daughter to ensure that her feelings and concerns are respected and that these are translated to the health care team. Any matter relating to sex is normally taboo to anyone other than between husband and wife (Dahmi & Sheikh 2000). She will become dependent on her carers once she is admitted to hospital and this dependency will vary during the perioperative period until her discharge home and postdischarge.

Factors affecting sexuality

Beliefs about how her body works will be an important aspect for the nurse to determine as this will in turn influence how the intended surgery and its outcomes will be understood by Razia Bibi. We have already seen (p. 355) the beliefs of Asian women in regards to the menopause and undergoing a hysterectomy will expose her to potentially stressful situations in many areas or daily living activities. For example, personal cleansing and dressing and elimination.

The psychological impact of having a hysterectomy on her as a woman who could still have more children will need to be considered as well as her understanding of the short- and long-term impact of cervical cancer. Her home circumstances (environmental factors) will need to be considered in order to be able to plan effective discharge. How she will manage when she leaves hospital will be an important issue to consider. Her religious and cultural beliefs will also be an important factor in her care.

Assessment of Razia Bibi's needs

Using this knowledge of her background and potential influencing factors you can now assess her individual needs on admission to hospital (use the questions on pp. 361–362 as a framework).

Collection of data on admission

> **Exercise**
> Using the 12 Activities of Living as a framework identify Razia Bibi's actual problems on admission to the ward.

McQueen (2000, p. 242) states that:

> " *The patient who is to have a hysterectomy for carcinoma of the cervix will be admitted to the ward with enough time to allow for necessary medical investigative procedures to be carried out before the operation. She is likely to be physically fairly independent of the nurse for her personal care but will need to be introduced to the new surroundings of the ward.* "

Ensuring a safe environment in which to carry out the initial assessment of Razia Bibi's needs will be an important aspect of the nurse's role. You will need to ensure that privacy is maintained as well as ensuring comfortable seating for both Razia Bibi, her daughter and the nurse. Ensuring confidentiality during the assessment interview is also an essential aspect of care (see NMC 2002 Code of Professional Conduct – Chapter 2). The assessment of her needs at various stages of her care will now be explored using an evidence-based approach.

Activities of Living – evidence-based approach
Expressing sexuality

It is important that the date of the last menstrual period is determined as Razia Bibi could be pregnant. She has tried to use an intrauterine coil and may no longer be taking precautions. Sensitive questioning will be required in relation to sexual activity between her and her husband. Her daughter who has been interpreting may not wish to know about this aspect of her parents' lives and it may be that another interpreter unconnected with the family might be recommended. It is also important to know what kind of vaginal discharge she has been having and how she has been managing to cope with it. This can be either physiological (i.e. normal) or pathological (Sutherland 2001). Physiological discharge can increase in certain circumstances, such as during pregnancy (leucorrhoea), sexual arousal or premenstrually. Pathological discharge is caused by either infective (e.g. chlamydia, *Candida albicans* (thrush) or gonorrhoea) or noninfective causes (e.g. cervical polyp, cervical cancer, 'lost tampon' or condom).

Sutherland (2001, p. 323) suggests the following questions might be asked of a woman to determine its origins:

- How is it different from normal?
- Why is she worried about it?
- Are there any other associated symptoms (dysuria, soreness, intermenstrual bleeding, pelvic discomfort)?
- Has anything happened to make her vagina less acidic (is she overwashing with strong soaps using disinfectant in the bath, douching, is she menopausal)?

- Does it have a characteristic smell?
- Does she have any reason to be worried about sexually transmitted infection?
- Has she treated herself unsuccessfully with an over-the-counter preparation?

It is apparent from these possible questions that not all of them will be applicable to Razia Bibi, given her overall history and her personal circumstances and cultural background. Sensitivity will be required in both the questioning approach taken and the phrasing of the questions themselves.

Most importantly will be Razia Bibi's understanding of the surgery to be undertaken, i.e. the hysterectomy, and its outcome. This is essential for consent to surgery and for postoperative care. Rodgers (2000) states that:

> " *The nurse has an important role to play in obtaining consent prior to surgery. For a patient to give valid consent she must comprehend fully what she is consenting to, i.e. her consent must be informed. The nurse can provide the team with knowledge of the patient's individual need for information and her comprehension of the information given. The nurse will also provide the patient with information about the procedure and the recovery period and may be able to clarify points previously discussed between the patient and the doctor. However the nurse cannot and must not be the provider of information in order for the doctor to obtain informed consent for surgery. This is a medical staff responsibility.* " (Rogers 2000, p. 804)

Actual problem Razia Bibi has cervical cancer and requires surgery for its removal.

Communication

From the case study information it can be seen that Razia Bibi does not speak much English and needs her daughter to interpret for her. She will however not be able to interpret throughout Razia Bibi's stay in hospital as she has her own commitments. Other alternatives will have to be found to ensure her communication needs are met. It can also be seen that she has been unable to talk to her husband about her health problems and their effect on herself and her family. It is important that nurses do not rely on families interpreting for their relatives, as this can cause both embarrassment for the patient and also can lead to misinterpretation (Gerrish et al 1996). Trained interpreters/translators, familiar with medical terminology and the health service as well as language should be available in these circumstances. However these are not always available when needed (Robinson 2002).

Actual problem
- She is unable to communicate her self-concerns.
- She is unable to converse in English with the nurse and other members of the health care team.
- She is unable to talk to her husband about her problems.
- She is visibly distressed on her admission to the ward.

Working and playing

She normally works in her husband's shop but as her illness has become problematic she is no longer able to do this. This may have caused an increase in her stress, especially following the diagnosis of cervical cancer and its implications for the future. Her health problems, especially the offensive vaginal discharge, may also have affected her going out and meeting with other women in her community. These have also begun to affect how she takes care of her family. An understanding of how important all these are to women in an Asian culture is essential if care is to be individualised and culture specific.

Actual problem

- She is unable to play an active part in her family's care.
- She is unable to take an active part in her husband's business.

Personal cleansing and dressing

Razia may be dressed in traditional Muslim clothes – either a shalwar (trousers), kameez (long shirt) and a chuni or dupatta (long scarf) which covers her head, mouth and nose (Holland & Hogg 2001), or if a Bangladeshi woman, a 'sari worn over a waist-length blouse and a long underskirt' (Karmi 1996, p. 56). She will need to be reassured that she can continue to wear these during her stay in hospital. She may be very concerned that she will have to wear a hospital gown that exposes parts of her body that she normally keeps hidden. Again reassurance on admission is crucial.

Razia is very upset by her symptoms, in particular the offensive vaginal discharge. As a Muslim woman she will already have a washing and cleansing routine, and will need to be assured that there will be running water available for her daily needs. Alternatives will have to be found when she is recovering postoperatively.

Actual problem

- Razia has concerns regarding removal of her clothes for examination and going to theatre.
- Razia has an offensive vaginal discharge.

Dying

It is important to determine on admission what she has been told about her illness and what she understands about it. Even though death is seen as marking 'the transition from one state of existence to the next' and inevitable as part of our acts of living (Sheikh and Gatrad 2000), Razia may still be fearful for her family and her children – as she is a relatively young woman. She will need to maintain her daily prayers and may also wish to do this in the company of her family.

Actual problem Razia is anxious regarding opportunities and facilities for daily prayers.

Elimination

Razia has recently begun to experience urinary incontinence problems, which have added to her distress and concerns she has for the impending surgery. An explanation that she may well have a catheter in place may be necessary, exposing her to further personal distress due to invasion of her body and dignity.

Actual problem Razia has urinary incontinence when she sneezes or coughs.

Summary

The above problems in some Activities of Living can be determined from the information offered in the case study. However, during the admission assessment and obtaining further information from Razia Bibi and her daughter, other actual problems may become apparent in the other activities. The kind of questions which will highlight these can be found in the other specific chapters, e.g. breathing. It is also important to acknowledge the involvement of the multidisciplinary team in her care, and how an integrated care approach would be an appropriate way of managing her stay in hospital and postdischarge. Following the assessment stage, care planning would be undertaken, along with the setting of patient and nurse goals (see Chapter 1). Priority for the nurse will be to prepare Razia for theatre (see Chapter 3 for a more detailed account of preoperative preparation of a patient).

Preoperative care of Razia Bibi

Exercise

1. Using the 12 Activities of Living as a framework identify Razia Bibi's needs and potential problems prior to going to theatre. (**NB.** We cannot predict her actual problems as she is an individual with her own life history – reality would be different – we can only offer some potential problems that she may experience.)

Potential problems in the preoperative period will take account of the actual problems already identified on admission and will focus mainly on physiological and psychological needs.

Razia will:

- need to know what the surgery is going to mean to her afterwards in order to ensure that her consent to the surgery is based on all the facts (informed consent)
- need to know that removing her uterus will mean that she is no longer able to have children
- need to be reassured about her privacy and dignity during the operation
- need to be physically prepared for going to the operating theatre for surgery.

2. Using the model for nursing and the Activities of Living identify the physical preparation Razia Bibi will require prior to surgery.

The following may have to be considered.

- preoperative fasting
- skin preparation, e.g. shaving (as above)
- elimination – suppositories/bladder
- personal care
- medication – writing in notes
- baseline observations – temperature, blood pressure, pulse, urinalysis and weight.

3. Determine what care she will receive during the intraoperative period – from her leaving the ward to returning. You need to consider the following stages: Operating theatre transfer; receiving the patient in the anaesthetic room; anaesthesia; patient care in the main theatre; patient care in the recovery area; immediate postoperative management and transfer back to the ward.

4. Using the 12 Activities of Living framework identify the potential problems Razia Bibi is likely to experience following an abdominal hysterectomy (again it is difficult to predict actual problems – but we can offer all potential problems in the postoperative period).

The following may also have been considered.

Continuing postoperative care

Razia will have had major abdominal surgery with all that it entails (Table 12.2 indicates the type of patient problems that could occur in the postoperative period).

1. *Maintaining a safe environment*
   - postoperative observations
   - pain relief
   - handover from theatre nurse
   - wound care.

2. *Communication*
   - reduce anxiety
   - interpreter service
   - talk to relatives.

3. *Elimination*
   - urine output (catheterised for 1–2 days)
   - bowel movement.

4. *Breathing*
   - maintaining clear airway
   - deep breathing exercises – physiotherapy
   - pulmonary embolism, etc.

5. *Personal cleansing and dressing*
   - oral hygiene and inability to meet own hygiene needs
   - pressure area care.

6. *Mobility*
   - restricted mobility.

7. *Sleeping*
   - interrupted sleep pattern due to surgery.

8. *Controlling body temperature*
   - postoperative stress
   - risk of infection.

9. *Dying*
   - concerns regarding the cervical cancer and its removal
   - need to take account of religious/spiritual practices.

10. *Working and playing*
    - concerns regarding her inability to be at home helping the family.

11. *Expressing sexuality*
    - concerns re: future sex life, inability to have children, perceptions of her womanhood, etc.
    - body image.

12. *Eating and drinking*
    - fluid intake/output
    - bowel action
    - dietary needs – cultural preferences.

Nursing interventions during this period can be summarised as follows:

1. 'promote comfort and control pain
2. maintain fluid and electrolyte balance and adequate nutrition
3. assist a return to normal patterns of elimination
4. encourage increasing levels of activity
5. promote wound healing
6. maintain ventilation
7. maintain circulation
8. decrease patient anxiety
9. prepare patient for discharge and self management' (Brown 2002, p. 182)

Evaluation of postoperative care

Brown (2002, p. 190) suggests the following criteria may be included in determining successful outcomes of care:

1. The patient is free from pain and discomfort, as shown by verbal expression and participation in physical activities and ability to rest and sleep.
2. The fluid intake and electrolyte concentrations are normal for the patient.
3. The patient is taking a nutritionally balanced diet.
4. Urinary and bowel elimination are re-established and normal for the patient.
5. The patient is ambulatory, active and participating in care.
6. The incision is clean, dry and intact.

Table 12.2 Potential problems common to the patient after operation (Walsh 2002, p.183)

Problem	Causative factors	Goals
Pain	Surgical intervention Nausea and vomiting Abdominal distension Anxiety	The patient will state he or she is free from pain
Dehydration and electrolyte imbalance	Decreased oral intake Fluid loss during surgery via drainage tubes Altered gastrointestinal activity	Minimum fluid intake of 2.4 litres per day Electrolytes within normal limits
Alternation in patterns of elimination	Decreased fluid volume Immobility Pain Surgical intervention Altered sensation	Patient will return to normal pattern of elimination once bowel function returns
Reduced mobility	Pain and discomfort Weakness Immobility	Short term. Patient will sit out of bed within 4–12 h; will not develop complications of immobility (deep vein thrombosis, pressure sores, chest infection); will walk to the bathroom within 4–12 h (with assistance)
Potential for infection	Decreased level of consciousness Inadequate airway clearance Decreased sensations Impaired skin integrity Decreased mobility	No infection will occur and wound will heal without complications
Inadequate respiration	Respiratory irritation from anaesthesia Pain and discomfort Decreased mobility	Respiratory rate 12–20 per minute; breathing to be of normal depth and pattern
Inadequate circulation	Effects of anaesthetic Surgical intervention Increased fluid loss Decreased mobility	BP systolic > 90 mmHg; pulse regular, within range 60–90 b.p.m
Anxiety	Fear of unknown Lack of knowledge Pain and discomfort Diagnosis	The patient is able to talk about concerns and fears
Insufficient knowledge about health care	Lack of knowledge and skill	The patient will verbalize an understanding of the factors involved in improving health after discharge

7. Vital signs are normal for the patient.
8. No manifestations of complications are present.
9. The patient and family demonstrate an understanding of the required care during convalescence and the resources available.

It is important to remember, however, that every patient is an individual and Razia Bibi's pathway following a hysterectomy, and any potential problems she might experience, will be unique to her.

Discharge home and follow up

Well-planned and effective discharge planning will be essential in ensuring Razia Bibi's postoperative recovery and wellbeing (Rodgers 2000, p. 827). Patients who have had major surgery no longer have a prolonged stay in hospital.

A referral may need to be made to the district nurse team and she will need a follow-up appointment to return to the out-patient clinic, e.g. 6 weeks following discharge home from hospital.

Exercise

1. Consider your clinical practice experience to date. How many of the health problems seen in Box 12.12 have you come across?
2. How did you assess, plan, implement and evaluate care in the AL of expressing sexuality for individuals who were experiencing these health problems?
3. Focus on one of these and identify what you did well and what you found difficult to deal with in your care of the patient.

Summary points

> 1. An awareness and understanding of cultural needs is essential in ensuring culturally appropriate care in relation to expressing sexuality and sexual health.
> 2. Health problems affecting the Activity of Living expressing sexuality can be seen to be interdependent on other Activities of Living.
> 3. The nurse needs effective assessment and communication skills to be able to plan care and implement care that is evidence based.

Case study 12.4

Myocardial infarction and expressing sexuality

This will focus on a health problem not directly connected to the AL of expressing sexuality – but one which has major implications for assessment of need in relation to the individual's specific sexual functioning: a patient who has experienced a myocardial infarction.

Case study
Mr John Eaves is a 55-year-old man, recovering from a myocardial infarction and he is transferred to a ward from the Coronary Care Unit (CCU) where he has been a patient for 3 days.

Health history
He is overweight and has smoked 20 cigarettes a day prior to admission. His wife is 40 years of age and they have three children – aged 18, 14 and 12. His wife uses the contraceptive pill but she now wants to stop and to use other means instead. He is worried that she could get pregnant again and this together with worrying about not having sex in case he puts more strain on his heart is already creating some tensions between them. He has been transferred to the ward after spending 3 days in the Coronary Care Unit. During his stay there he had one cardiac arrest but was successfully resuscitated. He has a vague memory of the event but realises he is vulnerable to further cardiac arrests.

Exercise
Before assessing his needs on admission to the ward consider what knowledge you will need with regards to myocardial infarction (MI) and the care of patients following MI.

The following may have been considered.

- knowledge of the anatomy and physiology of the heart
- knowledge of what happens when a myocardial infarction occurs – to the heart itself and to the rest of the patient's physiological systems
- current evidence-based practice in caring for patients who have had an MI
- current medication and treatments for MI
- knowledge of care from admission to discharge home and rehabilitation programmes postMI.

Factors affecting expressing sexuality following an MI

Rutter (2000c, p. 216) points out that:

> ❝ *Myocardial infarction (MI) is often thought of as a male illness but more post-menopausal women die each year from MI than from breast cancer. Sudden death during sexual intercourse is often a great anxiety for men and women with a diagnosis of heart disease or hypertension, but such death is very rare. However many people who survive MI suffer psychological damage that affects the quality of their lives by affecting self-confidence and their sexuality. Some patients are still anxious and depressed and have sexual problems 1 year following the heart attack. They feel fragile and vulnerable and this dampens sexual arousal and contributes to a fear of resumption of sexual intercourse which will have an impact on the partner and may lead to frustration.* ❞

Mr Eaves may well experience similar feelings and thoughts as he begins to recover from his MI. Other factors such as his beliefs about his age and his wife's may add to his concerns – she no longer wants to take precautions by taking the contraceptive pill which means that he has to take more responsibility to prevent further pregnancies. Given his illness and the need for a period of rehabilitation following his MI the added fear of becoming dependent on his wife could add to the tensions, i.e. there will be a period of time when he is unable to go to work. Worries about this together with when to safely resume sexual activity will need sensitive discussion with Mr Eaves, and his wife, before he is discharged home from hospital. Muller et al (1996) undertook a major study examining the sexual activity of post-MI patients and concluded that 'although baseline risk of MI is increased, sexual activity has now been documented to have a low likelihood of triggering an MI' (see Box 12.14 for details of study).

Assessment of needs on transfer from CCU – directly related to the AL of expressing sexuality

Expressing sexuality may not be the priority problem that Mr Eaves identifies – he has been near to death in the CCU

Box 12.14 Sexual activity and myocardial infarction – an abstract

Synopsis

A total of 1774 patients with myocardial infarction (MI) served as the basis for this study. In this group 858 (48%) were sexually active in the year prior to their MI. Nine percent reported sexual activity in the 24 hours preceding the MI and 3% reported sexual activity in the 2 hours preceding the MI. The relative risks of an MI occurring in the 2 hours after sexual activity were 2.5. That risk decreased from 3.0 for those who did not exercise heavily and to 1.2 for those who exercised heavily three or more times a week. There were too few women who reported sexual activity in the 2-hour hazard period preceding MI to determine if the relative risk varied by sex.

The authors concluded that sexual activity can trigger the onset of an MI. The relative risk is low. The absolute risk caused by sexual activity is also extremely low (one chance in a million for a healthy individual).

Commentary

The present study provides information of great value for counselling more than 500 000 patients who survive an MI each year and the 11 million patients with existing cardiac disease. Counselling has often been ineffective in decreasing the fear of triggering a cardiac event. With these data, health care professionals counselling patients can reassure them that although their baseline risk of MI is increased, sexual activity has now been documented to have a low likelihood of triggering an MI. The risk is particularly low for patients who engage in regular exercise. Based on these data physicians should encourage patients with known coronary heart disease to participate in a cardiac rehabilitation programme and perform regular exercises. Such exercise can decrease the cardiac work required for sexual activity and reduce the risk of triggering the onset of an MI.

From: Muller et al 1996, p. 10. (www.ingenta.com).

---

and suffered a cardiac arrest – although he does not remember much about the event. His main problems may arise from a realisation that he could have prevented the onset of the MI, by not being so overweight and not smoking. The nurses will have to cope with withdrawal symptoms of not being able to smoke, resulting in further tension and stress because he is unable to smoke.

As can be seen in his health history, Mr Eaves has already expressed some concerns regarding sexual activity postMI which could be linked to concerns that his wife is much younger than him and that he should still be sexually active.

Exercise

What are the nursing priorities in caring for Mr Eaves with regards to his wellbeing and his concerns regarding sexual activities?

In order to consolidate learning to use the model for nursing as a framework for care undertake the following exercise.

Exercise

1. Identify a patient/client with a health problem directly related to the AL of expressing sexuality.
2. Devise a care plan for this patient – using the documentation found in the appendices or one that is familiar to you.

Conclusion

Expressing sexuality and sexual health is essential for well-being, but how this is managed will depend on the culture and society in which we live. The case studies in this chapter have demonstrated some of the issues and problems facing patients who have illnesses that have either a direct or indirect impact on sexuality and sexual behaviour. Using a framework for care, such as the Roper et al (1996, 2000) model of living and model for nursing, has ensured that a holistic approach was taken to identifying actual and potential problems in a systematic way.

Summary points

1. Sexual activity can be affected by indirect health problems in other Activities of Living, e.g. myocardial infarction.
2. Professional counselling might be necessary for some patients who experience either short- or long-term problems in expressing sexuality as a result of illness.
3. It is important to remember that partners need support in coping with illnesses that affect their sexual relationships.

References

Adams G 1976 Recognising the range of human sexual needs and behaviour. American Journal of Maternal Child Nursing 6: 166–169

Abernathy K 1997 The menopause. In: Andrews G (ed) Women's sexual health, pp. 336–364. Baillière Tindall, London

Alexander MF, Fawcett JN, Runciman PJ (eds) 2000 Nursing Practice Hospital and Home – The Adult, 2nd edn. Churchill Livingstone, Edinburgh

Atkinson J 2000 The person with HIV/AIDS. In: Alexander MF, Fawcett JN, Runciman PJ (eds) Nursing practice – hospital and home (the adult). Churchill Livingstone, Edinburgh

Baltes PB, Staudinger UM, Lindenburger U 1999 Lifespan psychology: theory and application to intellectual functioning. Annual Review of Psychology 50: 471–507

Brown A 2002 The patient undergoing surgery. In: Walsh (ed) Watson's clinical nursing and related sciences, 6th edn. pp. 65–192. Baillière Tindall/Royal College of Nursing, London

Burnet KL 2000 The reproductive systems and the breast: Part 2 The breast. In: Alexander MF, Fawcett JN, Runciman PJ (eds) Nursing practice – hospital and home (the adult), pp. 278–311. Churchill Livingstone, Edinburgh

Carlisle D 1998 HIV and breast feeding: a global issue for midwives. RMC Midwives Journal 1(3): 78–80

Cifford D 2000 Professional awareness in psychosexual care. In: Wells D (ed) Caring for sexuality in health and illness. Churchill Livingstone, Edinburgh

Davis DL 1986 The meaning of menopause in a Newfoundland fishing village. In: Morse JM (ed) Qualitative health research. Sage, London

Dhami S, Sheikh A 2000 The family: predicament and promise. In: Gatrad AR, Sheikh A (eds) Caring for Muslim patients. Radcliffe Medical Press Ltd, Oxford

Department of Health 2000 National sexual health and HIV strategy. DoH, London (www.doh.giv.uk/nshs)

Gerrish K, Husband C, Mackenzie J 1996 Nursing for a multi-ethnic society. Open University Press, Buckingham

Golub S 1992 Periods: from menarch to menopause. Sage, London

Greer G 1991 The change, women, ageing and the menopause. Hamish Hamilton, London

Henley A, Schott J 1999 Culture, religion and patient care in a multi-ethnic society. Age Concern England, London

Hinchliff SM, Montague SE, Watson R 1996 Physiology for nursing practice. Baillière Tindall, London

Holland K, Hogg C 2001 Cultural awareness in nursing and health care. Arnold, London

Jamison JR 2002 Maintaining health in primary care – a guide for wellness in the 21st century. Churchill Livingstone, Edinburgh

Karmi G 1996 The Ethnic Health Handbook. Blackwell Science, Oxford

La Fontaine JS 1985 Initiation. Penguin Books, Harmondsworth

Mayor V 1996 Asian women and the menopause. In: Webb C (ed) Living sexuality – issues for nursing and health. Baillière Tindall, London

McCann E 2000 The expression of sexuality in people with psychosis: breaking the taboos. Journal of Advanced Nursing 32(1): 132–138

McQueen ACH 2000 The reproductive systems and the breast: Part 1 the reproductive system. In: Alexander MF, Fawcett JN, Runciman PJ (eds) Nursing practice – hospital and home (the adult), pp. 219–278. Churchill Livingstone, Edinburgh

Mok J 1993 HIV-1 infection, breast milk and HIV-1 transmission. Lancet 341: 941

Muller J, Mittleman M, Maclure M, Sherwood J, Tofler G 1996 Sexual activity and myocardial infarction. ACOG Clinical Review 1(5): 10

Nursing and Midwifery Council 2002 Code of professional conduct. NMC, London

Robinson M 2002 Communication and health in a multi-ethnic society. The Policy Press, Bristol

Rodgers SE 2000 The patient facing surgery: In: Alexander MF, Fawcett JN, Runciman PJ (eds) Nursing practice – hospital and home (the adult), pp. 799–831. Churchill Livingstone, Edinburgh

Roper N, Logan W, Tierney A 1996 The elements of nursing, 4th edn. Churchill Livingstone, Edinburgh

Roper N, Logan W, Tierney A 2000 The Roper, Logan, Tierney model of nursing. Churchill Livingstone, Edinburgh

Rutter M 2000a Becoming a sexual person. In: Wells D (ed) Caring for sexuality in health and illness, pp. 151–170. Churchill Livingstone, Edinburgh

Rutter M 2000b Life experiences and transitions in adolescence and adulthood. In: Wells D (ed) Caring for sexuality in health and illness, pp. 189–206. Churchill Livingstone, Edinburgh

Rutter M 2000c The impact on illness on sexuality. In: Wells D (ed) Caring for sexuality in health and illness. Churchill Livingstone, Edinburgh

Schott J, Henley A 1996 Culture, religion and childbearing in a multi-cultural society. Butterworth-Heinemann, Oxford

Selfe L 2000 The urinary system. In: Alexander MF, Fawcett JN, Runciman PJ (eds) Nursing practice – hospital and home (the adult), pp. 313–348. Churchill Livingstone, Edinburgh

Sheikh A, Gatrad AR (eds) 2000 Caring for Muslim patients. Radcliffe Medical Press Ltd, Oxford

Stewart D 1999 The attitudes and attributions of student nurses: do they alter according to a person's diagnosis or sexuality and what is the effect of nurse training? Journal of Advanced Nursing 30(3): 740–748

Stuart GW, Sundeen SJ 1979 Principles and practice of psychiatric nursing. CV Mosby, St Louis

Sutherland C 2001 Women's health – a handbook for nurses. Churchill Livingstone, Edinburgh

United Nations Programme on HIV/AIDS 2002 Children on the brink 2002. UNAIDS (www.unaids.org/youngpeople/index.html)

Waugh A, Grant A 2001 Ross and Wilson anatomy and physiology in health and illness. Churchill Livingstone, Edinburgh

Walsh 2002 (ed) Watson's clinical nursing and related Sciences, 6th edn. Baillière Tindall/Royal College of Nursing, London

Wells D 1999 Transitions: healthy ageing – nursing older people. In: Health H, Schofield H (eds), Healthy Ageing: Nursing Older People. Churchill Livingstone, Edinburgh

Wilson EW, Rennie PIC 1976 The menstrual cycle. Lloyd-Luke, London

World Health Organisation 1998 Reproductive health: meeting peoples needs. WHO/RHT/98.17

World Health Organisation 2000 Working with street children – module 4 – understanding sexual and reproductive health including HIV/AIDS and STDs among street children. World Health Organisation, Geneva. www.who.int/substance_abuse/PDFfiles/module4.pdf

Further reading

Andrews G 2001 Women's sexual health. Baillière Tindall, London

Davidson N 2000 Promoting men's health – a guide for practitioners. Baillière Tindall, London

Sutherland C 2001 Women's health – a handbook for nurses. Churchill Livingstone, Edinbugh

Useful websites

www.doh.gov.uk/sexualhealthandhiv/index
www.bbc.co.uk/health/sex
www.who.int/reproductive-health
Family Planning Association Sites (examples)
www.fpaindia.com (India)
www.fpa.org.uk (United Kingdom)
www.ifpa.ie (Ireland)
www.brain.net.pk/~fpapak (Pakistan)

Sleeping

Jane Jenkins

Introduction

Roper, Logan and Tierney (1996 and 2000) highlight that sleeping is vital for everyone and is therefore an important Activity of Living. All human beings have periods of activity and inactivity and adults spend up to a third of their lives asleep. These periods of activity and inactivity are regulated by a sleep–wakefulness cycle controlled by the hypothalamus. A 24-hour sleep–wake cycle is learnt through experience and is called the 'Circadian' rhythm and is produced by the 'Biological' clock (Rutishauser 1994). Babies learn this sleep–wake pattern over the first few months of life and mothers are always overjoyed when their baby has 'learnt' to sleep through the night and be awake in the daytime with short periods of rest and sleep throughout the day. The greatest amount of rest is produced when the person is asleep but body functions do still continue during this time but at a reduced level. Roper et al (2000, p. 48) define sleep as a 'recurrent state of inertia and unresponsiveness, a state in which a person does not respond to what is going on in the surrounding environment'.

Sleeping is very different to stages of unconsciousness leading to a coma, and unconsciousness produced by anaesthesia, as although consciousness is lost during sleep, it is for a short time only and new stimuli will wake the person. According to Roper et al (1996, 2000), sleep can be recognised by a person closing their eyes, lying still for some of the time, moving at intervals, relaxing so that the mouth opens and breathing is noticeably slower.

However, the quantity and quality of sleep may be affected by a person's health status and the quantity and quality of sleep that a person has may affect their health and wellbeing. Sleeping can, certainly, be affected by health problems which relate to other Activities of Living, such as suffering from acute or chronic pain linked to minor or major health problems, being stressed, anxious or depressed, or suffering from a marked loss of weight linked to anorexia, bulimia or cancer. It is important to remember that we are all individuals with life activities that are interlinked and when illness causes one or more activity to be affected then most of the activities can become compromised. This may then result in physical, emotional or social problems.

To enable an insight to be gained into both the normal and abnormal patterns of sleep, exercises and case studies have been introduced, as previously noted, which will incorporate evidence-based practice and cultural issues.

The aspects to be covered in this chapter are:

1. **The model of living**
   - sleeping activity in health and illness across the lifespan
   - dependence and independence in relation to the activity of sleeping
   - factors which influence the activity of sleeping.
2. **The model for nursing**
   - nursing care of individuals with health problems which affect their activity of sleeping.

It is important to be able to answer the question: Why do we need to sleep? Roper et al (1996, p. 375) state that the function of sleep 'is still not fully understood'. However, there appear to be two theories in relation to the function of sleep. One is that sleep is needed for restoration. Shapiro and Flanigan (1993) consider that the primary function of sleep is to preserve energy and allow the body to restore itself. Restoration and growth of all body cells are promoted by sleep. This is based on the fact that adrenaline, noradrenaline and corticosteroids are produced during wakefulness and they inhibit the formation of protein in tissues, whereas, in sleep, all of these are produced in small quantities only, therefore allowing protein to be formed, aided by the production of human growth hormone during the night. This may be the reason that children go to bed and appear to have grown overnight. The other theory is in relation to conservation. The energy used during the day must be balanced by a sleeping/resting phase to recuperate energy used up (Roper et al 1996).

It may be necessary to review knowledge of the normal anatomy and physiology of the central nervous system (CNS) and sleep patterns before continuing with this chapter.

MODEL OF LIVING

Activity of sleeping in health and illness, across the lifespan

Reet (1998) identifies that the need for sleep varies through life according to the person's age, but generalities can be made and these generalities will be discussed in relation to the lifespan. (N.B. It is important to note that the need for sleep can differ from these ranges.)

Birth and childhood

Babies usually sleep for 18 hours in any 24 hours and have up to 6–8 periods of sleep during this time and these periods tend to be between feeds. At about the age of 3, then they will have about 13 hours of sleep per night and a short nap in the day time, decreasing at the age of 10 to about 8–10 hours (Rutishauser 1994).

Adolescence

The need for sleep temporarily increases during teenage years and at least 10 hours of sleep per night is needed; still teenagers may be sleepy in the day time. By the time the child is 17, they will usually sleep for 7–8 hours and very little will wake them during this time (Lavery 1997).

Adulthood

Adults have developed their pattern of sleeping and resting by now and sleep between 7–8 hours per night. From the age of 30 onwards sleep becomes shallower and doesn't last as long and individuals may wake up far easier. Sleep patterns begin to change from the age of 40–45 in men and 50–55 in women.

Women sleep longer than men but tend to complain more of insufficient sleep. Hormonal levels affect women's sleep and those who suffer from premenstrual tension do have less sleep at this time than those who do not. Pregnancy can affect sleep patterns for a variety of reasons, such as movements of the baby and needing to micturate more frequently due to increased pressure on the bladder, particularly in the later stages of pregnancy. Daytime naps may then be taken to try to overcome this disturbed sleep pattern. The menopause can also be a time for sleep disruption as a result of hot flushes and night sweats, however the amount of deep sleep is higher and this may provide some rationale for the fact that women live longer than men (Lavery 1997).

The elderly

Older people tend to sleep for shorter periods at night, maybe only 5 hours and they tend to wake up more frequently and have periods when they are awake during the night and feel less refreshed in the morning. This lack of night time sleep is complemented by a daytime nap or naps. Many factors have been identified to explain why elderly people appear to sleep less. Physical factors may be influential, e.g. needing to get up to go to the toilet as their bladder function changes, disordered breathing, pain and discomforts. Psychological factors may also be responsible, in relation to simple matters, such as, after the death of a spouse the concerns of living and sleeping alone, or actual changes in mental states as shown in depression and dementia. Environmental and economic factors, relating to safety and possible inability to heat their houses properly can also affect their sleeping habits (Rutishauser 1994). It is important to be alert to the reasons for changes in the sleep pattern of older people and consider how sleep can be promoted.

Exercise

1. Observe the sleeping patterns of different age groups, if possible, for example, a baby or child, an adult or an older person (aged 65 and above) during the daytime.
2. What did you notice about their pattern of sleeping?
3. Ask individuals about the sleeping patterns of a baby or child, an adult and an older person during the night.
4. Are they able to identify changes in their sleeping patterns or needs in relation to sleep?
5. Did they have any health problems which may have affected their sleeping, if so, what did they notice as different.

Some differences in observations of people may have been noted. This may depend on the level of activity (mental or physical) they have been involved in during the day. People who exercise more tend to sleep for longer times, this may be due to the effect of the rise in temperature produced by exercise, which seems to promote sleep (Lavery 1997). The environment may have had an effect on whether they take daytime naps, particularly in the afternoon or evening. Mothers will have been overjoyed when their babies sleep through the night but don't seem to be as pleased when their offspring sleep for hours as a teenager and will not get out of bed. Sleep may have been affected by colds, coughing, snoring of partners or transient pain such as toothache and people may well have complained of broken sleep. When individuals go on holiday they frequently complain of poor sleep on the first night, but with a change in daily routine this problem is usually short-lived.

Dependence and independence in relation to the activity of sleep

Each individual is, according to Roper et al (1996), independent for the activity of sleeping and their independence level is related to their position on the lifespan.

Babies are dependent on others for the maintenance of their environment and their safety, but spend most of their time asleep while the older person may spend a lot of time in bed, although not always asleep (Roper et al 1996).

Children and adolescents can also be dependent on others for sleep, for they are affected by tension and noise. Childhood sleep problems, such as nightmares, night terrors and disturbed sleep, may need specialised support. Adults can become dependent on others to ensure that the noise levels are low, for instance, when they work shifts.

The main issue of dependency in adults relates to the use of hypnotic drugs, as Roper et al (1996) identify. Drugs may be used when other remedies have not been successful in aiding sleeping problems. Morin et al (1999) concluded that temazepam (a hypnotic drug), on its own or combined with cognitive behavioural therapy, improved short-term outcomes for older adults with persistent insomnia. However, these hypnotic drugs produce a different form of sleep to natural sleep and can create dependency. The drugs reduce the amount of restorative sleep but can aid the onset of sleep, reduce wakenings and increase the overall amount of time spent asleep and for these reasons, individuals take sleeping pills.

Different drugs can be prescribed such as hypnotics (benzodiazepines or anxiolytics or tranquillisers) which act on the central nervous system by depressing brain function to induce sleep, e.g. chlordiazepoxide, nitrazepam, temazepam and diazepam or barbiturates which depress nervous system activity, e.g. amylobarbitone. Barbiturates are no longer prescribed due to their addictive and overdose risks as well as the high risk of depressing respiration rates. Two new nonbenzodiazepine hypnotic drugs, a cyclopyrrolone such as zopiclone and zolpidem imidazopyridines, have been introduced and have shown some advantages with less dependency levels (Rutishauser 1994, Lavery 1997, Morgan & Closs 1999, Closs 2000).

Holbrook et al (2000) concluded that benzodiazepines do improve sleep duration but can lead to adverse effects in adults with insomnia. The pharmacological effect of hypnotics wear off after 2 weeks as the body learns to tolerate them and they produce physical and psychological dependence. Withdrawal from these pills may result in even worse insomnia.

> **Exercise**
> 1. Find out why people started taking sleeping tablets.
> 2. Find out if any of them have tried to quit and, if so, how successful they have been.
> 3. Ask patients who have taken sleeping tablets for the first time, whilst in hospital, what effect they had upon their sleeping habits and how they felt the next day.

There are many reasons why individuals start taking sleeping tablets. This may have been as a result of bereavement, hospitalisation, illness, worry over unemployment, financial, domestic or employment problems. They may well have described problems when they tried to stop taking sleeping tablets, depending on the length of time they have been taking these medications. They may also describe different coping strategies used, support they had and whether the initial sleep problem had been alleviated. The 'hangover' feeling, insomnia and nightmares may well have been described.

A 'hangover' feeling on the next day is based on the residual effects of the drugs taken. Rebound effects can occur, when the person tries to stop taking the sleeping tablets, such as insomnia which may last for 3–7 nights after just a 3-week course, nightmares may occur as the person often wakes up in the part of the sleep cycle when vivid dreams take place and anxiety levels can be raised. Impaired judgement, poor coordination and memory, reduced work performance, road traffic accidents and falls may occur when the individual stops taking the sleeping tablets. All of these effects are increased by the use of alcohol (Rutishauser 1994, Morgan & Closs 1999).

Depending on the absorption, distribution and elimination rates of the drugs used, drug accumulation and dependency can occur. Halfens et al (1994) consider that dependency can result from a short exposure to these drugs, e.g. short hospitalisation when sleeping tablets are offered as a routine measure.

For these reasons, it is better to promote nonpharmacological aids to sleep, such as a quiet dark room with a comfortable bed, mattress and appropriate pillows, relaxation therapy, taking food and drink which aid restful sleep, ensuring correct temperature to provide sufficient warmth yet be cool enough to allow sleep.

> **Exercise**
> 1. Ask adults what they do if they are unable to sleep.
> 2. Go to a health food store, and find out what nonpharmacological remedies are available for individuals with sleeping difficulties.

Adults may have developed their own remedies for sleep problems. Ensuring that the room temperature is correct for them, wearing comfortable night clothes, being in familiar, quiet surroundings, reading a book and having warm milky drinks may be offered as solutions. Counting sheep is always laughed at but this does provide the person with a task to focus on, which is monotonous and not stressful, and may work for some people.

Natural alternatives are considered by Lavery (1997) and nonaddictive sleep remedies, such as tryptophan, can be used. This is an amino acid which is good for protein repair and converts to melatonin which aids sleep. At present, this is available on prescription only but is found in milk and carbohydrates, so a hot milky drink with a biscuit may be just what is needed. Melatonin, the sleep hormone produced by the pineal gland, is beneficial for improving sleep, but it is not fully understand and therefore is not recommended for anyone who is pregnant or below the age of 35. It is being manufactured as a food supplement. Another product, Kava Kava root, which is a herb, can depress the central nervous system and relax muscles, so it can help to relax the individual and if taken before bedtime it can allow the individual to initiate sleep.

There are different levels of consciousness – from being fully alert and awake through to being unconscious and comatosed with natural sleep somewhere in-between. Temporary loss of consciousness may occur due to fainting or syncope. Hinchliff et al (1996) point out that this occurs when there is a temporary reduction in blood flow to the brain, which is quickly rectified by ensuring that the head is lower or is at the same level as the heart. Heat syncope is caused due to pooling of blood in the periphery and the extremities especially in hot climates in an attempt to lose heat. Consciousness is restored when the individual is moved to cooler areas.

Unconscious states, however, are not as easy to rectify and can lead to death. Coma states may result from brain tumours, head injuries, overdoses or metabolic disorders. The outcomes vary because of the differing causes but it is essential that you are able to assess levels of consciousness accurately and this will be discussed in the model for nursing section. General anaesthetics will also render the individual unconscious but when the anaesthetic is reversed, their conscious levels will be restored to normal. Individuals can be frightened at the thought of surgery because they are aware that their conscious level will be compromised and that they will not be able to control this.

Factors influencing the activity of sleep

Roper et al (1996, 2000) state that sleeping is influenced by many factors. In a healthy individual such things as exercise, food, drink, mood, noise, housing and work practices can affect the quantity and quality of sleep. These factors will be explored individually but include:

1. anatomy and physiology related to sleep (biological factors)
2. emotional issues related to sleep (psychological factors)
3. practices, associated health beliefs and habits in different cultures related to sleep (sociocultural factors)
4. environmental factors and how these relate to sleep (environmental factors)
5. policies, laws and economics related to sleep (politicoeconomic factors).

Anatomy and physiology related to sleep (biological factors)

In order to promote health and to care for people who have sleeping problems it is necessary to understand certain body rhythms, the normal cycles of sleep and the anatomy and physiology of relevant parts of the nervous system.

Sleeping is influenced by circadian rhythms. These rhythms are influenced by external factors or zeitgebers (exogenous) such as meal times, light, dark, noise, silence, sleep and rest patterns and internal factors (endogenous) such as cell function. These two sets of factors usually coincide if a normal routine is maintained, i.e. go to bed at a regular time, eat at regular times, respond by waking when it is light and sleeping when it is dark. However, air travel and shift work can upset this rhythm and can cause health problems (Rutishauser 1994).

Exercise
1. Ask different people what they consider may happen to sleep patterns when individuals:
   • fly to and from Australia or stay in Iceland or Greenland
   • work shifts.
2. Find out how these changes may affect their daily lives.

Individuals who have visited Australia may complain of 'jet lag'. This only occurs when people fly in an easterly or westerly direction and occurs because the circadian rhythm is affected. Flying from the UK to Australia takes 24 hours but, due to the time difference between the two places, it makes arrival time 36 hours later than departure time, there is therefore a 12-hour difference. For example, when a person leaves the UK at 8 pm, i.e. night time, they will arrive in Australia at 6 am, i.e. morning. The person will be ready for bed as his 'internal body clock' says it is evening and ready for bed whereas people around him will be ready to go to work and it is daylight (see Fig. 13.1). So the external clues (zeitgebers) are confusing, resulting in the symptoms of 'jet lag'. These symptoms last a few days, whilst the circadian rhythm readjusts itself, and include difficulties with sleeping, decreased alertness and ability to concentrate, gastrointestinal upsets and general fatigue. When the internal clock resets to its new schedule then the symptoms disappear (Rutishauser 1994).

The amount of light also affects the sleep–wake cycle, so in Iceland or Greenland the external clues in relation to daylight and darkness are different to those in the United Kingdom. In Iceland and Greenland, there are long periods of darkness every day in winter with very short periods of daylight and long periods of daylight and short periods of darkness in the summer (Roper et al 1996). As darkness indicates to the body it is time to retire to bed and sleep, problems arise if the time is actually still daytime and the individual is at work. Equally, when daylight is predominant, then the clues of needing to go to bed are lost. Yet people living in these countries still sleep at 'night' and work during the 'day' and learn to use other external clues, such as meal times to ensure their sleeping and waking cycle is in keeping with their lifestyle.

Practice nurses working in Travel Clinics need to give appropriate advice to individuals to minimise these problems, such as taking a night-time flight and trying to sleep during the flight, eat only a small amount, avoid alcohol and drink plenty of water. It is then advisable to take on the

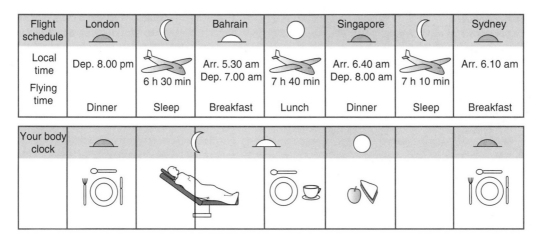

Fig. 13.1 Changes in circadian rhythms when flying from London to Australia (from Rutishauser 1994, with permission).

routine of the new time zone as soon as possible and to do some exercise rather than sleeping on arrival. Herxheimer and Petrie (2002) reviewed evidence assessing the effectiveness of oral melatonin for alleviating jet lag. Nine out of the ten trials reviewed found that melatonin can prevent or reduce jet lag and may be used as part of a sleep education programme for adult travellers, flying through five or more time zones in an easterly direction.

Individuals who work shifts also complain of problems and again this is due to disturbances in their circadian rhythm. Sometimes this may not be resolved and may lead to illness. When individuals work days then nights, their sleep–wake patterns are reversed, so they are active at night and asleep in the day. Outside influences, e.g. daylight and noise, affect the ability to change the 'internal body clock' so the person may present with the same symptoms of jet lag but of a long-term nature.

It is probable that when a person works nights, they will lose some sleep. If they are unable to make up this sleep loss, then various problems can occur, such as poor concentration, reduced efficiency, poor decision making, thereby increasing the risk of accidents and errors. Individuals themselves may become very irritable and 'touchy' (Rutishauser 1994).

Being on permanent days or nights is better than swapping from one pattern to the other as the body can develop a regular sleep–wake pattern. Brooks (1997) debates the future of permanent night shifts for health care personnel and concludes that choice and ability to adapt circadian rhythms influences the person's likelihood of developing health problems, absenteeism, job satisfaction, social and domestic disruption. It appears generally, from an employee's perspective, that working permanent nights is preferable to working internal rotation. However, internal rotation gives greater flexibility of rostering and there may be a conflict between these two different facets in the National Health Service (NHS) today.

Legal action may be faced by organisations, such as hospitals and nursing homes, if they fail to take steps to combat the ill effects of disrupted sleep patterns as a result of employees working irregular shift patterns. Employers should minimise the potential effects of poor health when working nights (Rajaratnam & Arendt 2001). The use of a risk assessment tool, before introducing internal rotation, is advocated by Martell (2001). Rutishauser (1994) considers that it is advisable to take a nap before beginning a night shift, take regular exercise, abstain from drinking alcohol before work, work in bright light and all this may help the nurse to promote a good sleep routine, but the latter element may affect the patient's sleep routine.

The circadian rhythm is greatly influenced by internal factors, such as the sleep–wake cycle, body temperature and cortisol secretion. Various physiological changes occur when individuals go to sleep and wake up which they are generally unaware of. When lying down and resting, the metabolic rate is lowered, the cardiovascular and renal systems are affected, resulting in temperature, pulse and blood pressure being lowered and the rate of urine formation is slowed. When going to sleep, further changes occur, noticeably the secretion of blood cortisol decreases and growth hormone increases. When getting up again then the growth hormone levels fall, cortisol levels rise, blood pressure and urine formation increase and heat is generated thereby increasing body temperature (Rutishauser 1994). It is important to note these changes are normal and therefore when on night duty it must be considered whether changes in vital sign measurements are due to normal changes related to sleep.

These internal or endogenous factors (cell functions) are set by an internal clock. This internal clock is set by cells in the hypothalamus which provide the impetus for the sleep–wake cycle. The biological clock within the hypothalamus and specifically in the suprachiasmatic nucleus drives special cells in the reticular formation within the brain stem, known as the raphe nuclei and nucleus locus coeruleus to determine the level of consciousness (see Fig. 13.2).

If individuals were left without any outside clues to time, then this sleep–wake cycle would occur every 25 hours but

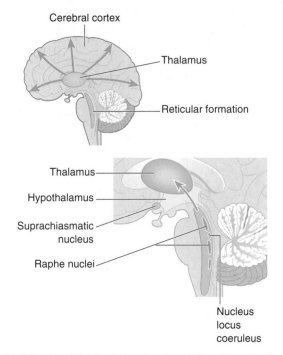

Fig. 13.2 Parts of the brain involved in determining the level of consciousness (from Rutishauser 1994, with permission).

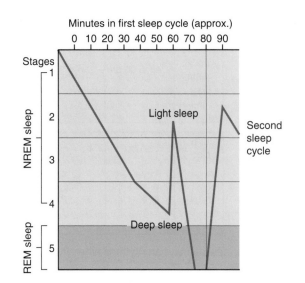

Fig. 13.3 One sleep cycle (from Roper et al 1996, with permission).

social habits, meal times, alarm clocks keep this cycle to a 24-hour time span. Sensory impulses enter the cells in the reticular formation and this triggers the person to wake up. It is then difficult to get back to sleep as sensory information reaches the brain easily now. Conversely when stimuli are low then sleep is easy (Rutishauser 1994).

Certain hormonal levels, such as adrenaline and corticosteroids are responsible for wakefulness and activity. Individuals go to sleep in the late evening when adrenaline and corticosteroid levels are at their lowest. The growth hormone level rises during the night and, at about 5 am the temperature level starts to rise, as does adrenaline and corticosteroid levels which initiate waking. The pineal gland, as previously discussed, secretes a hormone called melatonin during darkness. Levels of melatonin, the sleep hormone, fluctuate daily, depending on the amount of light entering the eye. When it is dark, or the individual closes their eyes, there is a lack of light entering the eye and so melatonin is released, which tells the body it is time to prepare for sleep (Lavery 1997). Research carried out by the Royal College of Psychiatrists, as reported in the Clinical Research highlights in *Nursing Times* (1998), has identified that people with myalgic encephalomyelitis (ME) have unusually high levels of melatonin which may be a reason for their chronic fatigue problems.

There are two different types of sleep, namely non-REM (nonrapid eye movements) and REM (rapid eye movements) and these types of sleep combine to form a sleep cycle which lasts for about 90–100 minutes. According to Roper et al (1996) an adult has between 4–6 cycles per night (see Fig. 13.3).

Non-REM sleep is sometimes classed as orthodox sleep and comprises 70% of adult sleep. Non-REM sleep can be noted by the use of an electroencephalogram (EEG) because when an individual falls asleep the electrical activity in the brain changes and these changes may be recorded on a graph. Alpha waves can be seen on an EEG when the individual relaxes but remains awake, the beta waves which are associated with waking and being alert disappear and delta waves of inactivity appear. Many body systems take a rest and therefore the heart rate and blood pressure fall and the body relaxes. There are four stages of non-REM sleep, with Stage 1 and 2 being classed as light sleep and Stage 3 and 4 as deep sleep with REM sleep having just one stage, Stage 5 (Rutishauser 1994, Hinchliff et al 1996, Roper et al 1996).

Exercise
1. Ask individuals what they think happens and how they feel when they are falling asleep.
2. Ask individuals what they remember about being asleep and what they remember when they wake up.
3. Compare your experiences of sleep with that of colleagues.

Individuals will recollect different experiences. Individuals may have described a feeling of floating, falling, drowsiness, disturbed sleep, being woken up, dreaming, not being able to remember a dream, talking in their sleep, grinding their teeth and others may talk about someone snoring.

All of these recollections are part of sleep and the different stages of the sleep cycle. Each stage has certain characteristics. Stage 1 or 'just dropping off' stage can be noted by the fact that eyes close and roll, the person feels relaxed and drowsy, a drifting or floating sensation may be felt, especially falling, and individuals can sometimes hear voices or see pictures. They are easy to wake during this stage.

However, if they are woken up at this time they cannot remember being asleep. This stage only lasts for 15 minutes and only occurs on the first cycle of the night's sleep. Stage 2 lasts for about 15 minutes, and is characterised by greater relaxation, dream-like thoughts, and individuals may remember dreams if they wake up now. They can still be woken easily.

Stage 3 lasts for about 20 minutes and is a period when there is complete relaxation of muscles, the pulse slows and the temperature falls. Individuals are not easy to wake during this stage and have no conscious thoughts. Although they may dream, they do not remember dreams if they wake up now. The growth hormone is released during this stage and it is therefore a time when blood cells and body tissues, especially skin can be rebuilt. Energy levels can be restored at this time. The final Stage 4 in non-REM sleep is when the individual is completely relaxed, rarely moves and is difficult to wake. Growth hormone continues to be released (Rutishauser 1994, Roper et al 1996, 2000, Closs 2000).

Stage 5 is REM (rapid eye movement) or paradoxical sleep and is characterised by light sleep, dreaming, where the eyes move rapidly from side to side, with little body movements. Vivid dreams are recalled if an individual is woken up during this stage. It is thought that this stage is used to update memories and integrate experiences with the past. Physiologically there is an increase in the blood pressure, pulse and respiration rate, with an increased blood flow, whereby protein levels can be renewed in the brain. Hormonally, there is an increase in the levels of testosterone and women have increased blood flow to vagina, whilst men can have erections. Individuals are easily woken at this time. The first episode of REM sleep lasts for only a few minutes, but as the night progresses, this time increases. Individuals change position in bed when they move from REM sleep to non-REM sleep (Rutishauser 1994, Roper et al 1996 and 2000).

Non-REM sleep is thought to be restorative for the body whereas REM sleep is thought to restore the mind. Within the cycles, there is a pattern throughout the night. The non-REM sleep becomes shorter and the periods of REM sleep become longer. Babies have more REM sleep than non-REM sleep, whereas adults generally have more non-REM sleep than REM sleep (Roper et al 1996).

The electroencephalogram (EEG) and the recordings of eye movements or electroculography (EOG) and chin muscle tone by electromyography (EMG) have provided the means to explore sleep. The five stages of sleep are shown in Figure 13.4 as noted on an EEG recording (Lavery 1997, Morgan & Closs 1999).

Different sleep problems are associated with the different stages of the sleep cycle. For example, Stage 1 problems may be enuresis (bed wetting) or teeth grinding, whereas Stage 2 problems often present as talking in their sleep, Stage 3 and 4 problems involve sleepwalking, night terrors, as well as sleep talking and bedwetting. Stage 5 problems are mainly related to nightmares.

The amount of sleep needed varies with each individual. Individuals can need anything between 2–15 hours of sleep a day, if they have more than that, it can cause the same problems as if they have too little. Individuals need to find a balance which suits them. Sleep deficits can build up over time but these deficits can be compensated if the individual takes a longer than normal sleep. Stage 3 and 4 non-REM sleep deficit is made up first, then REM sleep.

Hodgson (1991) identifies numerous physiological effects of sleep deprivation, e.g. falling body temperature, slight changes in cardiovascular, respiratory and hormonal levels. Emotionally, individuals become irritable, aggressive, depressed and may display antisocial behaviour but there don't appear to be any serious, lasting neurological problems. A research study by Wedderbum and Smith (1980), demonstrated that individuals who have been kept awake for over a week at a time, displayed the ability to walk even when they were in fact asleep. Care with driving and working whilst short of sleep is vital as there is an increased risk of being involved in a road traffic accident or having an accident at work. A current UK road safety campaign shows

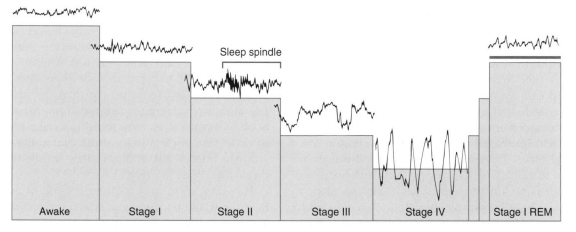

Fig. 13.4 Progressive changes in the electroencephalogram (EEG) following the onset of sleep, showing the patterns characteristic of each stage of sleep, non-REM (Stages I–IV) and REM (from Hobson 1995, with permission).

a horrific motorway accident involving a driver who is tired and falls asleep at the wheel. Individuals only need to lose 2 hours sleep to be tired enough to fall asleep whilst driving. Extra sleep does not appear to improve performance and may even make things worse.

Lavery (1997) suggests that lack of sleep will not only present with poor concentration, lack of judgement, irritability, depression, stress, dark circles under eyes, but fewer white blood cells are circulating and so there is a lowered resistance to infection. Recovery from surgery or illness is noted to be better if the individual is a good sleeper. Morgan and Closs (1999) consider that lack of sleep will impair tissue restoration. Equally, when patients are fasted or lacking in nutrition for other reasons, they may be tired as the metabolic rate falls in the night.

Apart from the external and internal factors influencing sleep patterns the lifestyle of an individual can affect sleep also. Bedtime routines appear to be useful in training the individual to sleep well.

Exercise
1. Ask different people what their routine is at bedtime.
2. Ask them if they can identify what aids or disrupts their sleep.
3. Discuss with colleagues the findings of these investigations.

Individuals may discuss their eating, drinking, smoking and/or reading activities before bedtime. Caffeine is a stimulant as it increases the amount of circulating adrenaline and its effects can last for 14 hours, so coffee is not advised prior to retiring to bed. Likewise, smoking stimulates the nervous system which raises the blood pressure and adrenaline and so should be avoided. Alcohol tends to send individuals to sleep quickly but they wake early in the morning. A lack of exercise or too much exercise late at night can delay sleep as can too much mental stimulation just prior to retiring to bed (Lavery 1997, Morgan & Closs 1999). It is, however, the routine that is important to the individual and not particularly the components of that routine.

Psychological factors

In everyday life, individuals talk about having a good night's sleep and equate this to feeling well. Equally, after what the individual considers to be a poor night's sleep, there is a feeling of not being on top form, not ill but not their usual self. It may well be a topic of conversation when in a strange place. It may be that certain individuals are more suited to employment involving shift work because of their individual personalities and their ability to adapt to sleep changes. A study done by Humm in 1996 did identify that toleration of night duty in 46 nurses was related to certain personality factors, in particular their 'rigidity and flexibilty of sleeping habits'.

Exercise
1. Ask individuals what affects their sleep in relation to their mood.
2. Ask them what effect different moods have on the amount and type of sleep they have.
3. What are their bedtime routines which they use to aid sleep?

Individuals recount many different moods which affect their sleep. They may be excited about a holiday or getting married and this nervous excitement may result in transient insomnia but the person is happy and generally feels well and is using the time of rest for reflecting on the preparations and thinking forward with anticipation to the events. They may also talk about times when life situations have not been good, for example, work difficulties, unemployment, family tensions or divorce. This may have interrupted their sleep patterns, where they experience difficulty getting to sleep, waking frequently and ultimately they feel worse on waking than they did before retiring to bed. A planned admission to hospital for investigations or surgery may affect the individual's sleeping habits even prior to admission.

Following bereavement, sleep patterns may be disrupted for several reasons, e.g. due to worry over safety, not being used to sleeping alone, as well as the grieving process itself. A leaflet by Health Facts (1996), launched by SLEEPtalk, was reviewed in the *Journal of Advanced Nursing,* and it advises people on how to get back to normal sleep routines as soon as possible to avoid long-term problems.

Insomnia is strongly related to depressive and anxiety-type illnesses. Depressed individuals may suffer from severe insomnia for several weeks where they complain of being awake for hours, difficulty in getting off to sleep, waking early and having disturbed sleep with frequent dreams (Closs 2000). People who suffer from anxiety states also complain of tension and this affects sleep. They may present with difficulty getting off to sleep and maintaining sleep throughout the night.

As it would appear that moods affect sleep, then individuals need to consider healthy living choices which include effective sleep routines. Simple measures may be all that is needed, especially going to bed when they feel tired and avoiding the temptation to sleep downstairs in a comfortable armchair. Some people may choose to listen to relaxation tapes, listen to their own favourite music, read a book or watch TV, go for a short walk, take a bath, or eat a snack or take a warm milky drink as it contains an amino acid which forms melatonin, to help soothe the mind and prepare the body for sleep (Lavery 1997).

However, some may consider the use of meditation to relax the whole body, or yoga which can provide a relaxing sequence ready for sleep, involving simple stretching and relaxation exercises suitable for all ages and levels of ability or biofeedback mechanisms whereby the visualisation of a relaxing place, perhaps on a beach or by a stream is conjured up in the mind and the individual concentrates on this picture (Lavery 1997).

Traditional Chinese medicine may be used, such as Shiatsu massage, hypnosis or T'ai'chi which can relieve muscular tension and mental stress. Certain herbal remedies, e.g. passion flower or hops are good for general insomnia, St John's Wort is used for depression, dill for jet lag, lettuce for restless and excitable people. The use of aromatherapy oils is increasing, whether they are inhaled or absorbed through the skin, e.g. jasmine, rose, lavender are found to be relaxing and soothing. Reflexology therapeutic foot massage is said to suit some individuals, whereas homeopathic remedies are available for a variety of sleep problems, e.g. for acute insomnia aconite can be used, arsenicum album is useful for early waking between 1–3 am due to overactive mind, nightmares may be lessened by nux vomica, whereas sepia can be used for individuals who find it difficult to fall asleep (Lavery 1997).

Sociocultural factors

Sociocultural beliefs and practices can influence sleeping and resting as these determine when, where, in what and with whom individuals sleep. Bedtime routines such as adopting a regular bedtime, where the individual has had a period of relaxation before bedtime and the avoidance of daytime naps, caffeine, alcohol and nicotine late at night may be socially orientated (Reet 1998). On a simple level, there are individuals who are classed as the 'Larks', these are morning people, who go to bed early, rise early and work best in a morning; whereas the 'Owls' are evening people, who go to bed late, get up late and work best in an evening. Rutishauser (1994) considers that some people are better suited to shift work than others. The 'larks' seem to have more difficulty in adjusting to shift work, whereas, the 'owls' seem to adjust better. Consider personal experience and whether this is the same for other family members. Are there conflicts between the 'Larks and the Owls'.

Roper et al (1996) identify that different cultures adopt different patterns of sleep. North European countries, predominately, sleep at night but Mediterranean cultures take a siesta in the afternoon and then retire for night-time sleep at a later time to the North Europeans. Siestas can improve the individual's mood, their concentration and productivity and doesn't affect sleep at night. Equally, the place in which people sleep is linked to their cultural roots. For example, Westerners sleep in a bed, whereas Japanese sleep on a bed roll on the floor and there are the 'cardboard cities' where the homeless sleep rough under and on cardboard. Sleeping alone or with a partner, in nightwear or nude is the norm for Westerners whereas people from Eastern countries often sleep with several people in the same place. Eskimos apparently sleep in the same clothes day and night, presumably linked to maintaining body temperature (Roper et al 1996).

Lavery (1997) discusses the influence Indian culture has on sleeping patterns. Indians believe in an Ayurvedic system which has three energy systems or doshas, namely 'pitta, vata and kaphas'. Individuals are seen as a mixture of all three energy systems but two predominate. 'Vata' people are thin, excitable, tire easily and are light sleepers with irregular sleeping habits and are prone to sleep problems. On the other hand, 'pitta' individuals are of medium build, get angry or irritable when stressed, tend to wake during the night feeling hot or thirsty but wake feeling alert. 'Kapha' people are calm, confident and slow moving. They love to sleep and they tend to sleep long periods and wake up slowly. Also, these energy phases occur at different times of the day, e.g. 'vata' occurs in the early morning, 'pitta' in the afternoon and 'kapha' in the late evening. Ayurveda advises people to go to sleep when it is 'kapha' time (between 6–10 pm) as sleep will be slow and then wake up in 'vata' time, before 6 am which is the active phase. To sleep well then these doshas need to be balanced. If they become imbalanced by illness then sleep is affected.

Dreams are also linked to these three doshas, as 'pitta' types usually have action and adventure dreams but if they are not balanced then these dreams can turn into anger and conflict. 'Vata' types have imaginative and action dreams but again if they are not balanced then become dreams of anxiety where the person is falling, running away or being chased. 'Kapha' types have tranquil dreams of lakes and oceans but unfortunately they are rarely remembered (Lavery 1997).

Chinese philosophy is different as they believe that individuals live between heaven and earth and the energies of these two, provide the energy for life. If the energies are balanced then they are in good health. 'Yin' and 'yang' energies are governed by three different forces, namely the spirit or 'shen', which is responsible for consciousness; energy or 'qi', which moves, warms and protects and essence or 'jing', which is responsible for growth and development. When a person is well, then all of these forces are in harmony and sleep is peaceful, growth and development takes place. If ill, then there are problems with 'shen' and 'jing' and growth and renewal cannot take place (Lavery 1997).

Sleep and dreaming are also influenced by the etheral soul or 'hun' and this is stored in the liver at night. If the person develops liver problems, then the 'hun' wanders, causing restlessness and exhausting dreams. If the person sleeps well then the 'hun' collects images and these images keep the person mentally, spiritually happy and creative (Lavery 1997).

Dreams that don't upset the person's sleeping pattern are normal but if they do affect the sleeping pattern, then these are related to some pathology. The type of dream is governed by balance of energy, when they occur as each hour of the day and night relates to different organs and emotions, e.g. 3–5 am is the start of the spiritual day and relates to lungs, sadness and grief, so dreams may cause breathing problems, loss and be of a spiritual nature (Lavery 1997).

These different aspects are important for you to consider when nursing patients from these cultural backgrounds.

> **Exercise**
> 1. If possible, speak to people who have lived in very different parts of the world, e.g Australia, Alaska, Iceland or India and find out about their sleeping habits.
> 2. Ask them what kind of sleep patterns they have and what affects them.

Environmental factors

For most people, sleep takes place in a specific room designed for sleep as environmental factors do influence sleep. Sleep is usually easier when individuals are in familiar surroundings, which are cool, dark, private and quiet. Roper et al (1996) and Reet (1998) identify that having their own belongings and being somewhere safe and quiet is important in aiding sleep.

However, these surroundings can change in life, e.g. following bereavement, moving to a smaller house or bungalow or changes in health which necessitate sleeping in a chair. Shift workers have to consider their environment and use thicker curtains to block out sunlight, lessen noise in the household. Homeless people have a very different environment to those who sleep in a house, as well as those who sleep in bed and breakfast houses or where multiple individuals share rooms and even beds and, therefore, their sleeping habits may well be affected.

The Government set a target to reduce rough sleeping by at least two-thirds by 2002 and this figure was met in December 2001, according to the Rough Sleepers Unit (RSU). The number of those individuals sleeping rough fell from 1850 in 1998 to 532 people in 2002, with some dramatic reductions, such as in Birmingham where 56 people slept rough in 1998 fell to just two in 2002 and 621 in London falling to 264 in the same timespan. This had been achieved by a variety of measures and the health and wellbeing of these individuals, including their sleeping habits would hopefully have improved (http://www.housing.dtlr. gov.uk/rsu/pn/rsu19.htm).

> **Exercise**
> 1. Ask individuals what type of environment they sleep in.
> 2. Ask them what environmental factors affect their sleeping habits.
> 3. Consider the differences and discuss findings with colleagues.

They may well describe a variety of settings but familiarity and safety issues may be prominent. They may say that the mattress and pillows are important yet some prefer a firm or soft mattress and pillow. According to Reet (1998), noise affects progression through the stages of sleep and increases the frequency of waking and body movements. Women and older people are more prone to waking due to noise, but it appears to be the significance of the noise and not the volume of noise which wakes them up. Traffic and aircraft noise is a problem for some yet others sleep well in this type of environment but wake easily when a baby cries or when they hear the sound of breaking glass. The temperature of the room is important and 18°C or 65°F is ideal, if above or below these temperatures then this affects sleep. It is for the same reason that fever affects sleeping. Exposure to bright sunlight in the day seems to promote sleep at night. Latitude does not seem to affect sleep, i.e. in Iceland where there is little night in summer and little light in winter individuals still sleep.

Home design takes particular note of the bedroom environment and Feng Shui, a traditional Chinese art and science of home design can be used to position furniture, rooms and buildings so that they are in harmony with individuals and lines of energy in the Earth. It is thought that, by placing the head of the bed against a wall, this will give the feeling of security and allow individuals to relax. The colour scheme may also be important and pinks, peach, pale yellow, blue or green, lilac are seen as restful colours (Lavery 1997).

Snoring (the noise produced from the soft palate and other parts of the upper respiratory tract) is another 'environmental' problem as the peace and quiet of a household can be disrupted by someone who snores and it can have major effects on the sleeping partners. Snoring is most common in middle-aged, older and obese men, although 40% of all adults snore (Morgan & Closs 1999).

Politicoeconomic factors

The link to politicoeconomic factors that affect sleep may not be immediately obvious as Roper et al (1996) identify. However, the type of housing, number of bedrooms and siblings have a link to economic factors which may impinge on sleeping habits. Employment practices may also link to economic forces and therefore shift workers may have a link to sleep. The Hours and Employment Act of 1936 controls the number of hours a person can work, in particular that of women and young people.

> **Exercise**
> 1. Look on the Department of Trade and Industry website http://www.dti.gov.uk.
> 2. Identify policies in relation to working time regulations and issues relating to hours of work and night duty.

Access to a document entitled 'Your guide to the working time regulations' formulated in 2000 by the Department of Trade and Industry may have been found. This document states that the working time limit is for a 48-hour week and sets out what constitutes working time, which includes working lunches, travel as part of the job, training related to job and working abroad. The average weekly working time is calculated over a 17-week period usually. The document states on page 4 that the 'average weekly working time is calculated by dividing the number of hours worked by the number of weeks over which the average working week is being calculated'. So a worker working 40 hours per week for 17 weeks and 12 hours overtime in the first 10 weeks, with no annual leave would have an average working limit of e.g. $(40 \times 17) + (12 \times 10) = 800$ divided by $17 = 47.1$ hours per week, so the limit of the 48-hour week is complied with. Workers can agree to work longer than a 48-hour week but they need to sign an opt-out agreement with their employer.

There are specific regulations in relation to working at night and these are outlined in this document. For example, a night worker is someone who works at least 3 hours a night and night-time is between 11 pm and 6 am. Night workers should not normally work more than 8 hours a night and night working time is calculated over 17 weeks. Average hours worked at night need to be calculated and these are worked out as follows:

> Number of hours worked in the 17 weeks divided by the number of days in the period (after rest days have been deducted), e.g. a night worker works 4×12 hour night shifts per week over 17 weeks. $17 \times (4 \times 12) = 816$.

> 119 days in 17 weeks minus 17 rest days = $119 - 17 = 102$.

> 816 divided by $102 = 8$ hours per day, as the average hours of work, which is within the normal working time allowed.

It may be interesting to review a qualified nurse's duty rota in the 1950s and compare it to today (with their permission). These are the rules for individuals working in the UK. In other countries these regulations may well be different and stories of 'sweat shops' where young people work long hours, in appalling conditions, with little time off are frequently retold.

In addition to ensuring working times are within the average limits, employers must offer night workers a free health assessment before they work on nights and on a regular basis whilst they remain on nights. It is, however, unusual that individuals are unable to work nights due to medical disorders. The employee does not have to take up this offer but if they do then they would need to complete a health questionnaire and undergo a medical examination, if there are any doubts about the employee's ability to work at night.

Workers are also entitled to have a period of 11 hours uninterrupted rest per working day and at least one full day a week off work. Whilst at work, workers are entitled to a 20-minute rest break, during the shift, if they work more than 6 hours at a stretch. Young workers have different rules regarding rest on a daily, weekly and shift basis. However, the night work limits, rights to rest periods and rest breaks don't apply in certain circumstances, for example, where the job requires round-the-clock staffing, such as in hospitals. It is therefore interesting to consider the effect of shift patterns and working hours in nurses.

Fitzpatrick et al (1999) investigated shift work and its impact on qualified nurses' performance and outcomes. They found that nurses working an 8-hour shift performed better than those working a 12.5-hour shift. They considered that mental and physical tiredness may well have affected the nurse and working several 12.5 hour shifts compounded the problems. Dingley (1996) attempted to define the optimum shift pattern for hospital night staff by comparing staff who worked permanent nights and those who worked internal rotation. The mental alertness of both groups was assessed at the beginning and end of each shift. Nurses felt they were more alert at the beginning of the shift and at the beginning of a span of nights than at the end. Yet, when tested, their performances were worse at the beginning than at the end of the shift and peaked after 4 nights. The need to conduct a risk assessment was also identified, by Dingley (1996), before any rotational system was put in place. Martell (2001, p. 7) quotes research in the *Lancet* and says that irregular shift patterns and night working 'outstrip our biological adaptation to the 24-hour cycle of light and darkness … sleep loss results in performance deficits, … slowed physical and mental reaction time, increased errors, decreased vigilance…'. To ensure that optimum and effective work patterns are maintained, it is necessary for employers to consider the length of a shift (8 or 12.5 hours) and the number of consecutive night duty shifts (four or eight nights).

Apart from employment regulations which relate to sleep and rest, there are driving regulations which have a link to sleep as, unfortunately, accidents at work and whilst driving have occurred when the individual is tired or has fallen asleep. Drivers need to comply with certain rules and alert the Driver and Vehicle Licensing Agency (DVLA) of any problems they may have which may affect their driving, e.g. epilepsy. Brugne (1994) identifies that road safety is dependent upon drivers being awake and vigilant at all times. A microsleep of 1 to 3 seconds could result in a driver missing a bend or going through a red light. Brugne (1994) identifies that, in the USA, 13% of road traffic accident fatalities were caused by people falling asleep at the wheel. It is, therefore, advisable that individuals are well rested before they set out on a long drive and that they don't drive on a motorway for longer than 2 hours before taking a break. Driving on motorways is monotonous and a long drive may be split up with some main road driving to lessen the monotony.

Numerous documents relating to drivers' hours and tachograph rules for goods vehicles in the UK and Europe may have been found. The rules are complex due to the nature of commercial driving in this country and overseas and are subject to change. However, the daily driving limit is 9 hours taken between two consecutive daily rest periods or between a daily rest period and a weekly rest period. Although there is no weekly driving limit, there is a 90-hour driving limit per fortnight. In the 9-hour daily driving limit, the individual must take a 45-minute break after 4.5 hours driving. It is the responsibility of the driver and employer to ensure that they comply with the drivers' hours and tachograph rules and records are made of both the driving and rest hours. A fine of up to £2500 for breach of drivers' hours and £5000 for failing to use a tachograph and if records are falsified, then, the £5000 fine is accompanied with 2 years imprisonment (http://www.roads.dtlr.gov.uk/roadsafety/tachograph/gv262/02.htm).

The reason why these regulations have been drawn up is that out of a total of 3600 road accident fatalities per year in the UK, it is estimated that between 800 and 1000 involve vehicles being driven for work purposes with another 80 000 nonfatal injuries. In addition to this, studies of the causes of road traffic accidents have demonstrated that tiredness and sleepiness are contributing factors in 10% of accidents overall and nearly 30% on motorways (http://www.roads.dtlr.gov.uk/roadsafety/research98/road/5c.htm.).

It was identified that sleep-related accidents peak at 2 am to 7 am and 2 pm to 4 pm when daily sleepiness is higher. These accidents are more evident in young male drivers in the early morning and older male drivers in the afternoon. Falling asleep at the wheel does not occur spontaneously without warning. Usually, individuals will be aware of their sleepy state and may open the window, stretch at the wheel and turn on the radio. These remedies are only effective for a few minutes and individuals should use the signs to prepare themselves for a break and a period of rest. In this rest time it is beneficial to have a caffeinated drink and a short nap. Specific data have been collated to ascertain relationships between sleep-related accidents on sections of selected trunk roads and motorways in the UK during 1995 and 1998. These data are being considered, with measures used overseas, to combat driver fatigue.

The Department for Transport, Local Government and the Regions is also conducting research relating to daytime fatigue linked with over-the-counter medications, alcohol consumption, elderly drivers and noting the effects on road safety. A report by Horne and Barrett (2001) identifies the over-the-counter medicines which potentially cause drowsiness and are therefore potentially hazardous to drivers and other road users. A total of 102 medicines may cause drowsiness, namely those belonging to the antihistamines, opioids and muscarinic antagonists groups. Older people are particularly vulnerable to the sedative effects of these drugs and the effects are enhanced when combined with alcohol.

Road safety research report No 25, produced by the Department for Transport, Local Government and the Regions (2001), presents the findings in relation to older drivers. Older drivers are increasing in number and particularly female drivers. The risk of an elderly person being killed or suffering serious injuries resulting from a road traffic accident is greater than a younger person because of their increased frailty. Some illnesses are associated with higher road accident risks, e.g. epilepsy, diabetes, heart disease, dementia, sleep apnoea, anxiety and depression and these may be more prevalent in older people. These findings, combined with the effects of drugs in older people, need to be considered from a health promotion perspective.

Another problem related to sleep and political issues is that of sudden infant death syndrome (SIDS) or cot death. SIDS claims seemingly healthy babies every hour in all countries of the world. The USA death rate from cot deaths is 5000–6000 per year, about one-third of all deaths in the newborn period, whereas four babies in 1000 die from cot death in New Zealand. According to Hinchliff et al (1996) there were about 1400 cot deaths in the UK in 1990 (1.7 per 1000) but this figure fell to 0.7 per 1000 by 1994. Infants who die from cot death are usually born with a chronic abnormality with undetected symptoms. However, infant, maternal and environmental characteristics are associated with an increased risk of cot death and the following exercise will help you to identify these characteristics.

There are numerous risk factors. Research in New Zealand identified that 73% of all cot deaths occurred when babies were lying on their stomachs, 63% were of babies of mothers who smoked, that babies were three times as likely to die if they slept in their parents' bed as opposed to sleeping in their own cot, and 33.6% were not breast fed (http://www.globalideasbank.org/BOV/BV-204.HTML).

There are various measures that can be discussed with Elizabeth to reduce the risk of cot death. For example, she could place her baby on its back to sleep as he is less likely to choke, by reducing smoking in the house and certainly not in the baby's bedroom, by ensuring the baby's room is kept at the correct temperature (about 18°C or 65°F), by leaving the baby's head uncovered, and ensuring that the baby sleeps on a firm, flat, well-fitting clean mattress (Department of Health 2000 leaflet available on http:www.gov.uk/cotdeath/). It was estimated that the UK cot death rate of 2000 per year could be cut to 500 a year if parents were informed of risk factors. Fortunately, this advice seems to have been successful with fatalities falling by two-thirds between 1988 and 1992.

Conclusion

The framework for the model of living has been used to demonstrate how the model can be used to guide understanding of health and everyday life in relation to the activity of sleeping. The final exercise will concentrate on the interrelatedness to the other Activities of Living and the factors which affect sleeping specifically through the use of a mini case scenario to demonstrate how individuality in living occurs.

Exercise

1. Read through the family scenario in Box 13.1.
2. Consider how the activity of sleeping may be affected in each of the family members.
3. Consider the effect on the other Activities of Living.

The following points may have been considered.

1. *Maintaining a safe environment*
   - safety of baby, position in bed at night, security of house.

2. *Communicating*
   - all family members need to be aware of the others' sleep needs and shift patterns.

3. *Breathing*
   - snoring and its effects on household.

Box 13.1 Family sleeping patterns

Mark, a policeman, and Patsy, a supply teacher, live in a four-bedroom house, with their two children. Their 20-year-old daughter has a 4-month-old baby and their son is working in the local supermarket, over the summer, until he goes back to college to study music (plays the guitar). Patsy's mother is recently bereaved and is living with them for a short time until she can move into a bungalow. She is depressed after the death of her husband and snores loudly. The baby is developing well but cries at night and still needs feeding. The daughter is breast feeding and has the baby in her room. Mark does not always sleep well when on nights and his son practises his guitar at any time of the day or night. Mark's sister is planning to visit the family, during the summer, flying from New York to London.

---

4. *Eating and drinking*
   - warm milky drinks and small snacks at night
   - avoidance of caffeine and alcohol at bed time

5. *Eliminating*
   - noise at night with regards to flushing toilets.

6. *Mobilising*
   - driving following night shifts. Moving house issues. Exercise habits during the day and prior to retiring at night.

7. *Expressing sexuality*
   - sexual activity of parents in this busy household.

8. *Maintaining body temperature*
   - temperature of the house at night and particularly the babies room.

9. *Working and playing*
   - music practice needs to organised around shifts.

10. *Sleep and rest*
    - sleeping habits, jet lag, sleep deprivation of family members such as Mark or the daughter.

11. *Dying*
    - coping with bereavement.

Summary points

---

1. Individuals spend one-third of their lives asleep.
2. Sleep is an essential part of health and wellbeing.
3. Individuals can learn to adopt a healthy sleep routine.

THE MODEL FOR NURSING

Introduction

This part of the chapter will link the components of the model of living (lifespan, dependency/independency and factors affecting sleeping) with the model for nursing in health and ill health in relation to sleeping. Exercises, mini case scenarios and one major case scenario will be used to allow you to apply the knowledge gained from the model of living section. The application of the model for nursing is based upon the integration of the model of living components and the four stages of the Nursing Process, as shown in Figure 13.5 (Roper et al 1996). (See Chapter 1 for further details relating to the Nursing Process.)

The initial stage of this process – assessing begins with the point of contact of the nurse and the patient and is the start of the nurse–patient relationship. The aim of the assessment stage in relation to sleeping is to collect information about how the individual relates to this Activity of Living when they are well and when they are ill.

Sleeping in health

In order to make this assessment, all the other aspects of the model should be integrated into the sleeping Activity of Living as shown in Box 13.2.

This Activity of Living in health is complex and the nurse needs to be aware of the normal health states of individuals before considering the activity of sleeping in ill health. This information needs to be integrated at each stage of the nursing process to identify individual patients needs and problems.

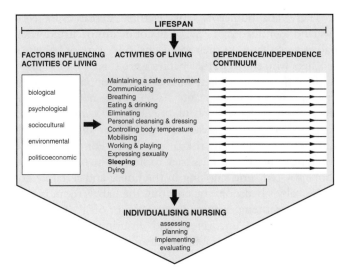

Fig. 13.5 Activity of sleeping within the model for nursing (from Roper et al 1996, with permission).

Sleeping in ill health

The components of the model will be used to show how a variety of ill health issues affect the activity of sleeping. It is estimated that 14–40% of the population of Europe and USA have sleep problems with 17% of these being serious problems (Roper et al 1996, Closs 2000). Insomnia is the most problematic disorder but the International Classification of Sleep Disorders as set by the Diagnostic Classification Steering Committee (1990) identified four different classes of sleep disorders with some 88 distinct sleep and wake patterns. Closs (2000) discusses research of 8000 sleep clinic patients who demonstrate a

---

Box 13.2 Summary of the model for nursing with the activity of sleeping in health

Lifespan
- Consider effect of age and gender on sleeping.

Dependence
- Dependency is linked to changes in the lifespan and health changes, e.g. security, environment, hypnotic drugs.
- Dependency is also linked to changes in health, e.g. fever, bereavement, pain, stress, conscious state.

Independence
- Independence linked to age and health.

Factors affecting sleeping
Biological
- Circadian rhythms, zeitgebers and cell function.
- Intact biological clock.
- Sleep–wake cycle.
- Degree of physical activity.
- Sleep hygiene/habits.
- Body's physiological responses to changes to circadian rhythms.

- Intact nervous system to enable effective sleep–wake cycles.
- Noted by observations of normal sleeping – stages, time asleep, dreaming, activity whilst asleep.
- Note any abnormal sleeping – snoring, insomnia, sleepwalking or talking, nightmares, night terrors.

Psychological
- Effects of emotional state on sleeping such as depression, anxiety, mood swings, excitement, bereavement.

Sociocultural
- Social issues relating to place of sleeping.
- Cultural aspects and beliefs may influence sleeping.

Environmental
- Surroundings, noise, temperature, safety, bedroom design.

Politicoeconomic
- Mechanisms to control working hours, shifts and accidents at work and on the roads.

wide range of sleep problems. The four classes are namely: dyssomnias (e.g. insomnias, excessive sleep), parasomnias (abnormal events which occur during sleep, e.g. sleep-walking), mental/psychiatric disorders and sleep disorders. Ill health, according to Lavery (1997) is one of the main causes of disrupted sleep as various disorders can affect sleep onset, quantity and quality of sleep.

Exercise

1. Using the components of the model (lifespan, dependency–independency continuum, factors affecting health – physical/biological, psychological, sociocultural, environmental, politicoeconomic) and your clinical experience to date, consider what illnesses patients may have which affect sleeping.
2. Check Box 13.3 for some examples.

Reflect on these conditions and identify learning needs following this exercise. It may be useful to discuss these learning needs with a qualified nurse and formulate action plans to address them.

Assessing the individual

The aim of this section, related to assessing an individual, in relation to sleeping, is to demonstrate how to utilise the components of the model of living to carry out the following three phases involved in assessment:

1. Collection of data when taking a nursing history in relation to the activity of sleeping and other related activities.
2. Interpretation of data collected to assess the degree of alteration in the activity of sleeping and the effect on other Activities of Living.

Box 13.3 Summary of illnesses affecting sleep patterns

Lifespan
- Childhood, e.g. difficulty establishing sleep routines in particular sleep onset, nightmares, night terrors, bedwetting, sleepwalking and talking.
- Adult, e.g. insomnia.
- Older person, e.g. difficulties staying asleep and complain of more disturbed sleep with early morning waking.

Dependence/independence
- Sleeping difficulties will affect many of the other Activities of Living and therefore the individual may become dependent on others, e.g. working and playing.

Factors affecting sleeping
1. Biological
  a. Disturbance with sleep–wake cycles, e.g.
    - Insomnia – dissatisfaction with sleep quantity or quality.
    - Hypersomnia – excessive daytime sleepiness or difficulty in waking.
    - Sleep apnoea – cessation of breathing during sleep due to obstruction of upper airway or loss of respiratory effort.
    - Narcolepsy – neurological syndrome, abnormal need to sleep.
    - Cataplexy – sudden temporary paralysis due to fright.
    - Sleep walking – somnambulism.
    - Nightmares/night terrors.
    - Night-time attacks of migraine and asthma linked to REM sleep.
    - ME (myalgic encephalomyelitis) a debilitating condition which presents with flu-like fatigue, depression and poor sleep. Fibromyalgia is similar but presents with muscle fatigue and multiple tender body parts. Alpha waves continue to be produced in their sleep so causing them to wake up.

  b. Damage to nervous tract
    - Brain damage, e.g. coma/head injuries.
    - Overdose of drugs.
    - Epileptic fits occur during NREM sleep and can be induced by sleep deprivation.
    - Parkinson's disease gives fragmented sleep and sleep apnoea can occur.
    - Neuromuscular disorders can affect sleep.

  c. Respiratory/cardiovascular disorders
    - Respiratory and heart problems can occur after dreams, especially if emotional dreams such as death and dying in men and separation in women.
    - Angina and myocardial infarctions are associated with REM sleep.
    - Asthma attacks due to bronchoconstriction occur frequently at night, between 4–6 a.m.

  d. Disorders where pain is present
    - Duodenal ulcers secrete more gastric juice during sleep so wake up with pain.
    - Fibrositis syndrome may be responsible for the generalised pain and stiffness in patients with rheumatoid/osteoarthritis who have sleep disrupted with joint pains.

  e. Disorders involving renal and endocrine systems
    - Diabetes mellitus
    - Myxoedema patient suffer from snoring and obstructive sleep apnoea.

2. Psychological
  - Link with depression and anxiety, e.g. insomnia.

Irwin 1992, Lavery 1997, Morgan & Closs 1999.

3. Identification of individuals' actual and potential problems related to the activity of sleeping and other related activities.

It is noted that assessment is a continuous activity but a thorough initial assessment is vital and this part of the chapter will describe how the components of the model can be integrated to support the assessment process. (For further details relating to assessment refer to Chapter 1.)

Collection of data when taking a nursing history in relation to the activity of sleeping and other related activities

The assessment stage is vital as all the other stages of individualising nursing are dependent upon it. Therefore, it is important to plan this activity and consider what may affect the collection of data, its interpretation and the identification of patient's problems.

Exercise

1. Consider that you have been asked to assess a patient who has been admitted to your clinical area who has been awake all night at home prior to admission in the afternoon.
2. Identify what physical, psychological, sociocultural, environmental and politicoeconomic factors may influence the collection of the data required.

Box 13.4 Factors influencing the activity of sleeping

Physical
- Actual physical state of person and energy levels.
- Actual conscious level of person.
- May be in pain which will affect their ability to sleep and rest.
- Facial expressions/behavioural characteristics such as swollen eyelids, yawning, slow speech.

Psychological
- Actual mental state due to sleep deprivation.
- Actual mental state due to fear and anxiety relating to illness and lack of sleep.
- Actual knowledge of disease and past experiences.

Sociocultural
- Different social/cultural backgrounds of patient and nurse which may affect their ability to communicate.
- Level of interpersonal skills of the patient and the nurse.
- Presence, attitudes and reactions of others.

Environmental
- Ward environment noisy and not very private causing distractions and repetition of answers.

Politicoeconomic
- Quality of the environment.
- Time available to conduct the interview.

Refer to Box 13.4 and consider how these influencing factors can be minimised. Reflect on how nurses can ensure that the collection of data is accurate and how these factors can be minimised so as not to influence the information collected. As noted, there are many factors that may affect the collection of the data and therefore there is a need to use a variety of skills when collecting data. Consider the skills needed in the following exercise.

Exercise

1. What skills will you need to develop to enable you to obtain a comprehensive nursing history with a patient who has difficulty sleeping?
2. Check in Box 13.5 with regards to these skills.

Reflect on these skills and consider why they are important. Then identify the skills which you may need to improve upon and consider how you can do this. Discuss this and write an action plan for this learning need.

Having identified that various factors may affect the ability to collect information and that a variety of skills are equally required, it may be useful to consider what data need to collect specifically and for what purpose these data will be used.

Box 13.5 Assessment skills

Interviewing skills
- Asking open and closed questions as appropriate so as not to tire the individual.
- Consider the length of the initial interview.
- Return and complete the interview when the patient has rested.
- Explain issues in lay terms and check understanding.
- Use of silence to allow individual to rest or think.
- Prioritise questions.
- Involve relatives.

Observation skills
- Verbal and nonverbal cues.
- Physical signs, e.g. desire to sleep, yawning, temperature, pulse rate, respiratory rate.
- Psychological cues, e.g. anxiety.

Writing skills
- Completion of accurate and specific report on patient's individual sleep routines, patterns and problems.

Listening skills
- Therapeutic relationship skills.
- Use own body language appropriately.

Exercise

1. Reflect upon a recent admission you have been involved with and identify potential questions that would help you collect specific data.
2. You may wish to check Box 13.6 for possible questions.
3. Reflect on how you feel about asking these questions and how you would ask them in a conversational manner.

Box 13.6 Questions for assessing the activity of sleeping

Lifespan and independence
- Does the individual sleep normally in relation to the expectations of the time of the lifespan?

Dependence
- Has the individual experienced any difficulties with sleeping in the past or do they have a longstanding difficulty with sleeping?
- How has the individual coped with these sleeping difficulties?
- How is the individual coping with these sleeping difficulties now?
- Could the individual experience difficulties with sleeping in the future?

Factors affecting sleeping
Physical
- What is the individual's normal presleeping, sleeping and waking routines?
- What time does the individual go to sleep?
- How long does it take to get off to sleep?
- What time does the individual wake up in the morning?
- How long does the individual sleep for?
- How many times does the individual wake up during the night?
- What wakes the individual?
- Does the individual take naps in the day time?
- Does the individual snore, talk or walk in their sleep fall out of bed, or have dreams or nightmares?
- What is the individual's usual sleeping position?
- Does the individual take any medication to aid sleep?
- Are there any signs of sleep deficits on admission?
- What specific difficulties is the individual experiencing in relation to sleeping and what are the causes?

- What specific problems are noted in the individual's sleeping pattern or habit?
- What other Activities of Living affect the individual's sleeping problems?
- What effect does the individual's sleeping difficulties have on the other Activities of Living?

Psychological
- What emotional responses affect sleeping?
- What is the individual's attitude to sleep, i.e. quantity and quality needed?
- Does the individual feel refreshed in the morning?
- Does the individual feel sleepy in the daytime?
- Is the individual able to concentrate on tasks in the day?

Sociocultural
- Does the individual normally share a bed or sleep alone?
- What type of clothing does the individual wear in bed?
- How many pillows, sheets, blankets does the individual normally use?
- Does the individual's work or lifestyle affect their sleeping habits, i.e. shift worker?

Environmental
- What factors may alter/inhibit the individual's sleeping pattern at home or hospital?
- Is the individual used to noise, lights or other disturbances during the night at home?

Politicoeconomic
- Are there any difficulties which may have long-term effects on sleep?
- What information and resources does the individual have or need to have in order to assist them in promoting sleep and healthy living?

Box 13.7 Three brief case studies to explore assessment in the AL sleeping

(A) A 22-year-old woman, who has recently been made redundant and has recently separated from her partner, is admitted with anxiety and depression. This is resulting in the woman complaining of insomnia and early morning wakening. She recently took a drugs overdose and was admitted to hospital.

(B) A 40-year-old businesswoman has been complaining of excessive amount of tiredness, fatigue, depression and poor

sleep and has been diagnosed, after some time, as having myalic encaphalomyelitis (ME).

(C) A 66-year-old retired schoolteacher has been diagnosed with Parkinson's disease. He has been complaining of difficulty getting off to sleep, waking up frequently through the night as the activation of muscle tone affects his ability to sleep. He is generally sleeping less than he did before, therefore making him feel tired through the day.

Exercise
1. Consider the brief case studies in Box 13.7.
2. Identify specific questions relating to the following patients with specific ill health sleeping problems.

1. *Case study A questions*
   - What is your pattern of sleep like now?
   - Do you have difficulty falling asleep?
   - How long does it take for you to get off to sleep?
   - When do you wake up in the morning?
   - What do you think keeps you awake or stops you from going back to sleep?
   - When did all these problems start?
   - What helps you to get to sleep or rest?
   - Do you fall asleep in the daytime?
   - Have the problems got worse?
   - How do you feel in the morning?

2. *Case study B questions*
   - What did you sleep like before you started being ill?
   - When did the problems with sleep start?
   - Where do you sleep?
   - What level of activity do you have in the daytime?
   - What is your pattern of sleep like now in the day and the night?
   - What preceded these problems?
   - What helps or makes the problems worse?
   - What are you able to do in your everyday life?
   - How are you coping at work and at home?
   - Have the problems got worse?

3. *Case study C questions*
   - What did you sleep like before you started being ill?
   - When did the problems with sleep start?
   - What is your pattern of sleep like now in the day and the night?
   - Do you have difficulty rolling over in bed or getting in and out of bed?
   - What level of physical activity do you have in the day?
   - What helps or makes the problems worse?
   - Have the problems improved since you have started treatment?
   - Have you noticed an improvement in yourself in the day time if you have a good night's sleep?

It is impossible to cover all feasible adult health problems and their associated sleeping difficulties in this chapter, but it is important to consider that the objective is to collect information to identify:

- the individual's usual habits when they are well
- whether there are any difficulties now in relation to their independence in sleeping
- previous coping strategies with sleeping and associated Activities of Living
- specific problems now.

However, there are common difficulties experienced by individuals with sleeping problems such as:

1. changes in sleep due to hospitalisation
2. changes in sleep patterns
3. changes in conscious levels.

It is useful to consider how each of these difficulties can be assessed and what observations would be required.

Changes in sleep due to hospitalisation

Research has identified that hospitalisation does indeed affect people's sleep habits and routines. Closs (1988) interviewed 200 patients on eight surgical wards to elicit their normal sleep patterns at home and then in hospital. Nurses' recordings of patient's sleep patterns were also recorded. The majority of patients thought that their sleep was worse in hospital than at home. The length of time taken to get to sleep was longer and they woke earlier and slept for less time during the night as they woke up more frequently. There were many factors which affected their sleep, e.g. sex (women slept better than men), ward design (slept better in small wards) and the type of mattresses (slept better on foam mattresses than horsehair ones). Pain or discomfort, noise, temperature and dissatisfaction with the beds disturbed their sleep.

In 1995, Southwell & Wistow conducted a survey of 454 patients and 129 nurses from three different hospitals on medical, surgical, elderly and psychiatric wards. A good response rate was achieved (75% and 84% respectively) and the results indicated that many patients consider that they didn't have sufficient sleep whilst in hospital. This was due to their own personal discomfort, worry and pain, the many disturbances on the ward and that they were woken early in the morning. There were discrepancies between what the patients and nurses viewed as disturbances. It is therefore important that information is collected, from the patients, in relation to sleeping habits and routines.

Interviewing patients is the main method of collecting data to identify changes in sleep due to hospitalisation. The nurse needs to consider what may affect the sleep of the patient due to them being in a strange environment and what may upset their usual sleep routines.

However, there are other subjective assessment methods which can be used to assess sleep as identified by Closs (2000). Sleep charts or diaries can be maintained or visual analogue scales can be completed on a daily basis, or rating scales can be completed throughout the day. Visual analogue scales (see Fig. 13.6) involve asking a patient to mark on a line which runs from 'best sleep ever' to 'worst night ever' and this can give a visual impression of the type of sleep the individual thinks they have had. On the other hand, rating scales involve asking the patient to rate numerically how they feel at that time, with 1 being 'very alert' to 7 being 'excessively sleepy'. These are discussed fully by Morgan and Closs (1999).

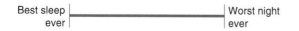

Fig. 13.6 Visual analogue for monitoring sleep (from Morgan & Closs 1999, with permission).

The nurse needs to develop skills, such as observation, questioning and listening as these are the main ways in which reliable data can be collected. However, Morgan and Closs (1999, p. 72) consider that '…nurses' written records of sleep tend to lack validity and accuracy'. The need to ask open questions, such as 'How did you sleep last night?' or 'Did you experience any problems with sleeping last night?' will elicit better information than if a closed question, such as 'Did you sleep well last night?' is asked. Although patients appear to underestimate the length of time spent asleep and overestimate the time taken to get to sleep, there appears to be a correlation between the patient's reports and their problems even if the estimation of time is inaccurate (Morgan & Closs 1999). Therefore, the accurate collection of data from patients is essential to identify the changes in sleep since their hospitalisation.

Issues relating to environmental aspects need to be clearly delineated, e.g. noise, mattress, bed, temperature and light, from illness issues, e.g. pain, confusion and sleep problems which stem from the actual illness. Reactions to being ill in hospital, such as anxiety, must be differentiated from anxiety as an illness. Changes in the patient's normal circadian rhythms and presleep routines should be identified as separate issues also.

Changes in sleep patterns

Apart from the subjective measures noted previously, there are further objective methods which can be used to assess the associated physiological and psychological events related to sleep. However, this data collection involves expensive and specialised equipment, for example, polysomnography and electroencephalogram (EEG) and these are usually only used in specialised sleep clinics. If there is a sleep clinic within the clinical area, it would be useful to discuss these objective measurements.

Changes in conscious levels

It is important that the nurse is able to differentiate between sleep and changes in conscious levels. Altered consciousness can be considered from what may be described as 'normal conscious level through (to) impaired attention, loss of alertness, drowsiness, sleep, stupor and finally coma' as Roper et al (1996, p. 389) identify.

Although the terms drowsy, stupor and coma are used, they aren't really helpful in identifying whether the patient's condition is improving or deteriorating, especially if different nurses undertake these assessments. Nurses need to be alert to any change in a patient's conscious level, as recognising this change, however small it may be, could be lifesaving and possibly prevent brain damage, if it is reported

and acted upon appropriately. In an attempt to standardise the assessment of conscious levels the Glasgow Coma Scale (GSC) is commonly used throughout the UK and the world (see Jamieson et al 2002, p. 369 and Chapter 3). This allows all health care professionals to utilise the same questions, the same stimuli in the same way and for these responses to be charted in a clear manner so that an accurate picture of the patient's condition can be easily seen.

Three aspects of the patient's behaviour are monitored independently, namely eye opening, verbal response and motor response and scored according to the best response. There are two versions of the Glasgow Coma Scale which can cause some confusion (see Fig. 13.7a and b, Roper et al 1996). There are a 14-point (original) and a revised 15-point versions. It is essential that all health professionals using this scale identify which scale they are using (see Frawley 1990, Roper et al 1996, Alexander et al 2000 for further details on these variations).

Depending on which point version is used, the best response for 'eye opening' is 4, the best response for 'verbal response' is 5 and the best response for 'motor response' is 5 or 6, with 1 being the lowest score for all three areas. The scores are charted and when the scores are combined then this indicates the conscious level. The score can therefore range from 3 to 14 or 15. A score of 7 and below indicates a coma, whereas a higher score indicates a higher level of consciousness.

> **Exercise**
> 1. Observe other health care professionals carrying out these observations.
> 2. What kind of charts were used to record the observation findings? Are they similar to the Glasgow Coma Scale chart?
> 3. How do they identify the best response for eye opening, verbal and motor responses?

It may have been possible to observe health care professionals using the Glasgow Coma Scale in Accident and Emergency Departments, Intensive Care Units, High Dependency Units, specialised Neurological Units or general medical or surgical wards. The charts used may have been single Glasgow Coma Scale charts only or they may have been modified to include observations such as temperature, pulse and blood pressure, pupils sizes and reactions.

To monitor the patient's response to the spoken word and the 'eye opening' activity, the health care professional may have observed noting whether the patient opened their eyes spontaneously because they felt the presence of someone at their bedside (score 4) or if they opened their eyes when the health care professional spoke to them without touching them or by shouting or shaking them gently (score 3). If no response is gained from talking to the patient in this way then the health care professional may have been observed applying a painful stimuli, such as

a 14 point version of the Glasgow Coma Scale

G L A S G O W C O M A S C A L E		
	Eyes open	spontaneously to speech to pain none
	Best verbal response	orientated disorientated monosyllabic response incomprehensible sounds none
	Best motor response	obey commands local pain flexion to pain extension to pain

b 15 point version of the Glasgow Coma Scale

	Eyes opening Score	Motor response Score	Verbal response Score
High score ↑		6 If command such as 'lift up your hands' is obeyed	
		5 If purposeful movements to remove painful stimulus such as pressure over eyebrow	5 If oriented to person, place and time
	4 If eyes open spontaneously to approach of nurse to bedside	4 If finger withdrawn after application of a painful stimulus to it	4 If conversation confused
	3 If eyes open in response to speech	3 If painful stimulation at finger tip flexes the elbow	3 If inappropriate words are used
	2 If eyes open in response to pain at finger tip	2 If the patient's arms are flexed and finger tip stimulation results in extension of elbow	2 If only incomprehensibe sounds are uttered
Low score ↓	1 If eyes do not open in response to pain at finger tip	1 If there is no detectable response to repeated and various stimuli	1 If no verbal response
	A normal person would score 15 on the scale; the lowest possible score is 3 which is compatible with, but does not necessarily indicate, brain death. A score of 7 is used as a definition of coma.		

Fig. 13.7 (a) 14 point version of the Glasgow Coma Scale, (b) 15 point version (from Roper et al 1996, with permission).

exerting pressure on the patient's finger nail bed, by rolling a pen over the nail bed (see Fig. 13.8, Roper et al 1996).

This is done to the third or fourth digits as they are the most sensitive but care must be taken to avoid pressure on the cuticle. If the patient opens their eyes at this point then 2 is scored but if the eyes don't open then a score of 1 is given. Difficulties may have arisen for the health care professional, when monitoring the patient's response to the spoken word, if the patient had impaired hearing. If the eyelids are swollen then the patient may not be able to open their eyes and C should be recorded for 'closed', equally the eyes may remain open and therefore are recorded as not responding to the painful stimuli.

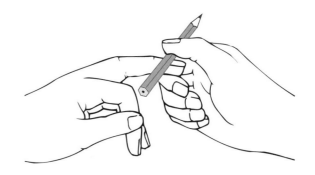

Fig. 13.8 Pressure on finger nail bed (from Teasdale et al 1975, with permission).

Any damage to the brain stem from trauma or raised intracranial pressure will affect the patient's ability to open their eyes as this ability is linked to being alert and awake. It must be remembered, however, that the patient may not be aware of their surroundings and therefore there is the need to continue with the assessment of the verbal and motor responses.

To assess the best verbal response, the health care professionals will have asked the patient various questions and on the basis of their responses will attach a score to the appropriate level achieved. To score 5 on the scale, i.e. orientation, the patient must be able to state their name, say where they are, i.e. which hospital and in which town it is and what month and year it is. The order in which these questions are asked may be altered but if answered correctly the person is said to be orientated to time, people and place.

If the person answers these questions incorrectly or inappropriately then the person is not orientated to time, people or place and is said to be confused and scores 4. The patient may be able to converse, in sentences, with the health care professional but it is a rambling conversation and this must be differentiated between being 'confused' and using 'inappropriate words', which scores 3. Inappropriate words are identified by the individual answering in one or two words only, quite often after painful stimuli have been exerted to assess the eye-opening section of the scale. The words will probably have made little sense and may have been obscene. Incomprehensible sounds score 2 and this should have been noted if the patient only makes a noise but no words can be identified and they moan, mumble or scream. If the patient didn't utter any noise, even with painful stimuli, then they would be said to have no verbal response and would score 1. However, there may be reasons why patients cannot answer questions or make noises, e.g. don't speak English, they are deaf, have a speech defect or an endotracheal or tracheostomy tube in situ. The health care professional should document these issues to clarify any of these issues, e.g. put E or T if the patient has an endotracheal or tracheostomy tube in situ.

If the scores obtained for verbal responses are decreasing then the patient's condition is worsening and this may be due to trauma to brain tissue, hypoxia, or raised intracranial pressure. These tests indicate whether the patient is able to receive and understand a variety of inputs (sensory, verbal or physical) and then their ability to respond verbally. The final area to be assessed is that of motor responses, in the upper limbs only, which tests the patient's abilities to receive and understand any of these inputs and then to coordinate a motor response (see Fig. 13.9 for the tests and the responses noted; Pemberton 2000).

The best motor response is scored at either 6 or 5 (depending on whether using the 15- or 14-point version) and is when the patient is able to respond to a command given by the health care professional, such as, 'Lift up your arms', or 'Stick out your tongue'. If the patient doesn't

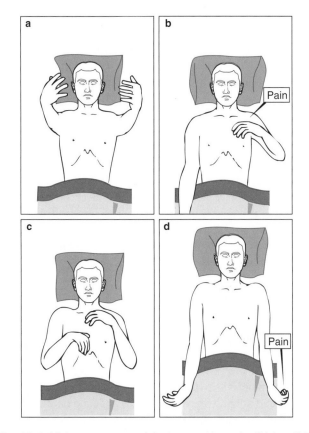

Fig. 13.9 Motor responses, (a) obey commands, (b) localising to pain, (c) flexing to pain, (d) extending to pain (from Alexander et al 2000, with permission).

respond to these commands then the health care professional must assess the patient's motor response to painful stimuli. The trapezium pinch is the safest method to use as the shoulders are easily exposed and the muscle can be grasped and pinched easily. If the patient lifts the arm purposefully towards the area being pinched, then the patient is said to be 'localising to pain' and scores 5 or 4 (depending on the scale used). If using the 15-point scale, then the score of 4 is given if the patient withdraws the finger after the painful stimuli has been applied but they don't try to remove the stimuli. Rubbing of the sternum and pressure applied to the supraorbital ridge is not advocated now due to the bruises left on the chest and the possibility of damage to the orbital structure. If the patient doesn't appear to localise to the painful stimuli then you should have observed the health care professional apply pressure to the nail bed again and if the patient flexes or bends the elbow and withdraws their hand but does not localise to the finger itself then they would score 3, as they have demonstrated their ability to flex to pain. If the elbows are straightened after the painful stimuli has been applied, then the patient scores 2, as they have shown their ability to extend to pain. If no movement occurs, then the health care professional will score 1 on the chart.

It is vital that the nurse ensures that she understands how to conduct a coma assessment using the Glasgow Coma Scale and that the findings are interpreted correctly and actions taken appropriately. There are others reasons, apart from head injuries, why a patient may experience changes in their conscious levels, e.g. fainting or syncope, during a convulsion or fit and when undergoing general anaesthesia. Therefore, it is important for you to consider the possible cause of any alterations in conscious levels.

Interpretation of data collected

Once the data have been collected it is necessary to utilise knowledge and decision-making skills to interpret the information prior to the identification of the individual's actual and potential problems. Using the assessment questions outlined in Box 13.6, consider the information that may be gathered from Case study 13.1 by considering the components of the model.

Case study 13.1

Emma Simmons

Emma Simmons is a 45-year-old married lady who has rheumatoid arthritis which is currently affecting her hands, wrists, knees and feet. She lives with her husband, two sons aged 13 and 17 years of age and is a secretary at the local school. She has been admitted because she is having pain when she types and when normal movement of the hands and feet is attempted. The joints are swollen, tender and warm to touch and she is aware that there is a loss of function in her hands and she is experiencing some stiffness especially in the morning. The pain in the joints is now affecting her ability to sleep at night with frequent awakenings which is causing more difficulties for her. She has noticed that she has lost weight over the last year and feels tired. She is currently taking aspirin as an analgesic and a nonsteroidal anti-inflammatory agent (NSAID). An assessment of her treatment regime is being carried out with a view to improving her quality of life. The possibility of surgery has been discussed with Emma.

It is now necessary to utilise the components of the model to interpret the information collected with Case study 3.1 relating to chronic systemic joint disease problems which are affecting her sleep patterns.

Exercise

1. Consider the factors which may have led to Emma's health breakdown.
2. Identify the effect on other Activities of Living.
3. Check your answers with those in Box 13.8.

Box 13.8 Health breakdown and its effects on other ALs

Factors leading to health breakdown

- Age and gender – usually affects women in 40–50 age range.
- Dependency continuum may be affected now as work and home activities are proving to be a problem.
- No known cause although:
  - infections, hormones and autoimmune factors (physical) and
  - familial factors (sociocultural) are being investigated.

Other activities being affected

Communicating
- Pain, in joints and on movement, is affecting her ability to socialise.
- Emma is anxious and depressed over the current exacerbation of her disease and the effects it is having on her life.

Eating and drinking
- Loss of appetite and weight loss due to pain, medications and systemic disease, difficulty using utensils.

Eliminating
- Finding it difficult to sit down on the toilet, especially in the morning when her knees are stiff. Constipating effect of medications.

Personal cleansing and dressing
- Skin is fragile and stretched over the joint surfaces.

Mobilising
- Fatigued easily, warm, painful, swollen stiff joints, especially in the morning. Loss of function in the hands and wrists.

Sleep and rest
- Wakes frequently during the night, feels tired and not rested.

Expressing sexuality
- Pain and impaired mobility may be affecting her sexual relationships with her husband.

Maintaining body temperature
- Mildly pyrexial.

Working and playing
- Tired, difficult to type at work and carrying out some of the household jobs, especially in the morning.

From this exercise it can be seen that Emma has:

- a longstanding chronic systemic joint disease
- an exacerbation of this disease which is affecting other Activities of Living
- an occupational problem
- a problem with completing housework
- alterations in socialisation and possible sexual relationships due to disease, pain, difficulty to mobilise and tiredness.

Following this interpretation of the data, it is then necessary to complete the final stage of the assessment process and identify actual and potential problems.

Identification of actual and potential problems

Actual and potential sleep problems will be specific to the individual's sleep difficulty and their health breakdown problem but common sleep problems can be identified in relation to:

1. changes in sleep due to hospitalisation
2. changes in sleep patterns
3. changes in conscious levels.

Changes in sleep due to hospitalisation

Sleep deprivation can occur due to hospitalisation affecting the amount, consistency and quality of sleep. The strange environment of the hospital ward, the numerous disturbances, discomfort, pain and worry, medications, illnesses and the need for nursing care all contribute to sleep deprivation in the patient. A variety of illnesses affect sleep, such as arthritis which disturbs a person's sleep due to joint pains and asthma which affects sufferers by increasing bronchoconstriction at night, especially around 4–6 am, which affects sleep at this time. The quality of life of Parkinson sufferers and their carers is often made worse, according to Crabb (2001), by impaired sleep. This is due to many reasons, such as the ageing process, the medications used and the disease itself.

Through the use of diaries, Schaefer (1997) identified the sleep problems of eight women who suffered with fibromyalgia and found that there was a relationship between muscle aches and pains with sleep and other issues such as the weather. Brostrom et al (2001) identified that sleep was affected in 20 patients suffering from congestive cardiac failure by their daily activities, the disease itself and the cardiac symptoms. The sleep disturbances then gave rise to fatigue, listlessness, loss of concentration and loss of temper. These effects then lead onto the need for daytime sleep and seclusion.

Whatever the disease, the resulting sleep deprivation may result in lack of concentration, irritability, fatigue and may pose safety risks. In addition to these psychological effects, sleep deprivation may have a negative influence on healing. Caution is necessary, according to Closs (1990), in making the direct link of healing and sleep deprivation as the studies to support this link are confined to animals. The promotion of sleep is, however, an essential factor to consider in the management of surgical patients, especially if this link was supported by research conducted on human subjects.

A pilot study conducted by Ersser et al (1999) identified that a marked proportion of older people reported sleeping well in nursing care settings and those in nursing homes slept better than those in a community hospital. However, disturbances in both settings were related to personal needs for micturition during the night, noise, discomfort and pain.

Snoring can also be a major problem for the snorer and those near to them, therefore this may cause other patients in a ward environment to have disturbed sleep patterns. Snoring is caused by an obstruction in the upper airways (nose or throat) and is found to be more common in men, those who are overweight, suffering from hypothyroidism or who have a nasal or tonsil problem. Snoring rarely causes serious health problems.

Night wandering, especially elderly people with Alzheimer's disease, may cause problems in a hospital or nursing home environment. Whilst night wandering is not sleepwalking (somnambulism), as the person is awake, they are confused about whether it is day or night and a change of environment can often trigger this wandering. The safety of the individual is of utmost importance and it is also important that they don't disturb the other patients around them.

A potential problem is that patients may be at risk of injury if they are restless in bed due to a variety of reasons. The patient may be dreaming, not used to sleeping in a single bed or alone, may wish to go to the toilet or the restlessness may be due to medications taken or brain stem irritation. Hospital beds tend to be much higher than ordinary beds and therefore the risk of injury is greater than at home if the patient was to fall out of bed. Cot sides are sometimes used to prevent restless patients from falling out of bed but the use of cot sides does raise ethical and legal issues, as they are classed as a form of physical restraint, and injuries can still occur.

In the UK, the use of physical restraints with older people is often classed as a form of abuse (UKCC 1999) and Dimond (1995) states that to impede a person's freedom (by the use of physical restraint) is unlawful. The Royal College of Nursing (1999) argue that nurses who use restraints with patients must be able to justify their actions. The use of restraints doesn't guarantee safety and can cause physical and psychological problems. However, patients may choose to have cot sides or side rails in situ to stop them rolling out of bed or to help them sit up and if so the cot sides are not noted as restraints. Gallinagh et al (2002) concluded that specific protocols are needed in relation to the use of physical restraints. An assessment would be needed to ascertain if restraints are necessary and to decide on which type is the best to use. If they are necessary, the restraint needs to be discussed with the patient and their relatives and if agreed upon, as a safety and short-term measure only, then the restraints need to be ordered by the medical team and documented fully.

Gallinagh et al (2002) conducted an observational study to investigate the prevalence and type of physical restraints used with older people on four rehabilitation wards in Northern Ireland. Most of the patients (68%) were subjected to some form of physical restraint and cot sides were the most commonly observed method of restraint. Those who were restrained were dependent on nursing care but no link to staffing levels or incidence of falls were found, even though nurses often cite the risk of injury from falls as the reason for using restraints. In this study, wandering and patient protection were the reasons why nurses used restraints. In a study by Karlsson et al (2000), they identified that nurses' decisions to use restraints in two nursing homes were affected by a variety of issues and although the patient's best interest were considered, the working conditions and the nurses' willingness to take risk when not restraining a patient were also factors used in deciding to use a form of restraint or not.

Another potential problem is that there is a risk that the patient may become dependent on night sedation medication or analgesia and this should be avoided at all costs. Halfens et al (1994) concluded that the administration of sleep medication is not without danger. This statement was as a result of a study of 233 patients who used sleep medication in Dutch hospitals. This medication was given to the patients for the first time and for at least 5 days. After discharge from the hospital, these patients continued to use sleep medication at home. On the other hand, those patients who did not receive sleep medication in hospital did not use it at home following discharge. Although prescribed by the doctor, the sleep medication was given by the nurse. An alternative to night sedation is needed to discourage patients from being given sleep medication for the first time in hospital and then finding it difficult to stop taking this when they are at home.

Changes in sleep patterns

Actual sleep problems include insomnia, sleep apnoea and narcolepsy and the nurse needs to have an understanding of these problems. Insomnia is the best known actual sleep problem but it can be divided into three types, namely sleep-onset problems, sleep maintenance problems and early-wakening problems. The main cause is often worry over a particular problem but it is also associated with depressive illness (Irwin 1992).

Sleep apnoea refers to the temporary cessation of breathing during sleep, in between snoring episodes. Obstructive sleep apnoea occurs when the pharynx closes during sleep and is accompanied by loud snoring as the person tries to breathe through a narrowed space. Eventually the space closes and respiration stops for up to 1 minute. The patient then clears the airway with a snort and is aroused and starts to breathe again. This cycle can occur many times each night. It is estimated that nearly 4% of the UK population suffer from sleep apnoea with corresponding excessive daytime sleepiness and complaints of insomnia. Breathing disorders can give rise to sleep apnoea also, as does hypothyroidism. It is more prevalent in older people, the obese, smokers and drinkers (Morgan & Closs 1999). Central apnoea occurs when the drive to breathe is abnormally reduced during sleep, as opposed to obstructed, but this again leads to asphyxia and arousal. According to Irwin (1992), it is associated with neuromuscular disorders, respiratory and brainstem disorders.

Narcolepsy is a serious but rare sleep disorder occurring in 0.04% of the population. It occurs between the ages of 15–25 and varies between being a mild inconvenience to being a severe, debilitating disease with excessive sleepiness and daytime sleep attacks. The overwhelming need to sleep, even in the middle of the day, is the main complaint. Narcolepsy sufferers may fall asleep when standing up, whilst talking, driving a car or whilst swimming. It can be accompanied by cataplexy, where the individual is unable to move, or the person may have hallucinations (Morgan & Closs 1999).

Problems related to waking behaviours (parasomnias) can cause actual sleep problems such as sleepwalking (somnambulism), grinding of teeth (bruxism) and bed wetting (enuresis). These problems tend to be found in children only and further information can be found in Morgan and Closs (1999).

Changes in conscious levels

Any alteration in the conscious level of a person indicates that there is a problem, some of which are extremely serious. Roper et al (1996, p. 389) identify that the stages of altered consciousness can be described as a '…gradual change from a normal conscious level through impaired attention, loss of alertness, drowsiness, sleep, stupor and finally coma'. The latter two descriptors are abnormal states compared to the others and the nurse would need to utilise observational skills to differentiate between the normal and abnormal states and act appropriately.

Exercise

1. Re-read Case study 13.1 on p. 396.
2. Using the Activities of Living as a framework, identify Emma's actual and potential problems.
3. Check your identified actual and potential problems with those in Box 13.9.

In this section how to collect data when taking a nursing history in relation to the activity of sleeping and other related activities will have been considered. In addition how to interpret the data collected in order to assess the degree of alteration in the activity of sleeping and the effect on other Activities of Living. It is also important to have identified how an individual's actual and potential problems related to the activity of sleeping affect other related activities.

Planning nursing activities

Planning nursing activities involves the following:

- identifying priorities
- establishing short- and/or long-term goals
- determining nursing actions/interventions required
- documenting the plan (refer to Chapter 1 for further information).

Box 13.9 Actual and potential problems that Emma may experience

Activity of Living	Actual problems	Potential problems
Communicating	Emma is experiencing pain in her joints and on movement due to the arthritis/inflammation and this is shown by limited mobility, some loss of function in the hands and wrists, facial expression and verbal complaints of pain. Emma is anxious and depressed over the current exacerbation of her disease and the effects it is having on her life.	
Eating and drinking	Emma is experiencing loss of appetite and weight loss due to pain, medications and systemic disease which made it difficult for Emma to hold and use utensils due to the painful swollen joints.	
Eliminating	Emma has difficulty with sitting down on the toilet, especially in the morning due to her knees being stiff.	Emma is at risk of developing constipation due to her restricted mobility and the medications she is taking.
Personal cleansing and dressing		Emma may have difficulty in meeting her hygiene needs due to the pain, tiredness, loss of function in her hands and morning stiffness.
Mobilising	Emma has difficulties mobilising because she tires easily, and the joints in her hands, knees and feet are warm, painful, swollen and stiff, especially in the morning. Emma is experiencing some loss of function in the hands and wrists.	
Sleep and rest	Emma is having difficulty sleeping due to the joint pains and this is shown by waking frequently in the night, and that she feels tired and not rested.	
Expressing sexuality		Emma may be experiencing difficulties in her sexual relationships with her husband due to the constant joint pains and sleep deprivation.
Maintaining body temperature	Emma may feel warm due to her being mildly pyrexial.	
Working and playing	Emma is having difficulty working (at home and school) and socialising due to the pain and her tiredness	

To ensure that the nursing activities are planned appropriately, it is necessary to review the individual's actual and potential problems and then consider the level to which the activity of sleeping can be helped. There are different levels of helping, such as:

- to solve or alleviate actual problems
- to prevent potential problems becoming actual ones
- to prevent solved problems from reoccurring

- to develop positive strategies for any problems which cannot be solved.

Exercise

1. Re read the three brief case studies in Box 13.7 (p. 391).
2. Identify the levels of helping that may be achieved in relation to these case studies.

The following levels of care may have been considered appropriate:

1. *Case study A*
   - to develop positive coping strategies for lifestyle changes to alleviate anxiety and depression
   - to alleviate insomnia and early morning wakenings by developing positive coping strategies to alleviate anxiety and depression.

2. *Case study B*
   - to develop positive coping strategies for lifestyle changes to alleviate fatigue, tiredness, poor sleep and depression.

3. *Case Study C*
   - to develop positive coping strategies for lifestyle changes to alleviate sleep problems and difficulties directly related to Parkinson's disease.

The focus must be on the individual's problems and wishes as opposed to the nurse's ideas. Therefore, involvement of the patient is crucial at this stage. However, this may be affected by the problems that the patient may have, e.g. pain, altered conscious levels, inability to communicate verbally, as noted previously.

Many factors may influence the nurse and the patient in the planning stage of nursing activities with a patient with sleeping difficulties. Consider this in relation to a patient with sleeping difficulties and check these in Box 13.10.

Identifying priorities

Following the assessment, the next stage is to plan the care. Determine priorities of care as this skill is a vital component of any nurse's repertoire. Determine which problem is the most important and grade it as follows:

- life-threatening – totally dependent
- urgent – mainly dependent but some ability to be independent
- semi-urgent – some dependency but mainly independent
- non-urgent – totally independent.

This priority status may change day by day, shift by shift or hour by hour and therefore the assessment stage must be a continuous activity to ensure that the nurse remains alert to possible changes.

Exercise

1. Re-read the actual and potential problems that have been identified for Emma Simmons in Case study 13.1.
   - Identify which problems are life-threatening, urgent, semi-urgent, and non-urgent.
   - Decide which would be the first three problems that need to be addressed, giving a rationale for this choice.
   - Check your decisions with those found in Box 13.11.

Box 13.10 Factors which influence planning care for a patient with sleeping difficulties

From the nurse's perspective
- Knowledge of normal physiology and specific pathophysiological processes in relation to sleeping disorders and disorders which affect sleeping habits of individuals.
- Knowledge of normal living and dependency across the lifespan in various cultures in relation to sleeping.
- Knowledge of sleeping difficulties specific to the patient's problem.
- Knowledge of nursing interventions available and evidenced-based practices.
- Knowledge of assessment methods and the accuracy of these methods.
- Skills in observing, assessment, interpreting and prioritising.
- Staffing levels and skill mix on night duty.
- Own sleep habits and sleep hygiene routines.

From the patient's perspective
- Ability and degree of involvement of the patient in the decisions related to care to be planned.
- Knowledge of sleeping difficulties specific to the patient's problem.
- Personal beliefs, attitudes, experiences and coping strategies.
- Enactment of the sick role.

It can be seen that Emma's problems are varied in relation to their priorities and involve many of the Activities of Living. A suggested priority order is:

1. Emma is experiencing pain in her joints and on movement due to the arthritis/inflammation and this is shown by limited mobility, some loss of function in the hands and wrists, facial expression and verbal complaints of pain.
2. Emma is having difficulty sleeping due to the joint pains and this is shown waking frequently in the night, and that she feels tired and not rested.
3. Emma is experiencing loss of appetite and weight loss due to pain, medications and systemic disease which made it difficult for Emma to hold and use utensils due to the painful swollen joints.

The rationale for the priority order is that the pain is the main difficulty which is directly affecting her ability to mobilise, sleep, work and socialise. If nursing actions are not planned then the pain will become worse. If, however, nursing actions are planned to alleviate the pain then the problems with mobilising, sleeping, working and socialising will be diminished if not solved.

The sleeping problems will be better if the pain is relieved but the change in routine and hospitalisation may also have an effect on Emma's sleeping habits and, if sleep

Box 13.11 Priority status of actual problems experienced by Emma

Activity of Living	Actual problems	Problem status
Communicating	Emma is experiencing pain in her joints and on movement due to the arthritis/inflammation and this is shown by limited mobility, facial expression and verbal complaints of pain.	Semi-urgent
	Emma is anxious and depressed over the current exacerbation of her disease and the effects it is having on her life.	Semi-urgent
Eating and drinking	Emma is experiencing loss of appetite and weight loss due to pain, medications and systemic disease which made it difficult for Emma to hold and use utensils due to the painful swollen joints.	Semi-urgent
Eliminating	Emma has difficulty with sitting down on the toilet, especially in the morning due to her knees being stiff.	Non-urgent
	Emma is at risk of developing constipation due to her restricted mobility and the medications she is taking.	Non-urgent
Mobilising	Emma has difficulties mobilising because she tires easily, and the joints in her hands, knees and feet are warm, painful, swollen and stiff, especially in the morning.	Semi-urgent
	Emma is experiencing some loss of function in the hands and wrists.	Semi-urgent
Sleep and rest	Emma is having difficulty sleeping due to the joint pains and this is shown by waking frequently in the night, and that she feels tired and not rested.	Semi-urgent
Maintaining body temperature	Emma may feel warm due to her being mildly pyrexial.	Non-urgent
Working and playing	Emma is having difficulty working (at home and school) and socialising due to the pain and her tiredness.	Semi-urgent
Personal cleansing and dressing	Emma may have difficulty in meeting her hygiene needs due to the pain, tiredness, loss of function in her hands and morning stiffness.	Non-urgent
Expressing sexuality	Emma may be experiencing difficulties in her sexual relationships with her husband due to the constant joint pains and sleep deprivation.	Non-urgent

deprivation occurs, then more problems arise which can affect her physical and mental wellbeing. Nutritional problems are very important to Emma's wellbeing. There are problems with the medications used for arthritis as they can cause gastrointestinal problems and Emma may be reluctant to take them because of this which, in turn, will affect her pain levels and subsequently her mobility, sleep, work and socialisation patterns.

Goal setting

Goal setting is based upon sound assessment and the identification of problems and priorities. Goals can be short term (hourly to generally less than a week) or long term (for a longer period). Many short-term goals may be needed to achieve long-term goals.

The goal statement is essential so that the process of evaluation can take place. It is therefore important that the goal is written in the terms of what the patient ought to be able or has agreed to achieve. The goals should be written in observable, realistic and measurable behavioural terms so that it is easier to monitor and evaluate the patient's progress (refer to Chapter 1 for further details on goal setting). This may be a skill that needs to be developed and practiced.

Exercise

1. Re-read Emma Simmons' actual and potential problems related to Case study 13.1, listed in Box 13.9 on p. 396 in the assessment section.
2. Choose three of these problems and set short- and long-term goals.
3. Check the example given in Box 13.12.

Box 13.12 Short- and long-term goals

Problem
Emma is experiencing pain in her joints and on movement due to the arthritis/inflammation and this is shown by limited mobility, facial expression and verbal complaints of pain.

Short-term goal
Emma will be able to verbalise her pain to nursing staff and assess the effect of medications given for the pain.

Long-term goal
Emma will be able to mobilise, sleep, work and socialise within the pain limits and be able to adapt her lifestyle to cope with the pain.

Once the short-term and long-term goals have been set it will be necessary to determine the appropriate nursing actions which will aid the alleviation of problems and the achievement of the short- and long-term goals.

Determining nursing actions

It is vital that the appropriate nursing actions are chosen to alleviate patient's problems. To be able to do this, the nurse must constantly update their knowledge and skills to ensure that care given is evidence-based and delivered in a safe, competent and professional manner. Nursing actions will be considered in relation to the factors which affect ill health (physical, psychological, sociocultural, environmental and politicoeconomic) and with patients who have 'difficulty with sleeping'. There is a need for the nurse to act as a health educator in relation to all of these nursing actions to ensure that the patient and their significant others are appraised of the problem, treatments and ways in which problems can be minimised and prevented.

Nursing actions associated with physical factors affecting ill health

The purpose of the nursing actions, associated with the physical factors related to sleeping difficulties, is that the nurse, provides specific care to individuals who are not able to provide for themselves to promote and maintain health and prevent disease. The place on the lifespan, the level of dependency and biological factors identified in the model of living will need to be considered when the nursing actions are planned.

There are many nursing actions, related to physical care, which affect sleeping but some of the main actions are described below.

Nursing observations of vital signs, conscious levels and sleeping habits

These observations have been noted earlier in this chapter and in Chapters 3, 5 and 9. However, it is important that you consider when and how often these observations should be carried out. This will depend on the severity of the patient's condition and whether the problems are acute or chronic. The initial assessment of vital signs, conscious levels (where appropriate) and sleeping habits can be used as a baseline for future evaluations. It may be that these observations are carried out continuously as the patient is in a critical care environment or a specialised sleep clinic, or they are carried out hourly, 4-hourly or daily.

Once the observations have been taken, they must be recorded accurately and the significance of the observations identified and reported to senior members of the health care team. Any alterations in the patient's conscious level must be reported immediately.

Sleep may well be affected by taking these observations and you need to plan the care so that patients are not disturbed during the night to have observations recorded, wherever possible. The timing of some treatments, such as blood transfusions and the observations needed with these, may need to be considered. It may be that the blood transfusion can be completed during the day so that the observations are not needed during the night to ensure that the patient's sleep patterns are not unduly disturbed (Cawthorn & Hope 1992).

Administration of drug therapies The administration of any medications is an important aspect of the nurse's role and professional, legal and local policies govern these actions. The professional practice of the nurse, in relation to the administration of medicines, is guided by the Nursing and Midwifery Council 'Guidelines for the administration of medicines' (NMC 2002a) document and further details can be found in Chapter 3 and on the Nursing and Midwifery Council website at http://www.nmc-uk.org. The nurse needs to have an up-to-date knowledge of pharmacology and needs to consider any ritualistic practices that may occur with 'drug administration rounds', such as the practice of a 6 am drug round.

In relation to sleep issues, the nurse must be aware of certain hypnotics and tranquillisers (benzodiazepines) which act on the central nervous system to promote sleep and reduce anxiety, such as nitrazepam (Mogadon), diazepam (Valium), temazepam (Normison), chloral hydrate (Welldorm), chlordiazepoxide (Librium) and the new non-benzodiazepine hypnotics which have less side effects. As all of these drugs can affect the activity of the central nervous system and breathing system, they must be monitored carefully as the patient is at risk from these medications.

Various problems have been identified when patients take hypnotics and tranquillisers. For example, the sleep is very different to normal sleep, patients may suffer from a hangover feeling, but the risk of dependency is the major problem, with drug accumulation and residual sedation, adding to safety issues as mobility and coordination can be affected, and all of these are compounded with withdrawal problems (Morgan & Closs 1999).

These types of drugs are often prescribed as 'prn' medications, i.e. 'when necessary'. The nurse, therefore, is charged with making the decision of when it is necessary to give the medication prescribed by another health care professional who is not present at the time. It is vital that the nurse discusses these issues with the patient and ensures that the appropriate treatment regime is maintained. The nurse and patient, therefore, need to have knowledge of the medication's action, side effects, patient's condition and other medications. A study by Duxbury (1994) identified that nurses who delivered care via a team nursing approach gave three times as much 'prn night sedation' as nurses who delivered care via a primary nursing approach. This difference may have been related to the beliefs held as the team nurses' views were more consistent with a medical approach of the advantages of night sedation and its continuing use.

Administration of complementary therapies There are many different forms of complementary therapies which may be useful for the patient with sleeping difficulties, such as aromatherapy, massage, reflexology and pet therapy. There is some evidence to support the claims made, as these therapies have been successful for some patients. Therefore, complementary therapies should be considered. Deakin (1995) identified that relaxation techniques were successful when used with clients who exhibited disruptive behaviour. Dunn et al (1995) identified that massage, rest and aromatherapy, when used in an Intensive Therapy Unit, proved to be beneficial to most patients and Cannard (1995) used aromatherapy with elderly patients successfully. Brownfield (1998) also used complementary therapies with patients suffering with rheumatoid arthritis. Relaxation, heat, therapeutic touch, light massage and acupuncture were found to be effective for the eight women in Schaefer's study in 1997. In this study, the writing of a diary was noted as a useful tool as it empowered the women. They were able to predict times when muscle aches and pains may be worse and therefore adapt their lifestyles accordingly.

The controlled use of essential oils to produce health and relaxation is offered and lavender and sandalwood have been found to be relaxing and promote sleep, whether put in a bath or inhaled in a burner. However, care is needed as this may affect other patients in a ward setting. Massage, with or without oils, is said to reduce anxiety and help sleep and that it is the touch that is important (Lavery 1997).

The use of complementary therapy has grown and the RCN has formed a specialist interest group for complementary therapies. Trevelyan and Booth (1994) discussing this specialist interest group reported, in 1992, that, providing nurses were appropriately trained, there were 'potentially acceptable therapies' that they could use. Acupuncture, reflexology, massage and aromatherapy were amongst those therapies identified. NHS Trusts are developing policies to clarify roles and responsibilities and to ensure good practice (Walsh 2002). Trevelyan and Booth (1994) discuss that nurses seem to be more aware of possible legal repercussions of their actions and highlight one District Health Authority's action in drawing up a local policy to cover the use of complementary therapies by nurses. Four criteria were set by them, namely consent by the patient, consultation with medical staff, authorisation as agreed between the nurse and the nurse manager and documentation in the patient's notes. Trevelyan and Booth (1994) saw that this type of policy could help to protect the nurse, patient and the organisation.

When nurses are involved in delivering complementary therapies, they are accountable under the Code of Professional Conduct (Nursing and Midwifery Council 2002b, Section 1.3) and answerable for their actions. Training is needed in relation to the use of these therapies or the patient may be put at risk due to lack of competence. The Code of Professional Conduct (Nursing and Midwifery Council 2002b, Section 1.4) clearly states that the nurse has a duty to care and the patients are entitled to receive safe and competent care. It is, therefore, important for the nurse to ensure that these therapies are in the patient's best interest and that the patient is safe. It must also be remembered that these therapies are 'complementary' and therefore will work along with other treatments, so the total package of care and therapy needs to be considered. Discussion with all members of the multidisciplinary team must take place and the patient must give informed consent prior to their use (Nursing and Midwifery Council 2002b, Code of Professional Conduct, Section 3.11).

The British Medical Association (1993) discuss the variations in the regulations governing nonconventional therapies in Europe. The Netherlands are liberal in their approach, whereas France, Belgium and Italy are more restrictive. In the UK, which is midway between these liberal and restrictive approaches, the Medical Act of 1858 allows qualified doctors to administer unconventional medical treatments to patients as long as they adhere to professional standards of care. Qualified doctors can also delegate the administration of complementary therapies to a nonmedically qualified practitioner, as long as certain criteria are satisfied. Nonmedically qualified practitioners of nonconventional medicine are free to practice, whatever their level of training, as long as they do not infringe the Medicines Act 1983, by implying that they are registered medical practitioners. They are also prevented from advertising treatments or remedies for a number of conditions (diabetes, glaucoma and epilepsy) but they are allowed to treat these patients.

Consumers of complementary medicine are protected under UK law in relation to the tort-based common law of negligence which protects people under the category of breach of duty of care. Other legislation relating to Trades Description Act 1968, Health and Safety at Work Act 1974, Control of Substances Hazardous to Health (COSHH) Regulations 1988, and Supply of Goods and Services Act 1982 may be used. At present there are no registering bodies to which complaints may be lodged for users of nonconventional therapies.

Specific actions related to the disease process Nasal clips or strips can be used for snorers. These clips or strips are fixed to the outside of the nose to open nostrils and improve breathing. Patients who suffer from sleep apnoea problems can use a continuous positive airway pressure device (CPAP). This is when a nasal mask is strapped to the face to deliver air at a slightly higher pressure than normal and so keep the airway open (Lavery 1997). Antisnoring surgery is available (uvulopalatopharyngoplasty) and this is when the soft palate is cauterised so that it is less likely to flap. However, according to the Royal College of Physicians Report into Sleep Apnoea (1993), this does not always work and is seen as experimental which carries a number of fatalities.

In disorders where sleep is affected, e.g. arthritis, the therapeutic regime may include the use of anti-inflammatory medication, rest, use of heat, appropriately planned exercise and night resting splints in order to reduce the inflammation and pain, preservation of joint function and prevent joint deformities (Walsh 2002).

Nursing actions associated with psychological factors affecting ill health

Stress and worry can affect the patient whilst in hospital and therefore the nurse needs to consider ways in which stress and worry can be minimised. This may simply be the provision of a call bell so that the patient feels safe, provision of a warm bath to help them relax, provision of light food and warm milky drinks at night and the use of relaxation tapes; all of these can help to minimise stress, fear of the unknown, their own worries and the death of others (Cawthorn & Hope 1992).

Specific relaxation therapies may include guided imagery, yoga, t'ai chi, or meditation, where the patients are shown how to use their mind and body to let go of tension which in turn can help to relieve muscle tension. When there is a need to reduce the tension in muscles and relieve pain, then progressive muscular relaxation techniques can be used. This is done by tensing each set of muscles then relaxing them, working up from the toe to the head (Cawthorn & Hope 1992, Lavery 1997).

Nursing actions associated with sociocultural factors affecting ill health

In a multicultural society, the nurse will be faced with patient's individual sleep routines and the need to maintain the patient's individual social, cultural, spiritual and religious beliefs is vital. The nurse will need to discuss these issues with the patient and consider how their needs can be met. It is unlikely that the patient will be used to sleeping with so many people in close proximity and they may not be used to sleeping on their own.

Nursing actions associated with environmental factors affecting ill health

The nurse will need to manage the ward environment to promote a therapeutic environment which enables patients not only to get off to sleep but one which allows them to remain asleep. The main environmental threat in hospitals is from noise (from the nurses, equipment and patients themselves). Nurses need to wear soft-soled shoes, ensure trolleys are well maintained, keep talking down to a minimum and ensure that the patients have a call light which is less noisy than a call buzzer.

Equally the nurse must ensure that patients are comfortable in the bed or chair when they are sleeping or resting. This relates to the pillows, bedclothes, mattresses as all should be appropriate for the patient and their condition. The temperature of the ward, the use of dim lights or blindfolds and the use of ear plugs need to be considered also (Morgan & Closs 1999).

Hogg (1998) discusses the problems of sleep deprivation and disturbances in a High Dependency Unit (HDU) setting and stresses that nurses have a key role to play in preventing these disturbances and ensuring quality sleep to promote recovery. Various strategies are put forward to limit or prevent sleep deprivation by Hogg (1998), such as noted earlier, regarding limiting noise, ensuring that the environment is conducive to sleep and the patient is comfortable, free from pain and anxiety. Consider the working environment and what aspects could disturb your patient's sleep. Consider ways in which these could be minimised.

Nursing actions associated with politicoeconomic factors affecting ill health

The nurse must be alert to the financial hardships hospitalisation and illness can bring to the patient and their immediate family. The ill health state may affect their ability to work, e.g. narcolepsy or exacerbation of the disease process as in arthritis. This may be a short-term problem and sickness benefits may cover the period of illness. However, patients may have to come to terms with changes in their employment status, need to retrain for different jobs or retire completely. The nurse will need to discuss the economic repercussions of the illness with the family and consider the support needed from health and social care professionals. Worry and anxiety over their illness and the effects this may have on the patient and their family can affect the sleep pattern of the patient at home and in hospital.

Documenting the nursing care plan

Once the nursing actions have been identified then the nursing care plan needs to be written. Nursing care plans should abide by the Nursing and Midwifery Council (2002c) 'Guidelines for records and record keeping' document and identify individualised actions and specify:

- who should be involved in the care planned
- what care should be given
- why that care should be given
- when the care should be given
- where the care should be given and
- how the care should be given.

Box 13.13 Nursing care plan–Emma Simmons

Problem

Emma is experiencing pain in her joints and on movement due to the arthritis/inflammation and this is shown by limited mobility, some loss of function in the hands and wrists, facial expression and verbal complaints of pain.

Short-term goal

Emma will be able to verbalise her pain to nursing staff and assess the effect of medications.

Long-term goal

Emma will be able to mobilise, sleep, work and socialise within the pain limits and be able to adapt her lifestyle to cope with the pain.

Care plan

- Observe pain levels and the link to treatment and mobility.
- Administer the prescribed anti-inflammatory medications.
- Ensure Emma's joints are rested and place supportive night splints on affected hands and wrists.
- Assist in the investigations ordered by the medical staff, e.g. full blood count and ESR levels, joint X-ray examination.
- Apply moist heat to joints affected.
- Encourage a planned range of movement exercises.
- Schedule daily care once morning stiffness has subsided, use of a warm bath may help movement initially.
- Listen to patient's worries and concerns about work, home life, etc.
- Plan a health education strategy with Emma when she is ready to participate in the activity.
- Discuss possible adjustments in relation to her lifestyle.

Exercise

1. Write the nursing care plan for the three priority problems identified on p. 401 in the previous exercise relating to Emma Simmons.
2. Check your answers with one of the problems as shown in Box 13.13.

It may be useful to consider the five factors (physical, psychological, sociocultural, environmental and politicoeconomical) when writing the nursing care plan also. Re-read the care plans and decide if all the factors are utilised. Once the nursing care plan has been written then this must be communicated to other health care professionals by verbal handover ready for the next stage – implementation.

Implementing nursing activities

Implementation of nursing activities involves three stages:

1. Preparatory stage of reading the nursing care plan, receiving handover report and ensuring that staff know what is required to accomplish the goals and decide on the skill mix needed.
2. Implementation where safe, competent practice is the key to successful care. The plan is then put into action and shows both the artistic and scientific side of nursing.
3. Postimplementation stage when nursing activities are communicated to health care professionals (written and verbally) via progress notes.

Success of the implementation depends on the initial assessment, quality of the care plan, organisation of care delivery and the competence of the care given. The written nursing care plan guides the implementation phase to help the patient achieve the goals set but the plan must be reviewed and updated according to changes in the patient's condition (see Chapter 1 for further information on implementation).

To ensure that this stage is both effective and efficient, there are numerous factors which can influence the care given. It is necessary to consider what influences care, what knowledge is needed and what skills are required to ensure that patients receive the best care.

Exercise

1. Re read Case study 13.1.
2. Consider what may influence the implementation of nursing activities planned.
3. Consider what knowledge you would need to implement this care.
4. Consider what skills you would also need.

Four domains were identified by the ENB in the Education for Focus (1999) document and these can be linked to the implementation stage. The four domains are:

- professional and ethical practice
- care delivery
- care management
- personal and professional development (see Chapter 2 for further details).

These will be explored in relation to sleeping difficulties and the three scenarios used previously in this chapter.

Box 13.14 Implementing nursing activities

Factors influencing the implementation of nursing activities:
- philosophy of care
- nursing model used
- assessment and planning stage
- care delivery system used
- resources available – skill mix, sufficient equipment and support services.

Knowledge required when implementing nursing activities:
- normal and abnormal anatomy and physiology of sleep cycles
- related psychological effects associated with sleeping
- social and cultural issues relating to poor sleeping, health or recovery
- environmental influences and concerns
- political and economic concerns.

Skills required when implementing nursing activities:
- caring skills
- interpersonal skills
- clinical psychomotor skills
- management skills – supervision, delegation, organising team/individuals
- counselling skills
- teaching skills
- research skills
- problem-solving skills
- leadership skills.

Exercise
1. Re read the three mini case studies in Box 13.7.
2. Identify issues, from these mini case scenarios, which relate to each of the four domains.

Professional and ethical practice
- *Scenario A:* Confidentiality regarding recently separated partner. Attitudes regarding overdose admission.
- *Scenario B:* Counselling regarding difficulty with diagnosis.
- *Scenario C:* Dopamine used from fetus.

Care delivery
- *Scenario A:* Key worker system.
- *Scenario B:* Empowerment approach.
- *Scenario C:* Multidisciplinary team approach, care delivered on a holistic basis, adaptations needed.

Care management
- *Scenario A:* Close observation due to previous overdose.
- *Scenario B:* Symptom controlled.
- *Scenario C:* Tertiary health promotion, community management, family involvement, Parkinson's Disease Society.

Personal and professional development
- *Scenario A:* Treatment of anxiety and depression, overdose care.
- *Scenario B:* Differences with fibromyalgia and ME.
- *Scenario C:* Action of dopamine, anti-Parkinson's drug therapy, parkinsonian crisis.

Having identified the potential aspects within these domains, it may be necessary to increase knowledge and skills relating to the aspects identified.

Evaluation of nursing activities

Evaluation of nursing care is integral to the professional accountability of nurses to their clients and is an essential stage of the process, yet, according to the Clothier Report by Clothier et al (1994), it is unfortunately a neglected part. The evaluation stage involves reflection on the degree of goal achievement, so that feedback on care can be gained. Evaluation should be ongoing to gain an insight into the patient's progress and effectiveness of nursing activities. Evaluation can be continuous, hourly, daily, on a shift basis or longer depending on the individual patient's problem and the goals set (for further information on evaluation see Chapter 1).

Again various factors can influence this evaluation stage and the number of skills which are required.

Exercise
1. Re-read Case study 13.1.
2. Consider the influencing factors which may affect the evaluation of nursing activities.
3. Consider the skills needed to evaluate nursing activities.
4. Check your answers in Box 13.15.

There are various steps which need to be followed when evaluating care:

1. Check goals against the patient's progress (discuss with patient if possible)
   - have the goals been completely or partially met?
   - have they been met at all?
2. Is the time scale realistic?

Box 13.15 Factors and skills influencing the evaluation of care

Factors which influence the evaluation stage:
- abilities of nurse and patient
- standards and quality assurance mechanisms
- assessment, planning and implementation stages
- goals set
- timing of evaluation.

Skills required in the evaluation stage:
- reassessment to include:
  - observation
  - interviewing
  - listening
  - identification of plan
  - time scale
  - plan of action
- analysis of patient's response to care
- auditing.

---

3. Record the findings and plan accordingly:
   - goal completely met, then state evidence for this and discontinue the problem
   - goal partially met, then decide if need to extend the evaluation time or modify the plan
   - goal not met at all, then decide if need to extend the evaluation time, modify the plan or reassess the problem.

Exercise
1. Read the following information in Box 13.16 and review the goals set for Emma's problems and evaluate her progress.
2. Consider what needs to be done in the next few days and write a revised plan of action if needed.
3. Discuss your plan with a colleague and agree its evidence base.

It can be noted that part of the long-term goal has been met, i.e. she is able to mobilise and is sleeping better and feels able to go home which may mean socialising more. However, part of the long-term goal relating to returning to work has not been met.

Box 13.16 Long-term goal review

Long-term goal previously set
- Emma will be able to mobilise, sleep, work and socialise within the pain limits and be able to adapt her lifestyle to cope with the pain.

Evidence available
- Emma is able to walk around ward area, her joints are still slightly swollen and tender but the morning stiffness and pain is less.
- Emma does not feel able to return to work as yet but feels able to go home and continue with her exercises.
- She is sleeping better and she has woken up less frequently with the aid of the night resting splints. If she does wake up then it is not due to the pain but due to a disturbance on the ward itself.

Where goals have not been met then the following questions may need to be asked:

- Is more information required?
- Should the plan be modified?
- Has the problem changed?
- Has the problem worsened?
- Should the goal be reviewed?
- Was the goal appropriate?
- Does the nursing plan need interventions from other health care professionals?

In Emma's case it may be that the plan needs to be continued for a short time discharge and be reviewed at a later date in the Outpatients Department and by her GP.

Summary points

1. A variety of skills are needed to deliver care to patients with sleeping difficulties.
2. Accurate, continuous assessment is vital as all other stages are dependent upon it.
3. Ensuring adequate sleep is essential for patient wellbeing.

References

Alexander MF, Fawcett JN, Runciman PJ 2000 Nursing practice hospital and home, 2nd edn. Churchill Livingstone, Edinburgh

British Medical Association 1993 Complementary medicine: new approaches to good practice. Oxford University Press, Oxford

Brooks I 1997 The lights are bright? Debating the future of the permanent night shift. Journal of Management in Medicine 11(2): 58–70

Brostrom A, Stromberg A, Dahlstrom U, Fridlund B 2001 Patients with congestive cardiac failure and their conceptions of their sleep problems. Journal of Advanced Nursing 34(4): 520–529

Brownfield A 1998 Aromatherapy in arthritis: a study. Nursing Standard 13(5): 34–35

Brugne J-F 1994 Sleep, wakefulness and the nurse. British Journal of Nursing 3(2): 68–71

Cannard G 1995 On the scent of a good night's sleep? Nursing Times 88(8): 52–54

Cawthorn A, Hope K 1992 Nursing intervention at night. In: McMahon R (ed) Nursing at night. A professional approach. Scutari Press, London

Closs SJ 1988 A nursing study of sleep on surgical wards. Report prepared for the Scottish Home and Health Department. Nursing Research Unit. Department of Nursing Studies, Edinburgh

Closs SJ 1990 Influences on patients' sleep on surgical wards. Surgical Nurse 3(2): 12–14

Closs SJ 2000 Sleep. In: Alexander MF, Fawcett JN, Runciman PJ (eds) Nursing practice hospital and home, 2nd edn. Churchill Livingstone, Edinburgh

Clothier C, MacDonald C, Shaw D 1994 Independent enquiry into deaths and injuries on the children's ward at Grantham and Kestevan General Hospital during the period February to April 1991 (Allitt Inquiry). HMSO, London

Crabb L 2001 Clinical. Sleep disorders in Parkinson's disease: the nursing role. British Journal of Nursing 10(1): 42–47

Deakin M 1995 Using relaxation techniques to manage disruptive behaviour. Nursing Times 91(17): 40–41

Department of the Environment, Transport and the Regions 1998 Road safety research. (http://www.roads.dtlr.gov.uk/roadsafety/research98/road/5c.htm)

Department of Health 2000 Reduce the risk of cot death. Leaflet available on (http:www.gov.uk/cotdeath/)

Department of Trade and Industry 2000 Your guide to the working time regulations. HMSO, London

Department for Transport, Local Government and the Regions 2001 Government meets target on reducing rough sleeping. (http://www.housing.dtlr.gov.uk/rsu/pn/rsu19.htm)

Department for Transport, Local Government and the Regions 2001 Road safety research report No 25 older drivers: a literature review. (http://www.roads.dtlr.gov.uk/roadsafety/research25/12.htm)

Department for Transport, Local Government and the Regions 2002 Drivers' hours and tachograph rules for goods vehicles in the UK and Europe (GV262) Part A and B. (http://www.roads.dtlr.gov.uk/roadsafety/tachograph/gv262/02.htm)

Diagnostic Classification Steering Committee (Thorpy MJ, Chairman) 1990 The international classification of sleep disorders: diagnostic and coding manual. American Sleep Disorders Association, Rochester, Minnesota (http://www.uni-marburg.de/sleep/ern/database/asdadefs/welcome.htm)

Dimond B 1995 Legal aspects of nursing. Prentice Hall, London

Dingley J 1996 A computer-aided comparative study of progressive alertness changes in nurses working two different night-shift rotas. Journal of Advanced Nursing 23: 1247–1253

Dunn C, Sleep J, Collett D 1995 Sensing an improvement: an experimental study to evaluate the use of aromatherapy, massage and periods of rest in an Intensive Care Unit. Journal of Advanced Nursing 21: 34–40

Duxbury J 1994 An investigation into primary nursing and its effects upon the nursing attitudes about and administration of prn night sedation. Journal of Advanced Nursing 19: 923–931

English National Board 1999 Education for focus. ENB, London

Ersser S, Wiles A, Taylor H, Wade S, Walsh R, Bentley T 1999 The sleep of older people in hospital and nursing homes. Journal of Clinical Nursing 8: 360–368

Fitzpatrick J, While A, Roberts J 1999 Shift work and its impact upon nurse performance: current knowledge and research issues. Journal of Advanced Nursing 29(1): 18–27

Frawley P 1990 Neurological observations. Nursing Times 86(35): 29–32

Gallinagh R, Nevin R, McIlroy D, Mitchell F, Campbell L, Ludwick R, McKenna H 2002 The use of physical restraints as a safety measure in the care of older people in four rehabilitation wards: findings from an exploratory study. International Journal of Nursing Studies 39: 147–156

Halfens R, Cox K, Kuppen-Van Merwijk A 1994 Effect of the use of sleep medication in Dutch hospitals on the use of sleep medication at home. Journal of Advanced Nursing 19: 66–70

Health facts 1996 Getting back to sleep after bereavement. Journal of Advanced Nursing 23(2): 218

Herxheimer A, Petrie KJ 2002 Melatonin for the prevention and treatment of jet lag (Cochrane Review). In: The Cochrane Library, Issue 3. Oxford, Update Software

Hinchliff SM, Montague SE, Watson R 1996 Physiology for nurses, 2nd edn. Baillière Tindall, Edinburgh

Hobson JA 1995 Sleep. Scientific American Library, New York

Hodgson LA 1991 Why do we need sleep? Relating theory to nursing practice. Journal of Advanced Nursing 16: 1503–1510

Hogg G 1998 Sleep deprivation in a high dependency unit. Professional Nurse 13(10): 693–696

Holbrook AM, Crowther R, Lotter A, Cheng C, King D 2000 Meta-analysis of benzodiozepine use in the treatment of insomnia. Canadian Medical Association Journal 162(2): 225–233

Horne JA, Barrett PR 2001 Over the counter medicines and the potential for unwanted sleepiness in drivers: a review. Department for Transport, Local Government and the Regions. (http://www.roads.dtlr.gov.uk/roadsafety/research24/01.htm)

Humm C 1996 The relationship between night duty tolerance and personality. Nursing Standard 10(51): 34–39

Irwin P 1992 The physiology of sleep. In: McMahon R (ed) Nursing at night. A professional approach. Scutari Press, London

Jamieson EM, McCall JM, Whyte LA 2002, Clinical nursing practices. Churchill Livingstone, Edinburgh

Karlsson S, Bucht G, Rasmussen B, Sandman P 2000 Restraint use in elder care: decision making among registered nurses. Journal of Clinical Nursing 9: 842–850

Lavery S 1997 The healing powers of sleep. How to achieve restorative sleep naturally. Gaia, London

Martell R 2001 Research shows dangers of rotational shift patterns. Nursing Standard 16(2): 7

Morgan K, Closs SJ 1999 Sleep management in nursing practice. Churchill Livingstone, Edinburgh

Morin CM, Colecchi C, Stone J, Sood R, Brink D 1999 Behavioural and pharmacological therapies for late-life insomnia. A randomised controlled trial. Journal of the American Medical Association 281(11): 991–999

New Zealand Cot Death Study http://www.globalideasbank.org/Bov/BV-204.html

Nursing and Midwifery Council 2002a Guidelines for the administration of medicines. Nursing and Midwifery Council, London

Nursing and Midwifery Council 2002b Code of professional practice. Nursing and Midwifery Council, London

Nursing and Midwifery Council 2002c Guidelines for records and record keeping. Nursing and Midwifery Council, London

Nursing Times, News Clinical Research Highlights 1998 Melatonin could be the key to ME generation. Nursing Times 94(26): 57

Pemberton L 2000 The unconscious patient. In: Alexander MF, Fawcett JN, Runciman PJ (eds) Nursing practice hospital and home, 2nd edn. Churchill Livingstone, Edinburgh

Rajaratnam SMW, Arendt J 2001 Health in a 24-hour society. The Lancet 358: 999–1005

Reet M 1998 Sleep and rest. In: Mallik M, Hall C, Howard D (eds) Nursing knowledge and practice. A decision making approach. Baillière Tindall, London

Roper N, Logan W, Tierney AJ 1996 The elements of nursing. A model for nursing based on a model of living, 4th edn. Churchill Livingstone, Edinburgh

Roper N, Logan W, Tierney AJ 2000 The Roper–Logan–Tierney model of nursing based on activities of living. Churchill Livingstone, Edinburgh

Royal College of Nursing 1999 Restraint revisited – rights, risk and responsibility. Guidance for nurses working with older people. RCN, London

Royal College of Physicians 1993 Sleep apnoea and related conditions. Royal College of Physicians, London

Rutishauser S 1994 Physiology and anatomy. A basis for nursing and health care. Churchill Livingstone, Edinburgh

Schaefer KM 1997 Health patterns of women with fibromyalgia. Journal of Advanced Nursing 26: 565–571

Shapiro C, Flanigan M 1993 Function of sleep. British Medical Journal 306: 383–385

Southwell MT, Wistow G 1995 Sleep in hospitals at night: are patient's needs being met? Journal of Advanced Nursing 21(6): 1101–1109

Teasdale G, Galbraith S, Clarke K 1975 Observation record chart. Nursing Times 71(19):972–973

Trevelyan J, Booth B 1994 Complementary medicine for nurses, midwives and health visitors. Macmillan, Houndmills

UKCC 1999 Practitioner–client relationships and the prevention of abuse. UKCC, London

Walsh M (ed) 2002 Watson's clinical nursing and related sciences, 6th edn. Baillière Tindall, London

Wedderbum Z, Smith P 1980 Sleep: its function and measurement. Nursing 1(20): 852–855

World Health Organisation 1980 International classification of impairments, disabilities and handicaps: a manual classification relating to the consequence of disease. WHO, Geneva

Further reading

Alexander MF, Fawcett JN, Runciman PJ 2000 Nursing Practice Hospital and Home, 2nd edn. Chapter 9, The Nervous System by Allan D; Chapter 10, The Musculoskeletal System by Jamieson L, McFarlane C, Brown J; Chapter 28, The unconscious patient by Pemberton L. Churchill Livingstone, Edinburgh

McMahon R (ed) 1992 Nursing at night. A professional approach. Scutari Press, London

Trevelyan J, Booth B 1994 Complementary medicine for nurses, midwives and health visitors. Macmillan, Houndmills.

Walsh M (ed) 2002 Watson's clinical nursing and related sciences, 6th edn. Baillière Tindall, London. Chapter 20, Caring for the patient with a disorder of the nervous system; Chapter 24, Caring for the Patient with a disorder of the muskulo-skeletal system.

Useful websites

National Sleep Foundation (NSF)
http://www.sleepfoundation.org

Nursing and Midwifery Council (NMC)
http://www.nmc-uk.org

Clinical evidence relating to insomnia and sleep apnoea
http://www.clinicalevidence.com

Dying

Debbie Roberts

CHAPTER 14

Introduction

According to Roper et al (1996, p. 395) 'Dying is the final Activity of Living and is normally (unless it is sudden and unexpected) preceded by a process (i.e. the process of dying) in which the individual actively participates'. It is because of this that dying is included as an Activity of Living. An understanding of death, dying and bereavement is essential if nurses are to undertake care that is holistic and takes account of individual beliefs and religious practice.

This chapter will therefore focus on the following:

1. **The model of living**
   - death and dying as an Activity of Living
   - lifespan and death and dying
   - factors influencing the AL of dying.
2. **The model for nursing**
   - nursing care of individuals with health problems affecting the Activity of Living: dying.

THE MODEL OF LIVING

Death and dying as an AL

What is death? Rutishauser (1994, p. 625) states that 'people die as a result of the failure of one or more body systems through injury, disease or ageing'. Death then is 'the stage when a person ceases to exist in their previous physical form' (Holland & Hogg 2001). Other types of death are 'clinical death' (the appearance of death signs upon examination) and 'social death' (when the individual is treated essentially as a corpse although still clinically and biologically alive) (Bond & Bond 1997). Death can occur at any age, and may occur suddenly, e.g. in an accident or suicide, or gradually, e.g. from cancer. How people cope with the aftermath of death will vary according to their cultural, religious and spiritual beliefs. They are often said to be 'bereaved'. 'Grief' or the feelings and emotion that 'may follow a bereavement' is also expressed in 'different ways according to the culture to which they belong' (Holland & Hogg 2001).

Dying in health and illness – across the lifespan

Childhood

Hindmarch (2000) argues that the death of a child is different from other forms of bereavement, and although a comparatively rare event in the Western world; the impact of child death is out of all proportion to its incidence. The death of a child is upsetting because it does not fit into our perception of 'the natural order of things'. This is true even when the *child* who dies is an adult with elderly parents. Roper et al (1996) highlight other issues associated with death in early childhood such as sudden infant death syndrome. In industrialised countries sudden infant death syndrome has become one of the major causes of infant mortality. However, Roper et al (1996) explain that if infants survive the first year, their life expectancy increases. Extensive research in recent years and subsequent education of the public has reduced the numbers of sudden infant deaths in the United Kingdom, but for a variety of reasons, infant mortality remains high in some developing countries (Roper et al 1996). The impact of childhood death is made evident to us in the number of children that die as a result of environmental and other health hazards. The World Health Organisation (2002) state that 'seven out of ten childhood deaths in developing countries can be attributed to just five main causes, or a combination of them: pneumonia, diarrhoea, measles, malaria and malnutrition' and that 'around the world, three out of every four children who seek healthcare are suffering from at least one of these conditions'. Prevention of death in children due to these illnesses is therefore a priority for the World Health Organisation.

The bereaved child

Children are perceptive, will often know when something is wrong and will want information. People often worry about how and when to tell children about an impending death. Ideally, when someone the child is close to dies, news of the death should be delivered by a parent or a close family member. If the death is expected parents will often forewarn children in advance. However, often these people are also bereaved themselves and may require the support of nursing staff. Initially, the information given to children should be short, clear and unambiguous. The words died and dead are easily understood. The age of the child will affect the child's perception of the event. Wright (1996) explains the impact of chronological age of the child on their perceptions of death (see Box 14.1). In order to develop an understanding of the reactions of children to the news of a death undertake the following exercise.

Exercise

Examine Box 14.1 and consider how the nursing interventions could be adapted for children of various ages and stages of development.

Children will dictate the amount of information they need by the questions they ask. Questions should always be answered truthfully. Children should be allowed to cry rather than being told to be brave, to scream, be angry or be silent. Wright (1996) explains that many children will be unable to remain still when discussing death and may find it comforting to walk around or continue to play with toys, or want food. Wright (1996) goes on to suggest that children should be encouraged to see, and if they wish, touch the person who has died. This process should not be forced or hurried, and similarly, the child should not be made to feel guilty for not wishing to do anything. When seeing the dead person, the child will require careful explanation of what they see and be helped to reach meaning and understanding (Wright 1996).

Box 14.1 Chronological age and perceptions of death

Below 5 years
- Lack of understanding about the finality of death.
- An inability to run through the events and arrive at a logical conclusion, 'Going round in circles'.
- A belief that they can cause what happens to them and around them (egocentricity).

5–10 years
- Concrete thinking, literal understanding.
- Understanding the physical causes of death, both internal and external.
- Concern with other people's feelings (empathy).
- An interest in the tangible expressions of grief: rituals, pictures, gravestones.

10 years and older
- A more abstract understanding.
- A great sense of justice/injustice, fate.
- Reflection on belief systems.
- Strong emotional reaction.

From Wright B 1996, p. 67.

Adolescence

As in childhood, death in adolescence can take place for many different reasons. However, Roper et al (1996) highlight the increasing suicide rates amongst adolescents within industrialised societies. In the UK the Government set out to reduce the numbers of people who commit suicide in the plan known as 'Saving Lives: Our Healthier Nation' (Department of Health 1999). However, the document does not distinguish between suicides at any particular age group. Death from suicide amongst adolescents may be more likely to be induced by drugs and/or alcohol. King (2001) demonstrates a number of key characteristics which are present in adolescents who attempt suicide. These include: experiencing stressful life events, being sexually active, poor family environment, low parental monitoring, marijuana use, recent drunkenness, current smoking and physical fighting (King 2001). The World Health Organisation (2001) report that at least 100 000 annual deaths in young people worldwide are attributed to suicide, whilst 'every year, almost 1.5 million adolescents die from substance abuse, reproductive ill health, suicide, injuries and violence' (WHO 2002).

Exercise

Access the World Health Organisation website www.who.int/en and find the latest policies and recommendations on adolescent health and deaths. Consider the implications for adolescents in your country.

Adulthood

Death in early adulthood is still likely to be perceived as untimely, i.e. happening before it should, especially in view of the fact that people are living longer (Roper et al 1996). The National Statistics site (official UK statistics) reports that 'in 1997 life expectancy at birth in the United Kingdom was approaching 75 years for men and 80 years for women compared with just 50 years for males and 54 years for females in 1911' (Office for National Statistics 2000). Death in adulthood is caused by a number of illnesses or traumatic events and the incidence of deaths between the ages of 45–75 is higher for men than women in the United Kingdom (Roper et al 1996). Roper et al (1996) suggest that death in later adulthood often serves to remind mankind of its mortality, making the possibility of death, and the process of dying more of a reality.

Exercise

Access the World Health Organisation website www.who.int/en and find the latest information on life expectancy in different countries. Consider the implications for health care of adults in various countries. Discuss with colleagues.

Old age

Perceptions about death in old age are often different to those concerning death at other times across the lifespan; death may be viewed as a natural event in old age. People tend to live longer and may have higher expectations of health in old age. Helman (1996) explains the concept of social death in old age whereby the person; although physically alive, will be seen as less alive socially in the eyes of society or even family members. Helman (1996) cites examples of social death as including those who have been confined to institutions for the rest of their lives, such as prisons, nursing homes, homes for the mentally handicapped and hospices. In some cases, during this transition between old age and death older people will lose the will to live and this concept is examined later in this chapter.

The maximum lifespan for humans seems to be approximately 100–115 years with the number of people exceeding 100 set to rise. According to the Health Education Authority (1998) the number of people aged 65 will increase by 30% between 1996 and 2021 and the numbers of over-90s will double in the same period; centenarians will quadruple by 2016. Further to this, Costello (2001) explains that the majority of patients who die in hospital are over the age of 65. Findings from Costello's study show that nurses working in elderly care wards demonstrate a lack of what he terms 'emotional engagement'; that is to say, nurses provide individual care to older patients who are dying, but the care is aimed at meeting physical needs (Costello 2001).

Before thinking about how to care for others it is important to understand the range of views associated with death and dying. Consider the following.

Exercise

Reflect on your personal experiences with people who are dying.

1. Do you feel differently about incidents involving children, adolescents, or people who try or succeed in taking their own lives?
2. Where do you think these personal ideas may have originated from?

The major causes of death differ in various parts of the world, and different stages of life. In the case of death in childhood it is not unusual for nurses to experience a sense of guilt and even failure following the death of a child. Costello and Trinder-Brook (2000) conducted a retrospective study of children's nurses and found that often the nurses could not provide any rational explanation for these feelings of guilt and failure. The study also showed that nurses experience great conflict when trying to foster hope with parents who are struggling to come to terms with preparing for the death of a child (Costello & Trinder-Brook 2000).

Brysiewicz (2002) explains that in South Africa, violent death due to interpersonal violence is a huge problem, with the majority of those involved being young adults 'in the prime of their lives'. Emergency nurses interviewed in Brysiewicz's study saw themselves as being engaged in a battle with death, fighting for victory. In this study violent and sudden loss of life resulted in the nurses feeling that they had failed the client when the battle was lost (Brysiewicz 2002). Feelings which are not dissimilar to those of the paediatric nurses in Costello and Trinder-Brook's study.

The origins of views on death and dying may be difficult to trace. Undertaking the reflective exercise may have been difficult to pinpoint feelings about particular life events. We inherit or learn certain guidelines through which we come to know how to live in our own social group or society. These guidelines are termed culture (Holland & Hogg 2001). Holland and Hogg (2001) suggest that our culture determines the pattern in which we undertake a variety of roles and responsibilities. In particular the beliefs, rituals and customs which we associate with death are deeply embedded. Personal experiences associated with death and dying may have a profound impact on how an individual nurse is able to support patients' families and colleagues in future situations.

Dependence/independence in the AL of dying

As in previous chapters the activity of dying sees people moving along a continuum between dependence and independence. Ultimately, throughout the activity of dying the person will move towards dependence, however, independence should be promoted for as long as possible or desirable by the person. Transition towards dependence may be a gradual or rapid process and is sometimes referred to as a dying trajectory. Each day may bring fluctuations along the independence/dependence continuum. Individuals may be aware of the gradual decline in the ability for self-care. Not all dying people will want or need nursing care. Roper et al (1996) suggest that, for those who do want or need care, it is the role of the nurse to help the dying person to balance the degree of dependence/independence in the Activities of Living up until death.

The onset of the process of dying is difficult to diagnose (see Biological factors). When medical treatment cannot halt the course of a disease, and can only alleviate the symptoms of the fatal illness the illness is referred to as terminal. However there may be a considerable length of time between terminal diagnosis and the rapid physical decline associated with the event of death; for example when someone who is HIV-positive develops AIDS, the illness may last many months or years. The dying trajectory is long. During the intervening period symptomatic relief becomes paramount and is known as palliative care (Roper et al

1996). Palliative care is the active total care offered to a patient with a progressive illness and their family, when it is recognised that the illness is no longer curable, in order to concentrate on the quality of life and the alleviation of distressing symptoms within the framework of a coordinated service (World Health Organisation 1990): Dougan and Colquhoun (2000, p. 963) state that the term palliative care 'is given to the approach adopted when cure is unlikely and it is expected that the patient will die in the foreseeable future'.

They state that 'palliative care has been developed to help those who are dying slowly, or as is often said, living with dying' (Dougan and Colquhoun 2000, p. 963). They offer a model for palliative care which supports the view of the patient on a dependence/independence continuum, whilst recognising the interdependence of the Activities of Living and holistic care.

Summary points

1. Death can occur at any time along the lifespan.
2. Attitudes towards death are often shaped by our personal experiences and cultural background.
3. Death may be expected, sudden, peaceful or violent. Bereavement may be affected accordingly.

Factors affecting the activity of dying

According to Roper et al (1996) there are core factors which have an impact on all the Activities of Living, and the activity of dying is no different. In the following section of the chapter each of the factors will be explored in relation to the activity of dying.

Biological factors

For most purposes it can be assumed that death has occurred when a person's pulse and respiration have ceased. However, throughout adulthood, cells throughout the body are dying. Rutishauser (1994) explains that cells die because they have come to the end of their natural lifespan, or because they have been fatally injured. For example, red blood cells are continually replaced, whereas other cells cannot be replaced if they become injured, as in the case of cells in the spinal cord. Rutishauser (1994) also states that death is a process which begins with the failure of one part of the body, thus altering the internal environment of the body, impairing the function of other organs and tissues. This leads to failure of the life of the body as a whole. But Roper et al (1996) suggest that sometimes a more elaborate diagnosis of death is required especially if there has been admission to hospital and sophisticated, artificial, 'life-support systems' are being used to maintain vital body functions. The concepts of 'clinical death' (death of the person), 'biological death' (death of the tissues) and 'brain death' (irreversible brain damage) reflect the different interpretations (Roper et al 1996, p. 404). Therefore, diagnosing the point at which a person is dying is difficult and problematic. The nervous system is often used as an indicator of status along the dying trajectory. Table 14.1 demonstrates the role of different parts of the nervous system and the consequences of loss of functions.

Loss of cerebral function (whilst the brain stem is intact) results in total loss of personality and absence of purposeful activity. The person may exist in this 'vegetative state' for many years; breathing occurs spontaneously, the heart beats, blood circulates and reflex movements occur. Rutishauser (1994) explains that the *person* has died even though the body remains alive and sometimes this may give the false impression that conscious awareness still exists.

Table 14.1 Role of different parts of the nervous system (CNS) in different behaviours and the consequences of loss of functions

Part of CNS	Role	Consequences of loss		
		State		**Features**
Cerebral cortex	Awareness Understanding Purposeful behaviour		Vegetative state	Eyes open and move Breathes spontaneously May grimace grasp and groan No voluntary movement
Brain stem	Maintains consciousness Controls breathing, swallowing Reflex control of muscles (e.g. eyes, face; larynx limbs) Autonomic control of circulation	Brain death		Coma Breathing stops Involuntary limb movement Incontinence
Spinal cord	Reflex control of muscles (e.g. limbs) Autonomic reflexes	Death		

Adapted from Rutishauser 1994.

Complete and irreversible brain death

There is medical agreement about the criteria indicating complete and irreversible brain death, requiring confirmation by at least two experienced doctors. A series of criteria is applied by the two experienced doctors on two separate occasions. The doctors will not be those assigned to care for the patient and have not usually met the patient prior to undertaking the tests. Roper et al (1996) suggest that the criteria include:

- fixation of pupils
- absence of corneal and of vestibulooccular reflexes
- absence of response within the cranial nerve distribution to sensory stimuli
- no response to bronchial stimulation when a catheter is passed into the trachea
- no spontaneous breathing movement when the patient is disconnected from a mechanical ventilator (Roper et al 1996, p. 404).

In order to understand the application of the brain stem death criteria it is useful to revise the anatomy and physiology of the brain.

The brain The brain lies within the cranial cavity and constitutes approximately one-fiftieth of the bodyweight (Waugh & Grant 2001). The brain is divided into five areas:

1. the cerebrum (the largest part of the brain)
2. the midbrain
3. the pons
4. the medulla oblongata
5. the cerebellum (situated at the back of the head; coordinates activities associated with the maintenance of balance and equilibrium of the body).

Together the midbrain, the pons and the medulla oblongata form the brain stem (see Fig. 14.1).

Vital centres lie deep within the medulla oblongata. These centres consist of groups of cells associated with autonomic reflex activity and their activities are seen in Box 14.2.

Having revised the anatomy and physiology of the brain you should have a better understanding of the brain stem

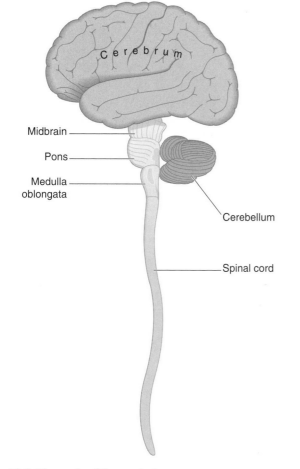

Midbrain
Pons
Medulla oblongata
Cerebrum
Cerebellum
Spinal cord

Fig. 14.1 The parts of the central nervous system (from Waugh & Grant 2001, with permission).

Box 14.2 Vital centres in the medulla oblongata

Cardiac centre
Controls the rate and force of cardiac contraction. Sympathetic and parasympathetic nerve fibres originating in the medulla pass to the heart. Sympathetic stimulation increases the rate and force of the heartbeat and parasympathetic stimulation has the opposite effect.

Respiratory centre
Controls the rate and depth of respiration. From this centre nerve impulses pass to the phrenic and intercostal nerves which stimulate contraction of the diaphragm and intercostal muscles, thus initiating inspiration. The respiratory centre is stimulated by excess carbon dioxide, and, to a lesser extent, by deficiency of oxygen in its blood supply and by nerve impulses from the chemoreceptors in the carotid bodies.

Vasomotor centre
Controls the diameter of the blood vessels, especially the small arteries and arterioles which have a large proportion of smooth muscle fibres in their walls. Vasomotor impulses reach the blood vessels through the autonomic nervous system. Stimulation may cause either constriction or dilation of the blood vessels depending on the site.

Reflex centres of vomiting, coughing, sneezing and swallowing
When irritating substances are present in the stomach or the respiratory tract, nerve impulses pass to the medulla oblongata, stimulating the reflex centres to initiate the reflex action of vomiting, coughing or sneezing to expel the irritant.

From Waugh & Grant 2001, p. 154.

death tests. Each of the tests relates to one of the vital centres inside the medulla oblongata. If no response is gained when the test is carried out it indicates that no autonomic nervous response is present, and the person is pronounced brain stem dead (see Table 14.1 above).

According to Gill (2000) death is not perceived by all as being merely a biological event. Brain stem death in particular, is not universally accepted, this is largely due to social, cultural and philosophical issues and values which are mostly Western in nature. In many societies Gill (2000) suggests that concepts such as intelligence and the soul extend beyond the brain. The common issues as to why brain death is rejected are complex and intermingled. Here are some examples.

- *Personhood:* Belief that a person is a unity of mind and body. From a Western philosophical perspective it is suggested that rationality is located in the brain, so when the brain is destroyed, so is the person. However, in some cultures such as Japanese, personhood is seen as more than rationality. The Japanese view the body and spirit as being connected, so whilst cardiorespiratory function persists the person is not seen as dead. The death of an individual's brain is not necessarily equated with the actual death of that individual. Death is seen as a long process, rather than as a single event. Helman (1996) explains that in Japan a death may sometimes only be recognised as final following a series of rituals conducted by the family and the community in which the person lived.

- *Death and the soul:* Many cultures, such as Muslims have firm beliefs about the existence of the soul or spiritual element of a person. Gill (2000) points out that it is medically impossible to establish the existence and location of the soul, although it is not perceived to be within the brain.

- *The significance of other organs:* There are cultural differences about which organs are most important. In particular the heart function seems crucial. Gill (2000) explains that for Jewish people, for example, it is the heart not the brain which is the 'seat of life'; therefore whilst the heart is beating (as in brain stem death) the person is still seen as alive (Gill 2000).

This Western concept of brain stem death may have particular significance when cadaveric organ donation is concerned. It would not be acceptable to remove organs from someone who is perceived to be alive by the family.

In order to explore the concept of brain stem death further please read Case study 14.1. In cases where brain stem death is diagnosed, families have little time to prepare; timespan from injury to diagnosis can be hours as opposed to days or months when someone is diagnosed as terminally ill. Whilst reading the case study consider the impact of this death on the family involved.

Case study 14.1

To illustrate and discuss brain stem death

20.00: John and Jane are 14-year-old twins who are out with a group of friends playing around the site of a disused factory. The football ended up on the roof and appeared to be easily accessible to both of them. Encouraged by his friends, John goes up to get the ball; he falls through the roof and falls awkwardly on his side some 3 metres below. John answers his name when one of his mates calls out to him. John got up and was helped out back through the roof. John was sure he was OK and swore Jane to secrecy, saying 'Mum will kill us if she finds out we were up on the roof!'.

21.00: John and Jane arrive home. John says that he feels tired and feels like an early night, so he goes to bed. Shortly after, Jane also goes to bed, keeping their secret safe.

23.00: Johns' parents, Madge and Reg are preparing to go to bed. As she had done for the past 14 years Madge put her head around Jane's door to make sure she was asleep. As she walked towards John's room she heard a strange noise which she later described as 'John sounded like he did when he had a cold as a baby; all snuffly, like he couldn't get his breath'. Madge went into the room to see if he was all right and give him a nudge but she couldn't rouse him.

'His breathing sounded really strange ..... . I called Reg .... we couldn't wake him ..... . we didn't know what to do ...... it was like it was happening in slow motion, not real somehow ..... . Reg must have called the ambulance'.

23.15: Ambulance arrives; John's right pupil is fixed and his left pupil is sluggish to react; the crew say something about a Glasgow Coma scale of 5, his pulse is 26 beats per minute, respirations shallow at a rate of 14 per minute; blood pressure is 160/40. John is intubated in the ambulance.

23.25: John is seen in Accident and Emergency and taken for a CT scan, Madge and Reg follow John's trolley but they feel almost invisible. The CT scan reveals massive extradural haematoma. John's left pupil becomes fixed. Madge and Reg sign something for John to have an operation, the words on the paper are long and technical, they hear what the Consultant is saying but don't really understand. They can tell by the look on the doctors' face that John is in a very serious condition. They wait in a small room with no windows for what seems like an eternity for some news of their son, the nurses do pop in from time to time but they are frightened to go outside in case they miss the doctor.

During the operation John undergoes a craniotomy and removal of the extradural haematoma, he is paralysed and sedated with drugs.

01.00: John is then transferred to another department (a neurological high dependency unit). Both pupils are fixed and dilated. Glasgow coma scale now 3. His intracranial pressure is monitored; the reading is 46 (normal is 10–15). Madge and Reg finally get to see John and watch the nurses come and go every few minutes. The neurosurgeon and the

consultant anaesthetist visit John and review his neurological state at 09.00.

09.00: Decision made to carry out brain stem criteria tests. The coroner is informed and the first set of tests is carried out at 09.30.

14.00: Second doctor performs the second set of brain stem tests and John is declared dead. Madge, Reg and Jane are there with John; each with their own feelings of loss, anger, guilt and love.

Exercise

1. What kind of support will the family need?
2. Develop some strategies to use in the clinical setting.
3. Will your support be different for different cultural groups?
4. How will you support a family during the decision to donate organs and beyond?

Transplant Law – United Kingdom

Wilkinson (2000) explains the legislation surrounding transplant surgery in the United Kingdom. The Human Tissue Act (1961) describes the circumstances in which organs may be removed. Only a designated person may authorise removal of organs once there is no reason to believe that the person had expressed an objection to their body being used in this way; or a surviving partner or relative objects; or there are religious objections. The Human Organ Transplant Act (1989) prohibits the sale of human organs and stipulates that living organ donors are genetically related to the recipient. Wilkinson (2000) goes on to say that unrelated live donation can take place if the Unrelated Live Transplant Authority approves the case.

Cultural and religious objections to transplant are explained by Holland and Hogg (2001). Jehovah's Witnesses do not receive blood transfusions and believe that human life should not be prolonged with another creatures' blood. The view of Muslims towards brain stem death is that it is accepted for the purpose of organ transplant. Holland and Hogg (2001) further explain the Muslim Law Councils' view that organ donation is supported as a means alleviating pain or saving life on the basis of the rules of Shariah (Holland & Hogg 2001, p. 155).

Exercise

1. Find out about the legislation concerning organ donation and transplant in your own and one other country, and make some comparisons.
2. Is there an organ donor register, and how do people make it known that they wish to donate their organs after their death?
3. Discuss your findings with tutors and colleagues.

Organ donation

Seriously ill or injured people will often be attached to a ventilator to allow the heart and lungs to continue to function, and for oxygenated blood to perfuse all the organs and tissues. However, when the person's condition is incurable a diagnosis of brain stem death is made and the time recorded for the death certificate. According to the British Organ Donor Society (BODY) there is no definite age limit for potential organ and tissue donors, the condition of the organs being a more significant consideration. However, generally donors may be up to 65 years old for heart, liver and lungs and 75 years old for kidneys. There is no age limit for corneas (BODY 2001). Organs used for transplant include: kidneys, heart, lungs, liver, pancreas and bowel. Usually one organ is transplanted, sometimes two, very occasionally three. Tissues used include: corneas, heart valves, bone, skin and connective tissue. (When skin is retrieved it is removed from discreet areas of the body resulting in a barely noticeable mark as only a thin sliver of skin is required. In the case of corneas, the eyes are retrieved and replaced with either cotton wool and plastic caps or glass eyes.)

All internal organs must be retrieved from what is known as a 'beating heart donor' (although kidneys can be retrieved after up to 1 hour of heart death). Currently there is a National Organ Donor Register within the UK, a national database of people who wish to donate their organs to help someone else when they die. Transplant coordinators are able to access information on a 24-hour basis to see if their potential donor has already expressed a wish to donate. However, BODY (2001) suggests that when medically and legally practical, families, or in some cases friends, should be approached concerning the possibility of internal organ and tissue donation. It is necessary to maintain artificial breathing and a beating heart until the donated organs are retrieved in the operating theatre (a beating heart donor).

Transplant coordinators will often meet donor families and explain what will happen over the next few hours and answer any questions or concerns a family may have. Some families are keen to have information about the outcome of the organ retrieval, often wanting information about the recipient's progress.

For further information about UK transplant law and becoming an organ donor see the British Organ Donor Society website at http://www.argonet.co.uk/body/DoH.html

Psychological factors

According to Ross (1994) the importance of hope to life can be seen not only in death caused by its absence, but also in healing produced by its abundance. Ross (1994) describes the work of Limandri and Boyle (1978) in examining hope or will to live. In her classic work Ross explains that often once an individual loses the will to live, a sense of hopelessness and helplessness prevails which can result in the rapid decline of the individual and subsequent death. This is sometimes termed 'passive suicide'. The following case study helps to illustrate what Ross (1994) is describing.

Case study 14.2

Marie

I had looked after Marie since she had been admitted to our medical ward with advanced carcinoma of her left breast, she had multiple metastases and was fully alert and aware of her diagnosis. Her carcinoma was now terminal. Marie knew she was dying and often remarked how lucky she was to be pain-free. One lunchtime I was caring for Marie and two other ladies in the same bay so I went to check if any of them needed any medication, in particular any analgesia. This is the conversation that took place:

Marie 'How long am I going to be here Nurse?'

Nurse 'I'm not sure Marie, why are you thinking about going home?'

Marie: 'Oh, no, I wouldn't manage at home …. I want to be here …. But there must be something you can do to help me. I want to go to sleep.'

Nurse: 'Are you tired Marie? Aren't you sleeping very well?,'

Marie: 'No, I'm not talking about being tired, I just feel so dreadful … the waiting is terrible …. . wondering if it will be today …. . I don't want to go on feeling like this, there must be something you could do? Can't you give me a pill? Please give me a pill; let me go to sleep.'

In this case study Marie is using the euphemism of sleep. The nurse seeks clarification from Marie by asking whether she is tired or having difficulty in sleeping, but in fact Marie is asking the nurse to help her to die. Marie is aware of her diagnosis and has reached the stage of accepting her imminent death. She has lost the will to live.

The following may have been considered.

Feeling some conflict between wanting to do something to help the patient, but being aware that in the United Kingdom, nurses may not shorten life. Just as there are psychological factors which affect patients with regard to death and dying, it is important to recognise that nurses also have psychological attitudes towards death and dying. The culture of the nurses also plays an important part in terminal care provision in hospital; or rather the enculturation or socialisation that the nurses have undergone. The following section examines some attitudes towards death and dying demonstrated by nurses, in particular some of the beliefs and rituals employed by nurses when someone is terminally ill or dies in hospital.

Attitudes to death and dying amongst nurses

Smith (1992) states that the emotional climate of a ward may be attributed to nurses' perceptions of whether death and dying are explicit components of the work. According to Smith's research study, nurses are able to manage their emotions by distancing themselves from the patient, particularly on wards where nurses encounter death more often. It seems that nurses become socialised into becoming hard or blasé about death. Although it is not clear from Smith's study how this change comes about. The study demonstrates that nurses employ certain strategies in order to manage the death; for example: nurses who know the patient well are allocated to care for the patient. The patient is also often removed from the main ward area to a side room.

It should be acknowledged that not all nurses have the opportunity to choose regarding whether or not to care for a dying person, this is particularly true of student nurses.

Smith (1992) demonstrates that qualified staff and student nurses develop a separate set of social relations with dying patients. The qualified staff being more likely to get to know dying patients and therefore invest in the deaths of patients whom they knew. The staff hierarchy also serves to separate technical from emotional nursing by assuming that at certain stages of nurse education students should be able to perform specific technical tasks surrounding death and dying.

It is generally assumed that the more experienced you are, the better you are able to cope with upsetting situations (Smith 1992). Experience shows that in practice, feelings are rarely acknowledged amongst nurses. Therefore, staff are likely to develop distancing strategies outlined by Smith (1992) which prevent nurses from personal involvement. Nurses package care, dividing the emotional from the technical labour. The process of dying is more difficult to define than the act of death; death requires clearly identified skills and tasks whereas the point at which patients are recognised as dying, and the skills required to care for them during their transition from life to death are less definable. However, according to Smith (1992) nurses feel that being present at a death enables them to conclude care. For many staff, performing last offices attains closure. Therefore, it seems that for nurses, learning about the emotional aspects of death is largely experiential.

Dealing with death and dying in the clinical setting is difficult. Holland and Hogg (2001) suggest that sometimes experiencing death and dying are part of an initiation into nursing for student nurses. They also state that after encountering death-related experiences student nurses' perceptions begin to change; and rather than worrying about how they will cope, student nurses speak of caring for and communicating with dying patients. In clinical practice, nurses are encouraged to reflect upon their experiences with a mentor or supervisor in order to make sense of what they have experienced in practice.

As previously illustrated, brainstem death can occur within a matter of hours and thus can have a devastating effect on the family. The following section will review sudden death from a different perspective. In particular, the role of the nurse in breaking bad news is discussed.

Sudden death

Sudden or unexpected death is always traumatic for those who are left behind. Families will not have time to prepare for the death and will often be shocked, angry or in a state of disbelief. It is suggested that experiences at the time of a sudden death have a powerful effect on the whole process of grieving (Wright 1996). Wright offers some valuable advice for staff who are faced with the situation of having to tell families that there has been a sudden death. In particular Wright (1996) examines the role of the nurse in making a telephone call to relatives and suggests

that this kind of telephone call will often cause acute distress to both the receiver of the call and the worker who makes the call.

Language used at the time of the call by the member of staff must be considered as it plays an important role. There should be an agreed and concise definition of words which are used to describe the condition of an acutely ill relative who arrives in an Accident and Emergency Department, words which will be clearly understood by most people. Wright (1996) suggests the examples of Critical, Serious, Fair and Good. He goes on to suggest that if the patient has already died, it may be preferable to tell the relatives at the hospital rather than over the phone because this allows relatives to actualise the information by seeing the deceased:

> *A dilemma will occur if the informer is asked over the phone if the patient has died, or is uncertain about whether to disclose over the phone that the patient has died ..... If the hospital is quickly accessible it is better to tell people at the hospital. If they have a long distance to travel, and believe that by rushing they can be with their loved one before death or at the time of death, then it is essential to be honest over the phone.*

(Wright 1996, p. 14)

Wright (1996) goes on to offer some guidelines concerning how to conduct such a telephone call (see Box 14.3).

The following case study demonstrates the impact of sudden death when the news of the death is not delivered well.

Box 14.3 Giving information over the telephone

- Clear, concise information must be given.
- Say who you are and from which hospital.
- Be clear about who you are speaking to.
- If it is not the most significant relative, where can he/she be found.
- Give the name of the ill/injured person and their condition.
- If there is doubt as to the identification, tell them you believe it is the person.
- After telling them all this, check they are clear about which hospital, how to get there, what you have said.
- Then advise them to get someone to come with them, to drive carefully or get someone else to drive for them, to inform other close relatives or friends where they are heading.
- Records of the time of the call, who responded and how are important. After a death some relatives will want to clarify details.

From: Wright 1996, p. 15.

Case study 14.3

Your father has died

Catherine is a student nurse in her second year of her course; she is on a placement in a large Accident and Emergency Department. She arrives on duty and is asked to accompany a doctor while he tells a woman that her father has died whilst in the department.

Doctor: 'Has your Father been ill recently?'

Woman: 'Well, he's old, and you know what old people are like ..... they always like to moan about something!. But of course he's suffered with high blood pressure for years; and last year he did have a small stroke.'

Doctor: 'Your Father has had another stroke today: I'm afraid there was nothing we could do ..... he died pretty quickly.'

At this the woman screamed at the top of her voice, over and over again. The doctor sat and watched her scream and said nothing. Catherine; the student nurse, didn't know what to do. She didn't know whether to hold the woman, to try and talk to her, or to watch; just like the doctor. After several minutes of screaming the doctor stood up and said: 'I'm very sorry'. He then left.

Exercise

1. Reflect on previous situations where bad news has been broken to you both in your personal and professional life.
2. How was the news delivered and received?
3. Can you identify any of the elements of good practice suggested in this chapter?

Breaking bad news is difficult for those who have to deliver it and is often unpleasant and difficult to hear. Therefore, information given needs to be delivered in a sensitive manner whilst being correct and honest. Nurses will often play a crucial role in delivering such news, they will often accompany doctors whilst the news is delivered. Use of euphemisms for death should be avoided; words such as dead or died are unequivocal (Wright 1996). In the case study whilst the information may have been correct, the doctor did not display any sensitivity. You may have questioned whether the setting was right. Many Accident and Emergency Departments have specific relatives' rooms, away from the bustle of the department and with comfortable furniture, so that the room appears less clinical. Other factors to consider include establishing what the relative already knows about the health of the patient. In this case the doctor did seek clarification by asking the woman if her father had been unwell recently. He did not allow the woman time for reflection. Catherine did not know what to do because she did not know what to expect and she had

not anticipated the woman's response. Breaking bad news requires great skill and practice (Holland & Hogg 2001).

Sociocultural factors

Culture plays an important part in how a person reacts to and behaves during the terminal phase of an illness. A person's culture may have a direct impact on their nursing care. For example, Neuberger (1994) explains that Jews have strict laws about not shortening a dying person's life. This may limit the use of opiate-type pain control that depresses respiratory function. Jews 'grip on to life' whereas Hindu's regard their death as insignificant. Holland and Hogg (2001) suggest that for Hindus and Muslims fasting is not uncommon even during the terminal stage of a disease. Devout Muslims do not take anything into their bodies by mouth, nose, injection or suppository during daylight hours for the holy time of Ramadan (Holland & Hogg 2001). This means that providing effective pain relief may be extremely problematic. Indeed, people observing a faith in hospital may have daily religious rituals which should be maintained in order to promote wellbeing. Obstruction in executing such rituals may serve to further compound feelings of anxiety and isolation.

Hindus and Muslims bathe many times a day often before prayer and will want to continue to practice this even when very ill and will require a lot of help in order to achieve this need. However it should be remembered that modesty is crucial to Muslims: men remaining covered from waist to knee and women from head to foot. Women must be treated by women and men by men, to do otherwise renders the person 'unclean' (Holland & Hogg 2001).

Attitudes towards health and illness then will have a subsequent impact on the meaning of death and bereavement which the individual experiences. Consider the following brief case study.

Case study 14.4

Cultural needs of the dying

Rifat Begum is a 68-year-old woman in the terminal stages of cancer and is aware of her condition. Staff on the ward want to move her to a side ward later because her condition is deteriorating. Her husband Mohammed Hafiz is unhappy about this.

Exercise

1. What knowledge of Rifats' culture would help you to communicate with her and her husband concerning the move into a side ward?
2. Are there any specific cultural needs which must be met?
3. Find out how other cultures view death and dying and consider how you could ensure that other colleagues are made aware of these.

Rifat is a Muslim. It will be important to her and her family, that her privacy and dignity are not compromised, e.g. that her body is not exposed unnecessarily, and that she may find it impossible to be nursed by male members of the health care team. Prayer will also be important to Rifat (Holland & Hogg 2001) and her family may read the Holy Qur'an to her (Holland & Hogg 2001). It is vital to maintain effective communication with the family and to ensure that visiting is facilitated. Nurses can enhance their care by talking to the family and the patient so as to provide individualised care (Holland & Hogg 2001).

Mourning and grief

Following a death, bereavement and the expression of grief is important. How people grieve is dependent upon the society in which they live and the culture in which they spent their formative years. Mourning and grief are surrounded in ritual and some of these will now be explored. One major theory which attempts to explain the emotional stages which people go through when facing death or during bereavement is that of Kubler-Ross (1969) and she identified five stages of grief (see Box 14.4).

The terms bereavement, grief and mourning are often used interchangeably but Costello (1995) explains that they have distinct definitions:

- bereavement being the fact of death which may result in grief
- grief being the feelings associated with loss
- mourning being the social expression of grief.

However, individual responses to grief may vary tremendously and according to Costello (1995) are dependent on a number of factors which includes the strength of the relationship, timing of the death, cause of death, and the age of the dead person.

The role of ritual in mourning is expounded by Helman (1996) as a standardised and socially acceptable mode of behaviour which helps to relieve the sense of uncertainty and loss. Excessive or pathological mourning is prevented by mourning rituals which encourage emotional display of grief and providing the mourner with a defined timeframe of mourning (Helman 1996). Therefore, mourning ritual provides a socially valid way of expressing and relieving unpleasant emotions. Cowles (1996) carried out an expanded concept analysis of cultural perspectives of grief and found that although cultural differences are perceived to exist in mourning rituals, traditions and behavioural

expressions of grief; in fact there are no particular differences in the individual, intrapersonal experiences of grief that can be attributed to cultural heritage or ethnicity alone. Cowles' findings indicate that the intrapersonal experience of grief is similar across cultural groups. Participants in the research study described grief consistently as being a process that occurs over time and does not follow any established linear pattern. The experience of grief is unique to every individual, and according to Cowles (1996) to assume that a client is experiencing grief in a certain manner or to attribute that behaviour solely to ethnic or cultural heritage, precludes any attempt to understand the very individual.

Summary points

> 1. Culture plays an important role in how individuals react to death, grief and loss. The nurse should have an understanding of a variety of cultural approaches to the activity of dying.
> 2. Nurses should remember to assess everyone as an individual and not allow labels of Christian or Muslim or other religion to dictate how to care for someone.
> 3. Effective communication is the key to supporting people during the grieving process.

Environmental factors

Roper et al (1996) reported that in 1991 in England and Wales between 1975 and 1987, most people died in hospital. However, given the choice it could be argued that most people would wish to die at home. In recent years there has been a steady decline in home deaths in the Western world. People are less exposed to death and dying than in years gone by and Laungani and Young (1997) suggest that in today's Western society, when death occurs most of the time in hospital, it is medicalised rather than viewed as a natural event. In the United Kingdom some specialist services have been developed to enable people to remain at home for as long as possible, and to provide an alternative environment to that of a hospital for terminal care.

Huda Abu-Saad and Courtens (2001) provide a useful chapter on the history of palliative care which includes the development and philosophy of the hospice movement. They suggest that the hospice can be seen as a place for care (as in the United Kingdom) or as a philosophy of care (as in the USA). In both cases the notion of the hospice is focused on an integrated, patient-centred approach to care. A hospice provides multidisciplinary team care that aims to meet the complex and changing needs of people with life-threatening disease, and their family; and offer a wide range of care including symptom relief, rehabilitation, terminal care, outpatient support, family counselling, day care and bereavement follow up (Huda Abu-Saad & Courtens 2001, p. 17).

Box 14.4 Kubler-Ross's five stages of grief

1. Denial
2. Anger
3. Guilt
4. Depression
5. Acceptance

Models of palliative care (see Dougan & Colquhoun 2000) include domiciliary services where the primary health care team plays a major role are of major importance to helping people to remain at home. The general practitioner has overall responsibility for the medical care of patients and coordinates the care, the district nurses play a key role in nursing care. Nursing care in the United Kingdom is also provided by Marie Curie Cancer Nurses and Macmillan Nurses, who are specialists in cancer care and are responsible for providing symptom relief, psychosocial support, information and support in bereavement (Huda Abu-Saad & Courtens 2001, p. 15).

Exercise

If hospice facilities exist near to where you live or work you may find it useful to try and negotiate an informal visit to discuss the services it offers patients, their families and friends.

1. Following your visit reflect on whether the hospice matched up to your expectations. Where did your preconceived ideas about the hospice originate?
2. Are there any support services existing in your locality which would enable someone to remain at home throughout terminal illness?

Summary points

1. In the United Kingdom most people die in hospital but would rather die elsewhere.
2. Specialist services exist which may help individuals to remain at home during a terminal illness.

Politicoeconomic factors

Roper et al (1996) highlight that the economic status of a country is reflected in the causes of death and the life expectancy of the population. In the UK the National Statistics Office produces data concerning infant mortality rates and causes of death. Refer back to the earlier table showing the main causes of death of different ages in England and Wales. The major cause of death for men and women is circulatory diseases. It is known that cardiovascular disease is linked to a high intake of saturated fat and low intake of dietary fibre (Rutishauser 1994), so-called Western disease, because the disease is not prevalent in developing countries. Furthermore, cardiovascular disease is environmentally determined as immigrant groups take on the incidence of their host country (Rutishauser 1994).

The death of a family member can also have economic consequences for those who are left behind. For example, in the UK on the death of a spouse the State pension falls. The Government also provides some financial assistance in the form of death grants, widows' pensions, widowed mothers' allowance. During the terminal phase of illness other monies may also be available but these may vary depending on where you live.

At the time of death and shortly after

Student nurses may worry about how they will cope with seeing someone who has died for the first time and are unsure about what to expect. Carrying out care of the deceased person (last offices) not having met before is difficult and does not allow the person to be placed in context. Therefore, if carrying out last offices is problematic, discuss concerns with a mentor or someone in practice who may be able to help with a therapeutic relationship with the person during their illness. Continuing to care for that person after they have died will seem a more natural thing to do, and will help ensure closure on the relationship.

In order to prepare for 'last offices' the following section of the chapter will examine some physical changes that occur at the time of death and offers some suggestions for carrying out care of the deceased person (see Jamieson et al 2002 – Chapter 12 for further details). Nurses are sometimes unsure of the family's needs at the time of death, and again some suggestions are offered.

Physical changes at the time of death

After death circulation ceases and the internal environment of the body deteriorates rapidly, the body cools, the tissues and muscles lose their tone and rigor mortis (stiffening of the body) sets in after 2 or 3 hours (Roper et al 1996). The face will stiffen before the hands and feet. The body is at its stiffest between 12 and 48 hours after death (depending on the environmental temperature), but then wears off over the next day or two. The skin may change colour and become purplish and mottled in appearance, blood drains from the surface structures of the body. Initially after death the person should be laid flat on his back with arms placed against his sides. False teeth must be correctly positioned and the mouth closed. If the lower jaw falls, it may be supported with a pillow or small sandbag whilst rigor mortis sets in. Likewise, the eyes should be closed, eyelids can be held shut with damp cotton wool or gauze. Sometimes the body is then left for up to an hour before being washed. The body is also usually screened from view during this time.

The body is usually washed. Some relatives may wish to be involved in this procedure. In particular, Muslims will expect to wash their relatives themselves, Jewish people may also prefer the nurse not to take part if they are not Jewish themselves. Remember that sometimes when the body is turned, air is sometimes forced out of the lungs and over the larynx, resulting in a groan coming from the deceased. Tubes, catheters and infusions are usually removed unless they are required for postmortem requirements. If leakage is apparent from wounds or orifices, use packing or padding according to your local policy. Permission to remove jewellery must be sought. Many cultures will wear jewellery which is of great importance, for example, Sikhs will often wear a steel bangle or Kara which should not be removed (Holland & Hogg 2001). Jewellery which remains on the body is usually secured with tape. The body should be appropriately dressed (some areas will use special shrouds, others encourage the use of nightwear) and a legible nameband is worn (some hospitals require a second nameband at the ankle). Policy may also require documentation to be placed on the chest. The body is then wrapped in a sheet. If there is a risk of infection, the body is placed in a cadaver bag, which is sealed and labelled 'Danger of infection', together with the name of the infection (Mallett & Dougherty 2000).

When someone dies in hospital relatives can often feel that they have given part of the deceased person to the organisation and as a result may be reluctant to state their own needs. Wright (1996) suggests that it is the role of the nurse to facilitate and encourage normal requests. Furthermore, Wright's research demonstrates that it is important for relatives to see the deceased where they died, even if this is the resuscitation or treatment room. Seeing the deceased where they died appears to allow the bereaved person to become closer to the event, which they have a strong need to feel part of. Therefore, nurses should actively encourage the bereaved to see the body, and make it a perfectly natural thing to want to do. More regrets and problems arise from not seeing the body and later, of course, the decision cannot be rectified, for example Wright (1996) states that:

> 66 *We have to state clearly what is possible in explicit terms:*
> - *You can hold his hand if you want to.*
> - *Feel free to talk if you have things to say.*
> - *I am sure you want to say goodbye.* 99
>
> (Wright 1996, p. 27)

It is important to remember that the need to hold the person is normal and should be encouraged. It is also suggested that after a death the relatives will often appear to be reluctant to leave the deceased and the hospital. After saying goodbye and being asked if there are any unanswered questions, people will need permission to leave (Wright 1996). However, relatives should be given adequate time and should not feel that they are being rushed out.

It should be acknowledged that not everyone wants or needs to view or touch the body. The need to do so will depend on the beliefs and attitudes associated with death and dying. Muslims believe that death is not the end of life

but rather as the time when an individual departs from this earthly realm to be closer to God. Burial practices are also affected by culture. Roper et al (1996) points out that in some instances ritual prior to burial or cremation carries great importance. Holland and Hogg (2001) explore this concept further and explain that for some cultures, such as Chinese, death is seen as a transition whereby the person moves from one social status to another. During this time, rituals, or rites of passage, take place. The rituals help those who are dying or bereaved to know what is expected of them (Holland & Hogg 2001). The nurse should also be aware of local information regarding registering a death. You may need to provide directions to your nearest Registrars Office, together with times when the Registrar will be present. Therefore, it may be useful to find out these details in advance so that relatives can be provided with this information (see Box 14.5 for responsibilities of the informant and the Registrar following a death in the United Kingdom).

Box 14.5 What to do after death

Registering a death
- It is important that what is written on the death certificate is explained to the next of kin, and that he/she knows how to register the death.
- Deaths must be registered within 5 days at the offices of the Registrar of Births, Marriages and Deaths for the district where the death occurred or the body was found.
- The informant must take the notice given by the doctor and also, unless forwarded by the doctor, the medical certificate of cause of death.
- The Registrar will need to know the deceased person's full name, maiden name (if applicable), sex, date and place of birth, last employment and marital status. For this reason, the deceased's birth and marriage certificates are useful to have to hand.
- The Registrar issues a certificate of registration of death (free) and death certificate (charged) and these are needed later for various purposes (e.g. claiming benefits).

Arranging the funeral
- A Funeral Director will make all the arrangements although the decisions (e.g. cremation or burial) are made by the family.
- Costs are determined by the choice of coffin and headstone (if required) the venue and form of the ceremony, the distances involved, notification, procedures and any gathering after the funeral. Relatives should request an estimate of the costs before agreeing arrangements.

From: Farrell 1990.

THE MODEL FOR NURSING

In this section of the chapter the model is applied to a case study and will examine the processes of assessment, planning, implementation and evaluation of the activity of dying. Reflect on the case study and consider the impact of the activity of dying on nursing practice. In addition reflect on some personal experiences throughout the section in order to consider beliefs and values in relation to the activity of dying. Engaging in the reflective exercises may also help to assimilate learning. This section will explore:

- issues associated with assessing the individual for the activity of dying
- identifying problems
- planning care in partnership
- some nursing interventions associated with Bobs' story
- evaluation: the good death.

Assessing the individual for the activity of dying

As with all the other Activities of Living outlined in this book, assessment has three phases (see Chapter 1). Knowledge about the person and his family or carers is gained through the process of assessment and the nurse aims to come to understand the person and his beliefs and values about the activity of dying. It is not possible to plan individualised nursing care without first having undertaken a careful assessment (Roper et al 1996). Roper et al (1996) remind us that assessment is not a once-only activity, assessment may take place on admission to hospital for terminal care, or be a reassessment of a patient whose condition has worsened and for whom terminal care is now required. Assessment takes place as the persons' condition changes and new problems emerge, or identified problems are resolved. When assessing an individual for the activity of dying the following questions in relation to the model should be considered:

Lifespan

- How old is the person?
- Has a terminal diagnosis been made?
- Are there any previous experiences which have affected the person's view of death and dying?

Dependence/independence

- Is the person experiencing any difficulties in relation to independent living?
- What future problems are they or you concerned about?

Factors affecting the activity of dying

- What specific health problem is the individual suffering from? Remember this is not the same as the 'medical diagnosis'.
- What does the person understand about their medical diagnosis and prognosis?
- What effect is their health problem having on their emotional wellbeing?
- Are there any cultural needs to be considered prior to undertaking assessment?
- Does the individual have any spiritual or religious needs?
- Are there any environmental needs which the person may have which will affect future care?

In some cases nurses may feel that the activity of dying is not appropriate to their clinical area and may decide to omit this Activity of Living from an individual's assessment. However, many people are frightened of dying when they come into hospital. For example, a general anaesthetic is not without risk and even if the surgery is 'minor', someone might still be scared when faced with a general anaesthetic. Similarly, some older people may view hospitals as places where people go to die. There may be any number of reasons why someone might feel worried about dying and these need to be explored, in order to help the person feel at ease. Nurses may also omit this Activity of Living from the assessment process because they feel ill-prepared to deal with any fears which the person may present.

Box 14.6 Assessing the individual for the AL of dying

Lifespan: relationship to dying
- Age group of dying person and family/friends.

Dependence/independence in dying
- Status in relation to all ALs.
- Status during grieving and bereavement.

Factors influencing dying
Biological
– terminal illness/cause of death
– diagnosis of death
– effects on other ALs
– effect on physical and mental health of family/friends.

Psychological
– beliefs about death and dying
– knowledge and awareness of approaching death

– whether or not significant others know prognosis
– fears, anxieties and feelings
– effect of loss on family/friends.

Sociocultural
– social customs surrounding death and dying
– religious/cultural rights.

Environmental
– home/hospital/hospice

Politicoeconomic
– causes of death and life expectancy as indicators of socioeconomic status.
– state support for the dying and the bereaved.

From: Roper et al 1996, p. 410.

Case study 14.5

Bob's story

Bob and Kevin have been partners for 4 years, they live together in an urban area. Bob is 28 whilst Kevin is in his early 30s. Bob contracted HIV as a result of unprotected sex. Bob has a good job in the travel industry and feels that he has everything to live for; a caring partner in Kevin, they own their home and have an active social life. Bob has a younger brother and an older sister who live near their mother some 150 miles away, Bob keeps in touch with his siblings. However, Bob's mother had not spoken to him since he declared his homosexual lifestyle to her when he was 17. Bob had lived with HIV for 6 years before developing AIDS.

Bob found that he was unable to continue working once his condition worsened. Bob is allocated a carer through Social Services, Bob has had the same carer since he was diagnosed with AIDS and Jean spends about 30 hours a week with Bob, taking him to hospital for appointments and supporting him through his low days. Bob had built up an excellent rapport with Jean. He did not like strangers to call on him at home and if his District Nurse was not on duty, Bob would instruct Jean not to let anyone else visit. Bob had been a patient on the District Nurses' caseload for about 12 months.

As time went on, Bob was feeling dreadful, he developed a chest infection and a sarcoma affected most of the right side of his face, his right arm and leg. As a result the District Nurse visits increased from weekly to daily, and by Friday of this particular week, the district nurse said that she would visit twice a day from now.

Visit one
Two nurses visited Bob on Friday evening to see if he would agree to them visiting in turns over the weekend.

Bob, although embarrassed, agreed that he needed care over the weekend and would allow them to call. In particular he was coughing especially at night. Jean was spending much longer periods with Bob and Kevin was there as much as his own work would allow. Bob spent most of his time in bed, which had been moved downstairs into the lounge to allow Bob to watch TV and for friends to call and talk. Bob was fully aware of how ill he was, and would remind Kevin constantly about the arrangements for his funeral. Everything had been arranged some 2 years earlier, when Bob was well. Bob had not eaten for 3 days and despite Jean's best efforts to tempt him to eat, he refused. Jean felt sure that Bob must eat and was very worried that he wasn't eating.

Visit two
On Saturday morning Bob was in a great deal of pain. Jean managed to sit Bob in a chair to have a wash and Bob saw himself in the mirror. He was shocked by his own appearance and asked Jean to remove the mirror. The sarcoma was increasing rapidly especially over his face and Bob was becoming very frightened. He asked the District Nurse questions about his future and desperately wanted Kevin to hurry home from work. The nurse assessed Bob's pain and felt that his regime of analgesia needed to be reviewed by the doctor (which she arranged). Bob liked to take a very low dose of his pain killers and took them at irregular intervals which often resulted in his pain not being controlled. However, Bob felt that at least this way he remained in control.

Jean was worried that she wasn't coping very well and felt responsible for the deterioration in Bob's condition. Jean had never been involved with anyone who was so ill and likely to die.

Case study 14.5 (continued)

The District Nurse helped Jean to make sense of what was happening. The Nurse also advised Jean to contact Bob's family and encourage them to visit as it was likely that Bob would die within 24 hours. The nurse talked to Jean about what to expect when Bob's condition got worse and who to contact should he die; or if she felt Bob was in pain. The nurse explained that the funeral director must be advised when a person dies from HIV or AIDS as not all undertakers will accept 'infected bodies'; any family or friends who wanted to pay their last respects would need to do so before the undertakers arrived because they would seal Bob's body in a body bag and this would not be reopened. Jean was not aware of this and was visibly shaken and distressed by the information.

Visit three

The District Nurse called again on Saturday evening. Bob and Kevin were lying on the bed, drinking whisky and chatting about past times. They were both cheerful and reminiscing about their life together. Jean was more relaxed with Kevin around. Kevin helped the District Nurse to wash Bob and change the sheets because Bob had been incontinent. The District Nurse talked to Kevin about whether the family would be visiting and reiterated that they should see Bob before the undertakers arrived, while Bob was still in the house.

Visit four

The District Nurse called on Sunday morning to find Bob dead in the bed. Jean and Kevin had followed Bob's instructions to the letter. He was dressed in his Scottish national costume and wearing Kevin's favourite aftershave. Bob's brother, sister and mother had all visited before Bob died and said their goodbyes. Kevin and Jean stayed with Bob but couldn't bring themselves to call the undertakers. Kevin looked numb but needed to talk, but Jean was inconsolably racked with guilt that she could have done more, and feeling that all her effort was to no avail.

Assessing biological factors

The following may have been considered. The nurse will need to be aware of Bob's underlying disease: that of HIV and subsequent development of AIDS. In Bob's case he has been aware of his diagnosis for some time and has lived with his disease for many months. However, it is only over the past 12 months that his disease has been at the terminal stage, where he has been dying from, rather than living with, AIDS. According to Waugh and Grant (2001) there are several key characteristics associated with the physical factor of dying associated with AIDS (see Box 14.7).

Assessing psychological factors

It is through an effective therapeutic relationship that assessment becomes possible. The emotional factors will vary, as will the nature of the problems experienced (Roper et al 1996). In order to assess Bob psychologically the nurse will need to establish a relationship. According to Peplau (1992) the nurse–patient relationship is the central feature of nursing practice, in that the nurse and patient act together to solve the patient's problems. Other therapeutic activities include the creation of partnership, intimacy and reciprocity; manipulation of the environment to include care delivery systems, familiarity (similarities to home, or previous experiences); teaching; providing comfort; use of complementary therapies and utilising tested physical interventions (McMahon & Pearson 1998).

According to Sundeen et al (1998) there are four stages to a therapeutic relationship.

Box 14.7 Complications of living with acquired immune deficiency syndrome (AIDS)

When AIDS develops the main complications are widespread recurrent opportunistic infections and tumours. Outstanding features include:

- Pneumonia may be present, commonly caused by *Pneumocystis carinii*, but many other microbes may be involved.
- There may be persistent nausea, diarrhoea and loss of weight due to recurrent infections of the alimentary tract by a wide variety of microbes.
- Meningitis, encephalitis and brain abscesses may be recurrent, either caused by opportunistic microbes or possibly HIV.

- There may be deterioration in neurological function characterised by forgetfulness, loss of concentration, confusion, apathy, dementia, limb weakness, ataxia and incontinence.
- Skin eruptions, often widespread, may be seen, e.g. eczema, psoriasis, cellulitis, impetigo, warts, shingles and cold sores.
- Generalised lymphadenopathy may occur, i.e. noninfective enlargement of lymph nodes.
- There may be malignant tumours: lymphomas, i.e. tumours of lymph nodes, Kaposi's sarcoma, consisting of tumours under the skin and in internal organs.

From: Waugh & Grant 2001, p. 386.

Preinteraction begins before face-to-face interaction whereby the nurse will begin to formulate ideas about the patient. It is suggested that planning is required for the first interaction. Before the first visit the nurse will be aware that Bob is reluctant to be seen by strangers and therefore, she will have to plan a careful introduction.

Orientation The first meeting which is said to influence the whole relationship. There is a need for careful introductions and explanations. During this meeting a contract can be developed which may be formal (the nursing care plan) or informal (a verbal agreement), which shapes the future of the relationship. The nurse must try to ensure that a good foundation is laid for their relationship so that she may continue to visit over the weekend and support Bob, Kevin and Jean.

Maintenance or working phase Here the relationship develops, nurse and patient can work together towards agreed goals. The relationship allows each party to express their feelings. The nurse is able to respond to feelings during this phase.

Termination phase Ending the relationship may be emotionally painful for both patient and nurse.

Exercise

Read Visit one in Bob's story. Here a new District Nurse is going to meet Bob for the first time. The nurse has to ensure that this first meeting results in a positive outcome so that Bob will allow her to visit over the weekend.

1. How should the nurse conduct this first interview?
2. What special considerations need to be made?

Consideration may have been given to how the nurse will start to develop the therapeutic relationship with Bob, Kevin and Jean. It will be important for the nurse to adopt an open posture and try to get to Bob's eye level, rather than standing over him. All questions should be directed to Bob, and he should be encouraged to answer for himself, rather than allowing Jean to respond on his behalf. Buckman (1988) outlines some practical tips on talking to someone who is dying.

Getting started with assessment: talking to someone who is dying

Assessment is essentially concerned with the collection of data, but traditionally nurses find it extremely difficult to discuss and document information related to the activity of dying. Indeed, some nurses who use the model ignore this section of the model suggesting that it is inappropriate to their clinical area.

Buckman (1988) suggests:

> *Most of us don't know what to say because nobody has told us. ... Most people don't know how to help, not because of their own failings but because serious illness and the threat of death are very powerful forces. They can – and often do – tear relationships apart, separating and isolating the patient from family and friends and making everybody confused and embarrassed.*
> (Buckman 1988, p. xiii).

Buckman (1988) provides some practical advice on how to support someone who is dying. He argues that as health care professionals we must learn how to improve our communication with individuals in difficult situations because talking about distress will ultimately help to relieve distress. According to Buckman (1988) the key to communication is effective listening.

- The setting is important, so you should ensure privacy, or try to engender an air of privacy by closing curtains around the bed.
- You need to establish if the patient wants to talk. Don't be afraid to ask the obvious question: 'Do you feel like talking?' and don't worry if the patient says 'No', but be prepared to ask again later.
- Remember to be an effective listener, don't interrupt but stop what you are saying if the patient interrupts.
- Use nodding and paraphrasing to encourage the person to talk. Reflect things back, 'Yes, I see, tell me more…'.
- Don't be afraid to say nothing. Just being with someone can be valuable in its own right.
- Remember you can be honest about how you feel in this situation: 'I find this difficult to talk about. … I'm not very good at talking about', or even, 'I don't know what to say'.
- Seek clarification to make sure you haven't misunderstood what the person is saying, but be careful not to change the subject.
- Avoid 'if I were you I'd…'. You are *not* him. Ideally you should not be giving advice at all.
- Encourage the person to look back on their life. Reminiscences serve as reassurance that life has meaning. You may both end up crying, but that's OK.
- Respond to humour. Humour serves as an important factor in our way of coping with major threats and fears, it allows us to ventilate, to get rid of intense feelings and to get things into perspective (adapted from Buckman 1988).

During the assessment process it is important to establish what the patient (and his family or carers) knows in terms of diagnosis and prognosis. Classic work undertaken by Glaser and Strauss (1965) identified four awareness contexts in terminal illness, each with its own difficulties (see Box 14.8).

It is important to establish the needs and wishes of the patient. However, this may not be as straightforward as it sounds. Hughes and Neal (2000) point out that needs and

---

Box 14.8 Four awareness contexts in terminal illness

Closed awareness
Similar to denial whereby the patient does not recognise his impending death, even though everyone else does.

Suspected/suspicion awareness
The patients suspects what others know and tries to confirm or refute his suspicion.

Mutual pretence awareness
All parties realise that the person is dying but everyone pretends that the other does not know.

Open awareness
Patient, family and staff recognise and accept that the person is dying and they act on this awareness relatively openly.

From: Glaser & Strauss 1965.

---

wishes are not necessarily synonymous as need may be identified by the health care professional on the basis of technical knowledge (normative need) or by the person on the basis of their subjective knowledge or experience (felt or expressed need). Furthermore it is suggested that family members will also have a view of the dying person's need which may not be easily separated from their own perceived needs. Establishing the patient's needs and wishes may be particularly problematic if the awareness context is one of closed awareness, suspicion awareness or mutual pretence.

Exercise

1. Reflect on your clinical experiences with regard to assessing the activity of dying.
2. How would each of the awareness contexts outlined in Box 14.8 impact on your assessment of someone who is dying?

Assessing the needs of dying patients: other tools which may be used during assessment

Dying patients have multiple needs and therefore, it is argued that palliative care needs assessment should cover a broad range to include psychosocial, spiritual, emotional and cultural needs, in addition to physical needs. Any assessment should also include input from patients and carers (Llamas et al 2001). It should be acknowledged that a number of tools exist which may be a useful aid in assessing the needs of dying patients. Llamas et al (2001) review a number of these tools which may be used in tandem with the Activities of Living (Roper et al 1996).

Consider if any of these tools are used in clinical practice. Discuss the tools with nurses and patients who use them to develop some conclusions about their effectiveness.

Actual and potential problems: identification and planning

The following section will explore the problems experienced by Bob, Kevin and Jean. At each visit the nurse will undertake an assessment to identify new problems or to ascertain if known problems have been resolved (reassessment). In order to identify and plan nursing needs and apply the model, the case study will be used to provide structure to ideas.

Actual and potential problems are assessed by the District Nurse each time she visits Bob. The Activities of Living are used as a framework to aid the assessment process. The actual problems could be things that Bob, Kevin or Jean tell the nurse, or they may be things which the nurse observes or can anticipate (potential problems). It is important to remember who has the problem. For example:

Visit one

Activity of Living: eating and drinking (see Chapter 6)
Bob has not eaten for 3 days. The problem here is that Jean is worried about Bob, not that Bob is not eating. However, if Bob had said that he was hungry, or felt sick, or had a sore mouth then Bob would be expressing a need.

Food refusal can often be a source of conflict between patients and their carers. Hughes and Neal (2000) suggest that if the seeking of food is a biological imperative, the giving of food also takes on a social imperative. They suggest that nutritional support may be justified if symptoms which diminish the quality of life, such as pressure sores, develop. Limited food intake should not necessarily be viewed as a problem to be rectified (Hughes & Neal 2000). Hughes and Neal (2000) explain that in many cases patients with terminal illness can experience comfort despite minimal, if any, food or fluid intake. They also point out that for some, a decision not to eat may be a direct attempt to hasten death, or acceptance of the inevitability of death. Food may also have a cultural significance at the end of life (Hughes & Neal 2000). As already discussed in this chapter many people will want to continue to observe cultural or religious rituals even during the terminal stages of an illness.

Nursing intervention
- to establish if not eating is a problem for Bob through careful interviewing
- to support Jean whilst Bob is not eating.

Activity of Living: sleeping (see Chapter 13)

Actual problem Bob is not sleeping well due to a cough caused by a chest infection.

Nursing intervention
- to help Bob and Jean adopt the position of most comfort which facilitates Bob's breathing.

In consultation with the general practitioner and Bob and Kevin, consideration may be given to obtaining a sputum specimen which may be sent to the laboratory for culture. Appropriate antibiotics may then be prescribed. However, Bob may decide to decline such treatment.

Visit two
Activity of Living: communication (see Chapter 4)

Actual problem 1 Bob has an altered body image which he is having difficulty accepting.

Actual problem 2 Bob is frightened about his future.

Actual problem 3 Bob has stated that he is in pain.

Exercise
1. From what you have read in this chapter write down some suggestions as to how you would address Bob's communication needs in relation to the first two problems he has expressed.
2. What would Jean's needs be in relation to these areas.

Nursing interventions Consideration may have been given to the elements suggested by Buckman (1988) earlier in the chapter. In addition the effects of fatigue and altered concentration span, as Bob may get tired very quickly and need to rest. Through careful dialogue, it may be discovered that Bob is frightened of being in pain, or that the pain will worsen and become unbearable. Of course, Bob may just be frightened of the unknown, and may ask you questions to which there is no answer. Do not be afraid to be honest, and tell the person what you are feeling; for example: 'I wish there was something I could tell you about that, so that you would be less frightened'. Remember that just being with an individual who is dying can be therapeutic in its own right. Some people may find it beneficial to speak with a priest or appropriate holy person.

Pain Pain is something which many nurses are concerned that their patients will suffer from. Symptoms of pain irrespective of their prevalence, seem to impact on daily functioning and quality of life (Huda Abu-Saad & Courtens 2001). Bob has expressed that he is in pain, therefore the nurse must make an accurate assessment of his pain. The following section will review some principles of pain management.

Pain management Huda Abu-Saad and Courtens (2001) suggest that the primary aim of symptom management in palliative care is to control the symptoms which are distressing to the patient, tailoring all therapy to the patient's needs. Huda Abu-Saad and Courtens (2001) also state that that treatment should be based on a logical approach, starting at the level most appropriate for the patient and progressing to the next step if the pain cannot be controlled. This system is often referred to as a pain ladder. The World Health Organisation (1998) developed the three-step analgesic ladder which is summarised in Table 14.2.

Roper et al (1996) suggest that the basic principle of pain management is that sufficiently potent analgesics are given regularly so that pain is not only relieved, but prevented and if pain does occur, then the dose should be increased or the drug changed (p. 412). *It should be remembered that increasing drug dosages or changing drugs is the responsibility of the Doctor.* However, the Doctor often relies on the nurse's assessment of the patient's pain (see Roper et al 1996 for information on tools for pain assessment and discussion of the physical and psychological aspects of pain).

According to Benner et al (1996) nurses influence medical decision making by the way in which they present information to the doctor. Experienced, expert nurses cue doctors in to what is important. Doctors also appear to get used to a nurse's reporting style and are able to utilise the expert nurse's judgements and are more likely to listen. Moreover experienced nurses can read when the doctor has understood her report of the salient facts whereas inexperienced nurses can not tell if the doctor has missed the relevant points. Therefore, developing a therapeutic relationship is vital in order for the nurse to assess the patient's pain and his response to it. Fear of pain should also be considered and acknowledged; such fear can be distressing and psychologically painful in itself.

The nurse will also need to understand the action of the drugs which she administers and be able to notice any undesirable side effects. In particular, the action and side effects of opiates needs to be considered. Huda Abu-Saad

Table 14.2 Three-step analgesic ladder

Level one		Level two		Level three	
Nonopioid. +/– Adjuvant	Pain increasing	Opioid for mild to moderate pain +/– nonopioid. +/– Adjuvant	Pain persisting or increasing	Opioid for moderate to severe pain +/– Nonopioid. +/– Adjuvant	Freedom from cancer pain

WHO (1998) Working Party on Clinical Guidelines in Palliative Care Guidelines for Managing Cancer Pain in Adults. National Council for Hospice and Specialist Palliative Services. London.

and Courtens (2001) provide a useful chapter on pain and symptom management across the lifespan.

Visit three

Activity of Living: personal cleansing and dressing (see Chapter 8)

Actual problem Bob is no longer independent in washing and dressing himself and requires assistance.

Nursing intervention

- to keep Bob's skin clean and dry at all times
- to educate Kevin and Jean of the importance of keeping Bob's skin clean and dry
- to demonstrate to Bob's carers how to care for Bob's skin, and how to help Bob to get dressed.

The interventions may require greater care to prevent causing pain and anxiety; and may take longer as a result. It should also be recognised that the activity of personal cleansing and dressing in particular gives the nurse the opportunity to utilise expertise in communication in order to further develop the therapeutic relationship.

Activity of Living: elimination (see Chapter 7)

Actual problem Bob is not able to control the flow of urine.

Nursing intervention

- to minimise the harmful effects of urine on Bob's skin by keeping the skin clean and dry
- use barrier cream in groins to prevent excoriation of the skin
- promote Bob's dignity by allowing him to do as much as he wants or is able for himself.

Visit four

During visit four the nurse must focus her attention to caring for Kevin and Jean. Providing care at home to someone who is dying places great strain on the carers. Roper et al (1996) acknowledge that in the first few days after a death, the family and/or carers will be physically and emotionally exhausted; particularly when the death has been protracted. At this time the nurse must offer practical comfort and support. The next section examines emotional support in relation to Bob's story.

Activity of Living: communication (see Chapter 4)

Actual problem 1 Kevin and Jean require support following Bob's death.

Nursing intervention

> **Exercise**
> How would the nurse support Kevin and Jean?

Think about the practical advice that Kevin might require, for example, where and when he might register Bob's

death. The nurse will need to encourage Kevin and Jean to talk, and be there to listen.

Planning care

According to Webster (1998) the patient is often identified by nurses as the key person in planning care, however, in practice patients play little or no part in this activity. Truly involving the patient in nursing care planning may be a skill which requires practice. One of the mechanisms suggested by Webster (1998) is to only document 'patient-centred information', however, in order to do this it is vital for the nurse to 'know the patient'. The concept of knowing the patient is relevant to therapeutic decision making and has two elements: the nurse's understanding of the patient and the selection of individualised interventions (Radwin 1996). Nurses appear to value treating each person as an individual and this concept appears to enable nurses to actualise a cherished value (Radwin 1996). The concept may be of particular significance to nurses working in community settings caring for terminally ill patients. Knowing about the patient and getting to know what the patient thinks about their situation helps the nurse to interpret concerns or anticipate needs (Luker et al 2000). Luker et al (2000) suggest that Community Nurses equate high-quality care with fundamental communication patterns which exist between nurses and patients, nurses and carers and/or carers and the patient. Furthermore, Luker et al (2000) go on to say that spending time in the home and ensuring continuity of care are seen as prerequisites to knowing the patient, and that nurses provided more than just physical care. By providing such care it is argued that nurses are able best to respond to individual needs (Luker et al 2000).

Evaluating care: the 'good death'

Roper et al (2000) suggest that like other Activities of Living, the activity of dying should be evaluated. Death should not be viewed as a failure by medical and nursing staff, indeed, a 'good death' can be achieved. It is suggested that there are 12 principles of a good death (Age Concern 1999) (see Box 14.9).

> **Exercise**
> Apply these principles of the good death to Bob's story.
>
> 1. Did he have 'a good death'?
> 2. Reflect on some of your other experiences. How do you feel about the notion of 'a good death'?
> 3. Can patients have a good death in different clinical settings?
> 4. Develop some strategies to ensure that patients in your care will have a good death.

Box 14.9 The good death

- To know when death is coming, and to understand what can be expected
- To be able to retain control of what happens
- To be afforded dignity and privacy
- To have control over pain relief and other symptom control
- To have choice and control over where death occurs (at home or elsewhere)
- To have access to information and expertise of whatever kind is necessary
- To have access to any spiritual or emotional support required
- To have access to hospice care in any location, not only in hospital
- To have control over who is present and who shares the end
- To be able to issue advance directives which ensure wishes are respected
- To have time to say goodbye, and control over other aspects of timing
- To be able to leave when it is time to go, and not to have life prolonged pointlessly.

From Age Concern, 1999

Roper et al (1996) suggest that the phases of the nursing process can be worked through rapidly, in an emergency, or quickly changing situation; such as cardiac arrest; or more time can be devoted to assessing, planning; as in Bob's story. However, all of the Activities of Living must be considered collectively (i.e. because of their interrelationships) although there may be some nursing goals that are specific to the AL of dying (Roper et al. 1996).

Summary points

1. The therapeutic relationship is crucial in communicating with someone who is dying. Developing such relationships requires practice and expertise.
2. The model can be applied to the activity of dying and provides a clear framework to help the nurse through assessment, planning, implementation and evaluation.
3. The activity of dying exists alongside all the other Activities of Living as defined by Roper et al (2000)

References

Age Concern 1999 Debate of the Age Health and Care Study Group. The future of health and care of older people: the best is yet to come. Age Concern, London

Benner P, Tanner C, Chesla C 1996 Expertise in nursing practice, caring, clinical judgement and ethics, 2nd edn. Springer Publishing Co., New York

BODY (British Organ Donation Society) 2001 (http://www.organet.co.uk/body/DoH.html)

Bond J, Bond S 1997 Sociology and health care. Churchill Livingstone, Edinburgh

Brysiewicz P 2002 Violent death and the South African emergency nurse. International Journal of Nursing Studies 39: 253–258

Buckman R 1988 'I don't know what to say': How to help and support someone who is dying. Macmillan, London

Costello J 1995 Helping relatives cope with the grieving process. Professional Nurse 11(2): 89–92

Costello J 2001 Nursing older dying patients: findings from an ethnographic study of death and dying in elderly care wards. Journal of Advanced Nursing 35(1): 59–68

Costello J, Trinder-Brook A 2000 Children's nurses' experiences of caring for dying children in hospital. Paediatric Nursing 12(6): 28–31

Cowles KV 1996 Cultural perspectives of grief: an expanded concept analysis. Journal of Advanced Nursing 23: 287–294

Department of Health 1999 Saving lives: our healthier nation. HMSO, London

Dougan HAS, Colquhoun MM 2000 The patient receiving palliative care. In: Alexander MF, Fawcett JN, Runciman PJ (eds) Nursing practice–hospital and home (the adult). Churchill Livingstone, Edinburgh

Farrell M 1990 What to do after bereavement. Professional Nurse 5(10): 539–542

Gill P 2000 Brain stem death – an anthropological perspective. Care of the Critically Ill 16(6): 217–220

Glaser BE, Strauss AL 1965 Awareness of dying. Aldine, New York

Health Education Authority 1998 Older people in the population. Fact sheet 1. HMSO, London

Helman C 1996 Culture health and illness, 3rd edn. Butterworth-Heinemann, Oxford

Hindmarch C 2000 On the death of a child, 2nd edn. Radcliffe Medical Press, Oxford

Holland K and Hogg C 2001 Cultural awareness in nursing and health care. An introductory text. Arnold, London

Huda Abu-Saad H, Courtens A 2001 Chapter 2. Developments in palliative care. In: Huda Abu-Saad H (ed) Evidence-based palliative care across the life span. Blackwell Science, Oxford

Hughes N, Neal RD 2000 Adults with terminal illness: a literature review of their needs and wishes for food. Journal of Advanced Nursing 32(5): 1101–1107

Human Organ Transplants Act 1989 (http://www.hmso.gov.uk)

Human Tissue Act 1961 (http://www.hmso.gov.uk)

Jamieson EM, McCall JM, Whyte LA 2002 Clinical nursing practices 4th edn. Churchill Livingstone, Edinburgh

King RA 2001 Psychosocial and risk behavior correlates of youth suicide attempts and suicidal ideation. Journal of the American Academy of Child and Adolescent Psychiatry 40(7): 837–846

Kubler-Ross E 1969 On death and dying. Macmillan, New York

Laungani P, Young B 1997 Conclusion I: Implications for practice and policy. In: Parkes CM, Laungani P, Young B 1997 Death and bereavement across cultures pp. 218–232. Routledge, London.

Limandri BJ, Boyle DW 1978 Instilling hope. American Journal of Nursing 78(1): 79–80

Llamas KJ, Pickhaver AM, Piller NB 2001 Palliative care needs assessment for cancer patients in acute hospitals: a review. Progress in Palliative Care 9(4): 136–142

Luker KA, Austin L, Caress A, Hallett CE 2000 The importance of 'knowing the patient': community nurses' constructions of quality in providing palliative care. Journal of Advanced Nursing 31(4): 775–782

Mallett J, Dougherty L 2000 The Royal Marsden manual of clinical nursing procedures. Blackwell Science, London

McMahon R, Pearson A 1998 Nursing as a therapy, 2nd edn. Stanley Thornes, Cheltenham

Neuberger J 1994 Caring for dying people of different faiths, 2nd edn. Mosby, London

Office for National Statistics 2000 (http://www.statistics.gov.uk/default.asp)

Peplau HE 1992 Interpersonal relations: a theoretical framework for application in nursing practice. Nursing Science Quarterly 5(1): 13–18

Radwin LE 1996 'Knowing the patient': a review of research on an emergency concept. Journal of Advanced Nursing 23: 1142–1146

Roper N, Logan WW, Tierney AJ 1996 The elements of nursing. A model for nursing based on a model of living, 4th edn. Churchill Livingstone, Edinburgh

Roper N, Logan WW, Tierney AJ 2000 The Roper, Logan, Tierney model of nursing. Churchill Livingstone, Edinburgh

Ross L 1994 Spiritual aspects of nursing. Journal of Advanced Nursing 19: 439–447

Rutishauser S 1994 Physiology and anatomy. A basis for nursing and health care. Churchill Livingstone, Edinburgh

Smith P 1992 The emotional labour of nursing. How nurses care. Macmillan Press, London

Sundeen SJ, Stuart GW, Rankin EAO, Cohen SA 1998 Nurse–client interaction. Implementing the nursing process, 6th edn. Mosby, London

Waugh A, Grant A 2001 Anatomy and physiology in health and illness, 4th edn. Churchill Livingstone, Edinburgh

WHO 1990 Cancer pain relief and palliative care. Report of a WHO expert committee (Technical report series No. 804. WHO, Geneva

WHO 1998 Working party on clinical guidelines for managing cancer pain in adults. National Council for Hospice and Specialist Palliative Services, London

WHO 2001 Adolescent crucial age for health of tomorrow's societies. WHO Press release No 3, 7 March. WHO, Geneva (www.who.int)

WHO 2002 Brief on the consultation on child and adolescent health and development. Press release. WHO, Geneva (www.who.int)

Wilkinson R 2000 Organ donation: the debate. Nursing Standard 141(28): 41–42

World Health Report 1997 (http://www.int/whr2001/2001/archives/1997)

Wright B 1996 Sudden death. A research base for practice, 2nd edn. Churchill Livingstone, Edinburgh

Webster J 1998 The effect of care planning on quality of patient care. Professional Nurse 14(2): 85–87

Further reading

Henley A, Schott J 1999 Culture, religion and patient care in a multi-ethnic society. Age Concern, London

Parkes CM, Laungani P, Young B (eds) 1997 Death and bereavement across cultures. Routledge, London

Sahberg-Blom E, Ternestedt B-M, Johansson J-E 2001 Is good 'quality of life' possible at the end of life? An explorative study of the experiences of a group of cancer patients in two care cultures. Journal of Clinical Nursing 10: 550–562

Smith-Brew S, Yanai L 1996a The organ donation process through a review of the literature. Part 1. Accident and Emergency Nursing 4: 5–11

Smith-Brew S, Yanai L 1996b The organ donation process through a review of the literature. Part 2. Accident and Emergency Nursing 4: 95–102

Wright B 1996 Sudden death. A research base for practice, 2nd edn. Churchill Livingstone, London

Useful websites

www.worldaidsday.org (World AIDS Day website)

www.avert.org (an AIDS education and medical research UK based charity)

www.who.int (World Health Organisation)

www.hospice-spc-council.org.uk (National Council for Hospice and Specialists Palliative Care Services)

www.argonet.co.uk/body/doh.html (British Organ Donor Society)

Appendices

Appendix 1

REFERENCE VALUES FOR THE MORE COMMON ANALYTES IN URINE

Analysis	Reference range	Units
Albumin	[See note 1]	
Calcium	1.2–3.7 (low calcium diet)	mmol/24 h
	Up to 12 (normal diet)	
Copper	Up to 0.6	µmol/24 h
Cortisol	9–50	µmol/mol creatinine
Creatinine	10–20	mmol/24 h
Hydroxyindole-3-acetic acid (5-HIAA)	<60	µmol/24 h
Metanadrenalines		
Normetadrenaline	0.4–3.4	µmol/24 h
Metadrenaline	0.3–1.7	µmol/24 h
Oxalate	80–490 (M)	mmol/24 h
	40–320 (F)	mmol/24 h
Phosphate	15–50	mmol/24 h
Potassium[2]	25–100	mmol/24 h
Protein	Up to 0.3	g/L
Sodium	100–200	mmol/24 h
Urate	1.2–3.0	mmol/24 h
Urea	170–600	mmol/24 h

Notes

Albumin/creatinine ratio (ACR) and urinary albumin excretion rate (AER) are used to detect microalbuminuria, i.e. excessive albumin excretion in patients with diabetes mellitus, which is of predictive value in identifying patients at risk of progression to diabetic nephropathy. The test should only be carried out in the absence of overt proteinuria (Dipstix negative).

ACR
Reference range:	<3.5 mg albumin/mmol creatinine
Borderline:	3.5–10 mg albumin/mmol creatinine
Sensitive test:	>10 mg albumin/mmol creatinine

AER
Reference range:	<20 µg albumin/min
Microalbuminuria:	20–200 µg albumin/min

The urinary output of electrolytes such as sodium and potassium is normally a reflection of intake. This can vary widely, especially on a cultural, worldwide basis. The values quoted are more appropriate to a 'Western' diet. Alexander et al 2000 (page 1071)

Appendix 2

COMMONLY USED FORMS	
(Section 1) **Patient's nursing records**	Biographical Data

PATIENT'S NAME: A

WISHES TO BE KNOWN AS:

ADDRESS:

POST CODE:
TEL NO:
AGE: D.O.B:
MARITAL STATUS:
LANGUAGE(S) SPOKEN:
OCCUPATION:

PRACTISING FAITH: B
CONTACT No:

NEXT OF KIN: C
RELATIONSHIP:
ADDRESS:

CONTACT Nos:
(DAY)
(NIGHT)
(EMERGENCY)
SIGNIFICANT OTHER:

AWARE OF ADMISSION? Yes/No

G.P. NAME + ADDRESS: D

TEL No:

COMMUNITY NURSE:
TEL No:

SOCIAL WORKER:
TEL No:

HEALTH VISITOR:
TEL No:

MEALS ON WHEELS:

HOME CARE TEAM:

DAY CARE:

OTHER AGENCIES:

HOSPITAL: E
WARD:
ADMISSION STATUS:
ADMITTED FROM:

DATE: TIME:
CONSULTANT:

REASON FOR ADMISSION: F

PREVIOUS MEDICAL HISTORY:

CURRENT MEDICATIONS:

ALLERGIES:

TYPE OF HOUSING/ACCOMMODATION: G

LIVES WITH:

DEPENDENTS:

PRIMARY/NAMED NURSE: H

ADMITTING NURSE:

INFORMATION OBTAINED FROM:

PATIENT'S VIEWS/FEELINGS ON ADMISSION: I

ADMISSION DEPENDENCY SCORE: J
PRESSURE ULCER RISK SCORE:
MOVING & HANDLING RISK SCORE:

VALUABLES: Retained/Sent home K

(Section 2)   Patient assessment

ACTIVITIES OF LIVING	NORMAL HABITS & ROUTINES (Physical, Psychological, Socio-cultural, Environmental & Economic)	ACTUAL & POTENTIAL PROBLEMS

Maintaining a safe environment

Communicating

Breathing

Eating & Drinking

Eliminating

Personal cleansing & dressing

Controlling body temperature

Mobilising

Working & playing

Expressing sexuality

Sleeping

Dying

Date: ....   Time: ....   Signature: ....

(Section 3a)	Patient care plan

PATIENT'S NAME .... **WARD** ....

ACTIVITY CONCERNED .... **DATE ASSESSED** ....

PROBLEM
The patient

GOAL
The patient

To be achieved by ....

NURSING INTERVENTION	

SIGNATURE ....

EVALUATION
The patient

DATE .... **SIGNATURE** ....

(Section 3b)   **Daily evaluation/communication/progress**   page ☐

PATIENT'S NAME ....   **WARD** ....

                                         A.L. ....

Date/Time	Remarks	Designation & Signature

| (Section 4) | **Medically-derived & collaborative care communication** | page ☐ |

PATIENT'S NAME .... **WARD** ....

Date/Time	Remarks	Designation & Signature

(Section 5a)   **Discharge planning**

RECORD THE PROBLEMS IDENTIFIED & THE ACTION & REFERRAL AGENCY REQUIRED

Date ↓   FACTORS AFFECTING HEALTH RECOVERY   ACTION   Signature ↓

Physical	

Psychological	

Sociocultural	

Environmental	

Economic	

(Section 5b) | **Discharge summary**

PATIENT'S NAME .... DISCHARGE DATE ....

DISCHARGE ADDRESS ....

....

....

COMMUNITY CARE ASSESSMENT   NO ☐   YES ☐   DATE ....

INFORMATION	✔	DATE	SIGNATURE
Patient aware			
Relative/carer aware			
Mode of transport			
Social worker/services			
Community nurse			
Physiotherapy			
Other			
Specific care instructions			
Aids/prosthesis			
Follow-up appointment			
Medication & education			
Equipment to take home			
Valuables/property			
Medical certificate			
G.P. letter/informed			

COMMUNITY CARE OUTCOME

(Section 6)

Patient dependency/independency progress

DATE																								
SCORE																								
0																								
1																								
2																								
3																								
4																								
5																								

Moving and handling risk score

DATE	
SCORE	

Pressure ulcer risk score

DATE	
SCORE	

Dependency scoring criteria

1. Completely self caring within the environment.

2. Is vulnerable to difficulties with the AL, due to altered state or medical intervention.
   Problems are potential.
   Minimal or occasional assistance is required.

3. Is unsafe in the AL.
   Lacks the necessary ability to carry out the AL without assistance/supervision.
   Other ALs affected.

4. Acute/chronic disturbance resulting in an increasing number of actual and potential problems.
   Disturbances in most ALs.
   Requires trained nurse assistance/observation.

5. Unable to manage the AL independently.
   Needs assistance from one or more trained nurses (total nursing/medical support).
   Example states: Unconscious/semi-conscious
   Very young/old
   Suicidal

Appendix 3

ASSESSMENT SCHEDULE USING ROPER–LOGAN–TIERNEY MODEL FOR NURSING
Possible questions to consider during the assessment stage of care planning

Activity of Living	Physical	Psychological	Sociocultural	Environmental	Politicoeconomic
Maintaining a safe environment	• Is the person able to prevent accidents or at risk from injury (day & night)? • Is the person at risk from infection, shock, haemorrhage, or unconsciousness? • Is the person aware or safe taking or receiving medications? • What are the vital sign baseline observations? e.g. pulse, blood pressure	• Does the person lack knowledge or ability to identify hazards or promote healthy living? • Does the person's mood, personality, behaviour or false perception put safety at risk? • Is the person under stress or anxious about safety/lifestyle?	• What are the person's beliefs and values concerning safety and healthy living? • Does the person require information or education regarding safety/ healthy living?	• Can the person recognise hazards within the environment hazardous to safety? • Are there any hazardous situations within the environment? • If in hospital – is the person aware of fire hazards and procedures, would they be able to leave the ward without assistance?	• Are there any lack of resources/ facilities compromising safety? • Are there any economic factors inhibiting the persons health/ lifestyle?
Communicating	• Is the person able to fully communicate – speech, hearing, vision, non-verbal, read & write? • Is the person in pain – location, intensity, type, and pattern? • What is the person's current conscious level recording?	• Does the person's mood, perception, personality or behaviour affect communication? • Does the person feel anxious or threatened about being in hospital or other care setting? • Does the person lack knowledge, information or intelligence? • What are the person's experiences of pain?	• What is the person's native language? • Are there any dialect difficulties? • Are there any social or cultural norms affecting communication, i.e. touch, clothing, relationships? • What are the person's beliefs about pain? • How does the person normally cope with pain episodes?	• Is the environment conducive to encourage good communications i.e. privacy, layout, lighting etc. • Are there any factors precipitating pain?	• Can the person use or access telephones, newspapers and other media resources? • Are there any economic difficulties affecting communication?

ASSESSMENT SCHEDULE *(continued)*
Possible questions to consider during the assessment stage of care planning

Activity of Living	Physical	Psychological	Sociocultural	Environmental	Politicoeconomic
Breathing	• Does the person have difficulty in breathing and what are the causes? • Are there any abnormalities in the person's breathing pattern or habit? • Are there any activities which affect breathing? • Are there any physical risks related to breathing? • What is the person's respiratory rate?	• Are there any emotional responses which might affect breathing? • Does the person require any information or advice to aid breathing or promote healthy lifestyle?	• What are the person's beliefs related to coughing, spitting and smoking?	• Are there any factors which might alter/affect the person's breathing i.e. O_2, temperature, ventilation position in bed, irritants, medications?	• Does the person have sufficient knowledge, information and resources to adopt a healthy lifestyle or overcome difficulties with breathing i.e. medication, housing, emotional support?
Eating and drinking	• Does the person have difficulty in shopping and preparing a nutritious diet? • Is the person having difficulty in taking in, chewing, swallowing or digesting food or drink? If so due to what cause? • How does the person describe their diet? • What is the person's current weight?	• Does the person understand what a healthy balanced diet is? • Does the person express any views on body image? • Does the person have knowledge about food handling and hygiene? • What is the person's attitude towards eating and drinking, likes and dislikes of certain foods and drinks? • Is the person stressed or anxious about eating and drinking?	• Does the person have any cultural influences regarding eating and drinking? • Does the person have any traditional or restrictive dietary habits pre/post meals? • Could the person make any necessary adjustments to the diet if required?	• What kind of environment does the person normally take meals in? • What factors are likely to affect the person's ability to eat or drink? • Does the person have facilities at home to shop, store, cook and eat food/drink?	• Are there any factors affecting the person's: Choice and availability of diet, malnutrition? Safe handling? • Does the person have sufficient knowledge and assistance to provide a healthy diet?

ASSESSMENT SCHEDULE *(continued)*
Possible questions to consider during the assessment stage of care planning

Activity of Living	Physical	Psychological	Sociocultural	Environmental	Politicoeconomic
Eliminating	• Does the person have difficulty in passing urine or having bowels opened – what is the cause? • Does the person have difficulty in using or reaching toilets, bedpans or commodes etc? • Does the person have any other devices in situ which alters normal urinary or defaecatory function? • What is the person's normal habit and routine?	• Does the person have any psychological or emotional problems altering normal function? • What is the person's concept of privacy and modesty? • Is the person anxious or concerned about eliminating? • Does the person express the need for self care/privacy?	• What is the person's normal language for eliminating? • What are the person's normal pre/posteliminatory routines? • Does the person understand the need for hygiene? • Are there any cultural/religious or social traditions to be followed?	• Does the person know where the toilet and hand washing facilities are situated and how to use them? • Are the facilities within reach, safe and sufficient for the person to use? • Are the facilities conducive to privacy?	• Does the person have facilities appropriate to their needs? • Does the person have sufficient knowledge to prevent the spread of infection and to use appropriate hygiene?
Personal cleansing and dressing	• What are the person's normal habits and routines related to masculinity/femininity? • What difficulties is the person currently or likely to experience – cause? • What changes can be detected in relation to: hair, mouth, teeth, hands, nails, feet, skin and overall dress and appearance? • Is the person at risk of any complications if unable to carry out this activity?	• What standards does the person normally achieve? • What knowledge does the person have – washing, bathing, dental care etc? • Does the person's anxiety, mood, perception or behaviour influence this AL? • Is the person likely to be embarrassed? • Is the person likely to be fearful, shocked or repulsed at the sight of skin trauma?	• What are the person's beliefs related to cleansing and dressing (day & night)?	• Are there sufficient facilities and resources to enable needs to be met? • Is the person worried about the facilities, privacy and dignity?	• Does the person have sufficient knowledge, finances and resources to meet their needs? • Does the person have essential items, i.e. clothing, footwear etc?

ASSESSMENT SCHEDULE *(continued)*
Possible questions to consider during the assessment stage of care planning

Activity of Living	Physical	Psychological	Sociocultural	Environmental	Politicoeconomic
Controlling body temperature	• Does the person have any difficulties with controlling body temperature, i.e. exercise, hormones, food and fluid intake or time of day? • Are there any difficulties/ disorders affecting normal body temperature – cause? • What is the person's body temperature on admission?	• Does the person's personality, perception, temperament or behaviour alter body temperature? • Does the person's mood alter body temperature?	• Are there any social or cultural influences affecting appropriate wearing of clothing etc?	• Is the person able to detect or control temperature changes and make appropriate choices/actions?	• Is the person vulnerable to changes in temperature?
Mobilising	• Does the person normally manage to mobilise unaided, i.e. without a stick, chair, frame or another person? • What physical or medical factors are inhibiting mobilisation? • How are other AL's affected by mobility difficulties? • Is the problem temporary or permanent? • Are there any risks/complications which might occur as a result of limited/reduced mobility?	• How does the person feel about problems or limitations, in mobility? • Is the person normally active/ adventurous? • Does the person understand the reasons for rest or exercise? • Is the person motivated towards appropriate recovery programme? • Does the person have sufficient information regarding mobility?	• How is the person likely to be affected socially as a result of temporary or permanent alteration mobility, n.b. social – family, friends, holidays, leisure activities, shopping, domestic activities? • Are there any social or cultural restrictions upon the person's mobility?	• What is the person's moving/ lifting risk factor score? • Are there any factors inhibiting the person's optimum mobility, i.e. walking and lifting aids, type of residence, visual/auditory impairment, temperature climate?	• Are there any factors affecting the person's ability to move around freely within the home environment? • Does the person have access to facilities/ resources/ adaptations to allow for optimum achievement of this AL?

ASSESSMENT SCHEDULE *(continued)*

Possible questions to consider during the assessment stage of care planning

Activity of Living	Physical	Psychological	Sociocultural	Environmental	Politicoeconomic
Working and playing	• What are the person's normal occupational and leisure activities and how physically demanding are they? • How does the person's current health status/ situation affect this activity?	• What are the emotional effects upon this activity caused by current health status? • Does the person have sufficient information to maintain safety and reduce harmful effects related to this activity, i.e. stress, overwork? • Does the person have sufficient intellect to receive and be motivated by appropriate information? • What are the person's reactions to hospitalisation, i.e. boredom, motivation, self-fulfilment? • What are the person's reactions to other life events, i.e. unemployment, redundancy, retirement, unpaid work?	• Has the person's social role been altered/ compromised as a result of current health status? • What moral and social obligations might be affected by a temporary or permanent change in this activity? • What support can the person expect from identified carers?	• Does the person have knowledge regarding Health and Safety at Work Act (1974) if appropriate? • Is the person aware of any environmental risks or hazards? • Can any environmental risks or hazards be identified?	• Does the person have any economic worries i.e. safety worries, employment worries? • Does the person have sufficient information and access to statutory and voluntary advice and support?
Expressing sexuality	• What is the person's gender? • Are there any physical changes in gender structure and function affecting the person's health status? • Is the person comfortable with interaction/ communication contact – touch, opposite sex, undressing, etc? • Does the presence of disease, illness or handicap, disabilities have any effect on this activity?	• What are the person's attitudes, normal habits, and routines in relation to expressing sexuality, i.e. dress, appearance, intercourse? • Does the person have any unusual or inappropriate sexual behaviour to be considered? • Does the person have any fears, anxieties or lack of information regarding maintaining this activity?	• Does the person have any cultural or religious influences which are to be considered?	• Are there any factors inhibiting the maintenance of this activity, i.e. hospital, home, lack of information?	• Does the person have sufficient information regarding safe and healthy sexual lifestyles? • Are there any ethical, legal or economic factors influencing this activity?

ASSESSMENT SCHEDULE *(continued)*
Possible questions to consider during the assessment stage of care planning

Activity of Living	Physical	Psychological	Sociocultural	Environmental	Politicoeconomic
Sleeping	• What is the person's normal sleep, awakening routine? • What are the person's normal presleep routines? • Does the person snore, sleepwalk, fall out of bed, have nightmares? • What is the person's normal sleeping position? • Does the person take medication to aid sleep? • Are there any sleep deficits present? • What are the causes of any sleep deficits, problems?	• Does the person have any fears or anxieties which may inhibit or reduce sleep? • What are the person's attitudes, beliefs about sleep and rest, i.e. quality and quantity?	• Does the person normally share a bed or sleep alone? • What type of clothing does the person normally wear? • How many pillows, sheets, blankets does the person normally use? • Does the person's work or lifestyle influence sleep in any way, e.g. shift work?	• How might the current environment alter or inhibit the person's sleep pattern? • Is the person used to noise, light or other? • Are there any safety aspects to consider?	• Are there any difficulties which are having long term or harmful effects on sleep deprivation? • Does the person have appropriate and sufficient knowledge related to sleep, rest and healthy living?
Dying	• Are there any confirmed or diagnostic factors threatening the person's life? • What are the physical effects upon the person, family and friends? • Is the person aware of the diagnosis, stage and progress of the life threatening disorder? • Is the possibility actual or potential?	• Is the person expressing a 'desire to know', anxiety or fear of dying? • Does the person desire that significant others 'know'? • What is the person's behaviour, mood, personality? • What is the person's understanding of their own dying/death?	• What are the person's attitudes, beliefs and life experiences about death? • Does the person have any specific cultural, religious, social or personal requests? • Who needs to be contacted on behalf of the person – family, partners, friends?	• Choice of environment to facilitate a peaceful death, i.e. hospice, home, hospital? • What resources will be required to meet the needs of the person, family and carers?	• Are there any economic, legal, ethical, resource, social or domestic factors inhibiting a peaceful death? • What is the effect of the death and reduced life expectancy of the person upon others? • Are there any sufficient and appropriate support services within the hospital and the home for the dying and bereaved? • Does the person wish to donate any organs, do the family know?

Index